Todd's Cardiovascular Review Book - Vol. 3:

Invasive Basics

6th Edition

by

J. Wesley Todd, BS, RCIS, RCES
Director, Cardiac Self Assessment
Spokane, WA 99216

ISBN 978-1-7326393-2-4

Self Published by:
Cardiac Self Assessment
1605 South Clinton Rd.
Spokane, WA 99216-0420
phone (509) 926-0344
Email w.t@westodd.com
Web Site http://www.westodd.com

ABOUT THIS SERIES

This book represents only one volume of a much larger series of 5 books. This vol. 1 combines material from the basic sciences, cardiovascular anatomy, physiology, and pathology. This book has been revised each time the author has taken one of the exams.

This book will serve those studying for all the cardiovascular registry exams for staff working in the cath lab, electrophysiology lab, ultrasound and vascular labs. Everyone needs knowledge of A&P, pathology, patient care, asepsis, BLS, and invasive lab protocols. Thus, volume 1 can be used to prepare for any of the CCI exams cardiovascular specialty exams or the ARRT exams (CI and VI). Those preparing for these cardiovascular invasive registries (RCIS, CI or VI) will also need additional books: Vol. 2, 3, 4 and 5 shown below:

INVASIVE REGISTRY - STUDY MATERIAL

Vol. #	Ch #	Chapter Content	Published	ISBN
Vol. I		Invasive CV Basics (this book) A. CV Science B. CV Anatomy & Physiology C. CV Pathology	2018	978-1-7326393-0-0
Vol. II		CV Diagnostic Techniques	2018	978-1-7326393-1-7
Vol. III		Hemodynamics	2018	978-1-7326393-2-4
Vol. IV		Interventions	2018	978-1-7326393-3-1
Vol V		Registry Practice Exams	2018	978-1-7326393-4-8

All 5 the above books and CD are available as a bundled set. See: www.westodd.com

DISCLAIMER

The author and the many reviewers have made every effort to insure the current accuracy of the material in this book. Where possible, recognized authorities are referenced and quoted. Due to the fast-moving nature of the cardiovascular field, and the changing nature of accepted practice, we cannot accept any responsibility for the errors or omissions or for the consequences from application of the information in this book. Although we have made every effort toward accuracy, you should always check with hospital standards and company literature such as drug package inserts, before applying the information in this book.

We have tried to include information that we believe will be on the national CV Invasive Registry examinations. But, since the examination agencies frequently update and change their test questions and formats, the questions included here will be similar but not identical to the ones you find on your national exam.

PREFACE to 6th Edition:

This edition of Todd's CV Review Books has been revised to include the new question formats given by CCI. CCI calls these new types of questions "innovative items." The exams are no longer just four item multiple choice questions, as in the past. New formats include matching, drag and drop, multiple response (checkbox) and hot spot questions. Although we have always used these formats in our Todd CV Review CDs & USBs we have modified many questions in this new edition to match these "innovative" formats.

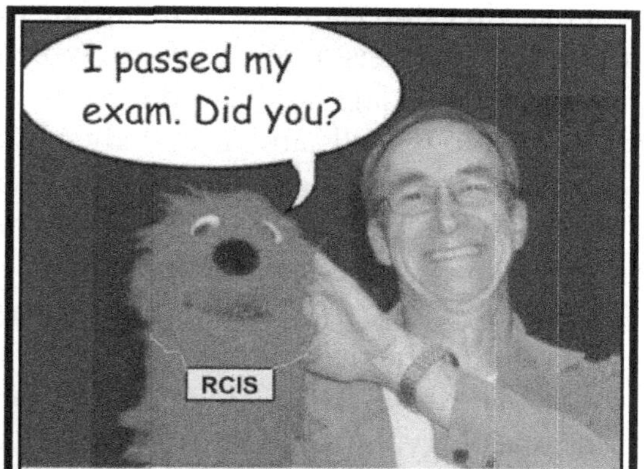

Wes Todd and his puppet Gomer.

Hundreds of new questions have been added. This 6th edition now includes new structural heart information and new devices like TAVR, Impella, and new diagnostic techniques like FFRct and iFR. Our new interactive CD & USB program will be available in 2019 to match the questions in this book and the current registry exams.

Wesley Todd, BS, RCIS, RCES 2018
Director, Cardiac Self Assessment

PREFACE to 5th Edition:

This edition of Todd's CV Review Books keeps pace with the field and changes in the national exams. In 2010 CCI eliminated the CV Science exam, and merged it with the registry exam. The RCIS exam was increased by 60 basic science questions, making the exam longer. Now, there is only one exam and everyone's invasive exam will include this basic material. This is essential background knowledge common to all invasive professionals. Because of this, we changed the name of this book from "CV Science", to "Invasive Basics." This volume will include anatomy, physiology, pathology and other basic skills common to the Cath lab, EP Lab, and Vascular Radiology Lab. As such, this volume contains core knowledge for all the invasive cardiovascular specialties.

CCI also changed the blueprint and weighting on the registry exams. The categories within the exam are now based on job skills and duties, determined by an extensive survey of working nurses and techs. These skills are grouped into categories such as, "Conducting Intra-Procedural Activities" and "Performing Therapeutic Procedures". Categories such as statistics and math were removed. That does NOT mean there are no math questions on the exam, only that the math questions should relate directly to the field, such as hemodynamic calculations. This should make the exam more relevant. Changes coming to the 2013 RCIS include removal of Pediatric cath, ergonovine, and Foley catheterization.

Several hundred new questions have been added and others removed, to keep pace with advancing medical technology and invasive job descriptions.

Wesley Todd, BS, RCIS 6/23/13

PREFACE to 4th Edition:

This edition of Todd's CV Review Books is designed keep pace with the latest changes in exams and the tremendous increase in cardiovascular technology. In 2000 CCI did a task analysis of the CV field, which resulted in changes in the CV exams. This material is based on the latest 2002 updates. New exams increasingly weight patient care and pharmacology skills and knowledge. In addition CCI's Science matrix has decreased emphasis on the CV specialties, with increased emphasis on basic concepts. For example, physical principles were removed - including ultrasound physics and pressure measurement. These specialized topics have been shifted into the specialty exams: RCS, RVS, and RCIS. CCI is also preparing to give EP and Vascular Interventions examinations sometime in the near future.

The 2002-2003 RCIS and CIT exams place increased weight on Patient Care, Pharmacology, Equipment, and Interventions.

What's new? Todd's CV Review CD 2nd Edition will be updated to include all this new material and continuing education material. We now offer online classes for cardiology professionals who need a systematic review of this material. These are based on Todd's CV Review CD. Wesley Todd, BS, RCIS 5/23/02

PREFACE to 1st Edition:

In my 23 years of teaching CVTs at the Spokane Community College I coached hundreds of CVT students through the national registry exams. With this experience I wrote this introduction to prepare them for the CV examinations. This book has hundreds of registry-quality multiple-choice test questions, answers, rationales, and reference material. It will also help **you** prepare for your national exam.

The students in our JRC-CVT approved CVT program have been tested with and helped refine many of the questions in this book. They have done very well on the RCVT examination. The RCVT exam has been in existence since 1973, when I first took it. I took the CCI/RCVT exam again in 1990, 1993, 1996, 1997 and 2002 and have ranked first in the country. In 1990 I started selling Self Assessment questions and answers by mail. Applicants taking the Science and RCVT exams around the country found it so helpful that I have refined it and expanded the number of questions and put them in this book.

Noninvasive (Echo) and Vascular technologists studying for the Basic CV Science Exam in preparation for their RCVT specialty exam also need this book. Although originally designed for those taking the Invasive RCVT exam, this book combines concepts of basic physical science that all branches of cardiovascular medicine need.

This book has become more than a review for the exam. It may also be used as a self study book and in-service education manual for working Cardiovascular Professionals of all types. Wesley Todd, BS, RCIS 1997, Director, Cardiac Self Assessment

INTRODUCTION

Volume III contains the hemodynamic background essential to all the CV registry exams taken by allied health and nursing staff. It is specifically designed for the Cardiovascular Invasive Exams (RCIS & CI).

I have organized this book around current exam content/matrix for the national CV exams, and designed it to be similar to the exam you will take. The content of each exam is detailed in this "Introduction to CV Exams." To prepare you for your exam, this book includes thousands of questions, answers, explanations, and references. It is up to you to match appropriate material from these volumes with the content of your exam. For example, RCIS and vascular candidates do not need the in depth EGM and action potential knowledge that EP candidates do.

GOALS OF THIS BOOK

Studying this book will improve your chances of passing the exam, but cannot replace formal education or clinical experience. This is not a "crash course." Neither can we cover all items that will appear on the exam. CCI's test bank includes more than 4000 test items, many more than in this book. If you have no formal training in your specialty, you will need extensive textbook study, tutoring, and clinical experience to gain the theoretical base necessary. These exams are difficult. Approximately 60-75% of the candidates pass these exams the first time. My experience shows that using this book to prepare for the exam can raise your exam score by as much as 20%.

This book will help you achieve your goal of passing the CV exams by helping you:

- evaluate your current Cardiovascular knowledge
- gain insight into your strengths and weaknesses
- form a directed plan of study to prepare for your exam
- gain confidence and reduce anxiety at test taking
- gain familiarity with the types of test items commonly used on these exams
- strengthen your test taking skills
- strengthen your problem-solving skills.
- Direct your study into recognized Cardiovascular references and textbooks.

References for each question are included.

REVIEWERS AND CONTRIBUTORS INCLUDE:

6th Edition Contributors:

Alan Bennett, RCIS
Director Invasive Cardiology School
Carnegie Institute
550 Stephenson Hwy, Suite 100
Troy, Mi 48083

Todd Ginapp, RN, EMT-P, RCIS. FSICP
Memorial Herman SE Hospital
Cardiology Manager
Houston, TX

Jay Andrews
Proof reader & technical services

Additional previous contributors:
Connie Marshall, RT(R), RCIS, M.A.
Anthony Williams, MSM, RN, RCIS
Sabrina Black, BS, RDCS, FASE
Patrick Hoier, BS, RCSA, RCIS, FSICP
Polly Keller MBA, RRT, RCIS
Kristy Schultz, M.Ed., RTRM, RCIS
Dan Sullivan, BSN, RN
Al Bennett, RCIS
Allan Mirehouse, RCIS
Christie Hodge, RCIS
Robert Howard, RCIS
Syed Mustafa Khundmiri, BS, RCIS
Esma Campbell RT, RCIS
Scott (William) Corson, RCIS
Lois Schaffer, MEd, RT®, RCIS
Marsha Holton, CCRN, RCIS, FSICP
Stephanie Ranck, BA, RCIS
Jeff Davis, RRT, RCIS, BS
Vicki Lemaster, BS, TR(R)(CV)
Richard Merschen, MS, RT(R)(CV)
Chuck Williams, BS, RCSA, RPA/RA, RCIS, RT(R)(CV)(CI), CPFT, CCT,

These knowledgeable reviewers have encouraged me and made suggestions throughout the years of book development. Although they have all proofed, critiqued, and edited my work I have not always taken their suggestions. And, they are not responsible for errors in the text. Full responsibility for the contents and accuracy of the book rests with the author.

Special thanks to all the others who have received advanced copies and made suggestions, whose names I have forgotten.

Chapters in 5 Volumes of Todd CV Review Books

CARDIOVASCULAR REVIEW BOOK
6th Edition

CARDIOVASCULAR INVASIVE DIAGNOSIS: Volume # III

Chapters E:

Pressure Introduction

INDEX: E1

Pressure Basics

Waveforms

1. **Normal cardiac waveforms resemble simple electrically generated waveforms. The normal cardiac waveform labeled #1 in the box (atrial) most resembles a/an:**

a. Sine wave
b. Square wave
c. Triangle wave
d. Impulse wave

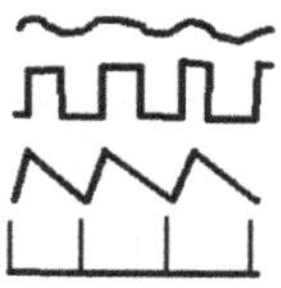

<u>Cardiovascular waves</u>
1. Atria (RA, LA)
2. Ventricle (RV, LV)
3. Arteries (PA, AO)
4. Pressure spike (snap)

ANSWER: a. Sine waves most resemble RA (CVP) or LA (PAW) tracings. Their A, x, V, y waves undulate slowly and smoothly like a sinusoidal wave. This is the simplest waveform to duplicate electrically.
BE ABLE TO CORRECTLY MATCH ALL ANSWERS:

1. Atria (RA, LA) ➜ Sine waves
   A, x, V, y waves undulate slowly and smoothly like a sinusoidal wave. A full cardiac cycle would take 2 complete sine wave cycles. This is the simplest waveform to duplicate electrically. It is composed of low frequencies that seldom show artifacts.

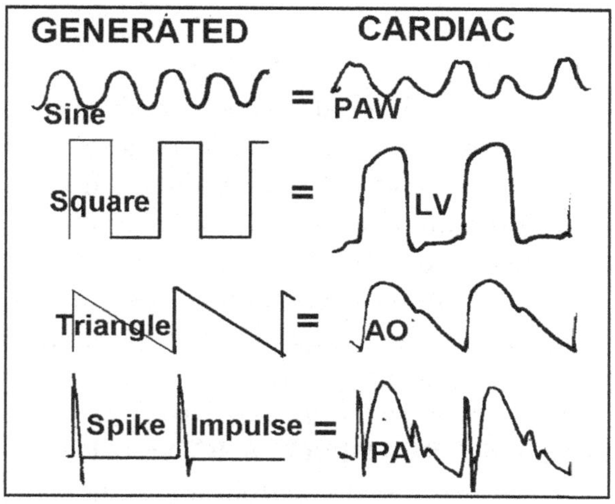

Simple electronically generated waves - analogous to cardiac waveforms

2. Ventricle (RV, LV) ➜ Square waves
   During systolic contraction the ventricular pressure rises rapidly and in diastole falls rapidly. These rapidly rising waves have the highest frequency components, and are the most difficult to duplicate electrically. That is why ventricular pressures often show resonance distortion which overshoots the true systolic pressure.

3. Arteries (PA, AO) ➜ Triangle wave
   Arterial pressures rise quickly to a peak and then slowly taper off, like a triangle. The dicrotic notch may sit on this down slope of this triangle. You can often see arterial resonance in early systole which overshoots the true systolic pressure.
4. Pressure Spike (snap) ➜ Impulse wave
   We occasionally see pressure spikes on PA pressure waves due to catheter fling, valve closure, or a valve opening snap. In pressure recording "spikes" are unwanted artifacts that contain high frequencies. ECG pacemaker spikes are also impulse waves. ECG recorders must accurately be able respond to higher frequencies (100 Hz) than pressure recording systems (20 Hz).

See: Personal Experience Keywords: sine, square, triangle, impulse wave

2. What pressure reading is normally taken at #1 in the box on the pressure shown?

a. Atrial mean
b. Atrial A wave
c. Atrial V wave
d. Arterial systole
e. Arterial diastole
f. Arterial mean
g. Ventricular beginning diastole
h. Ventricular end diastole
I. Ventricular systole

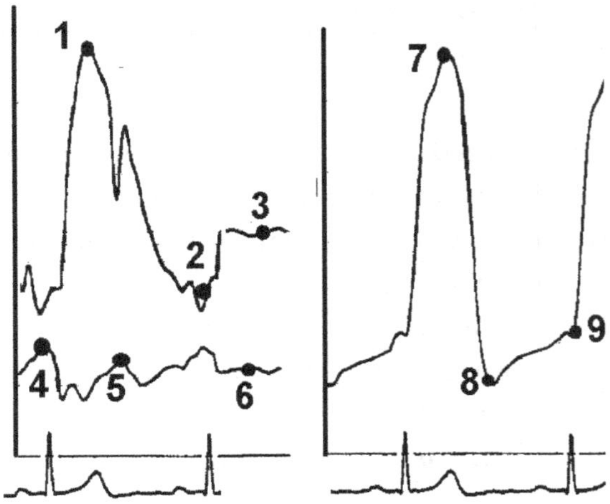

Arterial, venous and ventricular pressures

ANSWER: d. Arterial systole. The highest pressure on the systolic arterial pulse is the first number read in PA, AO, and all arterial blood pressure readings. This is actually PA recorded on x50. But both great vessel pressures (PA and AO) are read the same way (s/d,m). Just like all atrial pressures are read the same (a,v,m) ; and all ventricular pressures are read the same (s/bd, ed). MATCH ALL.

PRESSURE READINGS SHOWN ARE:

1. Arterial systole: highest reading
2. Arterial diastole: lowest reading
3. Arterial mean: average reading
4. Atrial A wave: wave after ECG p wave
5. Atrial V wave: wave after ECG t wave
6. Atrial mean: average venous reading
7. Ventricular systole: highest reading
8. Ventricular beginning diastole: lowest reading found in early diastole
9. Ventricular end diastole: atrial kick wave

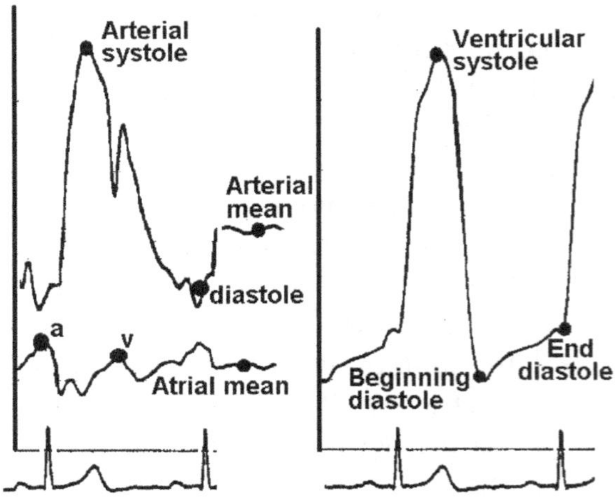

Reading PA, RA, and RV pressures

See: Kern, chapter on "Hemodynamics" **Keywords:** Where to read pressures

3. **Match #6 in the heart diagram with its usual pressure waveform below?**

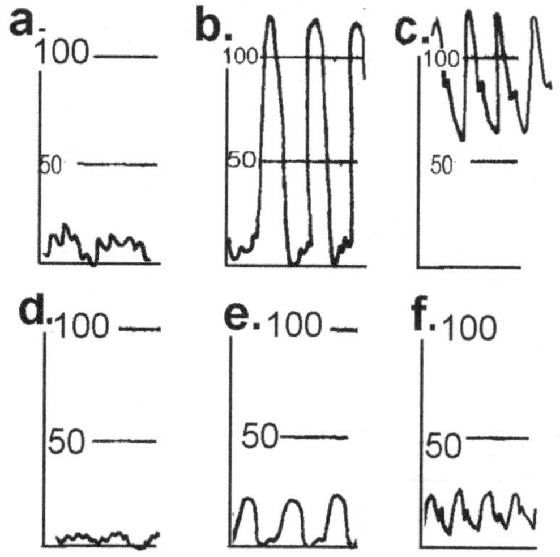

Cardiac pressure waveforms x 100

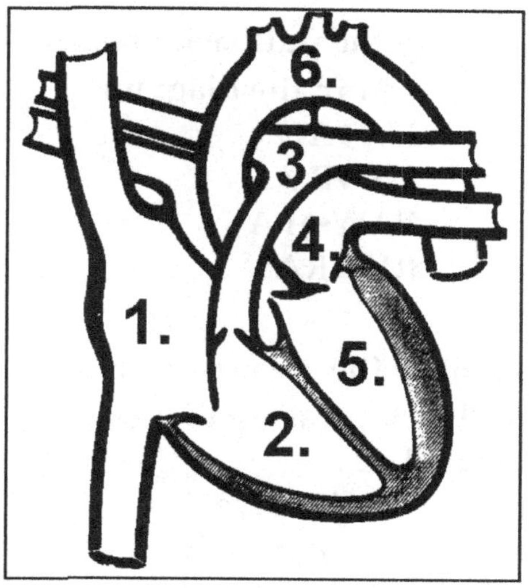

CV Pressures

ANSWER: c. #6 is the AO triangular waveform with dicrotic notch. Systolic pressure is usually over 100 mmHg. These are the only 6 pressure waveforms normally found in the heart. You should be able to identify them by their: shape, range, and three pressure readings.

BE ABLE TO CORRECTLY MATCH ALL ANSWERS:

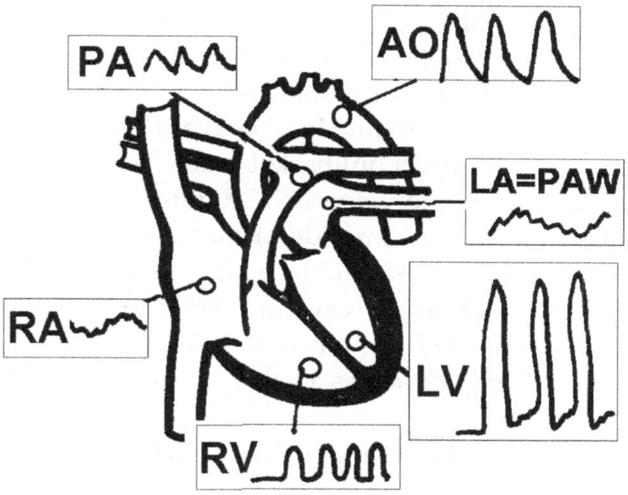

CV Waveforms

1. **RA:** wave shaped low pressure (0-5 mmHg)
2. **RV:** rapidly rising and falling pressure, systolic pressure usually around 25
3. **PA:** triangular waveform with dicrotic notch, systolic pressure usually around 25
4. **LA** (PAW): Sine wave shaped low pressure (5-10 mmHg)
5. **LV:** rapidly rising an falling pressure, systolic pressure usually over 100
6. **AO**: triangular waveform with dicrotic notch, systolic pressure usually over 100

See: Kern, chapter on "Hemodynamics" **Keywords:** shape of pressure waveforms

USE THIS DIAGRAM FOR BOTH QUESTIONS BELOW.

4. **Identify the pullback pressure labeled #1 in the diagram.**

a. LV→AO
b. PA→RV
c. PAW→PA
d. RV→RA

5. **Identify the area crossed in the pullback pressure diagram labeled #2 .**

a. **Aortic valve**
b. **Pulmonic valve**
c. **Tricuspid valve**
d. **Pulmonary capillary bed**

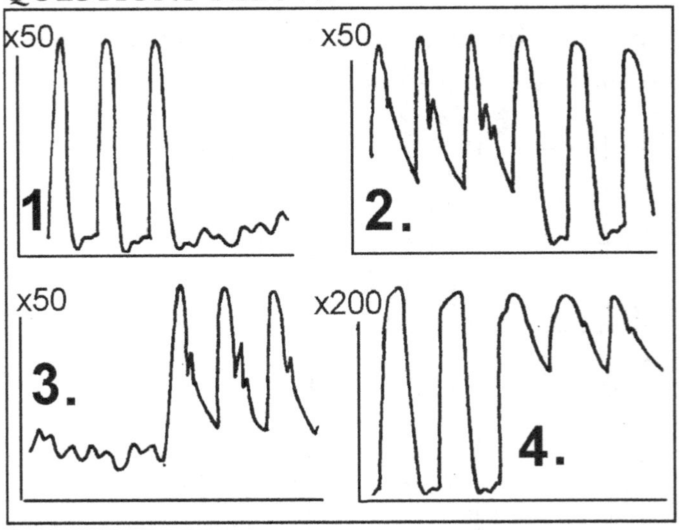

Pressure pullback tracings - across an area

BOTH ANSWERS APPEAR TOGETHER BELOW:

4. **ANSWER:** d. RV→RA is #1. Pullback across tricuspid valve. Note how a rapidly rising and falling ventricular pressure turns to a low sinusoidal atrial pressure. Pressure levels would be approximately RV = 25/5 mmHg to RA = (5) mmHg. The scale x 200 must be a left heart pullback, because only left heart pressures approach 200 mmHg. Although the scale provides a clue to the pressure site, you should be able to identify these pullbacks from waveform alone. Pullbacks are recording made as the catheter tip is pulled back across a valve.

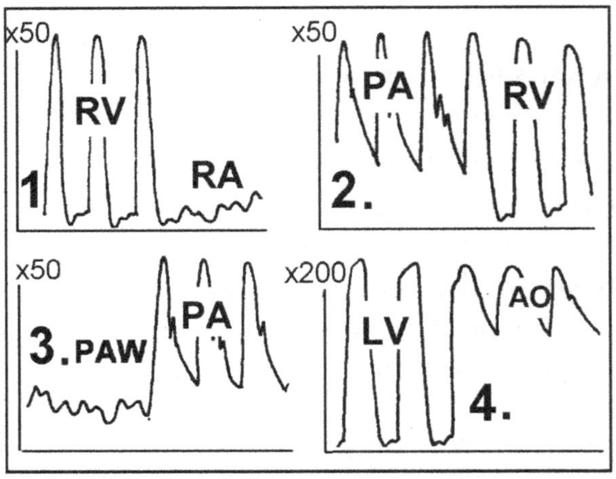

Pressure pullback tracings - across an area/valve

BE ABLE TO CORRECTLY MATCH ALL ANSWERS:

1. RV →RA
2. PA →RV
3. PAW →PA
4. LV→AO

See: Kern, chapter on "Hemodynamics" **Keywords:** ID pullback pressures

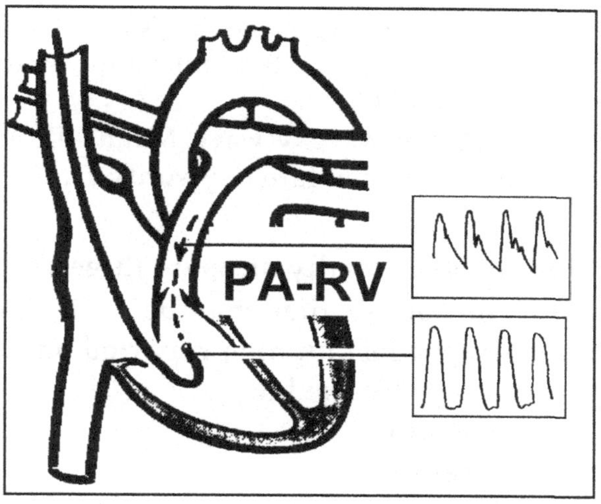

Pressure pullback tracings across PA valve

5. **ANSWER:** b. Pulmonic valve is #2. Pullback from PA →RV. Note how the waveform goes from arterial (triangular) to ventricular (square wave) shape. Right heart tracings are normally recorded on x 50 to expand the tracing for easier hemodynamic analysis. Pullbacks evaluate function of the valve or area crossed. A gradient at the time the valve is open indicates stenosis. This diagram shows a PA→ RV pullback. Note how the waveform changes from a triangular to a square shape. Pullbacks give hemodynamic information about the valve crossed. Note that right heart pullbacks are from an antegrade catheter pulled upstream. Left heart pullbacks are usually via a retrograde catheter pulled downstream.

CORRECTLY MATCHED ANSWERS ARE:

1. Tricuspid valve: RV →RA pullback
2. Pulmonic valve: PA →RV pullback
3. Pulmonary capillary bed: PAW →PA pullback
   Wedge pullback is not a valve crossing but *looks* like an LA to PA pullback (LV-EDP ≈LA≈PAW≈PA-EDP).
4. Aortic valve: LV→AO pullback

See: Kern, chapter on "Hemodynamics" **Keywords:** identify pullbacks

PRESSURE READINGS

6. **Cardiac waveforms are normally read at 3 points and those 3 numbers are reported. How is the right heart pressure labeled at #1 in the box (PAW) normally reported?**

a. A wave, V wave, Mean

b. Systolic/ Begin diastolic, End diastolic

c. Systolic /Diastolic, Mean

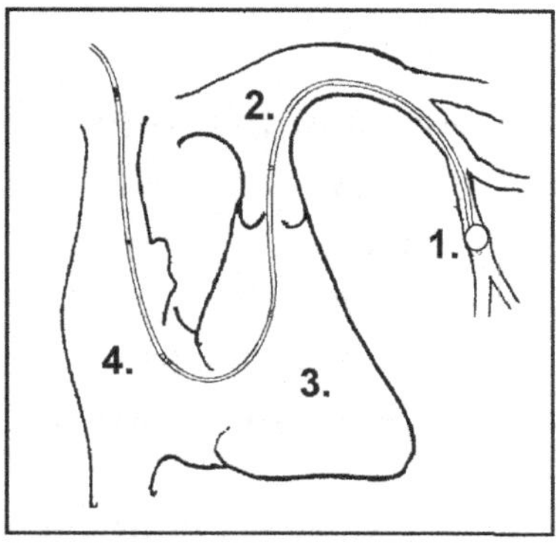

Right heart pressure sites

ANSWER: a. PAW = A wave, V wave, Mean. These 3 pressure points are read and reported on all atrial pressures (PAW, LA, and RA) - except in cases of atrial fibrillation or flutter where A waves are absent.

BE ABLE TO CORRECTLY MATCH ALL ANSWERS:

1. **PAW = A wave, V wave, Mean** - Read on all atrial pressures (PAW ,LA, and RA)

2. **PA = Systolic /Diastolic, Mean** - Read on all arterial pressures (PA and AO)
3. **RV = Systolic/ Begin diastolic, End diastolic** - Read on all ventricular pressures (RV and LV)
4. **RA = A wave, V wave, Mean**. - Read on all atrial pressures (PAW ,LA, and RA)

See: Company Literature **Keywords:** Three pressure numbers normally read

7. **Computers normally measure three pressure points on each cardiac chamber. What point is normally the last number reported on arterial pressures (#3 in the box)?**

> **Pressure Readings**
> ***Arterial (#1/ #2, #3)**
> Ventricular (#4/ #5, #6)
> Atrial or Wedge (#7, #8, #9)

a. **Systolic**
b. **Diastole**
c. **Begin diastolic**
d. **End diastolic**
e. **Mean**

ANSWER: e. mean. **BE ABLE TO CORRECTLY MATCH ALL ANSWERS:**
PRESSURE READINGS NORMALLY TAKEN ARE:

Arterial	=	(1. Peak Systolic/	2. End Diastolic/	3. Mean)
Ventricular	=	(4. Peak Systolic/	5. Begin Diastolic,	6. End Diastolic)
Atrial or wedge	=	(7. "a" Wave,	8. "v" Wave,	9. Mean)

Note that the slash (/) goes between peak systolic and minimum diastolic numbers. The commas are used to separate all other readings. Only arterial and ventricular pressures use "systolic peak". Only atrial and arterial pressures measure "mean." If it starts with the letter "a" measure its "average." Note also, that both sides of the heart are read the same. E.g., RV is read the same as LV (s/bd, ed), etc..
See: Kern, chapter on "Hemodynamics" **Keywords:** ID the 3 numbers read on pressures.

8. **On which of the following chambers is a mean pressure NEVER recorded?**

a. **PAW**
b. **LV**
c. **AO**
d. **Femoral artery**
e. **None of the above**

ANSWER b. LV. Ventricular pressures are never recorded with a mean. With ventricular pressures we only use the systolic and diastolic numbers. Mean ventricular pressure is not measured because it is of no use. Whereas, the LV-EDP is very useful. The "mean" pressures for all atrial and arterial pressures are used to calculate the vascular resistances.
See: Kern, chapter on "Hemodynamics" **Keywords:** no ventricular mean pressure read

NORMAL VALUES

9. What is the normal pressure found in the cardiac chamber labeled #4 in the diagram?

a. 6, 5, 3 mmHg
b. 120 / 0, 9 mmHg
c. 120 / 70, 85 mmHg
d. 25 / 0, 4 mmHg
e. 25 / 9, 15 mmHg
f. 10, 13, 8 mmHg

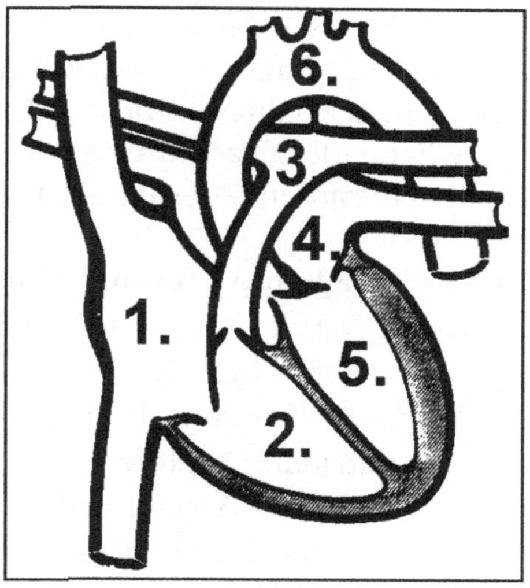

CV Pressures

ANSWER: f. LA = PAW = 10/13, 8 mmHg (a wave, v wave , mean) **BE ABLE TO CORRECTLY MATCH ALL ANSWERS:**

1. RA = 6,5,3 mmHg	(a, v, mean)
2. RV = 25/0,4 mmHg	(s/bd, ed)
3. PA = 25/9,15 mmHg	(s/ed, mean)
4. LA = 10,13,8 mmHg	(a, v , mean)
5. LV = 120/0,9 mmHg	(s/bd, e d)
6. AO = 120/70,85 mmHg	(s/ed, mean)

Right Heart	Pressures in mmHg	Left Heart	Pressure in mmHg
PAW =	12, 12, 10 (a, v, m)	LA =	12, 12, 10 (a, v, m)
PA =	25/10, 15 (s/d, m)	AO =	120/70, 85 (s/d, m)
RV =	25/0, 5 (s/bd, ed)	LV =	120/0, 10 (s/bd, ed)
RA =	5, 5, 5 (a, v, m)		

Kern's normal values are listed in the question. However, I teach the normal values listed in the box, because they are rounded off and simpler to remember. Note that those circled should be the same in adjacent chambers.
See: Kern, chapter on "Hemodynamics **Keywords:** Normal pressure

10. If the pullback labeled #4 (RV→RA) is normal, what two pressure readings should be approximately equal?

a. Arterial systole = → = ventricular systole
b. Ventricular systole = → = arterial systole
c. Ventricular diastole= → = atrial mean
d. Atrial mean = → = arterial diastole

<u>PULLBACK</u>
1. LV→AO
2. PA→RV
3. PAW→PA
*4. RV→RA

ANSWER c. Ventricular diastole ⇒ = atrial mean. If the tricuspid valve is normal, there will be no gradient during diastole. This diagram shows a normal right heart catheter pullback from PAW to RA, and what parts of each waveform should be equal in the absence of stenosis. KNOW THESE -

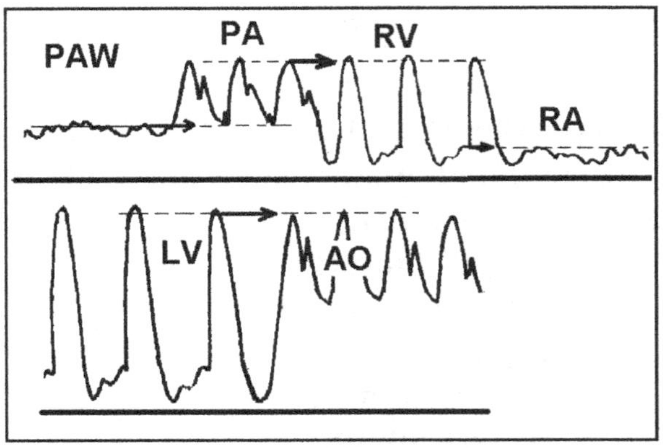

What pullback pressures should be equal?

PULLBACKS and pressure equalities:

1. LV➔AO: Ventricular systole =➔ = arterial systole
2. PA➔RV: Arterial systole =➔ = ventricular systole
3. PAW➔PA: Atrial mean =➔ = arterial diastole. This is not a pullback across a valve, but across the pulmonary capillary bed.

*4. RV➔RA: Ventricular diastole=➔ = atrial mean

See: Kern, chapter on "Hemodynamics." **Keywords:** ID pullback tracings

11. Match the normal MEAN pressure range with the chamber labeled #3 (PAW) in the box.

a. 1-5 mmHg
b. 5-13 mmHg
c. 9-19 mmHg
d. 70-105 mmHg
e. Not measured

MEAN PRESSURES
1. RA
2. PA
***3. PAW**
4. AO
5. LV

ANSWER: b. 5-13 mmHg. According to Kern, mean PAW pressure is 4.5-13 mmHg (average 9 mmHg). This diagram shows the normal range of pressures in the four chambers where "means" are recorded. [low mean - (average mean) - high mean range]. The average or mean numbers are marked with lines over them. Mean pressures are the most important numbers to remember.

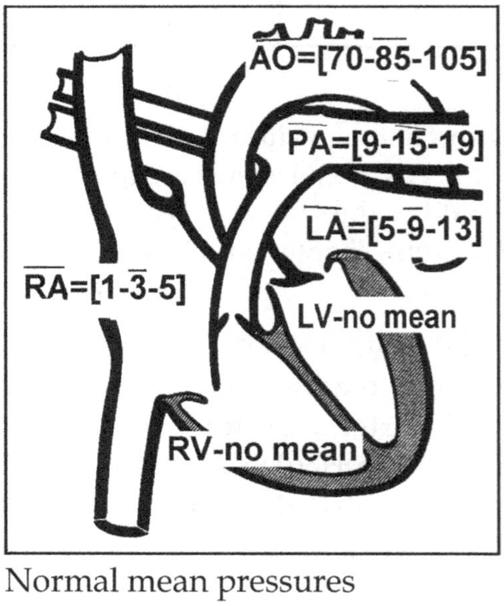

Normal mean pressures

BE ABLE TO CORRECTLY MATCH ALL:
NORMAL MEAN PRESSURE RANGES

1. RA = 1-(3)-5 mmHg
2. PA = 9-(15)- 19 mmHg
3. PAW = 5-(9)- 13 mmHg
4. AO = 70-(85) -105 mmHg
5. LV = Means not measured on any ventricle

See: Kern or Grossman, normal pressure chart in their appendix **Keywords**: Normal mean pressures

Respiratory Effects

12. Spontaneous breathing artifact is often present in right heart pressure tracings. At what time in the respiratory cycle should cardiac pressure readings be made for true resting transmural intracardiac pressure?

a. End inspiration (pre-expiration)
b. End expiration (pre-inspiration)
c. Through one complete respiratory cycle
d. With the patient holding a deep breath

ANSWER: b. The end expiration. Cardiac pressures we measure have the pleural pressure of respiration superimposed on top of them. The negative inspiration should be eliminated to get true transmural pressure. We want to know about the heart, not the lungs. Transmural pressure is defined as the pressure across the wall of a cardiac chamber or of a blood vessel. In the heart, transmural pressure is the resultant of the intracavitary pressure minus the extracavitary pressure (i.e., pericardial & pulmonary pleura).

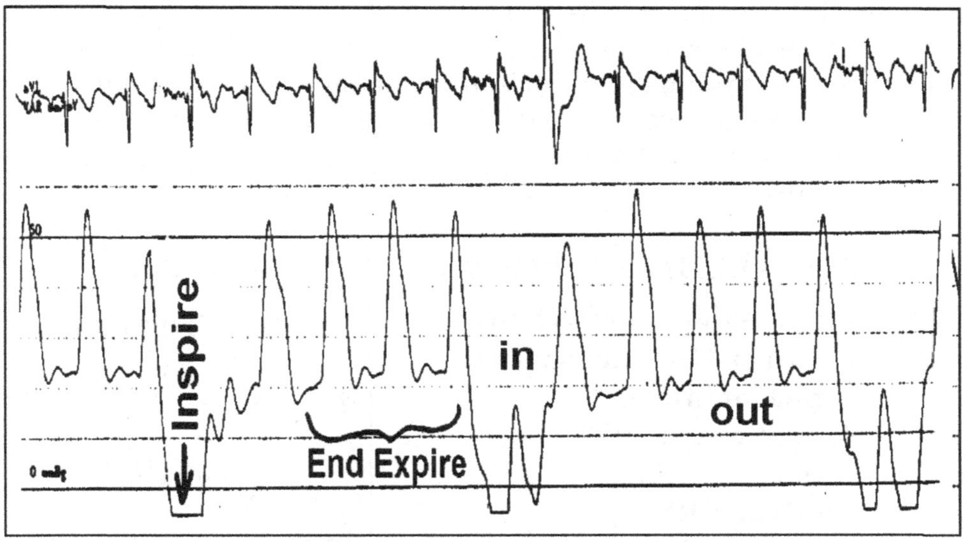

Effect of Spontaneous deep breathing on RV pressure

Since respirations are usually slow - perhaps 4-6 seconds apart, we can usually see the respiratory pattern. Rapid or deep inspiration shows as a drop in the pressure baseline, sometimes below-zero in labored breathing. A dip occurs in all intracardiac

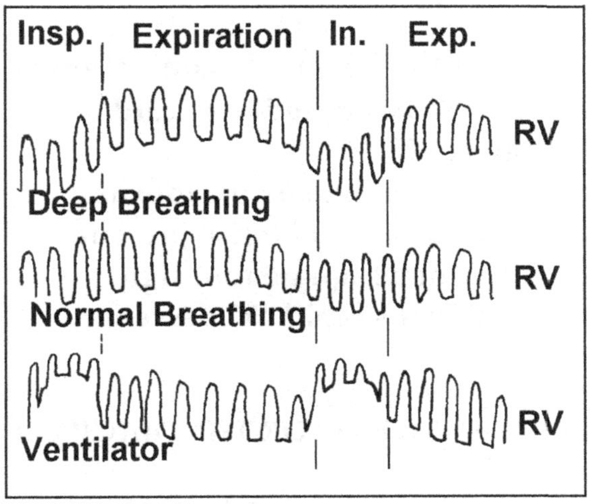

Respiratory effects on RV pressure

tracings as pleural pressure decreases with inspiration.

The best place to estimate "transmural pressure" is just before the inspiratory artifact (dip), where the pressures level out. At least one, preferably two complete respiratory cycles should be recorded to evaluate the end expiratory pressure. If respiration is rapid or labored it is best to tell the patient - **"let a normal breath OUT, hold it, and not bear down"** (without Valsalva) while recording. This lets the pleural pressure stabilize at the lungs naturally relaxed position. This RV-End expiratory pressure reads 55/20, 22 mmHg. (S/BD, ED). Ahrens says,

> *"In order to avoid incorrect readings, the clinician must approximate intrapleural pressures. This is most commonly done by reading pressure waves when intrapleural pressure is negligible or near normal. Intrapleural pressure is near baseline when no inspiratory or expiratory pressures are present. Gas flow at end expiration is, or should be, zero. End expiration is therefore the most commonly used approximation of a stable intrapleural pressure."*

When a patient is on a ventilator the inspiration artifact goes in the OPPOSITE direction. Because with a ventilator air is pushed into the lungs, pleural pressure goes positive with mechanical airway pressure. Again, pressure readings should be taken at the end of expiration where pleural pressure is most normal. But with a ventilator this is in the expiratory valley, just before the rise in pressure caused by mechanical inspiration.
See: Ahrens, chapter on "Respiratory Influence on Waveforms." **Keywords:** Read at end expiratory pressure

THE NEXT 2 QUESTIONS REFER TO THIS DIAGRAM:

13. Identify the respiratory effect on the pulses shown at #1 in the diagram.

- **a. Normal arterial (AO)**
- **b. Normal venous(RV)**
- **c. Normal artificial ventilation(RV)**
- **d. Pulsus Paradoxus AO)**
- **e. Kussmaul's sign (RV)**

14. Which of these hemodynamic signs is commonly associated with cardiac tamponade?

- **a. Arterial pulsus paradoxus**
- **b. Wide arterial pulse pressure**
- **c. Venous square root sign**
- **d. Venous rapid "Y" descent**

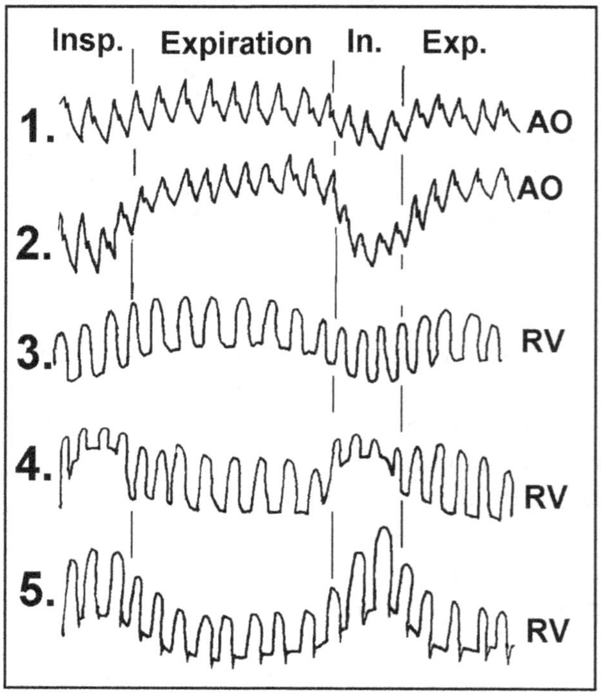

Respiration effects on RV & AO

BOTH ANSWERS FOR THE DIAGRAM ABOVE APPEAR TOGETHER BELOW:

13. ANSWER a. Normal arterial (AO).

BE ABLE TO CORRECTLY MATCH ALL ANSWERS BELOW:

1. **Normal arterial** (AO): Normally inspiration slightly encroaches on the LV preload and reduces the LV stoke volume. This normal 7% drop in stoke volume is reflected in a normal 3% drop in arterial pressure (3-6 mmHg). Labored breathing may increase this normal respiratory variation - e.g. heavy sedation.
2. **Pulsus Paradoxus** AO): is an exaggeration of the normal inspiratory decline of LV stoke volume. It is defined by a drop in systolic BP of MORE than 10 mmHg. It is associated with pericardial tamponade and occasionally with constrictive pericarditis, and restrictive heart disease.
3. **Normal venous**(RV): Venous and right heart pressures follow along with changes in the intrathoracic pressure. In the normal heart inspiration results in a fall in intrathoracic, intra-pericardial, and a fall in the diastolic baseline in all right heart pressures. However, it normally increases venous return and increases right heart pulse pressures. Expiration results in the opposite.
4. **Normal artificial ventilation** (RV): Positive pressure ventilators or manual bag ventilation increases the alveolar, pleural, and right heart pressures with inspiration. This is opposite to the **normal drop in pressure** with inspiration. Note the rapid rise in pressures from the ventilator pushing the air into the thorax. The systolic pressure will not rise as dramatically due to reduced venous return associated with the positive thoracic pressure.
5. **Kussmaul's sign (RV):** Increase in venous pressure and jugular vein distension on inspiration. This is opposite to the normal drop in venous pressure with inspiration. This is associated with Constrictive Pericarditis. Note square root sign (deep "y" wave) timed to early diastole when the RV rapidly fills.

See: Braunwald, chapter on "Pericardial Disease." and Ahrens, chapter on Respiratory Influence on Waveforms." **Keywords:** Pulsus Paradoxus

14. ANSWER a. Pulsus paradoxus. Note the dramatic BP drop with inspiration. The AO pulse pressure also drops. This is not really "paradoxical" because it normally drops a few mmHg with inspiration anyway. But Pulsus Paradoxus, seen in this AO tracing is an ***exaggeration*** of this normal phenomenon. Pulsus Paradoxus is a drop of more than 10 mmHg in the Aortic systolic pressure with inspiration. Also, note how the RV pressure moves oppositely in tamponade. It increases with inspiration (Kussmaul's sign).

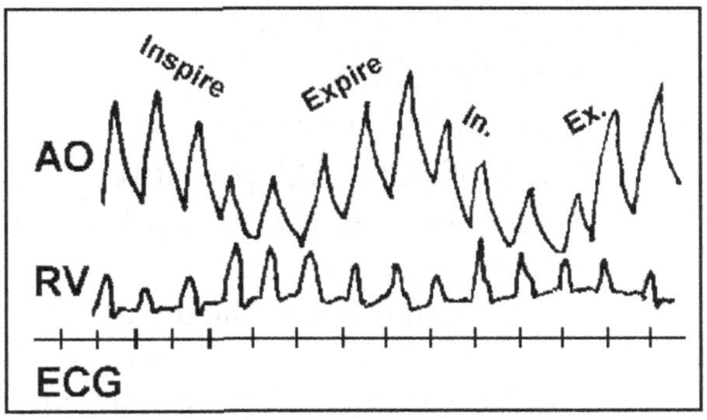

Pulsus Paradoxus/Tamponade

See: Braunwald, chapter on "Pericardial Diseases." **Keywords:** Pericardial tamponade exaggerates Pulsus Paradoxus

Normal Venous Pressures

15. Left ventricular end diastolic pressure (LV-EDP) readings are normally the same as the:

- a. **Right ventricular diastolic pressure**
- b. **Left atrial V wave pressure**
- c. **Pulmonary capillary wedge pressure**
- d. **Pulmonary artery systolic pressure**

ANSWER c. Pulmonary capillary wedge pressure or pulmonary artery wedge pressure (PCW or PAWP). The wedged catheter cuts off PA flow and measures pressures through the capillary bed to the LA. Since the mitral valve is open in diastole, PAW and LA both measure the important LV-end diastolic pressure. LV-EDP is one of the best indicators of left sided preload.
See: Daily, chapter on "Right Heart Catheterization" **Keywords**: Preload, Wedge, LA, PA-Edp

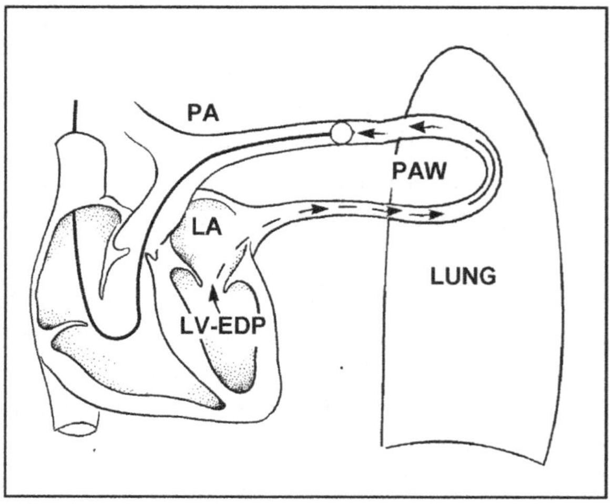

PA Wedge pressure = LA = LV-EDP

16. Which PAW measurement consistently approximates the LV-EDP?

- a. **Peak "V" wave**
- b. **Average "Y" wave dip**
- c. **Mean of entire PA pressure**
- d. **Mean between the top and the bottom of the PAW "A" wave**

ANSWER: d. Mean between the top and the bottom of the "a" wave. It is ½ the distance between the "a" and "x" descent. Here is how it is measured: add the top of a representative "a" wave to the bottom of that "a" wave ("x" or "x_2" trough). Then divide that sum by two, to get the "MEAN 'a' wave." The "mean 'a' wave" is then midway way between the top and bottom of the "a" wave. In the example shown the mean between 7 and 3 is 5 mmHg. Because it is so seldom seen, this measurement ignores any "c" waves.
Ahrens says,

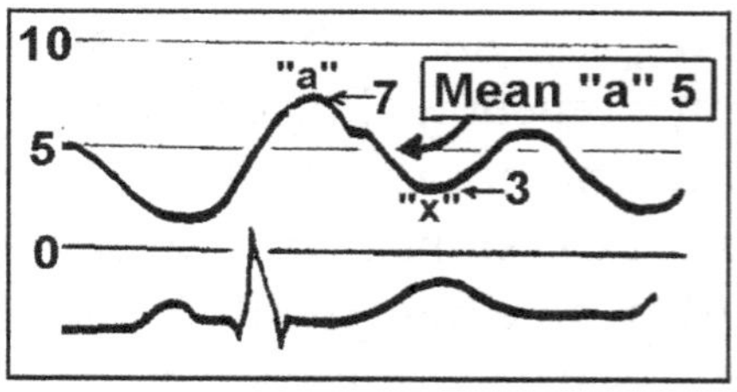

Measuring - mean "a" wave

"The primary method to ensure that all clinicians are consistently reading waveforms correctly is for all interpreters of waveforms to locate the A wave and determine its mean..."

The other measures that approximate the LA and LV-EDP are:

- "a" wave peak
- "z" wave (trough)
- PAW mean - (most commonly used)

The end expiratory point is the most consistent point to read all hemodynamic values. **See:** Ahrens, chapter on "Normal Pulmonary Capillary Wedge and Central Venous Pressure." **Keywords:** LV-EDP best approximated by mean A wave

17. What is the NORMAL relationship between PA wedge (PAW) pressure and PA-EDP?

a. **PAW mean usually 1-4 mmHg higher than PA-EDP**
b. **PA-EDP usually 1-4 mmHg higher than PAW mean**
c. **PA-EDP = PAW mean**
d. **PA-EDP = PAW "A" wave mean**

ANSWER: b. PA-EDP usually 1-4 mmHg higher than PAW mean. When evaluating LV preload with a Swan Ganz catheter it is often inconvenient to inflate the balloon each time you want to evaluate LV preload. It has been found that the blood flow through normal pulmonary capillaries is so slow at the end of diastole that only a small pressure gradient exists between PA and LA. So, normally PA-EDP is 1-4 mmHg higher than the PA wedge. This is consistent for any one patient. So measure the PA-EDP and subtract that difference to get the estimated mean wedge pressure.

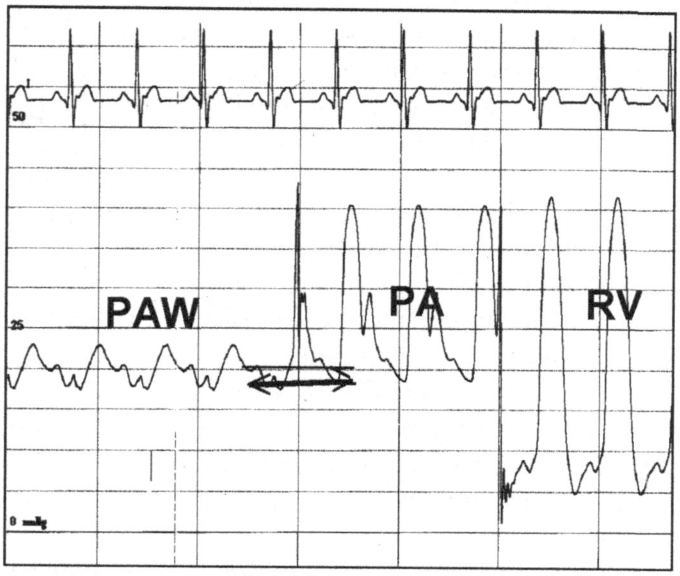

Simultaneous LV and PAW ➔ PA pullback x 50

Normally the resistance in the lung bed is small (around 1 Wood unit) and there is a very small gradient across the lung bed. But, for many patients the PA to LV-EDP gradient is higher than 4 mmHg. These:

PA-EDP significantly higher than LV-EDP (exceptions to the 1-4 mmHg rule):

- High CO.
- Primary pulmonary hypertension
- Pulmonary embolism, LA myxoma, Cortriatriatum, severe pulmonary vasoconstriction or mitral stenosis.
- Loss of pulmonary vasculature (such as in COPD).

See: Daily chapter on "PA Pressure monitoring" and Braunwald chapter on, "Pulmonary Hypertension."**Keywords:** Wedge= PA diastolic pressure-1-4 mmHg

18. In what condition is the PAWP usually EQUAL to the LV-EDP (or within 4 mmHg)?

- a. **Acute respiratory failure**
- b. **LA myxoma**
- c. **Cor-tri-atriatum**
- d. **Mitral stenosis**

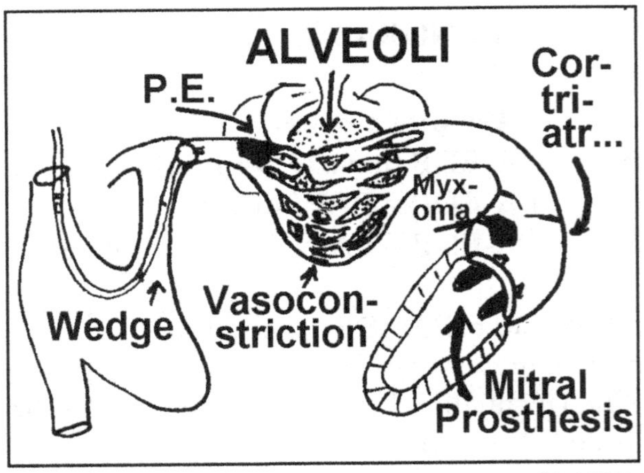

Conditions where wedge pressure (PAW) does NOT equal LV-EDP

ANSWER: a. Acute respiratory failure. In CHF there is not usually an obstruction between the pulmonary artery and the LV in diastole. However, with mitral valve stenosis, mitral valve prosthesis, Cortriatriatum, Pulmonary embolus, LA myxoma, and severe pulmonary vasoconstriction the PAW may NOT approximate LA or LV-EDP. In these cases some obstruction exists that creates a gradient between the PA and the LV. Note the types of obstructions noted in the diagram.

In mitral stenosis if it is essential to know both LA and LV-EDP, to evaluate the valvular gradient and valve area. If there are questions as to the accuracy of the PAW a transseptal heart cath may be required to get an accurate LA pressure.

Also, PCW pressure overestimates left atrial (LA) pressure in patients with acute respiratory failure, chronic obstructive lung disease with pulmonary hypertension, pulmonary Venoconstriction, or LV failure with volume overload. Here, a significant gradient exists between PAW and LA. This may be estimated from the PA-EDP to PAW gradient.

See: Kern chapter on "Hemodynamics." **Keywords:** PAW not = LV-EDP

19. Balloon floatation wedge pressure best reflects LA pressure when:

- a. **Low CO exists (CI < 2.0 L/min)**
- b. **The balloon completely blocks off distal PA flow**
- c. **The balloon is positioned in the anterior lung zone**
- d. **The balloon is positioned in the dependent lung zone**

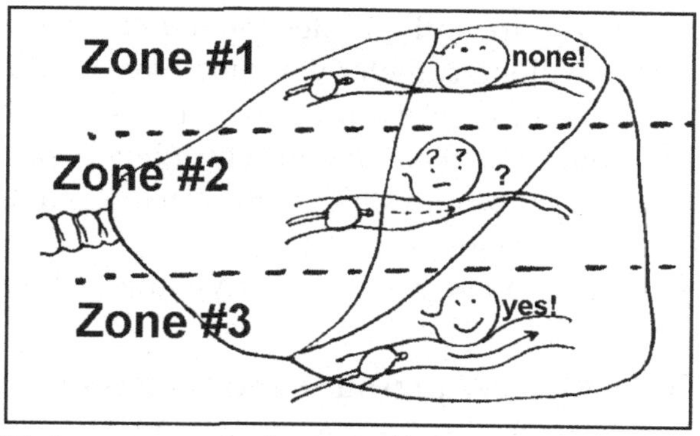

Pulmonary perfusion zones

ANSWER: d. The balloon is positioned in the dependent lung zone.

The three gravity dependent zones of perfusion in the lung are shown in the diagram. The dependent zone is nearest the ground. Blood tends to pool and expand vessels in this zone #3 (dependent). These open pulmonary capillaries assure transmission of LA pressure retrograde to the PAW. Because of this gravity effect, zone #1 (the superior aspect of the lung) has little or no pulmonary perfusion, so a wedge balloon positioned here is doomed to transmitting poor wedge pressure. When a PAWP is critical check the lateral X-ray view and reposition the balloon in zone #3.
See: Ahrens, chapter on "Normal Pulmonary Capillary Wedge and Central Venous Pressure." **Keywords:** Lung zone #3 (dependent) best for measuring PAW

20. In mitral valve disease, accurate measurement of the "wedge" pressure is critical. Which of the following can be used to confirm the accuracy of a "balloon wedge pressure"? (Check all that apply.)

- **a. Fluoroscopy (catheter tip advances to lung bed and stops moving)**
- **b. Make small contrast injections (contrast should not wash out)**
- **c. Properly timed "a" and "v" waves**
- **d. The O2 saturation of a "wedge"blood sample exceeds 80%.**
- **e. It is difficult to flush because it is wedged**

ANSWERS: a, b, & c.

- a. **YES: fluoroscopy (catheter tip advances to lung bed and stops moving)**
- b. **YES: make small contrast injections** (contrast should not wash out in 15 sec) Kern says this is 95% successful. A "fern" pattern contrast pattern also indicates "wedge."
- c. **YES: properly timed "a" and "v" waves assure that it is not just a "damped" PA tracing** (PA does NOT have a "v" wave component)
- d. NO: the O2 saturation of a "wedge" blood sample exceeds 80%.
- e. It is difficult to flush because it is wedged Kern recommends using a stiff, large-bore end-hole catheter. He says:

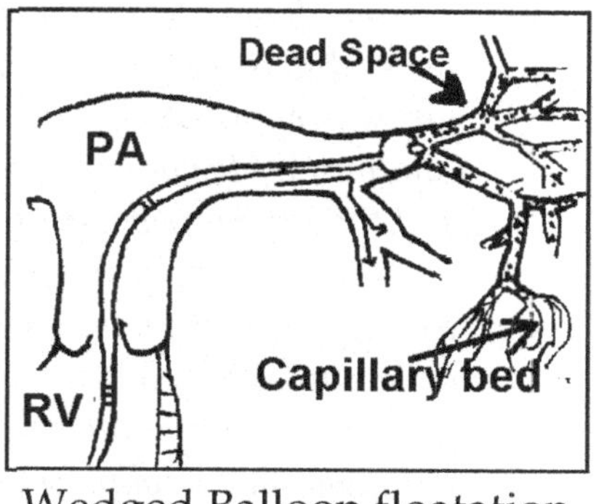

Wedged Balloon floatation catheter dead space

> *"Confirm the position of catheters (end-hole wedge) by oxygen saturation sample > 95% (obtaining this saturation not contaminated by low saturation pulmonary artery blood is difficult when the balloon is inflated)."*

With a balloon catheter 10-20 ml of trapped PA blood may remain between the balloon and the pulmonary capillary bed. This large unoxygenated dead space significantly dilutes the red Arteriolized blood that will be drawn back. With the balloon catheter you may have to draw back 20 or more ml. before you get the 95% saturation required for confirmation of the wedge.

Grossman also recommends checking that the wedge tracing "mean" is lower than the PA "mean," this assures the wedge tracing is not just a damped PA. Know these 3 indications of a good wedge pressure.

See: Kern, chapter on "Hemodynamics" **Keywords:** Wedge criteria

21. How do PAW pressure and transseptal LA pressures normally differ?

- a. **None - they are identical**
- b. **PAW has higher peak "A" and "V" waves**
- c. **PAW is delayed and slightly damped**
- d. **PAW shows increased respiratory variation**

ANSWER: c. PAW is delayed and slightly damped. For this reason when Wedge and LV are compared for mitral gradient assessment, wedge pressures must be shifted to the left .10 to .15 sec. so that the "V" wave coincides with the down stoke of the LV. Also, In PAW pressures the "a" and "c" waves often slur together and the "x" trough disappears. RA and LA have similar waveforms and are alike in having almost no delay. PAW and peripheral arteries are the most delayed due to the length of the transmitting fluid column. To reference these delayed PAW waves to the ECG : the "a" wave starts within or after the QRS complex. Whereas, the RA and LA "a" wave begins immediately after the P wave. Braunwald says,

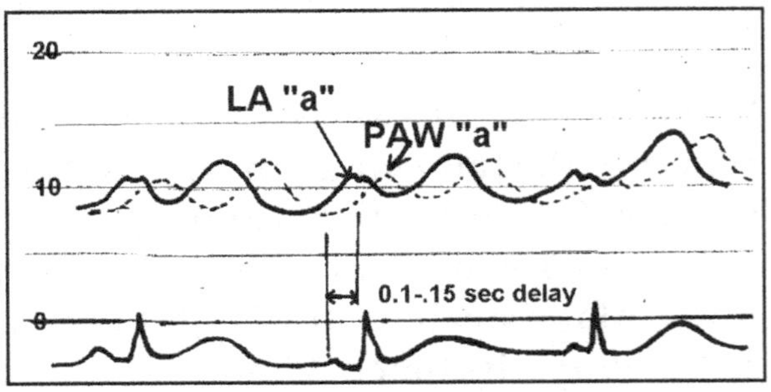

Superimposed LA and PAW tracings

> "*In the absence of mitral stenosis, left atrial and left ventricular pressures are equal during the mid-diastolic period (diastasis) and at end diastole. Because the pulmonary venous pressure approximates left atrial pressure in most circumstances, the mean pulmonary capillary wedge pressure provides a clinically useful estimate of mean left atrial pressure and the left ventricular filling pressure... The waveform of the pulmonary capillary wedge pressure also approximates the phasic left atrial wave pressure. However, the peak a and v waves in the pulmonary capillary wedge pressure are damped and delayed relative to the left atrial pressure. Accurate recording of pulmonary wedge pressures requires correct positioning of the catheter tip in the true wedge position to avoid recording a damped pulmonary arterial pressure. Failure to correct for the phase delay or mistaking a damped pulmonary arterial pressure for the wedge pressure may result in overestimating left atrial pressure.*"

See: Braunwald, chapter on "Left Heart Catheterization and Coronary Arteriography" and Kern, chapter on "Hemodynamics." **Keywords:** Difference between Wedge & LA pressures

USE THIS DIAGRAM FOR THE NEXT TWO QUESTIONS.

22. **What are the large waves seen in this PAW tracing?**

a. "A" wave
b. "V" wave
c. "X" descent
d. "Y" descent

23. **Estimate the end expiratory mean A wave of this PAW tracing.**

a. 15 mmHg
b. 18 mmHg
c. 22 mmHg
d. 27 mmHg
e. 44 mmHg

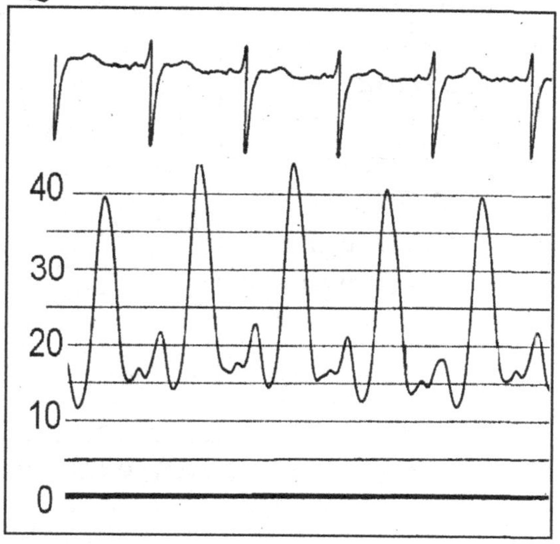

PAW tracing x 50

BOTH ANSWERS APPEAR TOGETHER BELOW:

22. ANSWER: b. "v" wave. The "a" wave is the small wave immediately following the QRS complex. Remember PAW "a" wave is normally delayed from P wave and starts IN or AFTER the QRS. The large wave seen is a "v" wave due to mitral regurgitation
See: Ahrens, chapter on "Normal Pulmonary Capillary Wedge and Central Venous Pressure." **Keywords:** ID "v" wave

23. . **ANSWER:** b. 18 mmHg. For the "MEAN A" select the 2 beats at end expiration where pressure is highest, just before the inspiratory dip. The "MEAN A" is the average between the top and bottom of that "a" wave, or (22 +14)/2 = 18 mmHg.

This "MEAN A" wave is supposed to be the best estimate of LV-EDP. LV-EDP in this patient was actually 20 mmHg.
See: Ahrens, chapter on "Normal Pulmonary Capillary Wedge and Central Venous Pressure." **Keywords:** Measure mean "a" wave

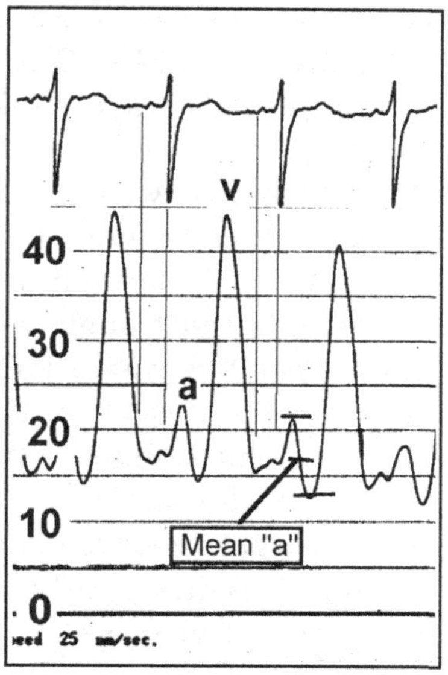

Mean "a" in PAW tracing x 50

24. **Identify the negative wave labeled #5 in this PAW tracing.**

a. **"A" wave**
b. **"C" wave**
c. **"V" wave**
d. **"X" trough**
e. **"Y" trough**

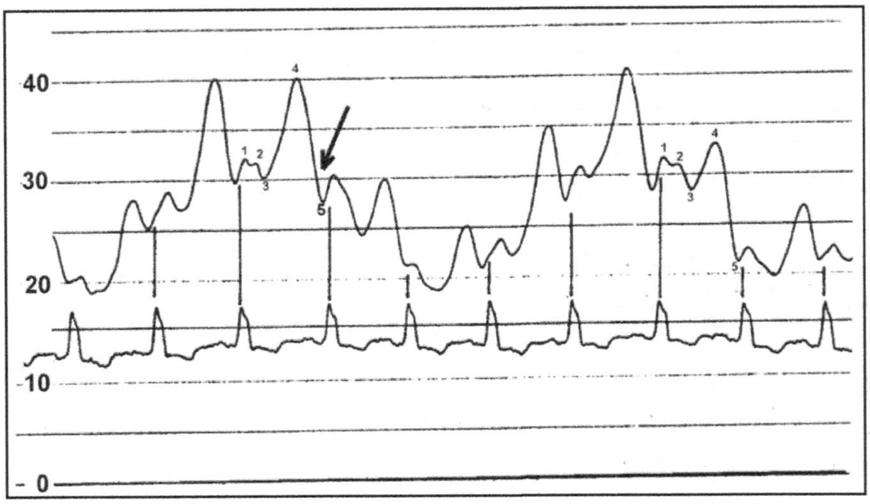

PA Wedge pressure x 50

ANSWER: e. "Y" trough. The "y" is due to early rapid diastolic filling. Note that it follows the positive "v" wave and preceedes the positive "a" wave. (To remember "Early" ends in "y"). **CORRECTLY MATCHED ANSWERS ARE:**

1. **"a" positive wave** - Follows ECG "p" wave, (Due to Atrial contraction)
2. **"c" positive wave** - Follows ECG "QRS" wave - often so small that it is not seen (Due to Closure of the AV valve and ventricular Contraction).
3. **"x" negative trough wave** - Follows "a" wave
4. **"v" positive wave** - Follows ECG "T" wave. Atrial pressure rises to a peak in late diastole due to Ventricular filling or "Villing" against a closed AV valve. (It peaks at AV valve opening.)
5. **"y" negative wave** - Follows ECG "T" wave. Remember the "y" is due to early rapid diastolic filling (Early ends in y).
6. **"z" negative wave** - Follows atrial "a" wave, and precedes "c" wave - not marked on this tracing.

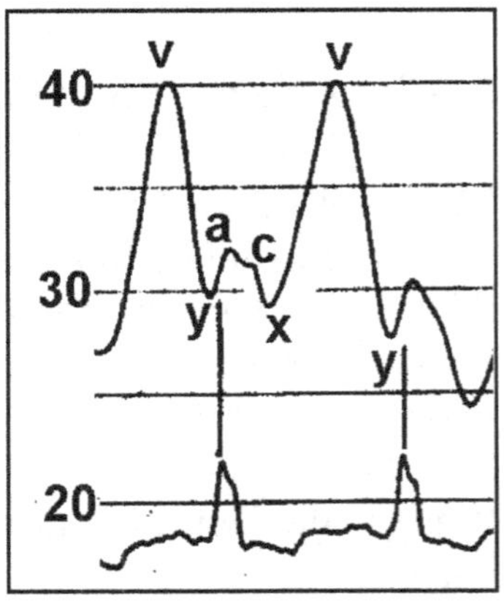

PA Wedge pressure x 50

Note that the PAW tracing is considerably delayed (0.1 sec) from the ECG. All the positive waves occur in alphabetic order: a, c, v. The negative waves also appear in alphabetic order: x, y, z. **See:** Kern, chapter on "Hemodynamics." **Keywords**: Venous waves: a, c, v, x, y, z

25. **Read the overall pulmonary artery wedge (PAW) pressure shown in mmHg as a computer would.**

a. 18,13,11
b. 18,11,13
c. 16,14,12
d. 11,16,20

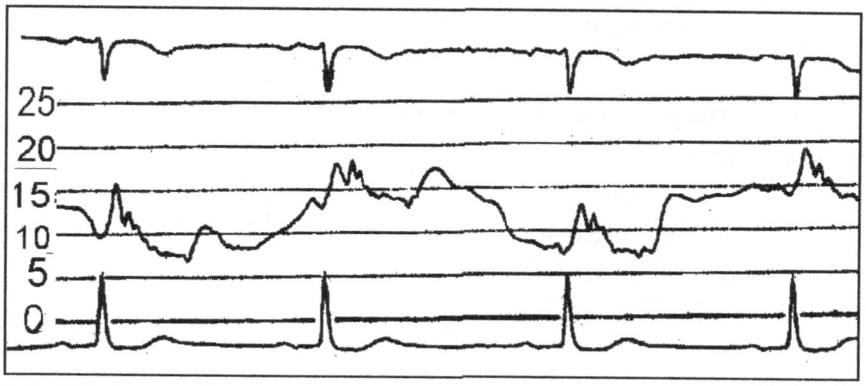

PA Wedge x 50

ANSWER: c. 16, 14, 12 mmHg. Remember that atrial pressures are read (a, v, m).

The notched wave is the "a" wave because it is the first wave to follow the ECG P wave. The time delay in the PAWP is about 0.1 sec (due to the long conduit through the lung bed). As the RV contracts in systole and the tricuspid valve slams shut it often vibrates the catheter, making a "c" wave closure" artifact. These A and C waves often imperceptibly join together. Overall average of the peak A waves is 16 mmHg.

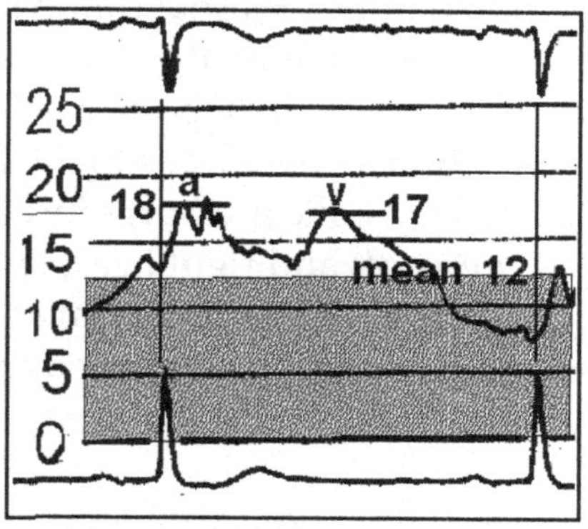

PA Wedge x 50 - End Exp.

The second rounded wave is the V wave, because it follows the ECG T wave.

The mean can be read by laying down a clear plastic ruler so that half the area is above and half below the straight edge. Overall readings through the 2 respiratory cycles shows gives 16, 14, 12 mmHg (a, v, m). This is how a computer would average the readings.

Considerable respiratory variation is present in all right heart pressures. Computers will read this "overall" mean pressure, throughout the sampling period. If the sampling period includes inspiration, as this one does, the averaged readings will be erroneously low. It is preferable to read pressures during the end of expiration or have the patient passively hold his breath. These expiratory plateau readings are 18, 17, 12 mmHg (a, v, m) as shown. Computers are only as accurate as the operator (Garbage In, Garbage Out).

See: Kern, chapter on "Hemodynamics." **Keywords:** LA pressure measurement

Normal Ventricular Pressures

26. **Measure the RV pressure shown in this diagram?**

a. **30 / 12 / 20 mmHg**
b. **30 / 18 / 22 mmHg.**
c. **33 / 12 / 20 mmHg.**
d. **35 / 18 / 22 mmHg.**

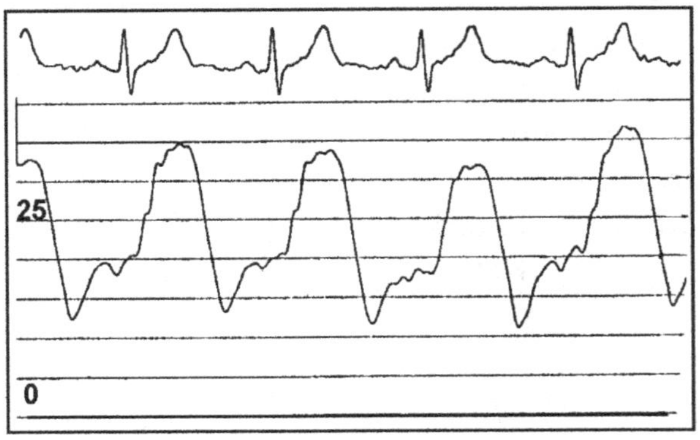

RV pressure x 50

ANSWER: c. 33/12/20 mm Hg.
Ventricular end diastolic pressure is measured after the atrial filling just before the ventricle begins its rapid contraction. Because the RV contracts slightly later than the LV, RV-EDP best correlates with the end of the QRS. The LV best corresponds to the peak of the R wave. The elevated diastolic pressures indicate probable elevated CVP (RA pressure) and right heart failure. Early diastole shows a "square root" pattern, associated with constrictive disease. **See:** Kern, chapter on "Hemodynamics." **Keywords:** LVEDP measurement

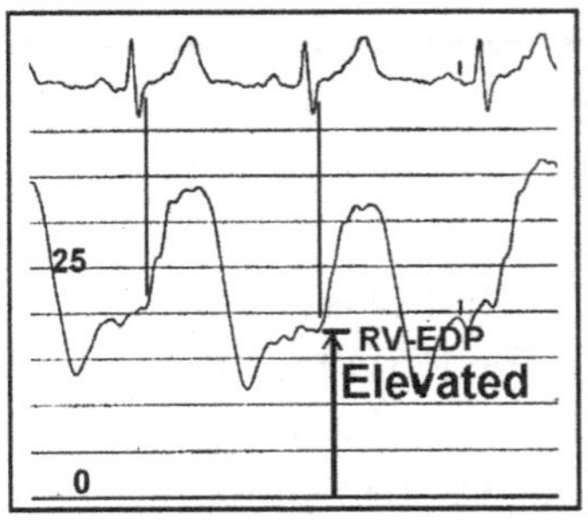

RV pressure x 50

THE NEXT 2 QUESTIONS REFER TO THIS DIAGRAM:

27. **How would you estimate and report the Beginning Diastolic LV (LV-BDP) pressures shown in this diagram?**

a. **- 5 mmHg**
b. **0 mmHg**
c. **12 mmHg**
d. **20 mmHg**

28. **How would you estimate and report the End-Diastolic LV (LV-EDP) pressures shown in this diagram?**

a. **15 mmHg**
b. **25 mmHg**
c. **32 mmHg**
d. **42 mmHg**

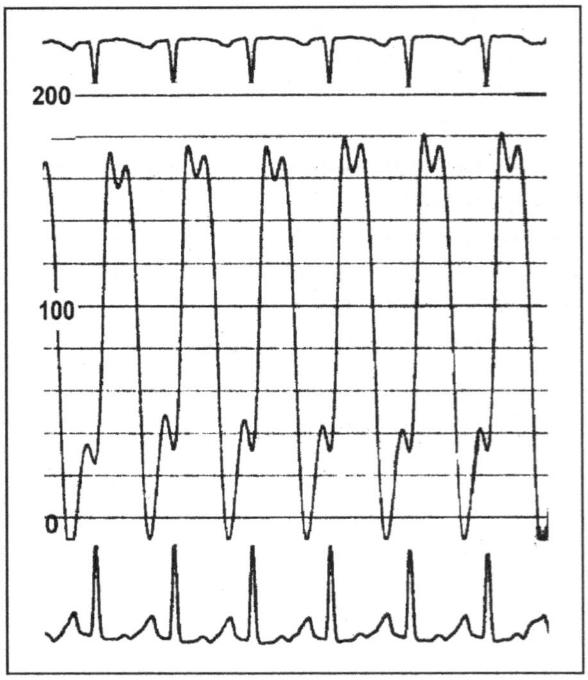

LV pressure x 200

BOTH ANSWERS FOR THE DIAGRAM ABOVE APPEAR TOGETHER BELOW:

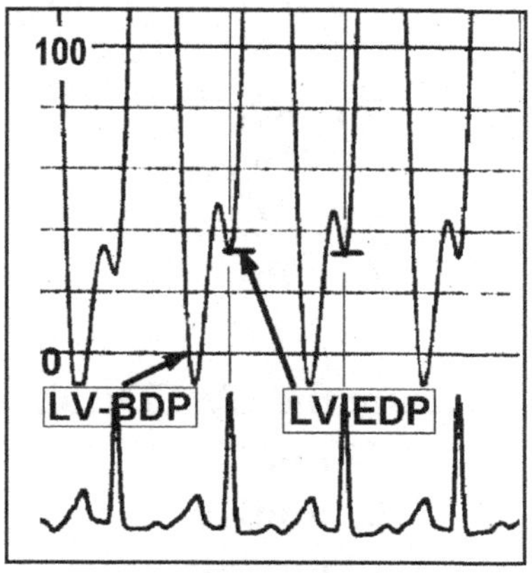

LV pressure x 200

27. ANSWER: b. 0 (zero) mmHg = LV-BDP. This beginning diastolic wave severely undershoots the true reading. ***Intracardiac pressure should normally never go below zero.*** This error is common in underdamped systems due to air bubbles or an excessively long pressure tubing. Negative computer readings should be corrected. When any pressure goes negative as seen here, edit the markers to make it read 0 mmHg.
See: Kern, chapter on "Hemodynamics" **Keywords:** LVEDP measurement

28. **ANSWER:** c. 32 mmHg. = LV-EDP. LV-EDP is a most important number used to evaluate LV function and preload. LV-EDP can be read either from the pressure tracing waveform (after the "a" wave), or by correlating it with the QRS complex on ECG (at the R wave).

• **THE TRACING METHOD**: look for the end of atrial contraction or a point from which the LV pressure rapidly accelerates - c wave. That is EDP. The atrial contraction wave is often evident on the LV curve at the end of diastole. The first beat shows a clear plateau EDP at 30 mmHg. All the diastolic dips average to 32 mmHg. Braunwald says,

> *End-diastolic pressure is generally measured at the c point, which is the rise in ventricular pressure at the onset of isovolumic contraction ... When the c point is not well seen, a line is drawn from the R wave on the simultaneous ECG to the ventricular pressure waveform, and this is used as the end-diastolic pressure."*

• **THE ECG METHOD**: the LV-EDP should normally align with the peak R wave. Lay a plastic ruler vertically between the 2 R waves shown and see how this electrical correlation gives the same EDP as reading the notch. Kern says,

> *"The left ventricular end diastolic pressure is measured after the A wave corresponding to the peak of the R wave (...follow the ventricular time line at the first R wave down to its crossing point on the left ventricular pressure)."*

The LV-EDP is more accurately measured on range X50 and 50 paper speed, where the diastolic values are magnified. Note that the systole also has a resonant notch, which should be averaged at 166 mmHg. Overall pressures average 170/0/32 mmHg.
See: Pepine, chapter on, "Pressure Measurement..." **Keywords:** LV-beginning diastolic pressure measurement

USE THIS DIAGRAM FOR THE NEXT 5 QUESTIONS BELOW:

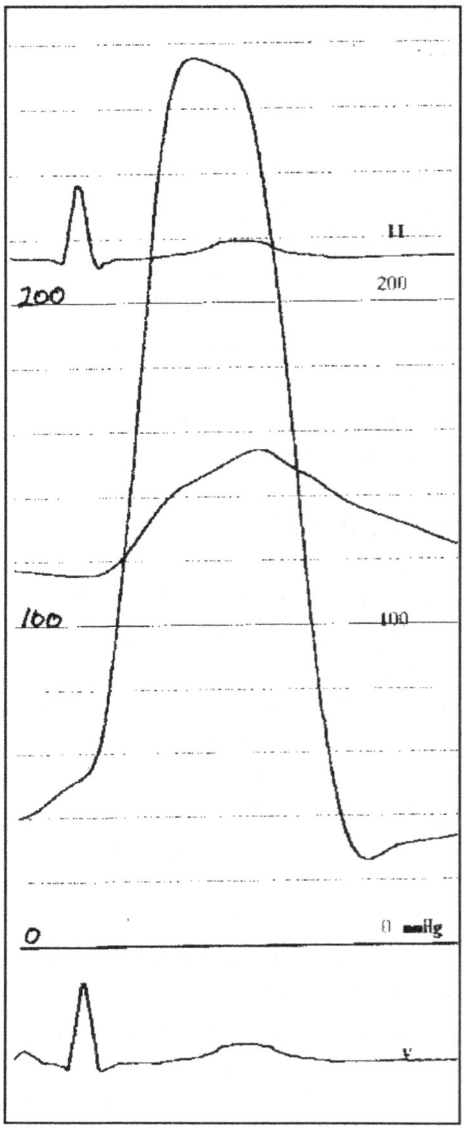

Simultaneous pressures recorded x200

29. What two simultaneous pressures are recorded here?

a. RV, RA
b. LV, PAW
c. LV, AO
d. AO, PA

30. Measure the LV-EDP shown.

a. 52 mmHg
b. 62 mmHg
c. 72 mmHg
d. 82 mmHg

31. Measure the peak-to-peak LV-AO pressure gradient shown.

a. 100 mmHg
b. 110 mmHg
c. 120 mmHg
d. 130 mmHg

32. Measure the maximum instantaneous LV-AO pressure gradient shown.

a. 100 mmHg
b. 110 mmHg
c. 120 mmHg
d. 130 mmHg

33. These two pressures are normally recorded simultaneously to evaluate the:

a. Aortic valve
b. Mitral valve
c. Pulmonic valve
d. Tricuspid valve

ANSWERS FOR THE DIAGRAM ABOVE APPEAR TOGETHER BELOW:

29. ANSWER c. LV, AO. LV is identified by the rapidly rising high systolic pressure with a slowly rising diastolic slope. AO is identified by the triangular high pressure with descending diastolic slope. See: Grossman, chapter on "Pressure Measurements"
Keywords: Identify simultaneous LV - AO pressures

30. ANSWER a. 52 mmHg = LV-EDP. Atrial kick "a" waves are seen immediately prior to LV systole. The junction of this triangular "a" wave and the rapid isometric contraction is the LV-EDP = 52 mmHg. It can also be identified as the point on the LV curve timed to the ECG R wave. See: Grossman, chapter on "Pressure Measurements" Keywords: Measure LV-ED pressure

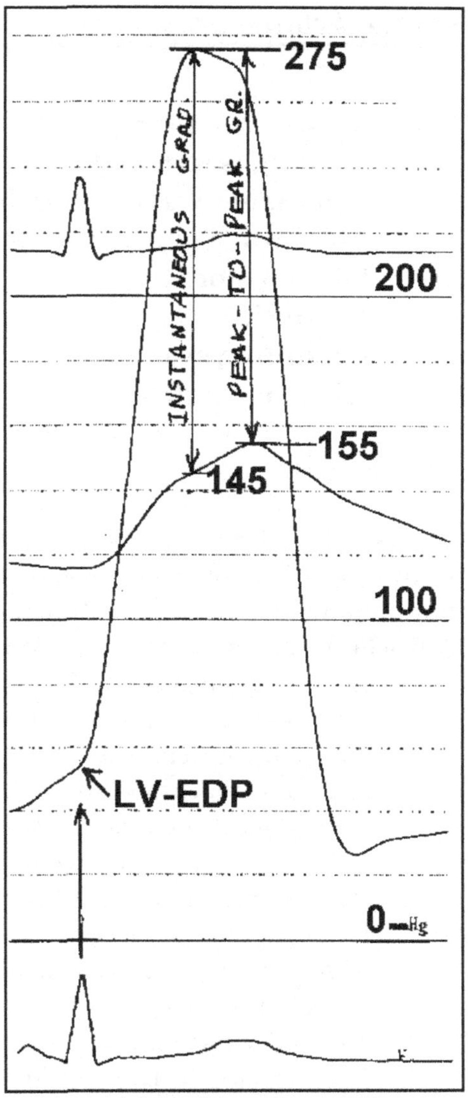

Simultaneous LV & AO gradients x 200

31. ANSWER c. 120 mmHg. The peak LV is 275 mmHg. The peak AO is 155 mmHg. Peak-to-peak gradient is the difference between these 2 peaks. Peak to peak gradient = 275-155 = 120 mmHg. Note that the peak AO is later in systole than the peak LV. So horizontal lines must be drawn at the 2 peak pressures, and the peak-to-peak gradient measured between them. Peak-to-peak gradient is the most commonly measured gradient in the cath lab. It can be easily identified on LV→ AO pullback as the difference between the 2 peak pressures. The peak-to-peak pressures need not be correctly aligned for transmission delay. However, instantaneous peak gradients must be exactly aligned to compare with echo and catheter tip manometer readings. See: Braunwald, chapter on "Echocardiography." Keywords: peak-to-peak aortic gradient

32. ANSWER d. 130 mmHg. The instantaneous gradient is the greatest gradient that can be found between LV and AO. It occurs prior to the peak-to-peak gradient - usually straight down from the peak LV pressure. These pressures must be correctly aligned for transmission delay. Usually the AO is delayed from the LV and needs to be shifted to the left. This tracing is properly aligned. Measure straight down from the peak LV (275) to where a vertical line intersects the AO (145). The peak instantaneous gradient is then 275 - 145 = 130 mmHg. This is important because echocardiographic gradients are measured instantaneously and are expected to be larger than the peak-to-peak gradient measured at cath. With skilled echocardiographers the echo/Doppler may becoming the gold standard for valvular hemodynamics. See: Braunwald, chapter on "Echocardiography." Keywords: Instantaneous aortic gradient

33. ANSWER a. Aortic valve. The aortic valve lies between the LV and AO. Simultaneous pressure gradients are taken across it to assess for aortic stenosis. Large valvular gradients usually require intervention, E.g., valve replacement or valvuloplasty. This gradient is excessive for demonstration purposes.
See: Grossman, chapter on "Pressure Measurements" **Keywords:** simultaneous LV-AO evaluates aortic valve

Normal Arterial pressures

34. The arterial blood pressure wave shown at #5 in this arterial tracing is termed the ________ wave/phase.

a. Percussion wave (rapid systolic ejection)
b. Tidal wave (slow systolic ejection)
c. Dicrotic notch
d. Diastolic
e. Beginning systole
f. Anacrotic notch

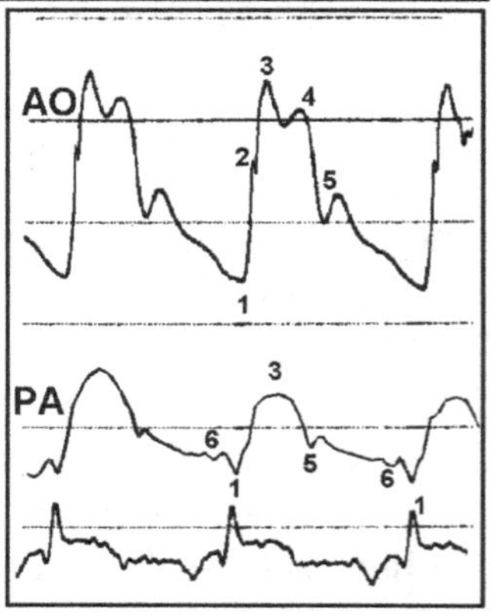

Arterial BP

ANSWER: c. Dicrotic notch is an important point marking the end of systole and the beginning of diastole (isometric relaxation). This notch is an important landmark in balloon pumping, where the IABP is timed to inflate at the dicrotic notch.

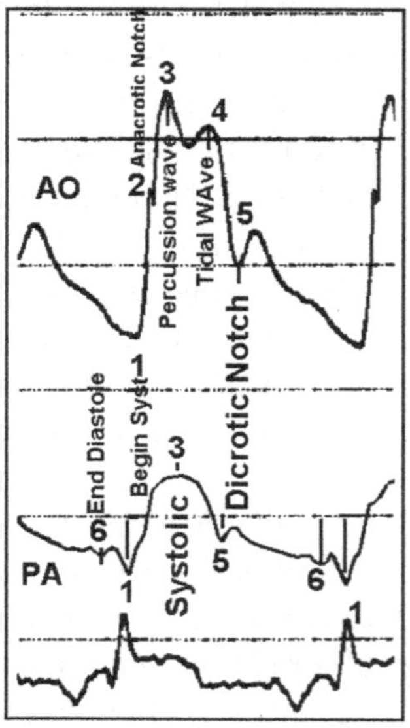

Arterial BP

CORRECTLY MATCHED ANSWERS ARE:

1. **Beginning systole**: Initial upstroke of the pulse associated with opening of the semilunar valve.
2. **Anacrotic notch:** occasionally seen on the upstroke of the arterial wave, associated with semilunar valve stenosis and slowed ejection. It is seldom seen except in aortic stenosis and in underdamped recording systems..
3. **Percussion wave or systole:** (rapid systolic ejection) - the highest point is "systole."
4. **Tidal wave (slow systolic ejection):** The tidal wave is the reflected percussion pulse returning after bouncing off the aorto-iliac bifurcation. It is not always seen.
5. **Dicrotic notch:** The dicrotic notch or "incisura" is the slight back-flow of aortic blood that occurs with aortic valve closure, resulting in a rebound in aortic pressure when the back-flow of blood bounces off the slammed aortic valve. This notch is the critical landmark for inflation of aortic counter pulsation devices.
6. **End diastole:** ends ventricular filling associated with closure of AV valves. It is chiefly seen on PA tracings as closure of tricuspid valve on the antegrade catheter - seldom seen on aortic tracings.. **See:** Kern's Chapter on "Pressure measurement."

35. The numeric difference between arterial systolic and diastolic pressures is termed the:

a. Driving pressure
b. Trans valvular pressure
c. Peak to peak pressure
d. Pulse pressure
e. Gradient

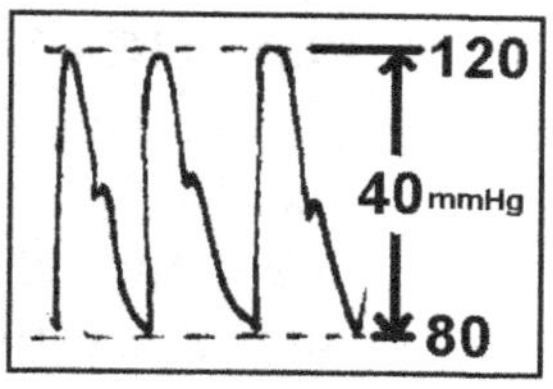

AO. Pulse Pressure

ANSWER: d. Pulse pressure is the difference between systolic and diastolic pressures. In a BP of 120/80 the pulse pressure is 120-80 or 40 mmHg. Aortic insufficiency may result in a wide aortic pulse pressure. What we feel when we palpate a pulse is this pulse pressure difference.
See: medical dictionary. Keywords: Arterial pulse pressure

THE NEXT 2 QUESTIONS REFER TO THIS DIAGRAM:

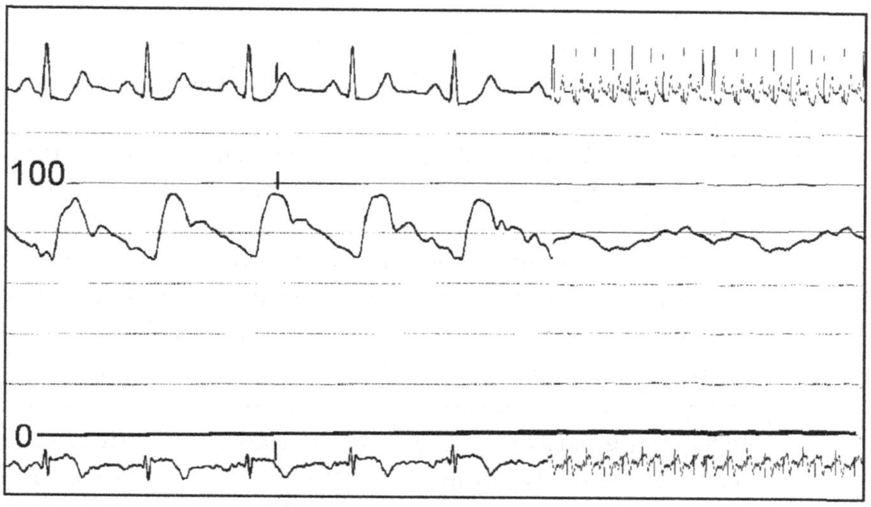

Arterial pressure with mean recorded x 200

36. **Measure the aortic pulse pressure on this recording.**
- a. **25 mmHg**
- b. **30 mmHg**
- c. **70 mmHg**
- d. **95 mmHg**

37. **Measure the "mean"arterial pressure from the "mean" recording shown.**
- a. **70 mmHg**
- b. **77 mmHg**
- c. **85 mmHg**
- d. **93 mmHg**

BOTH ANSWERS LISTED TOGETHER BELOW:

36. ANSWER: a. 25 mmHg. The first part of the tracing is recorded on "phasic" and shows the characteristic triangular waveform of AO on x 200. Systolic pressure here is 95 mmHg. Diastole is 70 mmHg. The pulse pressure difference 95-75=25 mmHg.
See: Kern, chapter on "Hemodynamics."

37. ANSWER: b. 77 mmHg. The last part of the tracing shows a recorded "mean." The "mean switch" was turned on and the recorder speed reduced to 10 mm/sec. The three methods of measuring mean are: Plastic ruler method, formula method, and computer integration.

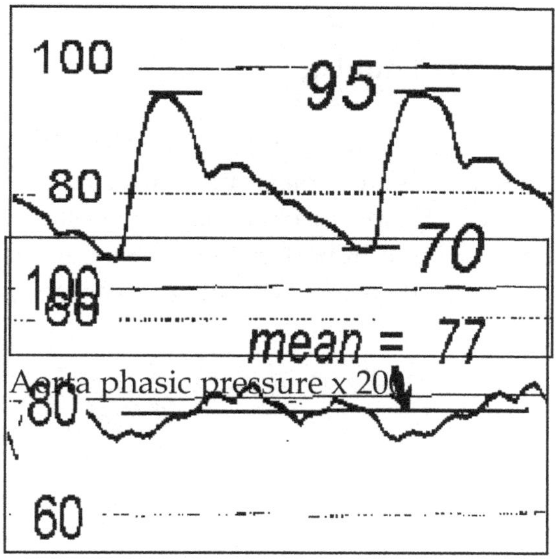

Reading a "mean" arterial pressure

- **PLASTIC RULER METHOD**: the "mean" is measured through the middle of at least one complete respiratory cycle. Lay a clear plastic ruler down horizontally over that mean and adjust it so there are equal amounts of the sine wave above and below the ruler edge. Read the mean pressure at the edge of the ruler. The average "mean" is estimated at 80 mmHg.
- **FORMULA METHOD:** another, ***less accurate*** method to estimate an arterial mean is the formula:

$$\text{mean AO} = \frac{\text{systole} + (2 \times \text{diastole})}{3}$$

  This places the mean 1/3 of the distance up, between diastole and systole, and is closer to diastole than systole. As you see the formula gives 78 mmHg - a close estimate.
- **COMPUTER INTEGRATION METHOD:** modern computers normally automate this averaging process. They can integrate the phasic curve, so a separate recording mean does not need to be run, like we did here. This computer method is quite accurate if you want the overall mean throughout the respiratory cycle. Ahrens favors this method for peripheral arterial line pressure. He maintains that ***peripheral arterial pressures (BA & FA) should be measured through one complete respiratory cycle, and NOT at the end of expiration.*** Since peripheral arterial pressures are not measured inside the chest, pleural pressure fluctuations have little effect. In the periphery, the slow fluctuations in arterial pressure are more related to changes in stroke volume, compliance, and peripheral resistance. However, since all right heart, LV pressures and thoracic aorta are measure within the chest, they should be measured at the *end of expiration*. Computerized recorders use an overall average since they cannot tell where the end of expiration is. You are smarter than a computer. **See:** Kern, chapter on "Hemodynamics."

38. Estimate mean arterial pressure of a patient with a BP of 200/100 mmHg.

a. **133 mmHg**
b. **140 mmHg**
c. **150 mmHg**
d. **160 mmHg**

Answer: a.133 mmHg. (S + 2 D)/3 = (200 + 2x100)/3 = 133.3 mmHg. This formula estimates that the mean BP is approximately 1/3 of the pulse pressure above diastole. True mean BP is closer to diastole than systole depending on the shape of the arterial pulse. That's why in hypertension measuring diastolic pressure is more important than systole. This formula is less accurate than actually measuring it by digital integration.

39. At what point int the respiratory cycle should brachial and femoral artery pressure be measured?

- a. **Through one complete respiratory cycle**
- b. **At end of expiration**
- c. **At end of inspiration**
- d. **At peak respiratory cycle**

ANSWER: a. Through one complete respiratory cycle. This is different than cardiac pressure measurement. ***Peripheral arterial pressures (BA & FA) should be measured through one complete respiratory cycle, and NOT at the end of expiration as cardiac pressures are.*** Since peripheral arterial pressures are not measured inside the chest, pleural pressure fluctuations have little effect. In the periphery, the slow fluctuations in arterial pressure are more related to changes in stroke volume, compliance, and peripheral resistance. However, since all right heart, LV pressures and thoracic aorta are measure within the chest, they should be measured at the *end of expiration*. Computerized recorders use an overall average since they cannot tell where the end of expiration is. **See:** Kern, chapter on "Hemodynamics."

40. Which arterial site will normally have the highest systolic blood pressure? (Consider the effects of harmonics and wave reflection.)

- a. **Ascending AO**
- b. **AO arch**
- c. **Descending AO**
- d. **Femoral artery**
- e. **Popliteal artery**

ANSWER: e. Popliteal artery. As arterial pulse waves propagate down the elastic aorta, reflection waves bounce back and increase the systolic components of distal pressures. As the distal vessels get smaller and further from the aortic valve, the systolic pressure increases (up to a point). This is termed "peripheral amplification" of the systolic pulse. In the periphery it may increase by as much as 20-40 mmHg. During LV →AO pullback, if AO is sampled low in the aorta, its higher systole may resemble a "reverse peak-to-peak gradient" (E.g. LV=120/8, AO=130/80)

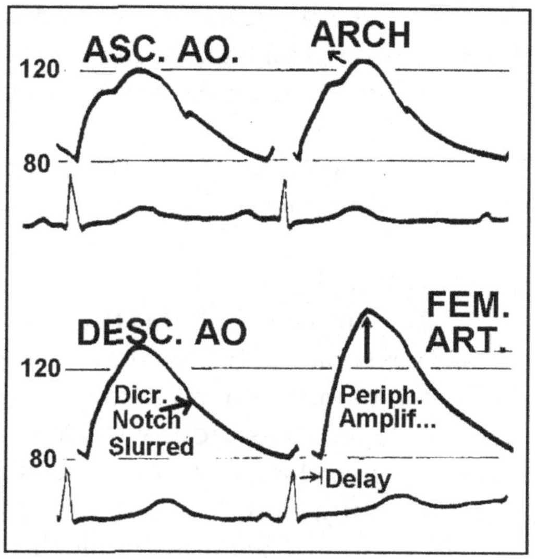

Arterial pressure - different locations

In addition to systolic increase, distal pulses show a more delayed and steeper upstroke. The amount of systolic amplification varies greatly depending on the elasticity of the AO and other factors. Braunwald says,

"As the systemic pressure wave is transmitted through the length of the aorta, the systolic wave increases in amplitude and becomes more triangular in shape, while the diastolic wave decreases until it reaches the midthoracic aorta and then increases. The mean aortic pressures, however, are usually similar, with the mean peripheral arterial pressure typically < 5 mm Hg lower than the mean central aortic pressure. The difference in systolic pressures between the central aorta and the periphery (femoral, brachial, or radial arteries) is greatest in younger patients due to their increased vascular compliance."

See: Braunwald, chapter on "Left heart catheterization and coronary Arteriography" and Grossman, chapter on "Pressure Measurement."

41. What chamber or vessel is recorded here on x 50?

a. RA
b. RV
c. PA
d. PAW

42. Estimate the diastolic pressure of this PA tracing:

a. 5 mmHg
b. 8 mmHg
c. 10 mmHg
d. 14 mmHg

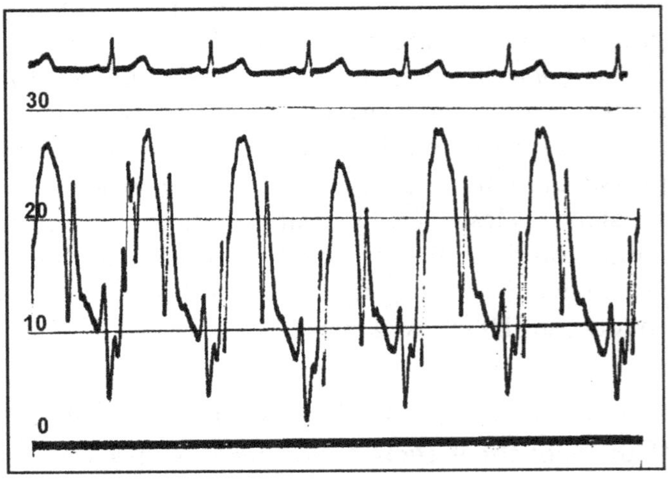

Pressure x 50

BOTH ANSWERS LISTED TOGETHER BELOW:

41. **ANSWER:** c. PA. This is Pulmonary artery shows the characteristic triangular waveform on x 50. Although, considerable resonance artifact occurs, the dicrotic notch is clearly seen. Systolic pressure here is near the normal value of 25 mmHg. Note the normally low PA-diastolic pressure near the PAW mean level.
See: Kern, chapter on "Hemodynamics."**Keywords:** Identify PA pressure

42. **ANSWER:** b. 8 mmHg.

The problem with this PA tracing is the excessive resonance that makes it difficult to read. This is commonly seen in PA tracings at the end of diastole. These pre-systolic vibrations may be due to tricuspid valve closure on the catheter or the RV's isometric contraction. A computer would incorrectly read the bottom of the pre-systolic dip. However, a skilled operator is able to "read through" the artifact and average the diastolic resonance to 8 mmHg. You must move the computer markers to a place

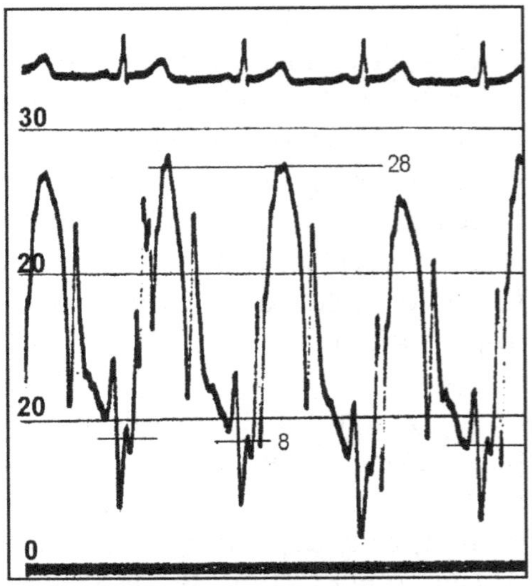

PA Pressure x 50

before the pre-systolic dip. Overriding computer sample points is essential for accurate hemodynamic results. In a clear PA tracing the end of RV diastole normally coincides with the end of the QRS.

Systolic peaks average between 25 and 28, with an end expiratory reading of 28 mmHg. Estimate the average peak by laying down a clear plastic ruler midway between the higher systolic peaks. **See:** Ahrens, chapter on "Normal Arterial Pressures."

REFERENCES:

Ahrens, and Taylor, *Hemodynamic Waveform Analysis*, 1st Ed., W.B. Saunders Co., 1992

Baim, D. S. and Grossman W., *Cardiac Catheterization, Angiography, and Intervention*, 7th Ed., Lea and Febiger, 2006

Braunwald, et. al. Ed., *Heart Disease, a Textbook of CV Medicine*, 9th Ed., Saunders, 2012

Berne R. M. and Levy, M. N., *Cardiovascular Physiology*, 8th Ed., Mosby Year Book, 2001

Daily, E. K., and Schroeder, J. S., *Techniques in Bedside Hemodynamic Monitoring*, 4th Ed., C. V. Mosby Company, 1989

Darovic, G.O., *Hemodynamic Monitoring: Invasive and Noninvasive Clinical Application*, WB Saunders, 1995

Kern, M. J., Ed., *The Cardiac Catheterization Handbook*, 6th Ed., Elsevier, 2016

PACEP.org Pulmonary Artery Catheter Education Project, sponsored by ASA

Pepine, J. C., and Hill, J. A., et. al., *Diagnostic and Therapeutic Cardiac Catheterization*, 2nd Ed., Williams and Wilkins, 1994

Ragosta, Michael, Textbook of Clinical Hemodynamics, Saunders, 1st Edition, 2008

Taylor, E. J. Ed., *Dorland's Medical Dictionary*, 27th ed., W. B. Saunders Co.,1988

Chapter Outline - INTRODUCTION TO CV PRESSURES

1. PRESSURE BASICS
   a. Waveforms
      i. Sine wave atrial
      ii. Square wave = ventricular
      iii. Triangle wave = arterial
   b. Pressure readings
      i. Venous = a, v, mean
      ii. Ventricular = s / bd, ed
      iii. Arterial = s / d, mean
   c. Normal values
      i. LA, LV, AO
      ii. IVC, RA, RV, PA, PAW
   d. Pullback pressures
      i. Valve crossing
      ii. Normal pullbacks
         (1) LV→AO
         (2) PA→RV
         (3) PAW→PA
         (4) RV→RA
         (5) Normal equalities
            (a) Vent. syst. = Art. syst.
            (b) Vent. EDP = Atrial "a"
   e. Push through pressures
      i. Inflated swan floating through
   f. Respiratory Effects
      i. Valsalva Effects on BP
      ii. Intrathoracic pressure
      iii. Pressures normally drop with inspiration
      iv. Pressures normally rise with expiration
      v. Ventilator effects are apposite (rise with insp.)
      vi. Transmural pressure
         (1) Eliminates pleural

pressure
- (2) True intracardiac pressure
- g. Expiration
  - i. Is passive
  - ii. End expiration is best place to measure pressure
  - iii. Do not let patient ValSalva
- h. Breathing patterns effect on pressures
  - i. Normal effect = mild insp. dip
  - ii. Pulsus Paradoxicus= excessive dip
    - (1) pericardial tamponade
  - iii. Kussmaul's sign
    - (1) opposite to normal dip
    - (2) Constrictive pericarditis
- i. Stenosis
  - i. Gradients

2. NORMAL VENOUS PRESSURES
   - a. Identify waves:
     - i. a,c,v,x,y
   - b. Read pressures
     - i. a,v,m
   - c. LVEDP = LA = PAW
     - i. If no stenosis between PA and LV
   - d. RVEDP = RA
   - e. Differences between RA, LA, PAW
   - f. Assessing PAWP
     - i. catheter tip advances to lung bed and stops moving
     - ii. contrast does not wash out
     - iii. Properly timed "a" and "v" waves
     - iv. PAW blood sample exceeds 95%
   - g. Lung zones: West 1, 2, 3
     - i. Dependent Zone 3 = best PAWP
3. NORMAL VENTRICULAR PRESSURES
   - a. Measure pressure levels
     - i. Never record ventricular mean
   - b. Identify & read LVEDP
     - i. Waveform method
     - ii. ECG method (R wave)
   - c. Identify and read LVBDP
     - i. never read below zero
   - d. Gradients
     - i. Peak-to-peak (LV-AO)
     - ii. Maximum (LV-AO)
     - iii. Mean gradient (for valve area)
4. NORMAL ARTERIAL PRESSURES
   - a. Arterial Waves
     - i. Percussion wave (rapid systolic ejection)
     - ii. Tidal wave (slow systolic ejection)
     - iii. Dicrotic notch
     - iv. Diastolic
     - v. Beginning systole
     - vi. Anacrotic notch
     - vii. Artifacts
   - b. Pulse Pressure = syst. - diast.
     - i. Ruler method
     - ii. Formula method
     - iii. Integration method
   - c. Peripheral amplification
     - i. Systole highest in periphery

READING PRESSURES

INDEX E2

1. ECG Related Pressures

43. **This hemodynamic tracing on x200 shows: (Beware the noisy ECG)**

a. Atrial fibrillation
b. Atrial flutter
c. Bigeminy
d. Large dicrotic notch

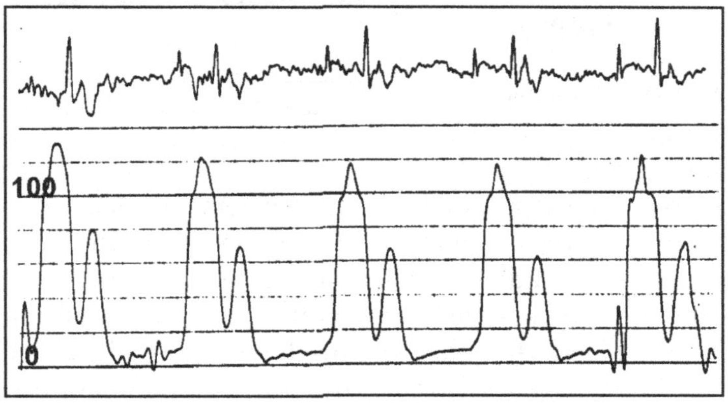

Hemodynamic trace with arrhythmia x 200

ANSWER c. LV in bigeminy. The catheter is in the LV with a systolic pressure of 120 mmHg. Note that the small contractions (associated with PVCs) have too short a filling time to generate significant LV pressure and may not result in any arterial pulse.

This ECG is noisy, but definite QRS complexes are seen between the last two ventricular systoles. PVCs coupled to sinus beats can be seen clearly in the last two cycles. A better ECG lead is added to clarify the second recording. Bigeminy refers to a pattern of normal and Premature beats, as follows:

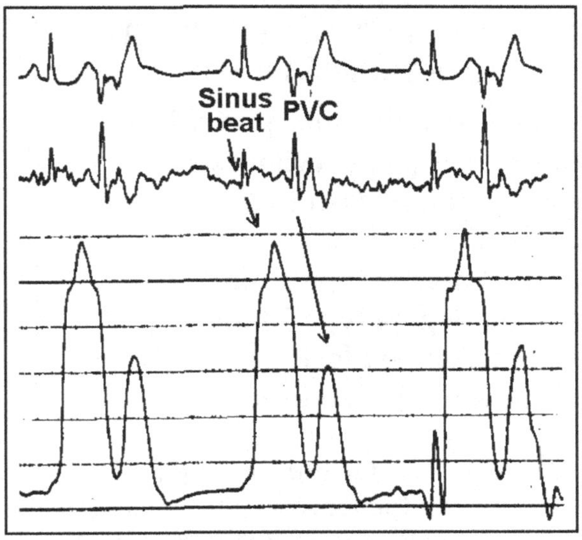

Hemodynamic trace in Ventricular Bigeminy x 200

- Bigeminy = a normal sinus beat followed by a PVC.
- Trigeminy = 2 normal sinus beats then a PVC or PAC.
- Quadrageminy = 3 normal sinus beats then a PVC or PAC...
- Couplet = Two successive PVCs
- Triplet = 3 successive PVCs
- Ventricular Tach. = more than 3 successive PVCs
- Sustained Ventricular Tach.. = more than 30 seconds of successive PVCs

See: Braunwald, Chapter on Specific Arrhythmias..." **Keywords**: Bigeminy

44. **This venous pressure tracing has no "a" waves because of:**

a. P mitrale
b. Atrial fibrillation
c. Atrial flutter
d. 3rd degree AV node block

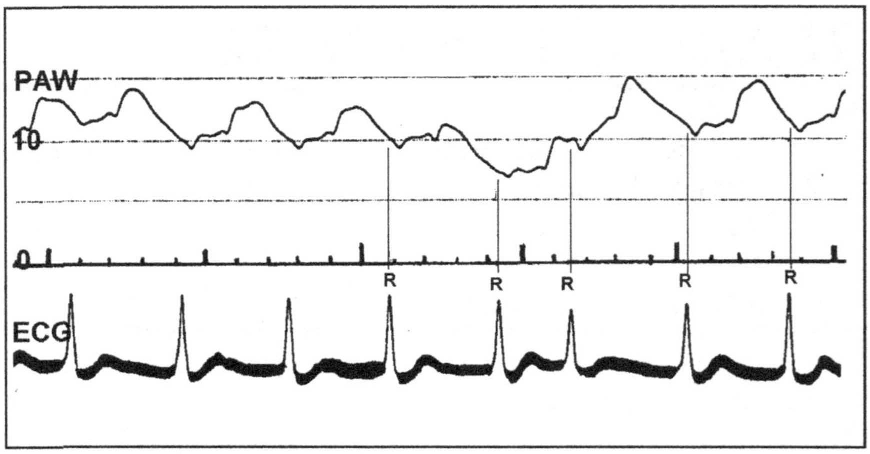

Absence of a waves PAW x 50

ANSWER b. Atrial fibrillation.
Since atrial contraction causes the hemodynamic a wave, loss of P waves on the ECG as in atrial fibrillation, results in loss of venous a waves. However, C waves are often seen, which normally immediately follow atrial contraction. Note the little "x" wave dips. Often fibrillation waves are not seen on ECG. In this example fine fibrillation was seen on a different lead. (It looks like muscle tremor on the baseline). The V waves will be the prominent venous wave in atrial fib. Computers often erroneously report "a" waves in atrial fibrillation. **See:** Braunwald, chapter on " Physical Exam."

THE NEXT 2 PRESSURE TRACINGS WERE RECORDED ON THE SAME PATIENT:

45. **This ECG helps interpret this RA pressure tracing. What ECG conduction pattern is seen?**

a. 1st degree block
b. 2nd degree type 1 block
c. 2nd degree type 2 block
d. 3rd degree block
e. Sick Sinus syndrome

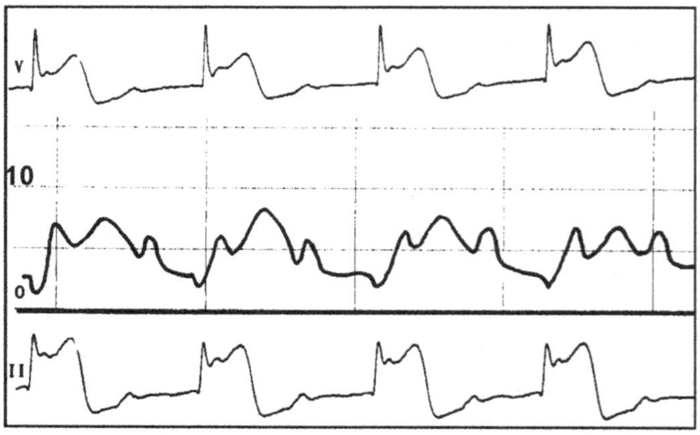

STEMI Patient, RA tracing x 25

ANSWER c. 2nd degree block type 2
with 2: 1 conduction. Note the small P wave sitting on top of the elevated ST segment between the R wave and the T wave. Also note the venous A waves corresponding to each P wave. These A waves sitting on both sides of the V wave indicate 2 atrial contractions for each ventricular contraction. Second degree - type 2 block is generally a fixed ratio block, where regularly occurring P waves are blocked at the av node. In this example every other P wave is blocked, in a 2:1 ratio. **See:** Braunwald, chapter on " Physical Exam.

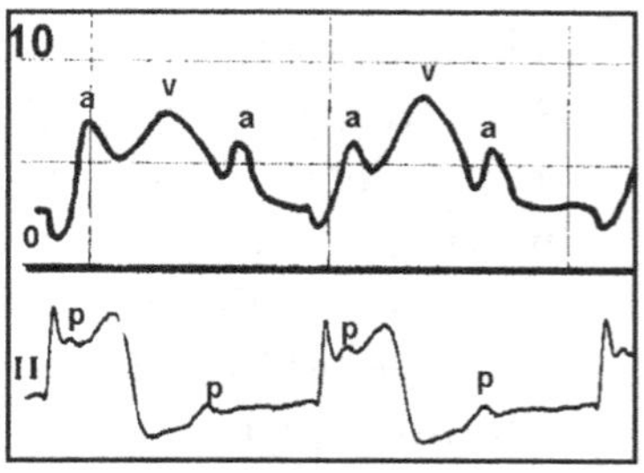

THIS LABELED DIAGRAM IS FROM THE SAME PATIENT DISCUSSED ABOVE.

46. Describe the conduction pattern shown in this ECG and RA pressure tracing?

a. 1st degree block

b. 2nd degree block

c. Sinus rhythm with conduction delay (LBBB)

d. VVI Pacemaker

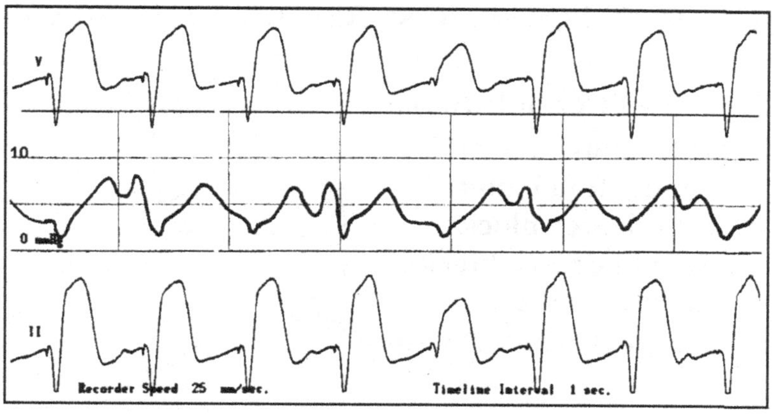

RA pressure x 50

ANSWER d. VVI Pacemaker, at rate of 68 ppm. Note the small "blips" or pacer "spikes" before each QRS. The second degree block seen in the previous question could have deteriorated to complete heart block. So a prophylactic temporary pacemaker was placed in this patient's RV. It was tested here to assure proper function. Biphasic "a" waves are still seen every other beat on the venous tracing.

See: Braunwald, chapter on " Physical Exam." **Keywords:** VVI Pacemaker rhythm

47. What are the large pressure waves marked in this RA pressure recording?

a. "V" waves in 2nd degree HB type I

b. "A" wave in 2nd degree HB type II.

c. "V" waves in complete heart block

d. "A" waves in complete heart block

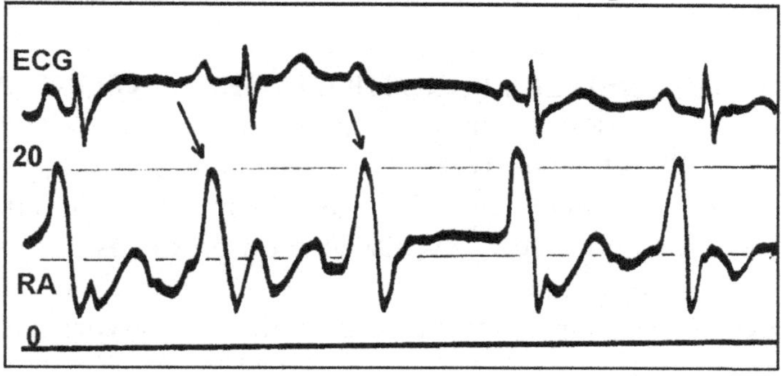

RA pressure x 50

ANSWER d. "A" waves in complete heart block. This patient is in complete AV block. Note that each marked pressure wave is preceded by an ECG "P" wave. And the ECG "T" waves are closely followed by the atrial "v" wave. Note that the electrical event always precedes the mechanical event:

- ECG p wave precedes a wave
- ECG r wave precedes c wave
- ECG t wave precedes v wave

See: Kern, chapter on "Hemodynamics."**Keywords:** recorded "a" waves in heart block.

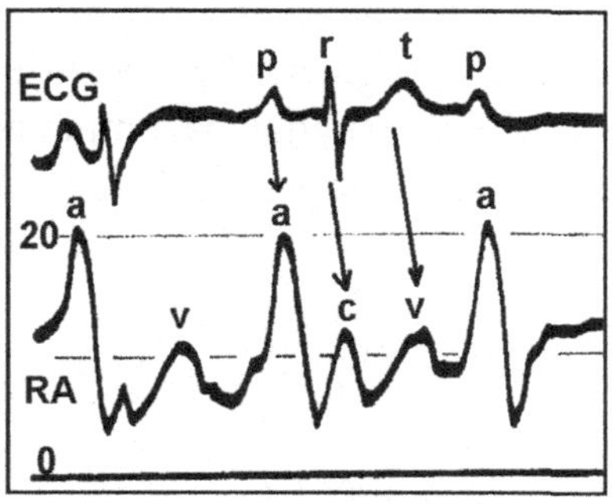

Venous waves in 3° block

THE NEXT 2 QUESTIONS REFER TO THIS DIAGRAM:

48. **From the ECG and arterial pressure shown, what is the conduction pattern?**
a. First degree block
b. Second degree block
c. Junctional rhythm
d. Ideoventricular rhythm

49. **Why is the aortic pressure in beats # 3, 4, 6 & 7 higher than in the other beats?**
a. Inspiration
b. Pulsus paradoxus
c. Pulsus alternans
d. Atrial kick

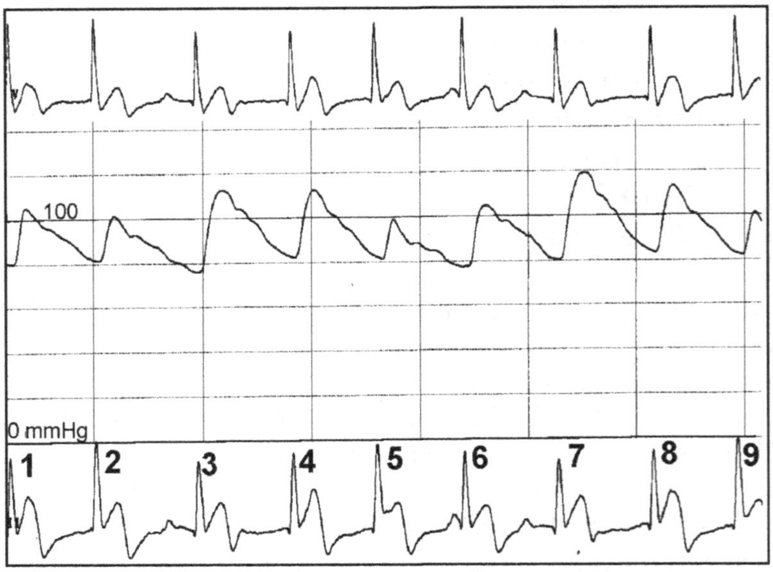

Arterial pressure x 200

BOTH ANSWERS FOR THE DIAGRAM ABOVE APPEAR TOGETHER BELOW:
48. ANSWER c. Junctional rhythm. There are no P waves except in front of beats 3, 6 & 7. The QRS is 0.10 sec wide indicating a narrow complex/supraventricular/ junctional rhythm. Unsynchronized P waves wander through the tracing. Most P waves are hidden in the QRS-T complex. AV dissociation produces inconsistent atrial contribution to ventricular preload.
See: Kern, chapter on "Hemodynamics."**Keywords:** junctional rhythm

49. ANSWER d. Atrial kick. When a P waves precedes the QRS the resulting arterial pulse is higher. This is a junctional rhythm where the AV junction triggers ventricular contraction. Atrial P waves wander through the tracing. When properly synchronized with the QRS these atrial contractions increase preload and the resulting arterial pressure according to Starling's law. This same atrial kick is why sinus rhythm gives the highest CO, and why dual chamber AV pacemakers are more physiologic than simple ventricular pacemakers.
See: Kern, chapter on "Hemodynamics."**Keywords:** atrial kick elevates arterial pressure

50. **Why do the pressures drop in the last part of this simultaneous LV & AO recording?**

a. Aortic regurgitation develops with pacing
b. Pacemaker malfunction
c. Loss of atrial kick with pacing
d. LV apex→LV out pullback in HOCM

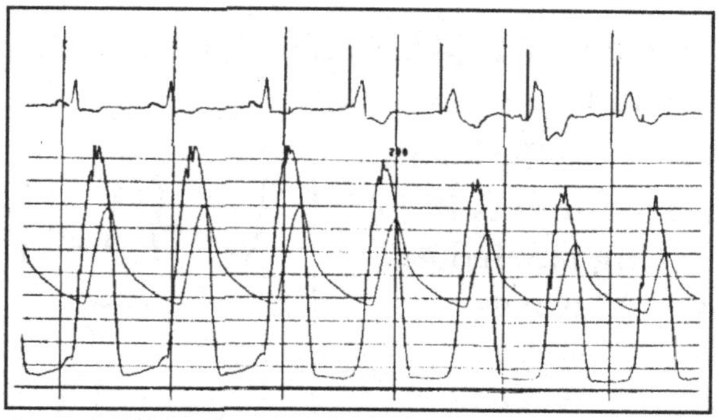
Simultaneous LV & AO x 200 (after Kern "Pacemaker Hemodynamics")

ANSWER c. Loss of atrial kick with pacing. Ventricular pacing spike precedes the last 5 beats. Atrial synchronization and atrial kick are lost. Note the loss of "a" waves on the pressure. This reduces the LV preload by 15-25% as well as the resulting systolic pressure.

Here the LV systolic pressure drops 25 mmHg and the AS gradient drops slightly. The valve area has not changed. But, the CO has dropped so pressure drop across the valve will also decrease. "Pacemaker syndrome" describes this reduction in atrial kick and CO in VVI pacing. Sinus rhythm gives the benefit of atrial kick and optimizes CO. This explains why dual chamber AV pacemakers are more physiologic than simple ventricular pacemakers. **See:** Kern, Hemodynamic rounds on, "Pacemaker Hemodynamics."
Keywords: Loss atrial kick with ventricular pacing

51. **The pressure tracing above shows a _____ pressure and _____ ECG rhythm.**

a. PAW, Atrial fibrillation
b. PAW, NSR with muscle tremor
c. AO, Atrial fibrillation
d. AO, NSR with muscle tremor

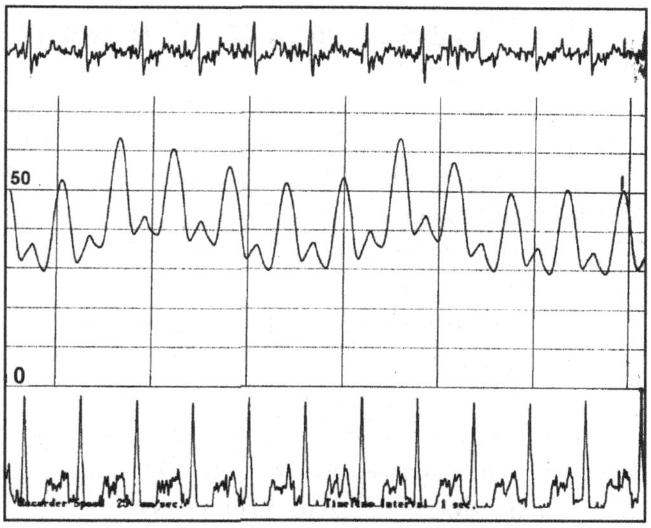

Cardiac Pressure x 100 , ECG leads I & II

ANSWER b. PAW, NSR with muscle tremor. The large pressure wave following the T wave must be the V wave. The small wave following the QRS is the venous A wave. It looks deceptively like a arterial pressure with a large dicrotic notch. ECG timing is essential for accurate wave identification. A noisy baseline often *looks like* atrial fibrillation waves. However, definite P waves are seen in the lower lead II ECG tracing with matching "a" waves on the PAW tracing. The QRS rhythm is very regular, another tip that this is NOT atrial fib. It is Normal Sinus Rhythm (NSR) with a noisy baseline. Noisy baseline is a sign of sloppy technique and should be cleared up before the case starts. Usually careful skin preparation or relaxing the patient will resolve muscle tremor.
See: Kern, chapter on "Hemodynamics." **Keywords:** ID Atrial fibrillation

THE NEXT 2 QUESTIONS REFER TO THIS DIAGRAM. Note the irregular rhythm.

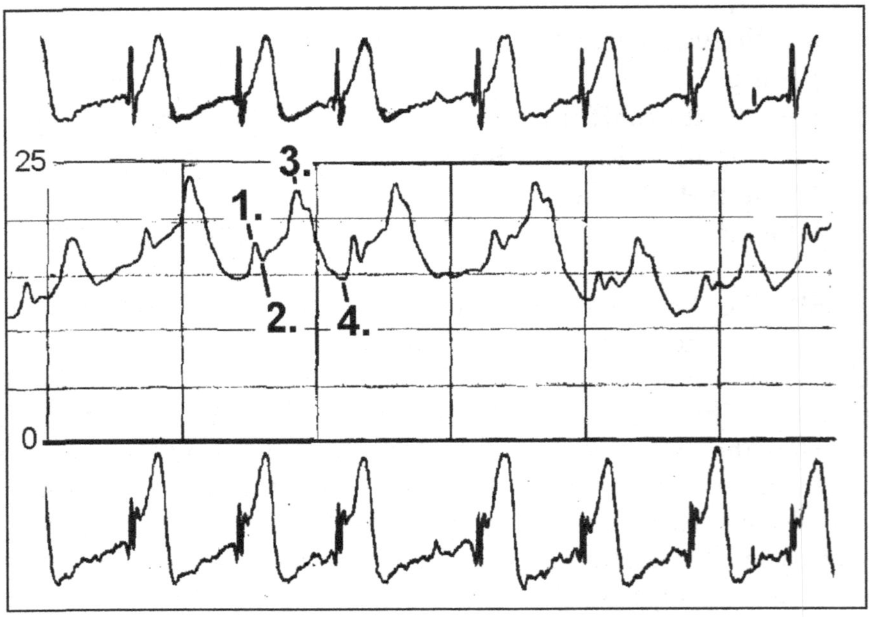

PA Wedge pressure x 50,

52. **What are the small waves on this PAW tracing labeled #1?**

a. "A" waves
b. "C" waves
c. "V" waves
d. "Y" waves

53. **From the ECG and PAW pressure shown, estimate the end-expiratory LV-EDP:**

a. 12 mmHg.
b. 15 mmHg.
c. 18 mmHg.
d. 23 mmHg.

BOTH ANSWERS APPEAR TOGETHER BELOW:

52. ANSWER b. "C" waves occur immediately upon ventricular contraction and closure of the mitral valve. A slight delay occurs in the PAW tracing due to the length of the conducting column. This ECG shows atrial fibrillation, so no "a" waves are seen.

WAVES SEEN ARE:

1. "c" positive wave - follows ECG "QRS" wave, (Due to **C**losure of the AV valve and ventricular **C**ontraction)
2. "x" negative wave - follows "a" wave
3. "v" positive wave - follows ECG "T" wave. It rises Due to **V**entricular filling against a closed AV valve. (It peaks at AV valve opening.)
4. "y" negative wave - follows ECG "T" wave, (Due to early **"Y"** rapid diastolic filling

See: Ahrens, chapter on "Normal Arterial Waveforms"
Keywords: identify & read atrial pressures

53. ANSWER b. 15 mmHg is the pressure measured at the beginning of systole (end of QRS on PAW due to transmission delay). This corresponds to the pressure immediately before the small "c" waves noted (labeled #3). The "mean a" wave cannot be used because there are no "a" waves in atrial fibrillation. As usual, end expiratory pressures best represent the most stable point to read pressures. Read this point (pre-C) as it levels-out during the expiratory cycle.

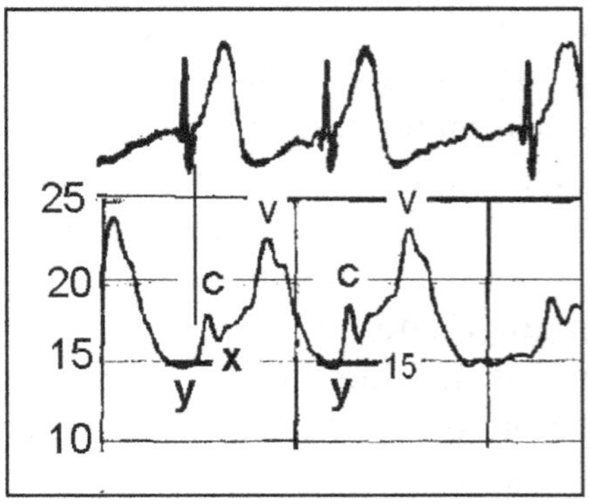

End QRS, Pre-V measurement, Estimate of LV-EDP in A- fib.

Ahrens says,

"The most common reason for loss of the A wave is loss of atrial contraction...including atrial fibrillation. If the A wave is absent, estimation of ventricular end-diastolic pressures can be attempted through ECG correlation. Considering that end diastole occurs near the end of the QRS complex, note the pressure at the end of the QRS should give an approximate value of ventricular pressure... This is referred to as the pre-V wave interpretation" (because the "c" wave is seldom seen).

Note that in MS, or when other obstructions exist between LV and PA, no PAW measurement accurately estimates the LV-EDP.

See: Ahrens, chapter on "Normal Pulmonary Capillary Wedge and Central Venous Pressure." **Keywords:** Reading PAW in Atrial fib.

THE NEXT 2 QUESTIONS REFER TO THIS DIAGRAM:

54. What pressure is shown recorded on X 50?

a. LV
b. PAW
c. PA
d. RV

55. Measure the 3 pressures normally recorded from this type of pressure tracing in the end expiratory phase:

a. 31/ 2, 12 mmHg
b. 31/ 5, 18 mmHg
c. 34/ 3, 18 mmHg
d. 34/ 5, 13 mmHg

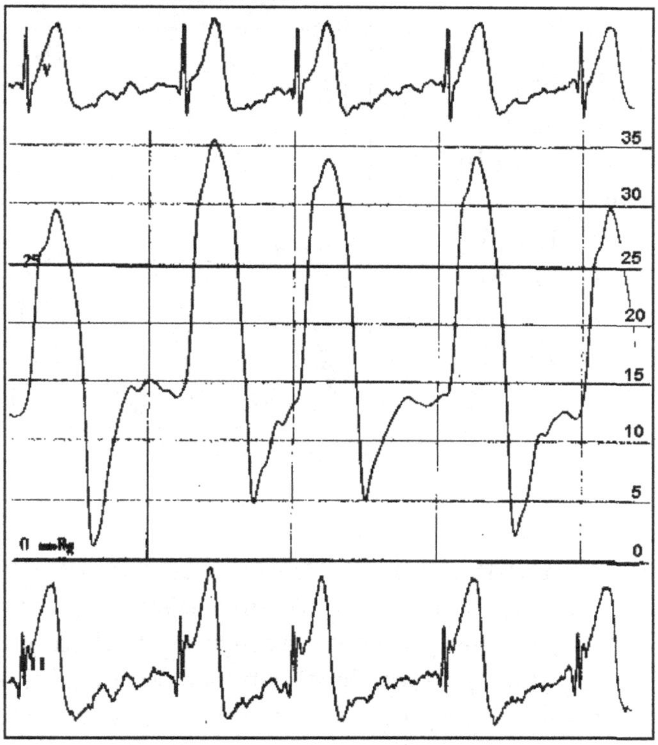

Pressure x 50

BOTH ANSWERS FOR THE DIAGRAM ABOVE APPEAR TOGETHER BELOW:

54. ANSWER d. RV. Several things distinguish this as an RV pressure:

- Rapidly rising and falling pressure waveform (square wave shape)
- Systolic pressure level between 30 and 35 mmHg on x 50 scale
- Marked respiratory variations (most prominent on right side of the heart)

See: Ahrens, chapter on "Normal Arterial Waveforms" **Keywords:** identify RV

55. ANSWER d. 34/ 5, 13 mmHg.(s/ bd, ed) The peak systolic pressure of the middle 3 end diastolic pressure is 34 mmHg. The lowest dip in early diastole for the middle 2 end expiratory beats average 5 mmHg. The end diastolic point measured at peak R wave is 13 mmHg. Due to the atrial fibrillation there are no "atrial kick" waves present.

See: Ahrens, chapter on "Normal Arterial Waveforms" **Keywords:** measure RV

THE NEXT 2 QUESTIONS REFER TO THIS DIAGRAM, on the same patient as above.

56. **What pressure is shown recorded on X 50?**
a. **AO**
b. **PAW**
c. **PA**
d. **RV**

57. **Read the end expiratory pressure from this tracing in mmHg:**
a. **31/ 15, 20**
b. **31/ 17, 25**
c. **34/ 19, 26**
d. **34/ 15, 22**

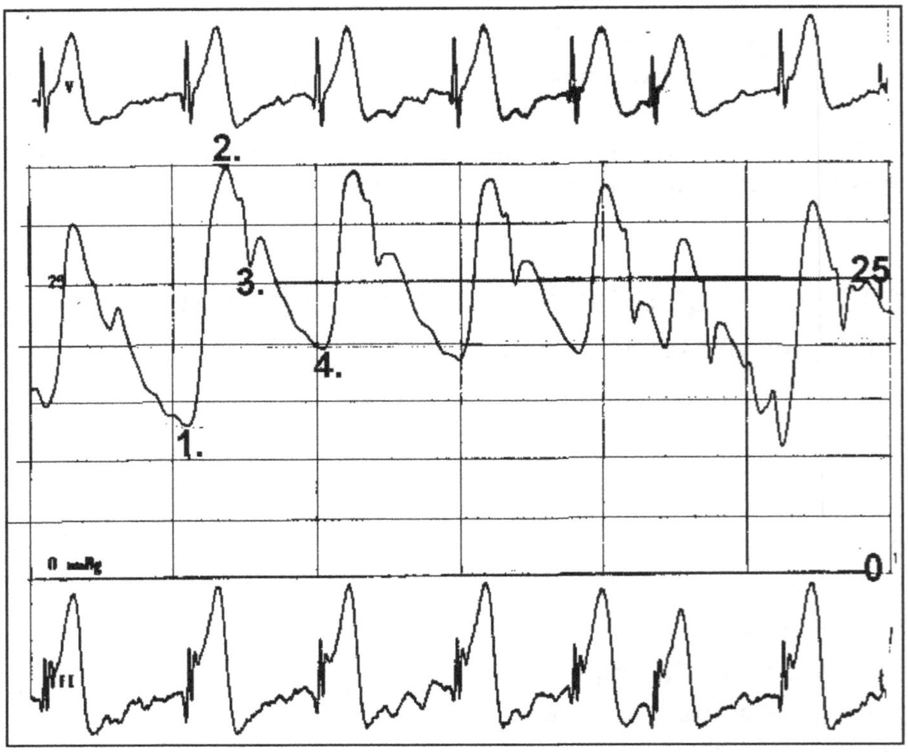

Pressure x 50

BOTH ANSWERS FOR THE DIAGRAM ABOVE APPEAR TOGETHER BELOW:
56. ANSWER c. PA. Several things distinguish this as a PA pressure:
- Triangular pressure waveform with dicrotic notch (arterial)
- Systolic pressure level between 30 and 35 mmHg on x 50 scale
- Marked respiratory variations (most prominent on right side of the heart)

The varying RR intervals affect the RV filling and the resulting PA pressure.
WAVES MARKED ARE:
- **#1**: inspiratory, end diastole - Do not measure.
- **#2**: expiratory, systolic PA - Measure and report.
- **#3**: expiratory, dicrotic notch - OK, but not usually reported.
- **#4**: expiratory, end diastolic PA - Measure and report.
- **#5**: mean, (not labeled) - should be estimated using the ruler method

See: Ahrens, chapter on "Normal Arterial Waveforms" **Keywords:** identify and read PA

57. ANSWER c. 34/ 19, 26 mmHg (s/ d, m). The middle 3 beats plateau and represent the end of expiration where the pressures should be read. These 3 systolic beats average 34 mmHg. The same 3 diastolic beats average 19 mmHg. The mean pressure can be estimated by laying a clear plastic ruler horizontally over those 3 end expiratory beats. Move the ruler up and down until equal PA area exists above and below the ruler.

See: Ahrens, chapter on "Normal Arterial Waveforms" **Keywords:** measure PA

USE THIS DIAGRAM FOR THE NEXT 2 QUESTIONS.

58. **What two simultaneous pressures are shown?**
- **a. RV, LV**
- **b. RV, PA**
- **c. RA, AO**
- **d. PA, AO**

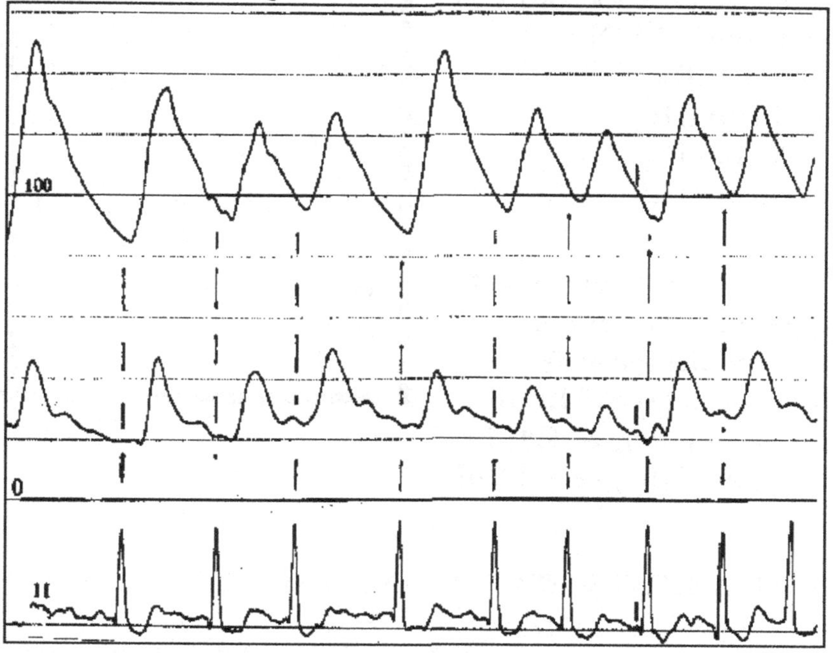

Simultaneous pressures recorded x 200

59. **This simultaneous pressure recording shows probable ____ hypertension with an ECG rhythm of _____.**
- **a. Systemic, complete heart block**
- **b. Systemic, atrial fibrillation**
- **c. Pulmonary, complete heart block**
- **d. Pulmonary, atrial fibrillation**

BOTH ANSWERS APPEAR TOGETHER BELOW:

58. ANSWER d. PA, AO Both waveforms are triangular indicating great vessel pressures. The two pressures shown are Aorta and PA both recorded on x 200. Although no dicrotic notch is seen in the upper tracing, it is consistent with the AO pressure level. ECG markers show a time delay in both AO and PA tracings. Atrial fibrillation is present. The varying RR intervals change the pulse from beat to beat.
See: Ahrens, chapter on "Normal Arterial Waveforms" **Keywords:** Identify simultaneous AO and PA

59. ANSWER d. Pulmonary hypertension in atrial fibrillation. Pressure readings are:

- AO: 125/93, 110 mmHg (s, d, m)
- PA: 42/22, 30 mmHg (s, d, m)

Normal PA systolic range is 17-32 mmHg. This patients systolic of 42 mmHg indicates that mild pulmonary hypertension exists. No P waves are seen on the ECG and the rate is irregular due to atrial fibrillation.
See: Ahrens, chapter on "Normal Arterial Waveforms" **Keywords:** Identify Pulmonary hypertension and atrial fibrillation

THE NEXT 2 QUESTIONS REFER TO THIS DIAGRAM:

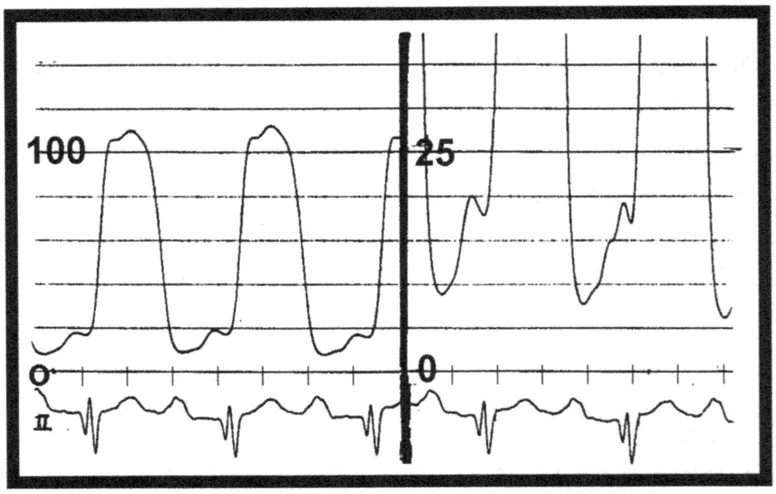

LV X200 LV X50

60. **This LV pressure was recorded on x 200 and x 50. Estimate LV-EDP:**

a. 9 mmHg
b. 15 mmHg
c. 17 mmHg
d. 20 mmHg

61. **Lead II ECG shows what types of heart block:**

a. First degree & WPW
b. First degree & LBBB
c. Second degree & WPW
d. Second degree & LBBB

BOTH ANSWERS FOR THE DIAGRAM ABOVE APPEAR TOGETHER BELOW:

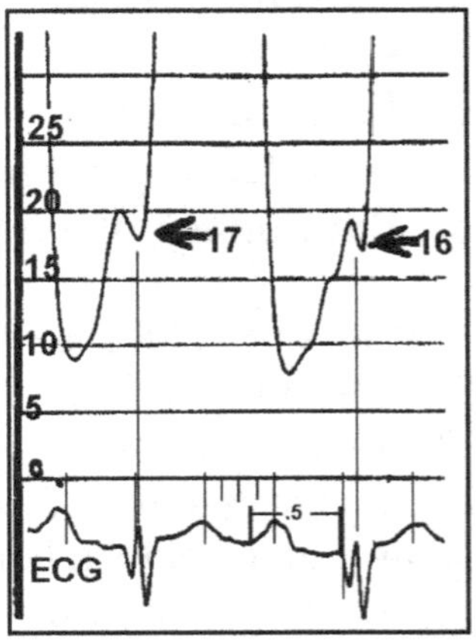

LV-EDP after "a" wave

60. c. 17 mmHg measured in the presystolic dip as shown, immediately following the a" wave and aligned with the ECG R wave. Kern says,

> "*The left ventricular end diastolic pressure is measured after the A wave corresponding to the peak of the R wave (...follow the ventricular time line at the first R wave down to its crossing point on the left ventricular pressure).*"

See: Kern, chapter on "Hemodynamic Data." **Keywords**: Measure LV-EDP at R wave

61. b. First degree & LBBB. The P wave is markedly early with a PR interval of 0.5 seconds indicating prolonged delay in the AV node and first degree AV block. The broad and notched QRS complex suggests a left bundle branch block (QRS duration = 0.2 sec). Other ECG leads such as V1 would be more helpful to diagnose the type of bundle branch block.

See: Ahrens, chapter on "Normal Arterial Waveforms" **Keywords:** measure LV-EDP

2. Practice Tracings

USE THIS DIAGRAM FOR THE NEXT TWO QUESTIONS

62. **Identify the dip labeled #4 in this tracing.**
a. **PAW "x" trough**
b. **PAW "y" trough**
c. **RA "x" trough**
d. **RA "y" trough**

63. **Measure the "a" waves on the RA tracing in mmHg.**
a. **6 mmHg**
b. **8 mmHg**
c. **13 mmHg**
d. **15 mmHg**

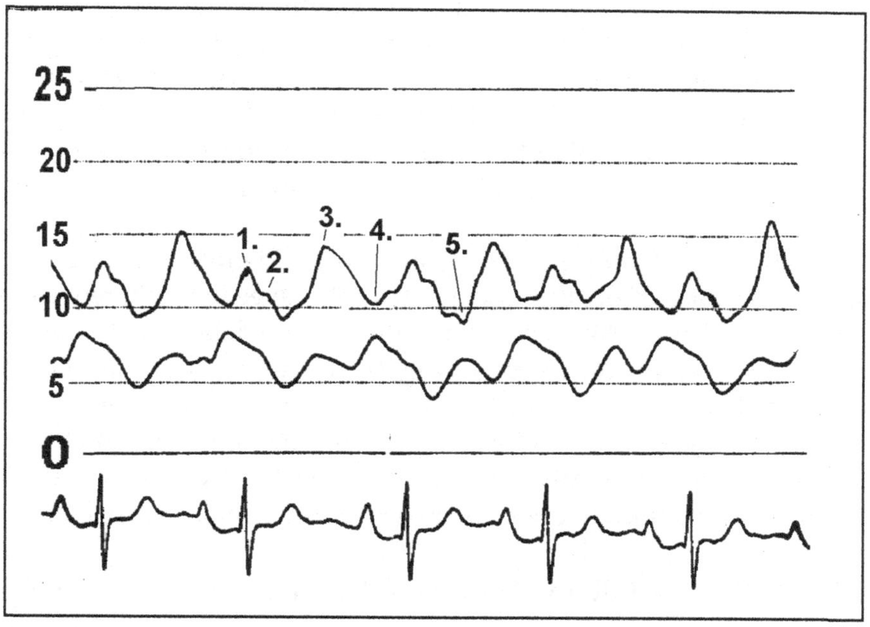

Simultaneous RA and PAW pressure x 50

BOTH ANSWERS APPEAR TOGETHER BELOW.

62. ANSWER b: PAW "y"trough is the early diastolic dip that caused by the "suction cup effect" rapidly sucking blood into the ventricle. The dips are called descents or troughs. They are "x", "y", and sometimes "z" in alphabetic order. The tiny dip between the "a" and "c" waves is seldom noted but is named the "z"or "x_1" wave. The "z" and "c" waves are both reported to be good estimates of ventricular end diastolic pressure. Both are close together.

Note that the RA "a" wave shows little or no delay from the ECG P wave. It usually begins during the P wave. Whereas, the PAWP "a" wave is usually delayed 0.1 sec or more from the ECG P wave, owing to the longer transmission distance through the lungs. It usually begins in the PR segment or during the QRS complex. In all cases "The electrical event (ECG) always precedes the mechanical event."

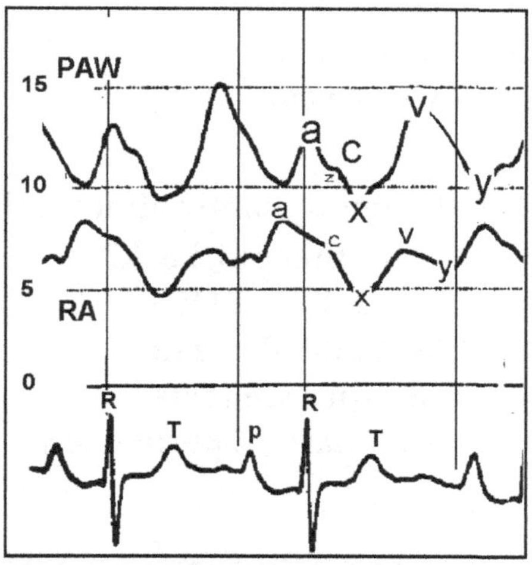

Simultaneous RA and PAW pressures x 50

CORRECTLY MATCHED WAVES ARE:
1. **"a" positive wave** - follows ECG "p" wave (Wedge "a" starts at end QRS)
2. **"c" positive wave** - at end of ECG "QRS" wave (Wedge "c" in ST segment)
   Wave between "a" and "c" is "z"or "x_2"
3. **"v" positive wave** - follows ECG "T" wave (Wedge "v" in T-P interval)
4. **"x" trough** - down slope of "a" & "c" waves

The dip following the "a" wave is termed "x" , "x' " (x^{prime}), or "z" trough.
The dip following the "c" wave is termed x' or "x_2" trough.

When the"c " wave is not seen, the dip following the "a" wave is simply termed the "x" trough. This makes for some confusion because, depending on whether or not you see a "c" wave the same dip could be labeled "x" or "x' " or "x_2"

5. **"y" trough** - dip follows ECG "T" wave, - follows the "v" wave.
The dip following the "v" wave is termed the "y" trough or descent.

See: Kern, chapter on "Hemodynamics." **Keywords**: Venous waves: a, c, v, x, y

63. ANSWER b. 8 mmHg. The RA tracing is identifiable because of the lower pressures and the absence of pressure delay. RA "a" waves immediately follow the ECG "P"wave. This is unlike the PAW which has considerable delay due to the distance the pressure wave travels through the lung bed. In the RA the "a" is usually larger than "v." (The opposite holds for PAW and LA.) To measure RA "a" waves, go though and mark the five a waves with a horizontal line (a colored pen would distinguish them from "v" waves). Then average these 5 "a" waves to 8 mmHg. Repeat this process for the "v" waves. **See**: Kern, chapter on "Hemodynamics." **Keywords:** measuring "v" waves

USE THIS DIAGRAM FOR THE NEXT 2 QUESTIONS BELOW:

64. What pressure sites are shown in this pullback tracing?
a. LV→ LA
b. LV→ AO
c. RV→ RA
d. RV→ PAW

65. What hemodynamic abnormality is shown on this pullback?
a. Elevated LV-EDP
b. Elevated RA mean
c. Tricuspid stenosis
d. Pulmonary hypertension

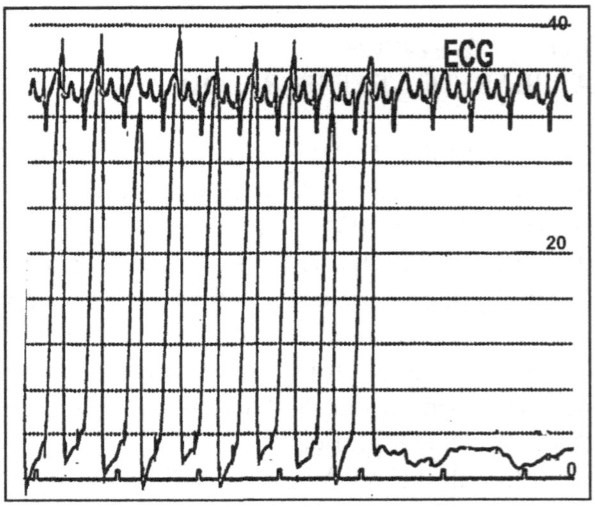

Pullback pressure x 40

BOTH ANSWERS APPEAR TOGETHER BELOW.

64. ANSWER c. RV→ RA. The range is x 40 so each horizontal line is 4 mmHg. The first pressure is ventricular in shape and peaks around 36 mmHg. So, it must be RV. A pullback from RV ends up in the RA. The RA pressure is 2 mmHg.
See: Kern, chapter on "Hemodynamics." **Keywords:** Normal RV - RA pullback

65. **ANSWER** d. Mild Pulmonary Hypertension. The RV pressure is elevated at 36 mmHg. Kern's normal values range from 17 to 32 mmHg. Since the RV pumps directly into the PA, the systolic PA pressures are also expected to be high. Pulmonary

hypertension suggests increased resistance downstream. This increased resistance (obstruction) can occur at any number of sites downstream including: PA, Pulmonary arterioles, pulmonary capillaries, venous outflow, LA, Mitral valve, and LV failure (most common). The RV diastolic pressures line up with the mean RA pressure levels. So NO tricuspid valve stenosis is present.
See: Ahrens, chapter on "Normal Pulmonary Capillary Wedge and Central Venous Pressure." **Keywords:** Normal RV - RA pullback with pulmonary hypertension

USE THIS DIAGRAM FOR THE NEXT 3 QUESTIONS BELOW.
These simultaneous pressures below were recorded during a right and left heart cath on a patient who is very short of breath.

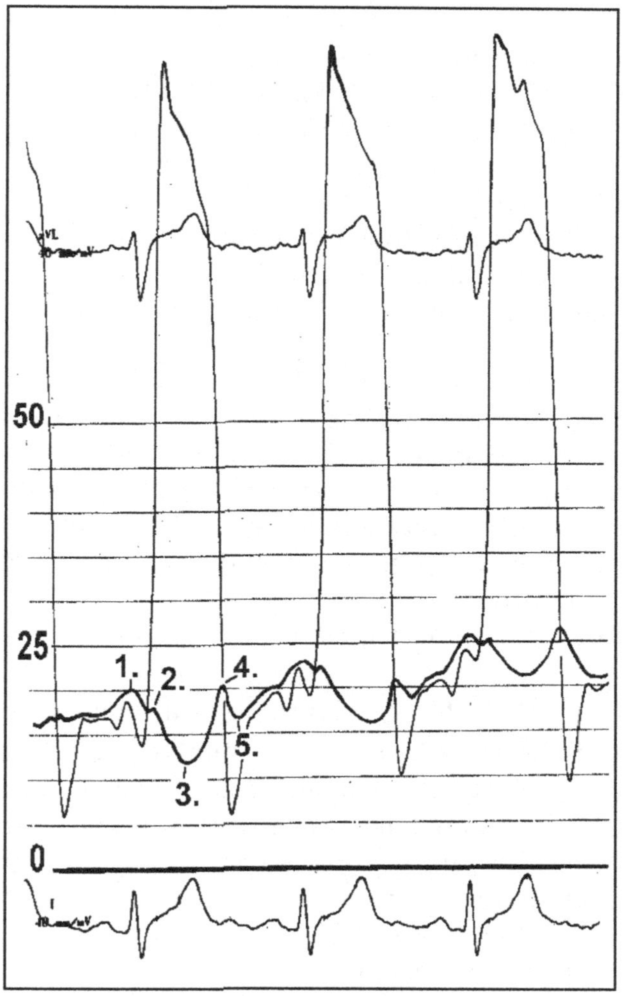

Simultaneous LV & LA recorded X50

66. **What intracardiac event is labeled #4 (diastolic pressure crossover) in the pressure recording shown?**
- **a. Mitral valve closes**
- **b. Mitral valve opens**
- **c. LA contraction ("a" wave)**
- **d. LA relaxation ("x" wave)**

67. **Estimate the average LV-EDP from the 3 LV beats shown in the diagram, as a computer would measure LV-EDP.**
- **a. 16 mmHg**
- **b. 19 mmHg**
- **c. 24 mmHg**
- **d. 28 mmHg**

68. **Average the LA "a" waves shown, as a computer would measure "a" waves .**
- **a. 10 mmHg**
- **b. 15 mmHg**
- **c. 19 mmHg**
- **d. 23 mmHg**

ANSWERS FOR THE ABOVE 3 QUESTIONS APPEAR TOGETHER BELOW.

66. ANSWER b. Mitral valve opens. Valve events always occur at these pressure crossover points. After atrial contraction the LA continues to fill although from the pulmonary veins. This causes the atrial pressure to build to a peak "v" wave.

At the "v" wave peak the mitral valve opens and the LV begins diastolic filling. The dropping atrial "Y" descent indicates rapid filling of the ventricle in early diastole. The ventricular rapid filling wave corresponds to the"y" trough, and appears exaggerated probably due to an underdamped recording system.

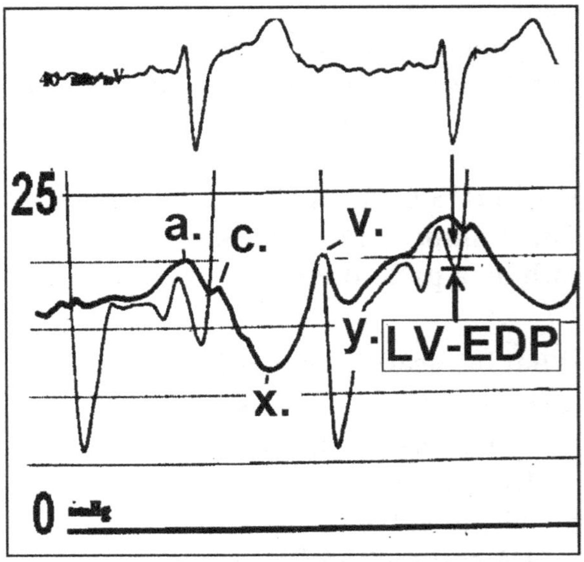

Measuring LV & LA diastolic waves x 50

CORRECTLY MATCHED ANSWERS ARE:

#1. LA contraction ("a" wave)

#2. Mitral valve closes ("z", "c" and LV-EDP waves)

#3. LA relaxation ("x" wave)

#4. Mitral valve opens ("v" wave)

See: Kern, chapter on "Hemodynamics." **Keywords**: mitral closure at pressure crossover

67. ANSWER b. 19 mmHg. LV-EDP is estimated from the dip in LV pressure immediately following atrial contraction. LV-EDP is the LV dip or hesitation that usually corresponds to the peak of the ECG "R" wave. LV- EDP readings from the 3 beats are 14, 19 and 23 which average 19 mmHg. Since the LV-EDP varies so much with respiration here, recording more beats or breath holding would provide a more accurate average. Reading LV pressures as a computer would: LA = 22 , 20, 20 mmHg. (a, v, m) LV = 95 / 6, 19 mmHg. (s, d, , m)

See: See: Kern, chapter on "Hemodynamics." **Keywords:** Read LV-EDP

68. ANSWER d. 23 mmHg = "a" wave peaks. The 3 "a" waves are 20, 23, & 26 mmHg. These average to 23 mmHg. Most hemodynamic computer recorders take the average of all the sampled peak "a" waves - just like this. This tracing shows how nicely the LA tracing follows ventricular diastole. Estimates of the LVedp can be made from the PAW using any of the following:

- mean "a" wave average
- "z" trough average
- "c" wave average
- mean of entire cycle

See: Ahrens, chapter on "Normal Pulmonary Capillary Wedge and Central Venous Pressure." **Keywords:** identify & measure LV-EDP

USE THIS SIMULTANEOUS TRACING FOR THE NEXT 2 QUESTIONS.

69. **What cardiac pressure is labeled #1 on the diagram?**

a. **LV-BD**
b. **LV-EDP**
c. **PAW "a" wave**
d. **PAW "v" wave**

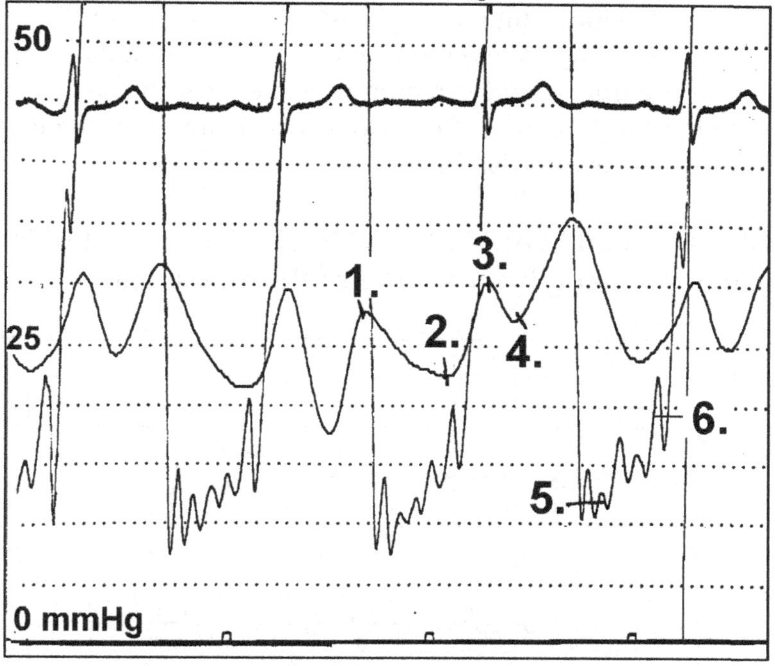

Simultaneous right and left heart cath pressures X 50

70. **These simultaneous pressures are usually recorded together to evaluate the function of:**

a. **The pulmonary capillary bed**
b. **The systemic capillary bed**
c. **The aortic valve**
d. **The mitral valve**

BOTH ANSWERS APPEAR TOGETHER BELOW:

69. ANSWER d. PAW "v" wave.

BE ABLE TO MATCH ALL BELOW:

1. **"v" wave** - follows the T wave
2. **"y" trough** - on the down slope of the "v" wave
3. **"a" wave** - delayed from P wave
4. **"x" trough** - on the down slope of the "a" wave
5. **"LV-BDP"** - lowest point in early ventricular diastole. LV-BDP = 12 mmHg. Note underdamping resonance in the tracing. These vibrations must be smoothed out for accurate pressure measurement.
6. **"LV-EDP"** - LV pressure following atrial contraction and immediately prior to LV contraction. LV-EDP = 19 mmHg. Note that atrial contraction seen on this PAW tracing is delayed due to transmission time through the lungs. .

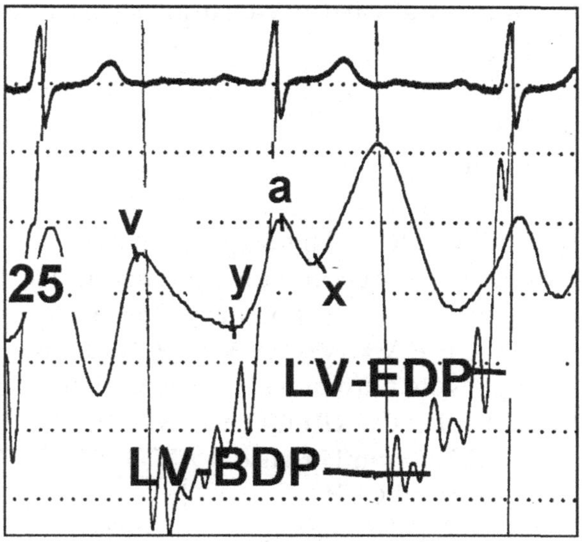

Reading PAW Pressures X 50

70. ANSWER d. The mitral valve. Simultaneous LV and PAW pressures are recorded to evaluate for mitral stenosis. Remember, the PAW approximates LA pressure, and the

mitral valve is between the LA and LV. This patient has a 10-15 mmHg gradient across the mitral valve indicating some degree of mitral stenosis.

Note that the LV tracing is underdamped with diastolic vibrations. You must smooth it out for accurate pressure readings. I averaged the last LV-EDP vibrations to give a LV-EDP of 19 mmHg as shown. **See:** Grossman, chapter on "Balloon-Tipped Flow-Directed Catheters" **Keywords:** Identify Swan Ganz pullback pressures

USE THIS DIAGRAM FOR THE NEXT QUESTION. Note it shows a Swan-Ganz catheter advance, not a pullback tracing.

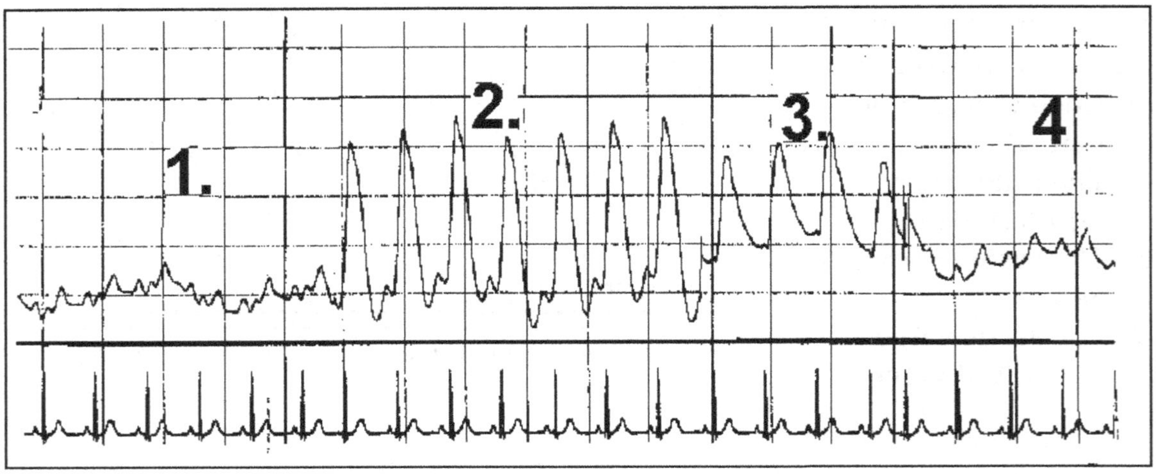

Right heart catheter **insertion** pressures X 50

71. What normal cardio-vascular pressure is recorded at #1 on the diagram above?

a. **RA**
b. **RV**
c. **PA**
d. **PAW**

ANSWER a. RA. This sequence shows normal pressures recorded as a Swan-Ganz catheter is inserted into the right heart. The balloon just floats with the current into the lungs until it hits a pulmonary arteriole too small to pass through. The total insertion sequence is RA→RV→PA→PAW. Note how the tracing begins and ends with a venous tracing. Note normal respiratory variations throughout the tracing.

BE ABLE TO CORRECTLY MATCH ALL ANSWERS BELOW:

1. **RA** (5 mmHg) also termed CVP
2. **RV** (23/5 mmHg
3. **PA** (20/10 mmHg)
4. **PAW** (10 mmHg) also termed PCW or just "Wedge"

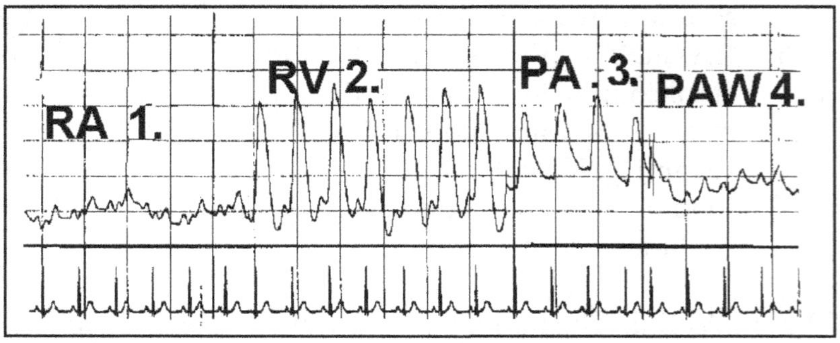

Right Heart catheter insertion Pressures X 50

See: Grossman, chapter on "Balloon-tipped Flow-directed catheters" **Keywords:** Identify Swan pullback pressures

THE NEXT 2 QUESTIONS REFER TO THE DIAGRAM BELOW:

72. **What cardiovascular pressure is recorded here on x 50?**
a. RA
b. RV
c. PA
d PAW

73. **Measure the pressures shown in mmHg.**
a. 38/15,24 mmHg
b. 38/15,29 mmHg
c. 40/28,24 mmHg
d. 40/28,33 mmHg

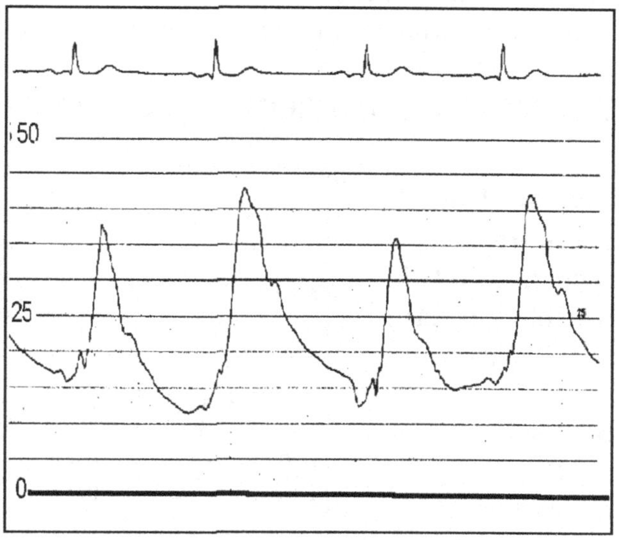

Right heart pressure x 50

BOTH ANSWERS LISTED TOGETHER BELOW:

72. ANSWER c. PA. This pulmonary artery tracing shows the characteristic triangular waveform on x 50.

Note the dicrotic notch on the down slope of each wave separating systole from diastole. There is slight pulsus alternans, with alternating high and low pressures- a sign of right heart failure. This pulmonary pressure is slight elevated with normal systole being around 25 mmHg. Left sided pressures are always higher and recorded on x 100 or 200. **See:** Kern, chapter on "Hemodynamics."**Keywords:** Identify PA pressure

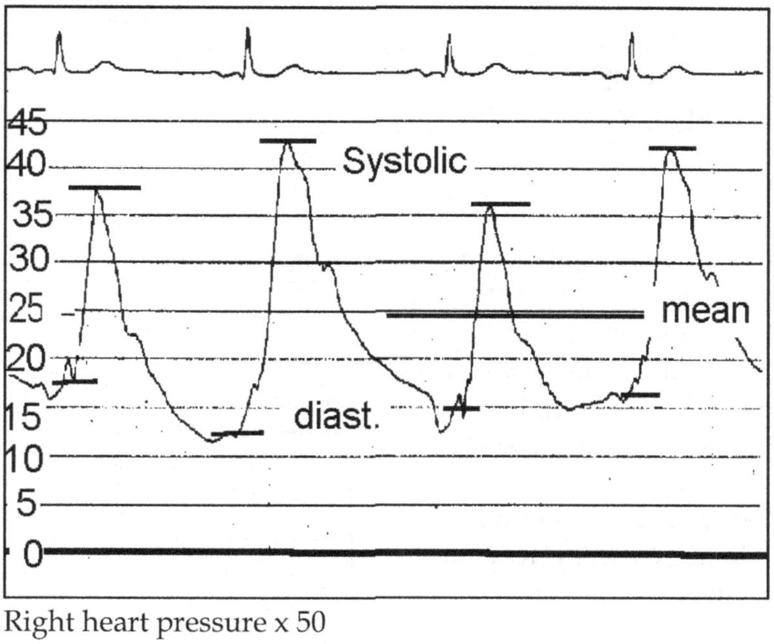

Right heart pressure x 50

73. ANSWER a. 38/15,24 mmHg. Systolic peaks are between 31 and 43 averaging 38. You can be very accurate by marking and reading each one, then average them. Or a quicker method is to estimate the average peak by laying down a clear plastic ruler midway between all systolic peaks. Diastolic valleys read the same way

average 15 mmHg. The mean of all the pressures is just under 25 mmHg. Again the plastic ruler method is easiest. Modern computerized monitors automatically calculate the mean. But they are no more accurate than the human eye. Your eye distinguishes artifact and respiratory variations.
See: Kern, chapter on "Hemodynamics."**Keywords:** read PA pressure

THE NEXT 2 QUESTIONS REFER TO THIS DIAGRAM:

74. **Identify the pressure recorded in this pullback tracing labeled #1.**
a. PAW
b. LV
c. RV
d. AO

75. **Measure pressure #1 in mmHg.**
a. 140/56,75
b. 140/56,92
c. 180/0,24
d. 180/-5,11

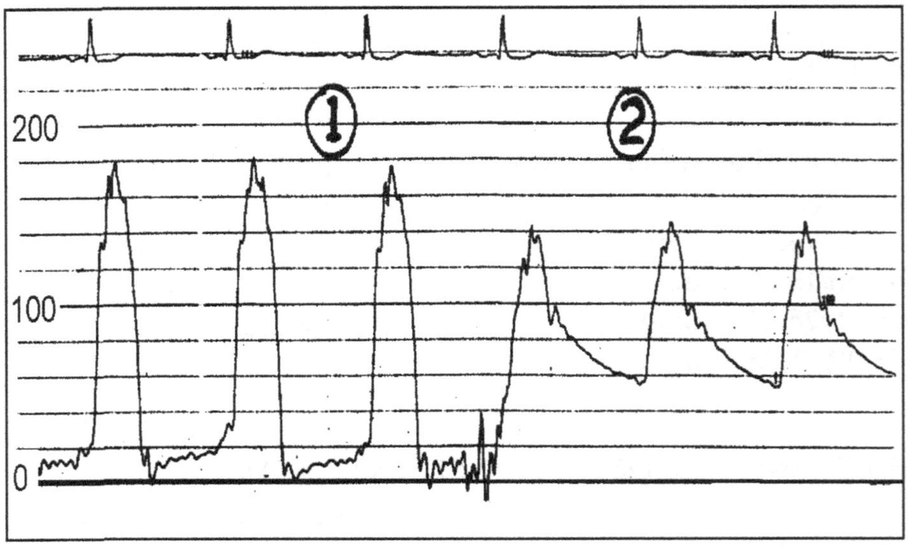

Pullback pressure x 200

BOTH ANSWERS LISTED TOGETHER BELOW:

74. ANSWER b. LV. This is a LV➔AO pullback across the aortic valve. Note a 40 mmHg peak to peak systolic gradient indicating aortic stenosis.
See: Kern, chapter on "Hemodynamics."**Keywords:** identify LV pressure

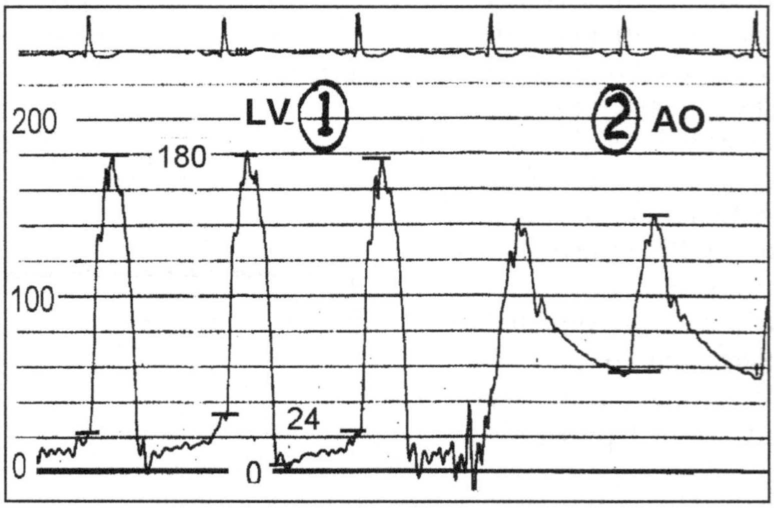

LV pressure x 200

75. ANSWER c. 180/0,24 mmHg = LV. Note that since the range is x 200 each grid line is 20 mmHg. Systolic peaks average 180 mmHg. The beginning LV diastolic touches the zero line, so LV-BDP = 0 mmHg. The LV-EDP varies from 20 to 30 and averages 24 mmHg. AO reads 142/56,92 (s/d,m). Note a peak to peak systolic gradient of

38 mmHg indicating mild aortic stenosis. Besides recording on x 200 as shown, you can run LV on x50 scale to magnify the diastolic numbers. This makes them easier to read. **See:** Kern, chapter on "Hemodynamics."**Keywords:** Read LV pressure

3. Pressures: Other

76. One of the best indicators of LV contractility is dP/dT, which is defined as:
- **a. Preload pressure / Isometric contraction time**
- **b. Digital LV peak pressure / Digital LV ejection time**
- **c. Differential LV pressure / Differential LV tension**
- **d. Delta pressure / Delta P wave**
- **e. Maximum slope of the LV Pressure curve**

ANSWER e. Maximum slope of the LV Pressure curve. The dP/dT comes from delta P/delta T, or change in pressure over change in time. It is a good index of LV contractility, but to be accurate must be measured with a catheter tip manometer and recorded at 100-200 mm/sec paper speed. A sloping line is drawn tangent to the steepest upward slope. Then a right triangle is constructed from this line with a "rise and run." The rise is measured vertically in mmHg, the run horizontally in seconds. The ratio in rise/run in mmHg/sec is the LV dP/dT.

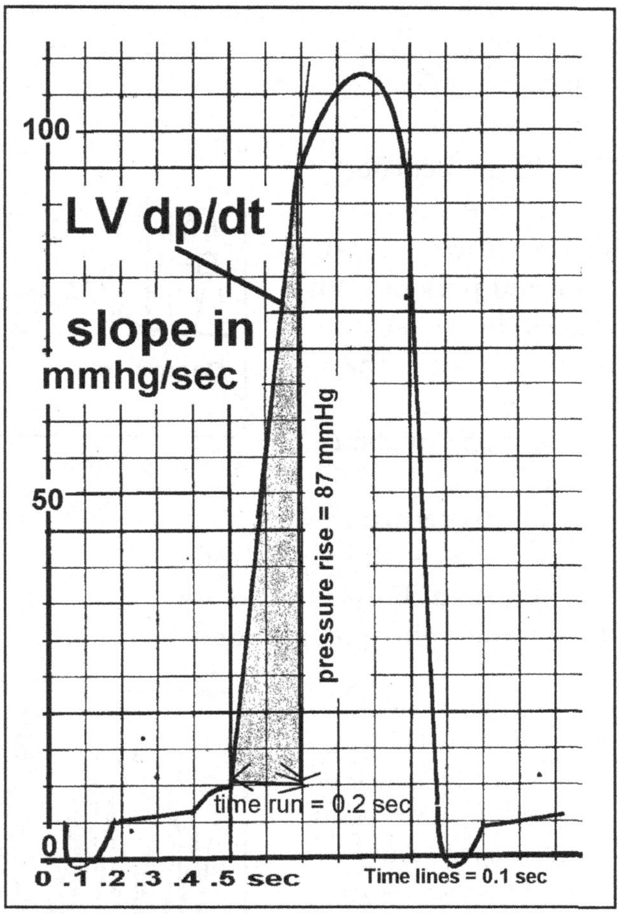

LV x 100 with measured dP/dT

This example shows a slope of 77 mmHg/.2 sec or 385 mmHg/sec. This means that if this LV was pressed to contract at its maximum for one entire second, the resulting BP would rise to 385 mmHg. This dP/dT slope is abnormally low for demonstration purposes. Normally this slope is very steep, with an LV dP/dT over 1200 mmHg/sec. Many computers calculate and report dP/dT.

The RADI pressure wire has adequate frequency response to measure dP/dT, but

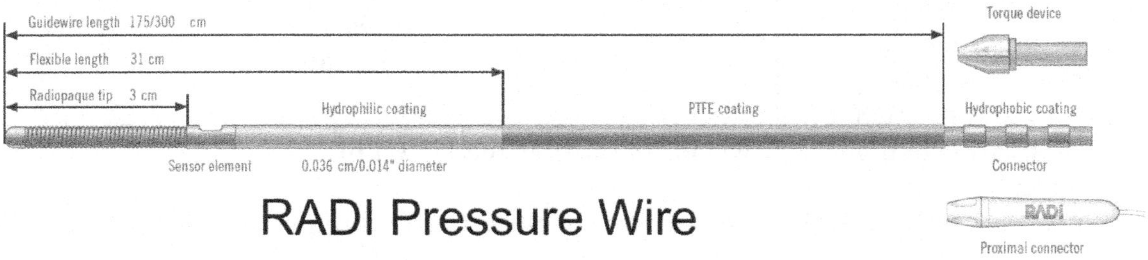

RADI Pressure Wire

most fluid filled measuring systems do not.
See: Braunwald, Chapter on "Evaluation of LV Function." **Keywords**: LV dP/dT

77. Accurate dP/dT measurement requires use of:
- **a. Blood in catheter (to eliminate air bubbles)**
- **b. A pressure wire**
- **c. A wire guide tipped with a Doppler velocity probe**
- **d. A critically damped fluid filled recording system**

ANSWER b. A pressure wire (best frequency response) or catheter tip manometer. This wire has a pressure transducer built into its tip. Its frequency response exceeds 25 cycles/sec, which is over 2 times a standard fluid filled system upper frequency limit. Grossman says that a flat frequency response greater than 20 Hz is needed for an accurate dP/dT. This is usually beyond the range of most fluid filled systems.
See: Grossman, chapter on "Pressure Measurements" **Keywords**: accurate dP/dT required cath tip manometer

78. This BP is recorded during Valsalva straining and release in a normal person. What causes the phase labeled at #2 in the box?

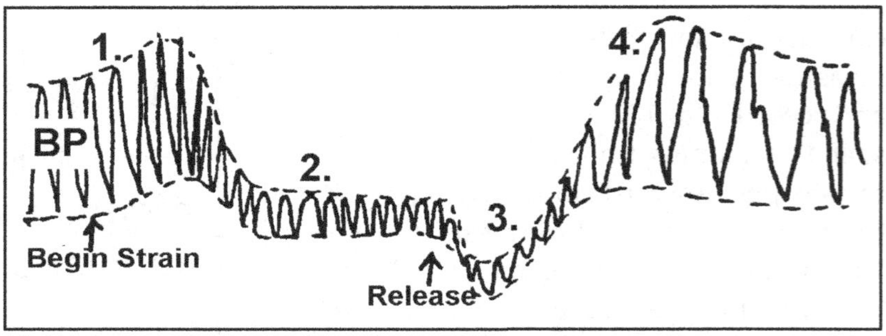

Effect of Valsalva maneuver on BP (exaggerated)

- **a. Thoracic pressure drops**
- **b. Venous return increases with inspiration**
- **c. Increased thoracic pressure**
- **d. Venous return is impeded.**

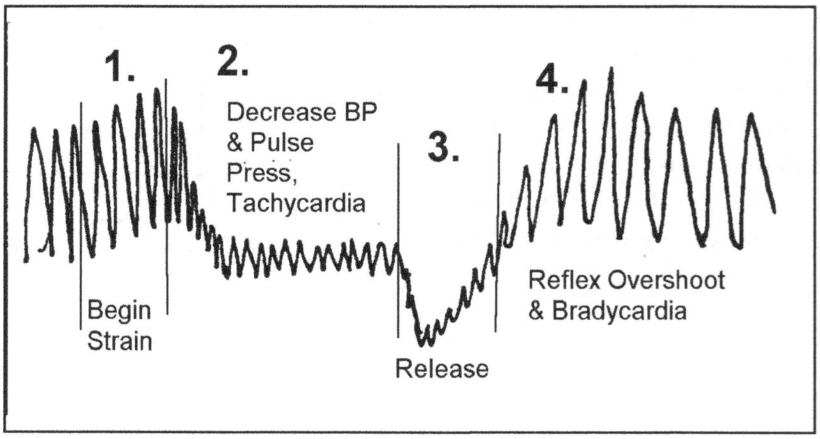

Effect of Valsalva maneuver on BP

ANSWER d. Venous return is impeded by the positive intrathoracic pressure. It compresses the vena cavae and inhibits venous return. This reduces preload, CO, and BP. The Valsalva test evaluates the patients baroreceptor reflex and Starling's mechanism. Phases #1 and #3 are not reflexes, but due to the changes in thoracic pressure. Phases #2 and #4 are reflexes due to altered venous return (Starling's effect). This normal Valsalva diagram is exaggerated for demonstration purposes. In severe LV dysfunction disease the Valsalva response is relatively flat. Here the Starling mechanism is already stretched to its limit, and Valsalva does not drop BP, but actually increases it.

CORRECTLY MATCHED ANSWERS ARE:

1. BP reflects increased thoracic pressure (straining)
2. Venous return is impeded. BP and CO fall (Starling's effect)
3. BP drops as thoracic pressure drops suddenly with release and inspiration
4. Reflexive overshoot of BP and bradycardia as venous return increases with inspiration
5. BP normalizes

See: Berne & Levy, chapter on "The Circuit." & Todd **Keywords:** Valsalva phases

79. Estimate the end-expiratory mean PAW pressure.

a. 10 mmHg

b. 15 mmHg

c. 20 mmHg

d. 25 mmHg

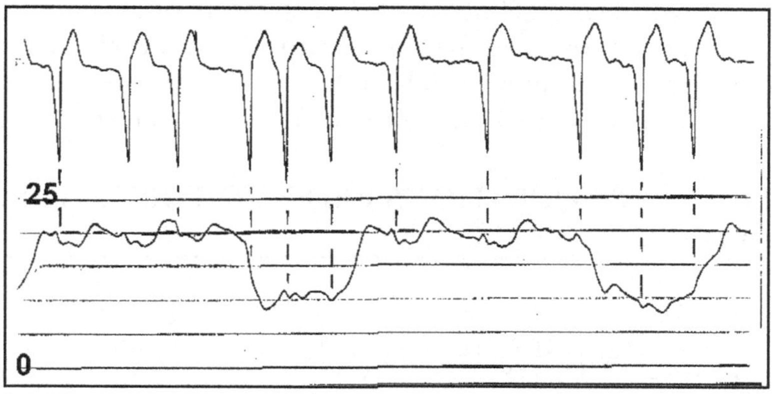

PAWP x 50

ANSWER c. 20 mmHg. Note the two dips in the PAWP. This is the negative pleural pressure of inspiration. Take your measurements on the plateau between the inspiratory dips. The mean through this expiratory plateau is 20 mmHg. This patient is in atrial fibrillation so there are no "a" waves. Note the "c" waves aligned with each QRS complex. The PAWP has small "v" waves following each ECG T wave.

See: Ahrens, chapter on "Normal Arterial Waveforms" **Keywords:** measure mean PAW

80. When the patient is breathing quietly, when is the best time in the respiratory cycle to measure the PA pressure?

a. **Just before the dip due to inspiration**
b. **Just before the rise due to inspiration**
c. **Just before the dip due to expiration**
d. **Just before the rise due to expiration**

ANSWER a. Just before the dip due to inspiration. This is the plateau at end expiration just before the next breath. Ahrens says: "In order to avoid incorrect readings, the clinician must approximate intrapleural pressures. This is most commonly done by reading pressure waves when intrapleural pressure is negligible or near normal. Intrapleural pressure is near baseline when no inspiratory or expiratory pressures are present. Gas flow at end expiration is, or should be, zero. End expiration is therefore the most commonly used approximation of a stable intrapleural pressure."
See: Ahrens, chapter on "Normal Arterial Waveforms" **Keywords:** resp cycle effect

THE NEXT 2 QUESTIONS REFER TO THIS DIAGRAM (SAME PATIENT AS ABOVE):

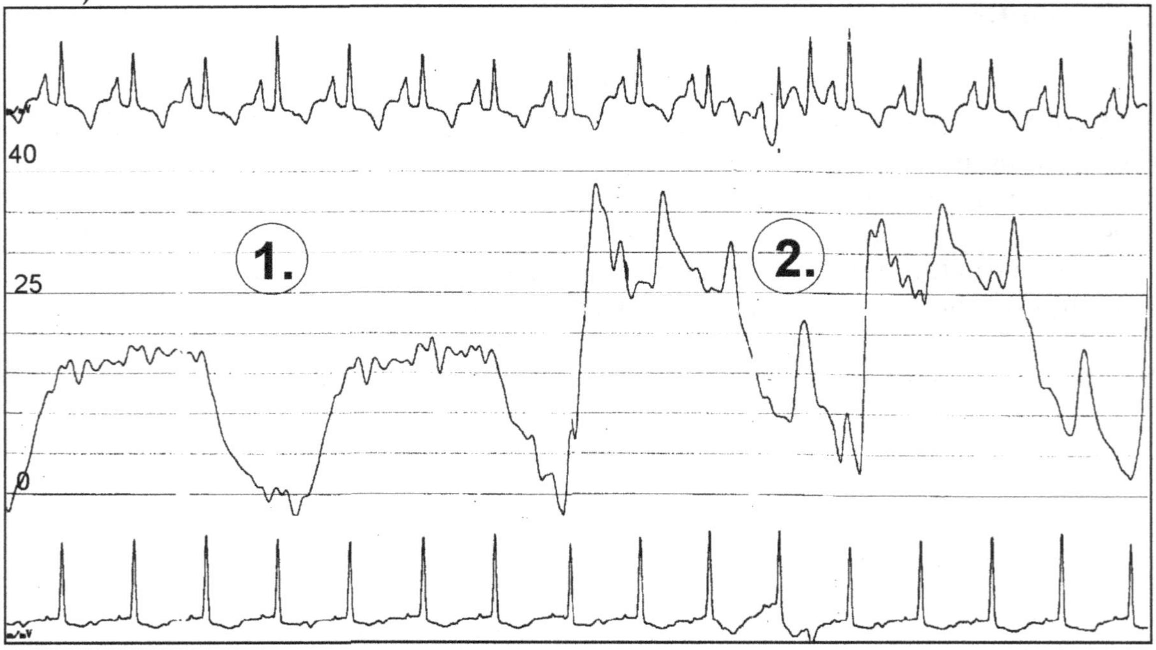

Pressure x 50

81. What pressure is shown recorded at #1 above?

a. **RA**
b. **RV**
c. **PA**
d. **PAW**

82. **On the tracing labeled #2 above read the end expiratory diastolic pressure in mmHg:**

a. 9 mmHg
b. 20 mmHg
c. 25 mmHg
d. 28 mmHg

BOTH ANSWERS APPEAR TOGETHER BELOW:

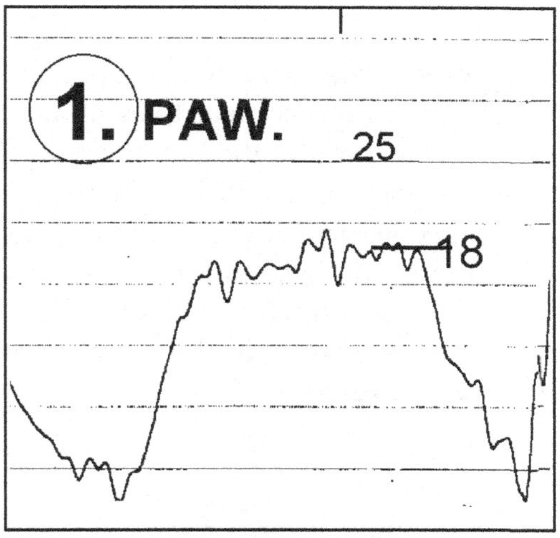

PAW x 50 increased respiratory artifact

81. ANSWER d. PAW. This is a pullback from PAW to PA. Several things distinguish #1 as a wedge pressure:

- Sine wave pressure waveform
- Low pressure level between 15 and 20 mmHg on x 50 scale
- Marked respiratory variations

Since tracing #1 does not rise to the same systolic peak as PA or RV, and is not rapidly rising in shape, this must be PAW.

The deep negative inspiratory waves suggest that this patient was short of breath. The PAW "a" and "v" waves are indistinct and of approximately the same height. To increase the accuracy of this tracing the patient should be asked to hold his breath in expiration.

See: Ahrens, chapter on "Normal Arterial Waveforms" **Keywords:** Identify PAW

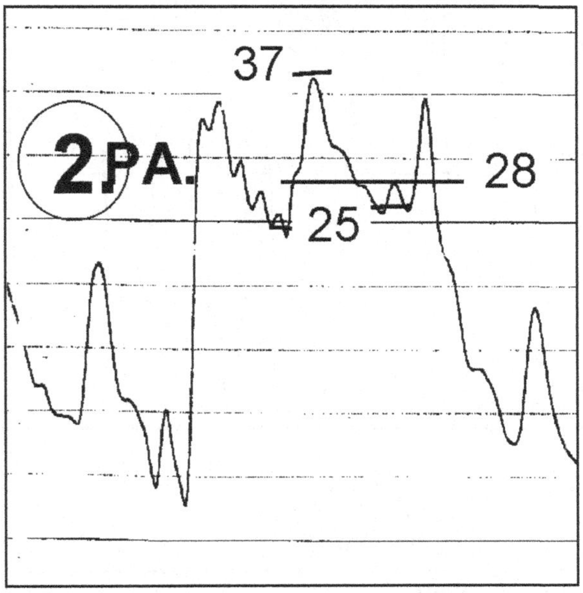

PA x 50 increased respiratory artifact

82. ANSWER c. 25 mmHg = Tracing (#2) PA diastolic. Read you pressures during end-expiration, on the plateau between deep breaths. The PA-EDP is seen clearly on only a few beats. It is just touching the 25 mmHg line. Pressure measurements shown are:

PAW: 18,18,17 mmHg (a,v,m)
PA: 37/25,28 (s/d,m).

Tracing (#2) is PA because it has a triangular waveform with dicrotic notch.
See: Ahrens, chapter on "Normal Arterial Waveforms" **Keywords:** measure PA

83. When a patient's breathing is labored and tachypnic how should you record and measure the wedge pressure?

a. Measure during the inspiratory dip
b. Measure during the expiratory hump
c. Have them let a normal breath out, then hold it
d. Have them take a deep breath and blow it all the way out

ANSWER c. Have them take a deep breath and let it out slowly at end of a normal expiration. The best place to estimate "transmural pressure" is just before the inspiratory artifact (dip), where the pressures level out. At least one, preferably two complete respiratory cycles should be recorded to evaluate the end expiratory pressure. If respiration is rapid or labored it is best to have the patient - let a normal breath OUT, hold it, and not bear down (without Valsalva) while recording. This lets the pleural pressure stabilize at the lungs natural relaxed position.
See: Ahrens, chapter on "Respiratory Influence on Waveforms." Keywords: Read at end expiratory pressure

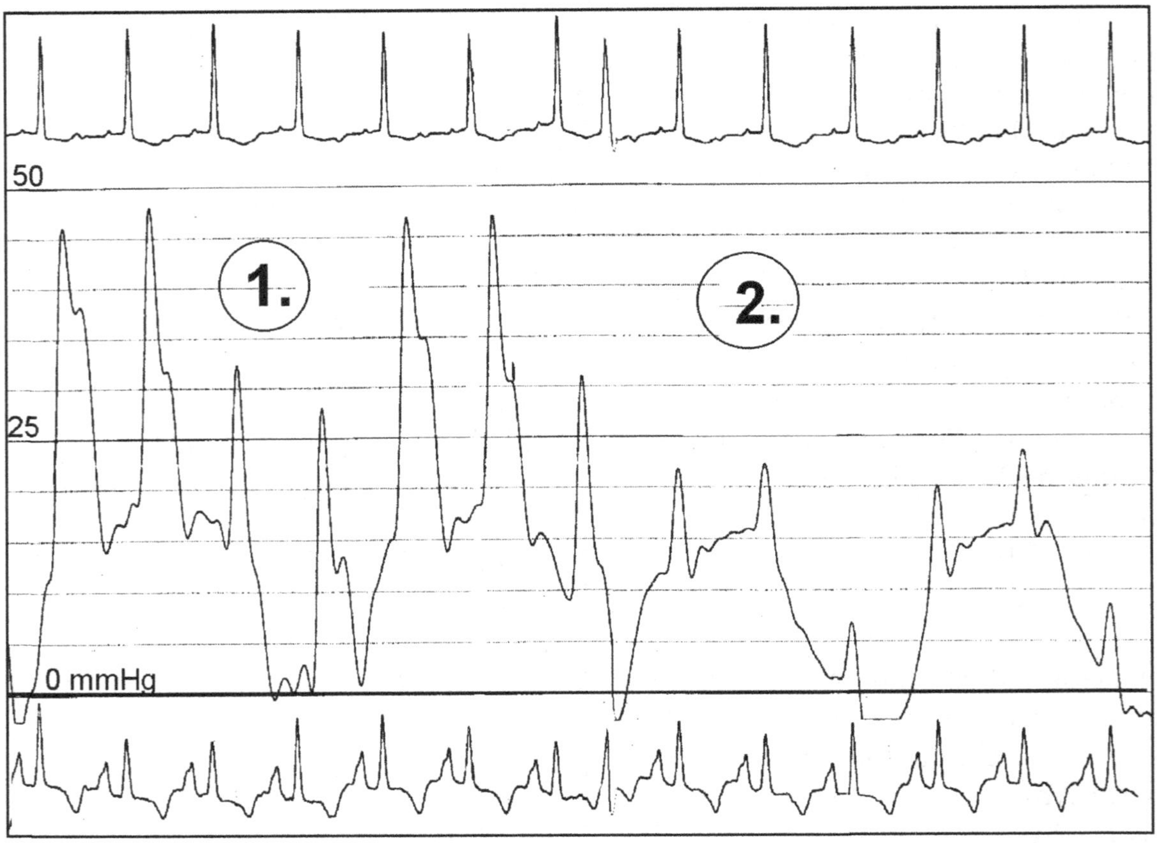

Pressure x 50

THE NEXT 2 QUESTIONS REFER TO THIS DIAGRAM (on the same patient as above)

84. **What pressure is shown recorded at #2 above?**
a. RA
b. RV
c. PA
d. PAW

85. **On the tracing labeled #1 above read the end expiratory EDP.**
a. 8 mmHg
b. 13 mmHg
c. 18 mmHg
d. 47 mmHg

BOTH ANSWERS APPEAR TOGETHER BELOW:

84. ANSWER a. RA This is a pullback from RV to RA. You can identify tracing (#1) as RV, by the rapid rise to a systole of 47 mmHg. Since the tracing is not marked with "pullback" or "insertion" you must decide what #2 is. Tracing #2 could be either of the adjacent chambers RA or PA. Since the #2 tracing does not rise to the same systolic peak as RV, and is not triangular (great vessel) in shape, this must be RA.

Note that all pressures are dramatically affected by rapid respiratory rate, as seen in the dramatic swings in the diastolic levels. The large positive waves on the RA (#2) tracing immediately following the ECG P wave are "a" waves. The RA is attempting to compensate the failing RV with atrial kick. These giant "a" waves increase RV preload. No "v" waves are seen so read it where it normally should be - after the T wave. **See:** Ahrens, chapter on "Normal Atrial Waveforms"
Keywords: identify RA

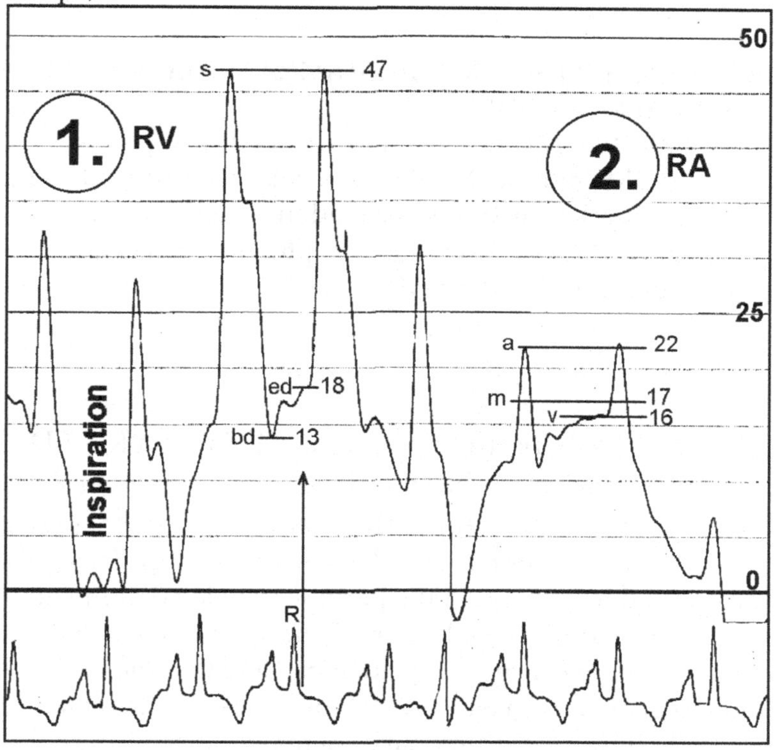

Right heart pullback pressure x50

85. ANSWER c. 18 mmHg. The pressures should be read at the end of expiration on the plateau between deep breaths. The RV-EDP is seen clearly on only a few beats. It is measured immediately prior to ventricular contraction, usually at the end of the ECG QRS wave. Pressure measurements shown are: RV: 47/13,18 (s/bd,ed) and RA: 22,17,18 mmHg (a,v,m). this patient should have been asked to hold his breath to get more stable end-expiratory readings.

See: Ahrens, chapter on "Normal ventricular waveforms" **Keywords:** measure RV-EDP

THE NEXT 2 QUESTIONS REFER TO THIS DIAGRAM:

86. Read the end expiratory RV-EDP recorded on the tracing shown.
a. 5 mmHg
b. 12 mmHg
c. 17 mmHg
d. 22 mmHg

87. This RV-EDP suggests that this patient may be having symptoms associated with:
a. Tricuspid valve stenosis
b. Peripheral edema
c. Chronic angina
d. Systemic hypertension

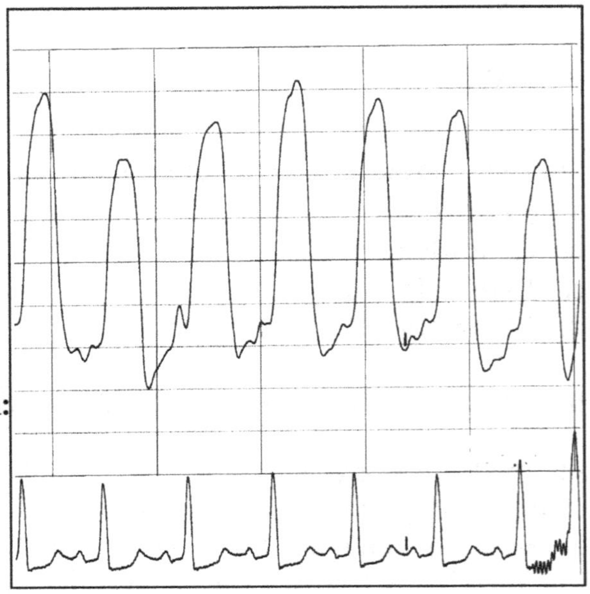

RV x 50

BOTH ANSWERS FOR THE DIAGRAM ABOVE APPEAR TOGETHER BELOW:

86. ANSWER c. 17 mmHg. Often, the RV tracing is delayed from the QRS and the RV-EDP is usually measured at the end of the QRS complex. It should be read in the dip following the presystolic "a" wave. **See:** Kern, chapter on "Hemodynamics." **Keywords:** Read RV-RV-EDP

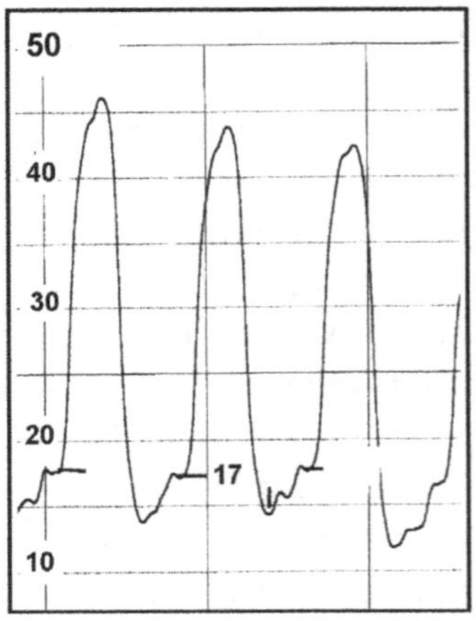

RV x 50 EDP measurement

87. ANSWER b. peripheral edema. This high RV-EDP indicates either right heart failure or volume overload. Since this RV-EDP is high, the upstream chamber (RA and CVP) will also be high (normal RA = 0-5 mmHg). This pressure causes fluid to back up in the peripheral veins dilating all venous structures. The fluid particularly gravitates to the feet and ankles and cause pitting edema. Note that the RV systole also is elevated at 42. This will translate into an elevated PA pressure downstream. The wedge and LV-EDP may also be elevated causing pulmonary edema.
See: Braunwald, chapter on " Physical Exam." **Keywords**: Elevated RV-EDP= RV Failure

USE THIS TRACING FOR NEXT QUESTION. Note the 2 different Ranges

.

88. **What pressures are shown in this simultaneous tracing? (Note that they are recorded on different scales.)**

a. **RV and PA**
b. **RV and PAW**
c. **LV and PA**
d. **LV and AO**

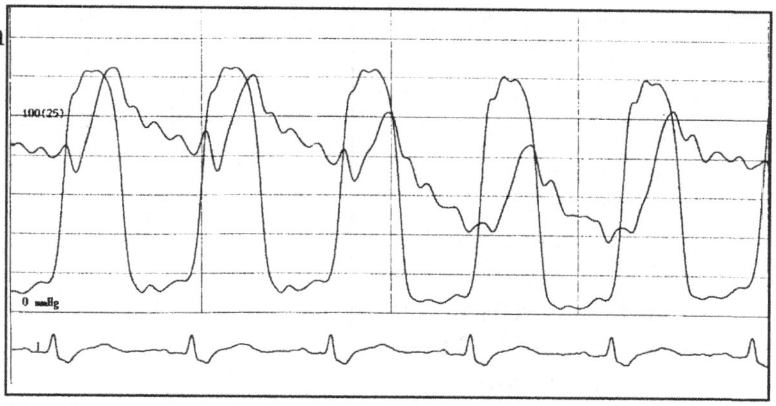

Simultaneous pressures x 200 and x 50

ANSWER c. LV and PA. The tricky pressure here is the triangular shaped one. Since it has marked respiratory variation and a presystolic artifact it is probably PA recorded on X 50 scale. The other tracings is LV recorded on x 200. At first glance these simultaneous tracings look like simultaneous LV and AO with an impulse type gradient. To avoid confusion it is best to record simultaneous pressures on the same scale. **See**: Personal experience **Keywords**: Record simultaneous tracings on same scale

:

USE THIS TRACING FOR NEXT QUESTION. Note the 2 different ranges or scales.

89. **What pressures are shown in this simultaneous tracing? (Note that they are recorded on different scales.)**

a. **RV and PA**
b. **RV and PAW**
c. **LV and PA**
d. **LV and PAW**

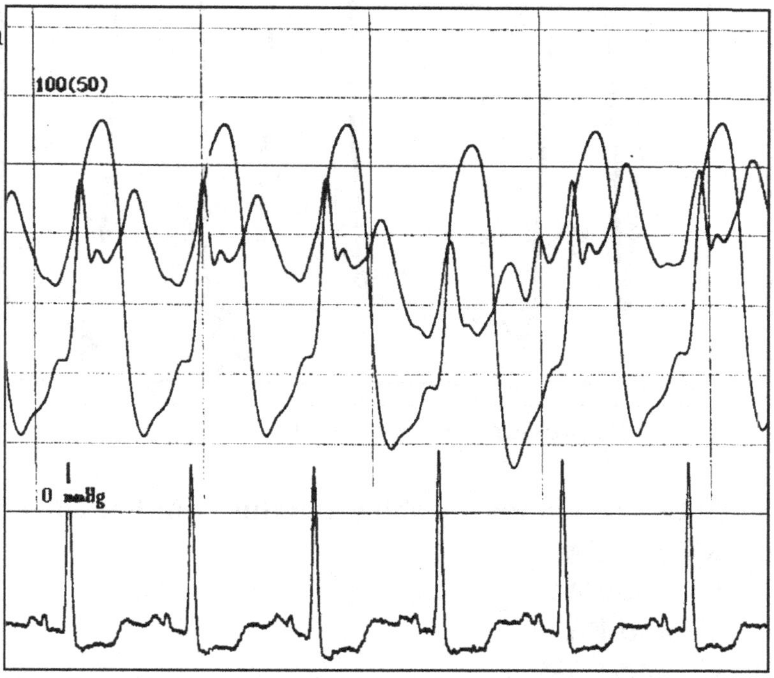

Simultaneous pressures x 200 and x 50

ANSWER d. LV and PAW. The tricky pressure here is the double humped one. Since it has marked respiratory variation and "a" and "v" waves it is probably PAW recorded on X 50 scale. The other tracings is LV recorded on x 200. This tracing is deceptive since for accurate LV-PAW comparison, they should be recorded on the same scale - usually x 50 to see the diastolic levels and planimeter for valve area. When properly recorded there is a small mitral stenosis gradient shown here. **See:** Kern, chapter on "Hemodynamics." **Keywords:** Record simultaneous pressures on same scale

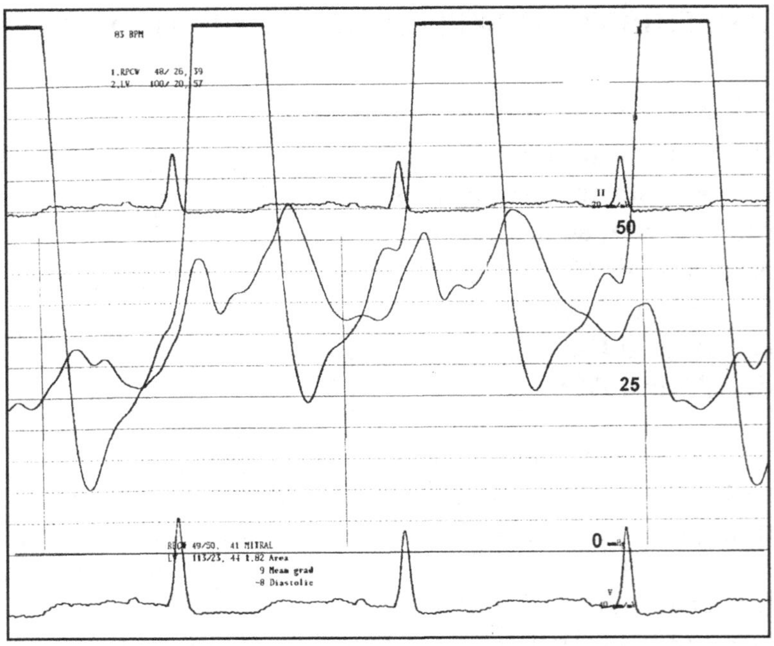

Properly recorded Simultaneous LV and PAWP x 50

USE THIS TRACING FOR NEXT 2 QUESTIONS

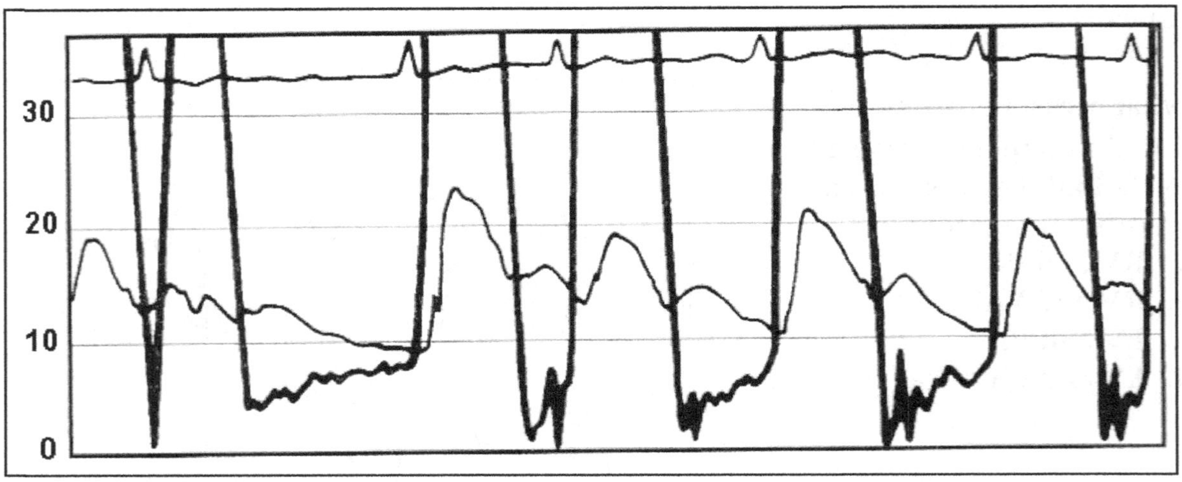

Simultaneous pressures x 50 (After Mark)

90. What two pressures are shown in this simultaneous pressure tracing above?

a. **RV and PA**
b. **RV and PAW**
c. **LV and PA**
d. **LV and PAW**

91. Estimate the average LV-EDP in the simultaneous pressure tracing above.
- **a. 7 mmHg**
- **b. 11 mmHg**
- **c. 20 mmHg**
- **d. Off the scale >30**

90. ANSWER c. LV and PA. The LV is in drawn thicker than PA. LV is off the scale, so systolic cannot be read. Note the dicrotic notch on the downslope of the PA tracing. Note also that PA-EDP nearly equilibrates with LV-EDP in the long cycle #2. Thus no mitral stenosis is present.
See: Ward, chapter on "PA and Wedge Pressure Artifacts"

91. ANSWER a. 7 mmHg. End Diastole varies from 6 to 8 mmHg depending on the length of the filling cycle. Atrial fibrillation is present which makes it difficult to find an accurate average. Grossman recommends recording at least 10 beats and averaging them.
See: Ward, chapter on "PA and Wedge Pressure Artifacts"

REFERENCES:

Ahrens, T. S., and Taylor, L.A., *Hemodynamic Waveform Analysis*, 1st Ed., W.B. Saunders Co., 1992
Baim, D. S. and Grossman W., *Cardiac Catheterization, Angiography, and Intervention*, 7th Ed., Lea and Febiger, 2006
Braunwald, et. al. Ed., *Heart Disease, a Textbook of CV Medicine*, 9th Ed., Saunders, 2012
Pappano & Wier, previously Berne R. M. and Levy, M. N., *Cardiovascular Physiology*, 10th Ed., Mosby Year Book, 2013
Daily, E. K., and Schroeder, J. S., *Techniques in Bedside Hemodynamic Monitoring*, 4th Ed., C. V. Mosby Company, 1989
Darovic, G.O., *Hemodynamic Monitoring: Invasive and Noninvasive Clinical Application*, WB Saunders, 1995
Kern, M. J., Ed., *The Cardiac Catheterization Handbook*,6th Ed., Mosby-Year Book, Inc., 2016
PACEP.org Pulmonary Artery Catheter Education Project, sponsored by ASA
Pepine, J. C., and Hill, J. A., et. al., *Diagnostic and Therapeutic Cardiac Catheterization*, 2nd Ed., Williams and Wilkins, 1994
Ragosta, Textbook of Clinical Hemodynamics, Saunders Elsevier, 2008
Taylor, E. J. Ed., *Dorland's Medical Dictionary*, 27th ed., W. B. Saunders Co.,1988
Ward, Johnathan B, Atlas of Cardiovascular Monitoring, Churchill Livingstone, 1998

OUTLINE: Reading Pressures

1. ECG RELATED PRESSURES
   a. Atrial fib. (no a wave)
   b. PVCs, bigeminy
   c. AV block
   d. Pacemaker rhythm
   e. Pacemaker syndrome
      i. loss of atrial kick
   f. ECG artifact

2. PRACTICE TRACINGS
   a. Hypertension (elevated systolic)
   b. Edema (elevated diastolic)
   c. Gradients
   d. Simultaneous tracings
      i. Record on same scale

3. OTHER
   a. Phases of Valsalva
      i. Increased thoracic pressure
      ii. Venous return is impeded.
      iii. Thoracic pressure drops with inspiration
      iv. Venous return increases with inspiration
   b. dP/dT
      i. Pressure Rise / time
      ii. Pressure wire or cath. Tip manometer
   c. Ventilator, effect on venous return

Pressure Recording Systems

INDEX: E3

System Electronics

92. When using standard disposable transducers with fluid filled catheters, where is the "Wheatstone bridge" located?

a. In the carrier amplifier (#1)
b. In the transducer (#2)
c. In the pressure manifold (#3)
d. Near the tip of the catheter (#4)

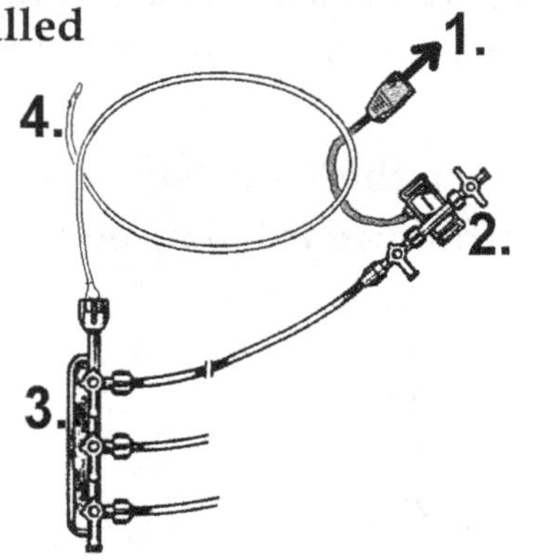

ANSWER b. In the transducer. The pressure sensors are within the transducers body and termed "strain gauges." These sensors are attached to a flexible diaphragm and arranged in a diamond configuration so that some stretch and some compress. This action imbalances the voltage dividers and creates a voltage output which is then amplified by the carrier amplifier.

Expensive "catheter tip manometers" are available and often used for research purposes. You can also get stopcock manifolds with pressure transducers built into them. This helps avoid the low frequency artifacts commonly induced by pressure tubes.

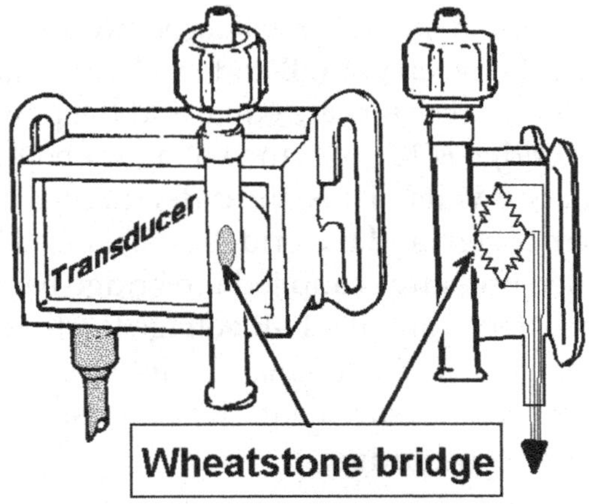

Transducer - Wheatstone bridge

See: Baim and Grossman's chapter on "Pressure recording." **Keywords:** Wheatstone bridge within a pressure transducer

93. **You are calibrating a non-computerized hemodynamic recorder. During a pressure transducer calibration, pressing the "zero" or "balance" button:**

a. **Opens the transducer to air and gives a 100-mmHg cal.**
b. **Adjusts the gauge or calibration factor**
c. **Adjusts the transducer to mechanical zero (mid chest level)**
d. **Balances the Wheatstone bridge resistors to give zero output**

ANSWER d. balances the Wheatstone bridge resistors to zero output. By varying the four resistances in the Wheatstone bridge, the output can be nulled to zero voltage. The baseline is then be set on the recorder and monitor screen. Then as the transducer is "strained" with pressure the output voltage changes and is displayed on the monitor. **See:** Baim and Grossman, chapter on "Pressure Measurement." **Keywords:** balancing the Wheatstone bridge to zero

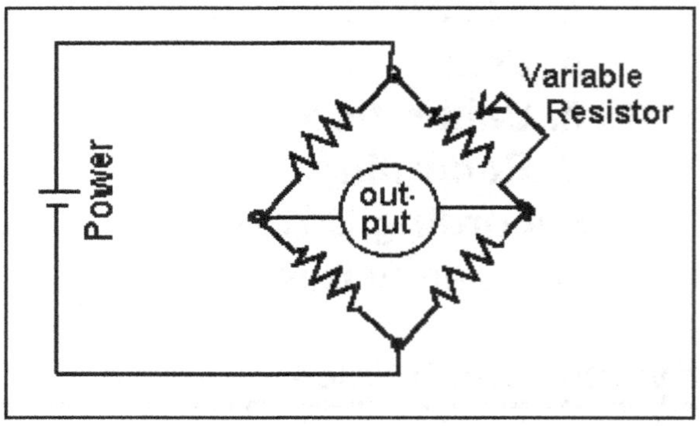

Wheatstone Bridge

94. **When the Wheatstone bridge is zeroed, what voltage difference is balanced to zero on the diagram?**

a. A-B
b. A-C
c. A-D
d. B-D
e. B-C

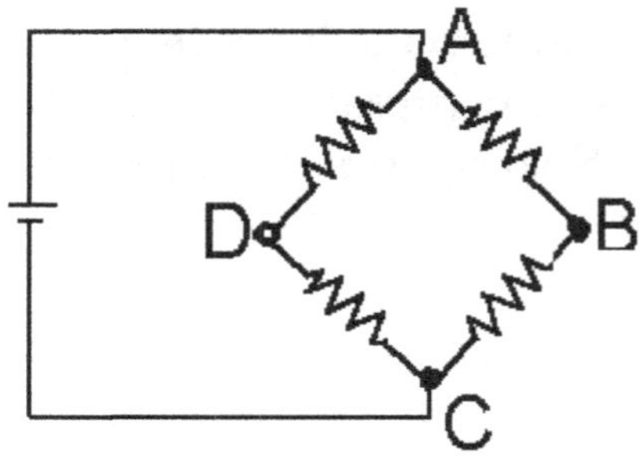

Wheatstone bridge circuit

Answer d. B-D. The voltage divides across the resistors so that when balanced no voltage exists between point B and D. As an example, if all four resistors are equal and the power to the bridge is 10 volts, the voltage at both D & B will be 5 volts. Thus, the difference between them is zero and the bridge is "balanced." When pressure is applied the bridge becomes imbalanced and the D-B voltage fluctuates. **See:** Baim and Grossman, chapter on "Pressure Measurements"**Keywords:** Balanced Wheatstone bridge

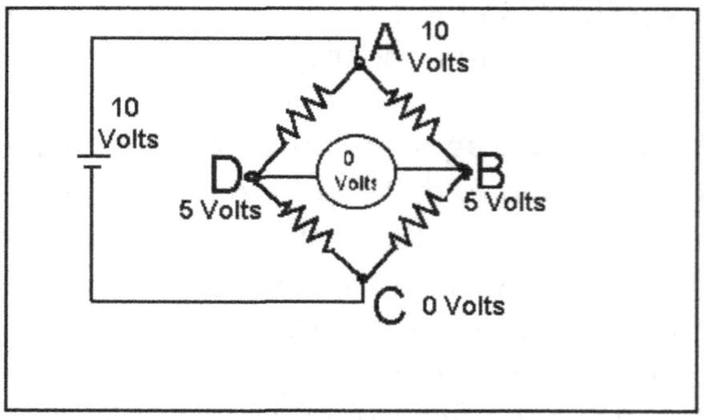

Wheatstone bridge circuit

95. **Another name for a hemodynamic physiologic PRESSURE RECORDING AMPLIFIER that is connected to a strain gauge transducer is a:**

a. **DC amplifier**
b. **Demodulator**
c. **Carrier amplifier**
d. **Analog to digital converter**

ANSWER c. Carrier amplifier. These are called "carriers" because they send a carrier signal to excite the transducer (#1). Here is how a transducer "piggy backs" the pressure information onto the carrier signal. When pressure is applied the strain elements imbalance the Wheatstone bridge and "modulate" the carrier signal. This is amplitude modulation (AM). It creates an envelope around the signal (#2). The signal is then "demodulated" by removing the AC carrier signal. Finally the envelope is displayed on the monitor screen as pressure (#3). **See:** Co. literature **Keywords:** Carrier amplifier

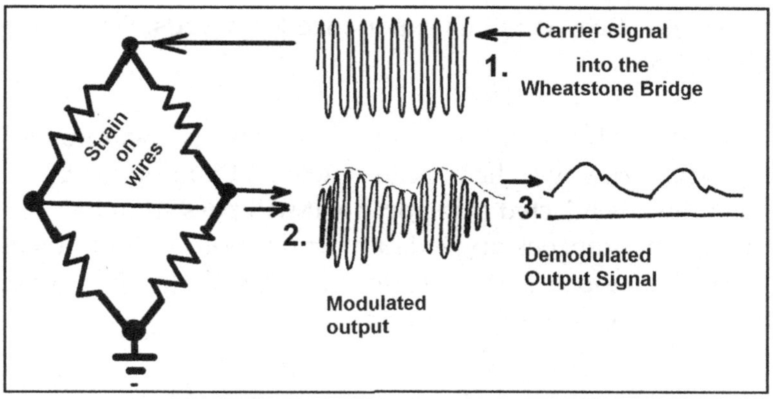

Carrier signal modulation/demodulation

Plumbing

USE THIS DIAGRAM FOR BOTH QUESTIONS BELOW:

96. **The upper stopcock (#1, 2, 3)drawn in the box is termed a:**

a. **2 way, handle OFF**
b. **2 way, handle ON**
c. **3 way, handle OFF**
d. **3 way, handle ON**

97. **If the handle of the lower stopcock is turned to position #6 as shown at the arrow, what will happen when you inject flush into port #6?**

a. **Nothing, blocked off**
b. **Flush will exit port #4**
c. **Flush will exit port #5**
d. **Flush will exit both port #4 and #5**

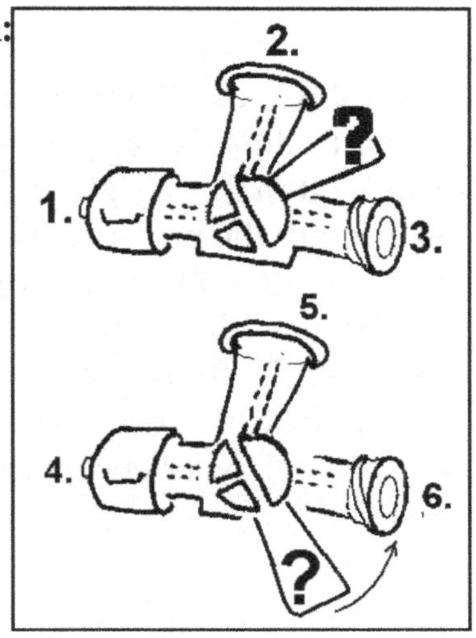

Handle off/on stopcocks

BOTH ANSWERS LISTED TOGETHER BELOW:

96. ANSWER c. 3 way, handle OFF. It is a 3 way stopcock because there are only 3 positions for the handle. The position shown is the not one of those 3. This is the "Panic Position" that turns everything off.

It is a handle-OFF stopcock because wherever the handle is turned, that port is closed. So if the handle is turned to the right (position #3) nothing can be injected through port #3. It is OFF. However, ports #1 and #2 are open, and blood may bleed back if it is connected to a catheter. Most stopcocks are of this type. **See:** Personal experience **Keywords:** Handle-OFF stopcock

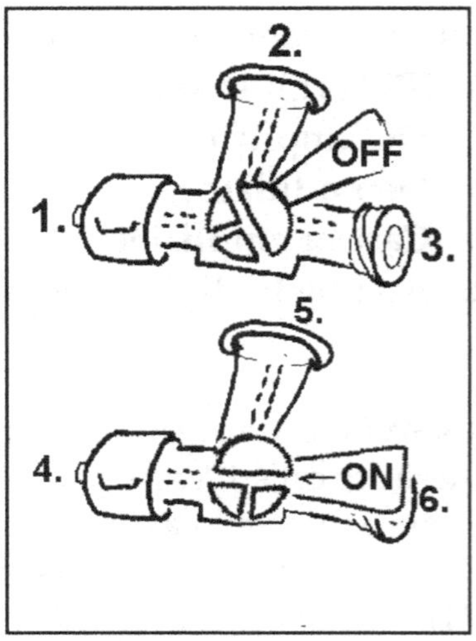

Handle off/on stopcocks

97. ANSWER b. Flush will exit port #4. This is a handle-ON stopcock. Wherever the handle is turned, that port is ON. When flush is injected into port #6, it will pass straight through the stopcock and exit at port #4. Some manifolds use this type of stopcock. **See:** Todd, Vol. II, Chapter on "Catheterization Equipment" **Keywords:** Handle-ON stopcock

98. The way the catheter /transducer system is set up in the diagram you can:
(Note the "handle-ON" stopcocks)

- **a. Get air zeros**
- **b. Flush the transducer to eliminate bubbles**
- **c. Measure arterial pressure**
- **d. Pump in 100 mmHg for a calibration**

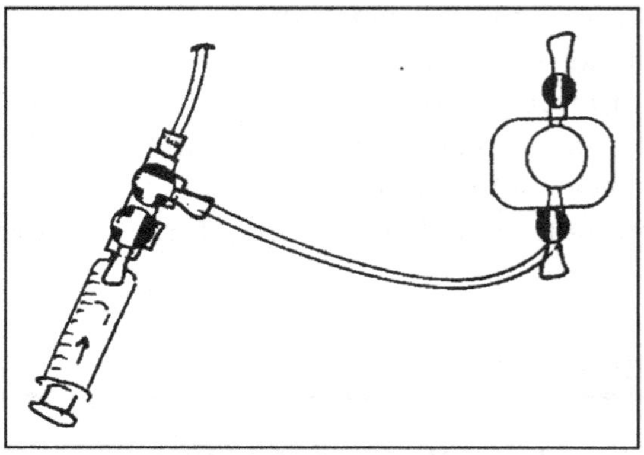

Manifold and transducer stopcocks

ANSWER b. Flush the transducer to eliminate bubbles. You inject saline through the proximal handle-on stopcock. It makes a right turn at the distal stopcock, goes through the pressure tube, through the lower stopcock (optional) and out the upper stopcock, taking any bubbles with it. While flushing the transducer and tubes, carefully for bubbles. While flushing snap your finger on the transducer to dislodge adherent bubbles. **See:** Personal experience **Keywords:** flushing transducer

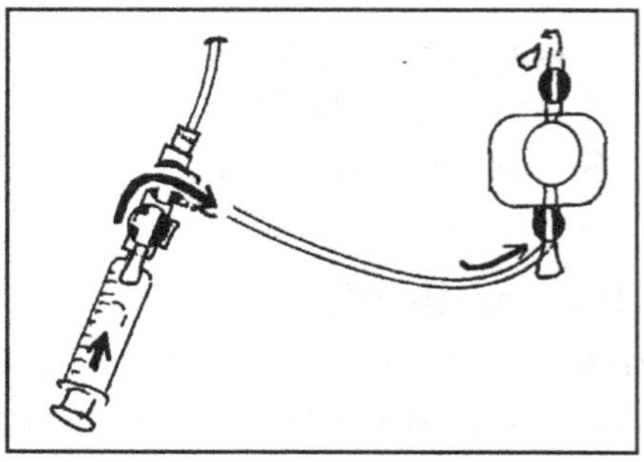

Manifold and transducer stopcocks

99. **This diagram shows a hemodynamic monitoring system with "handle-OFF stopcocks." With the stopcocks turned as shown, activating the quick-flush device (continuous flush) will:**

a. Not flush (the bag is not activated)

b. Flush the transducer

c. Flush the stopcock

d. Flush the catheter

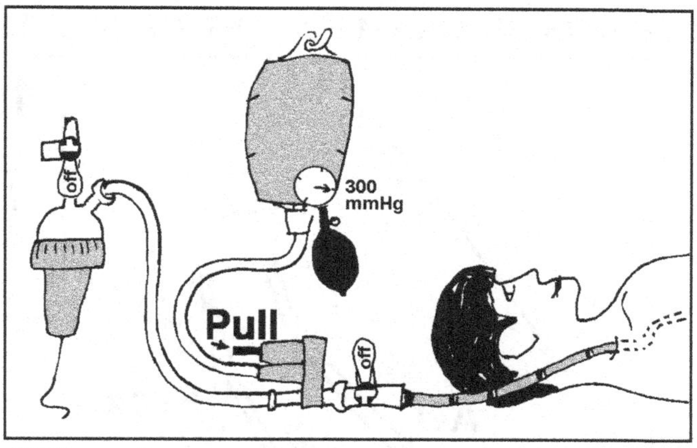

CVP monitoring catheter with quick/slow flush device

ANSWER d. Flush the catheter. The stopcock is handle-up which opens the catheter to the quick flush device. Since it is a "Y" device this will allow flushing and/or recording of RA pressure. You pull the rubber tail or squeeze the device to open the system to the pressurized bag of heparinized saline. This flushes the catheter. The transducer will sense sudden a burst of pressure as the "Y" adapter opens.

When you release the tail or stop squeezing the device flushes slowly, imperceptibly and continuously at 3-5 ml/hour. This is slow enough so it won't increase the recorded pressure. Unless you want to flush bubbles from the transducer, the transducer stopcock is always turned off, as shown. This way no pressure or saline can leak out. Some transducers come with built in continuous flow devices.

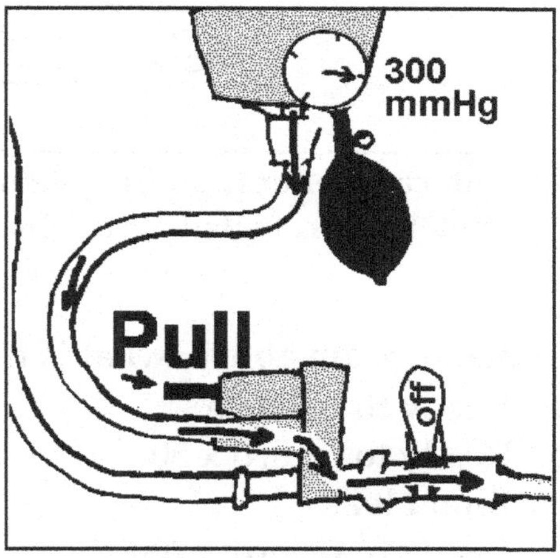

Quick flushing a catheter

See: TruWave transducers at edwards.com: http://www.edwards.com/devices/Pressure-Monitoring/Transducer and Quaal, chapter on "Bioinstrumentation of hemodynamic monitoring." **Keywords:** Continuous flush devices

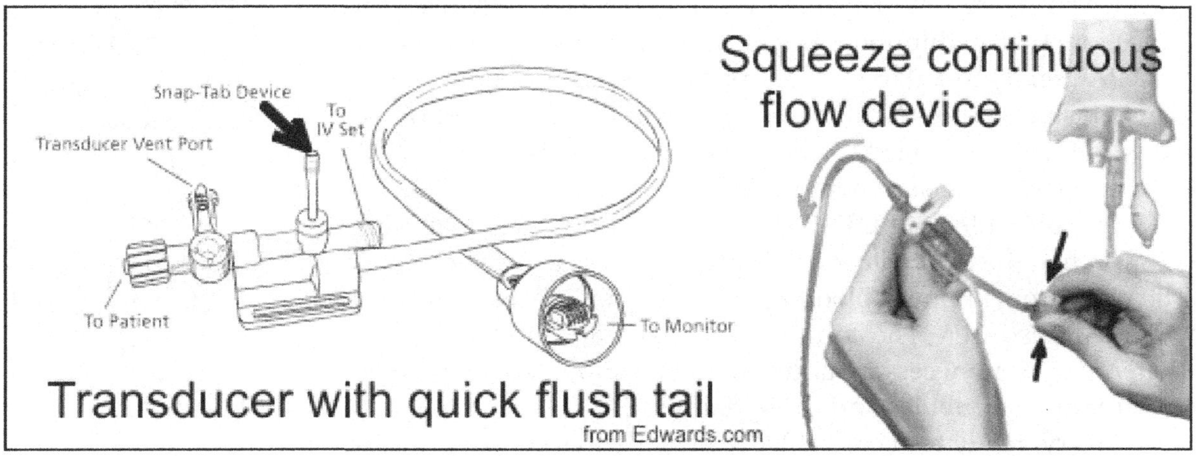

Transducer with built in quick flush (snap-tab) or squeeze device

USE THIS DIAGRAM FOR THE NEXT QUESTION.

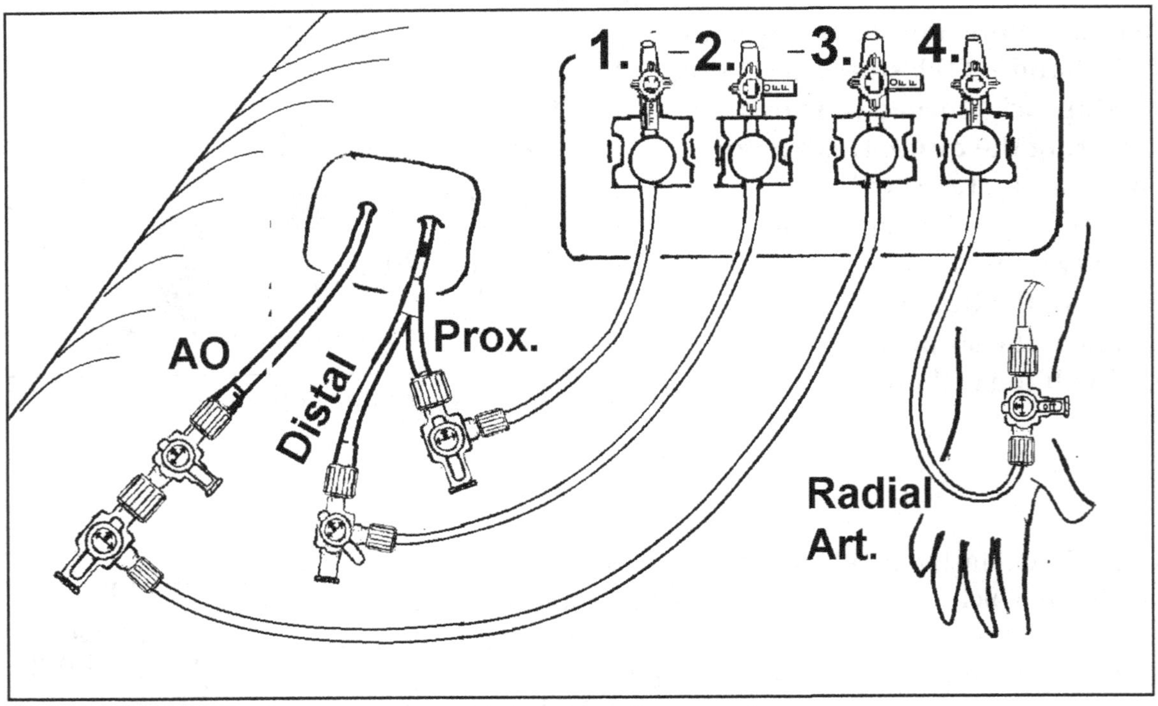

Four catheter transducer systems with handle-off stopcocks.
Catheters are: pigtail, 2 port Swan-Ganz, and radial artery cannula.

100. In the diagram above, what is the status of the transducer labeled # 2 ?

- **a. Ready to balance**
- **b. Ready to record x 50**
- **c. Blood leak**
- **d. Ready to record x 200**

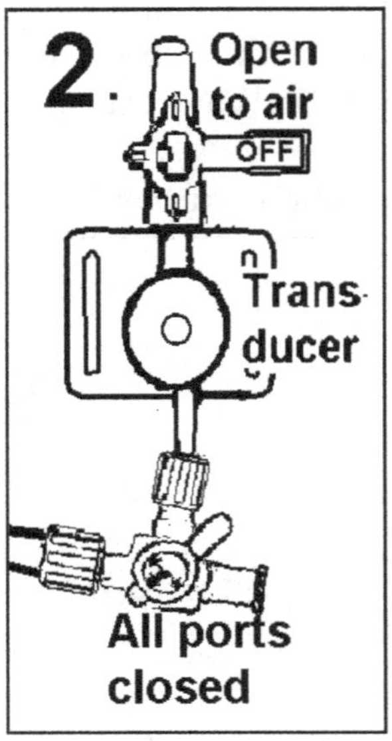

Zero PA line

ANSWER a. Ready to balance distal PA line. BE ABLE TO IDENTIFY STATUS OF ALL THESE TRANSDUCERS.

#1 RA, ready to record x 50: The transducer is closed; ready to record RA pressure x 50. This proximal RA port is usually used for IV injection, thermodilution injectate, or CVP measurement.

#2 PA , ready to balance: The upper stopcock is open to air ready to balance. The PA catheter stopcock is closed to all ports, so fluid will not leak from the system. This distal port is usually used for PA and PAW measurement x 50.

#3 AO, blood leak (OOPS!): The transducer is open to air - at the top. When the lower stopcock is open to pressure as shown, aortic pressure will pump blood up the pressure line and out the top of the transducer. The additional stopcock attached to the catheter may be unnecessary and should be eliminated as it is a source to trap air bubbles and cause damping.

#4 Artery, ready to record x 200: Currently measuring pressure from radial artery x 200. The additional stopcock may be unnecessary for this setup. **See:** Personal Experience **Keywords:** stopcock setup for air zeros

101. On the 2-stopcock coronary catheter manifold system shown, what stopcock port should be connected to the transducer?

a. **#1. Distal, rotating adapter**
b. **#2. Distal, side-arm.**
c. **#3. Proximal side-arm**
d. **#4. Proximal end female adapter**

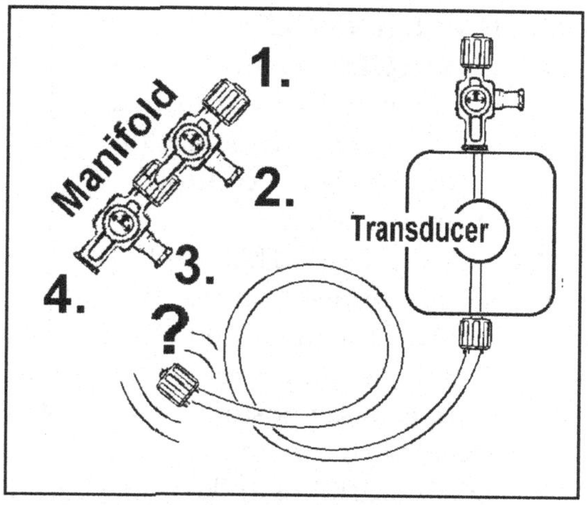

Coronary Manifold and transducer

ANSWER c. b. #2.-Distal, side-arm.
BE ABLE TO MATCH ALL ANSWERS:

1. Distal, rotating adapter (catheter)
2. Distal, side-arm (Pressure)
3. Proximal side-arm (contrast)
4. Proximal end female adapter (syringe)

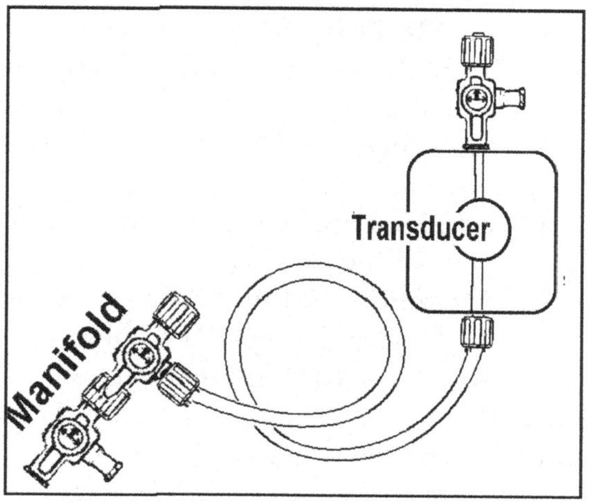

Coronary Manifold and transducer

The pressure transducer should be closest to the catheter for arterial pressure monitoring. Then the proximal stopcock can be used for closed-system bubble-free filling of the injection syringe. When angiographic injections occur, the pressure monitoring port must be closed. At all other times aortic pressure should be faithfully monitored.
See: Baim and Grossman, chapter on "Percutaneous Approach." **Keywords:** pressure monitoring stopcock → most distal side-arm

102. This is a four-stopcock coronary arteriogram manifold. Identify the port labeled #2 on the diagram.

a. **Dye**
b. **Syringe**
c. **Waste bag**
d. **Transducer**
e. **Flush**
f. **Catheter**
g. **Air Zero**

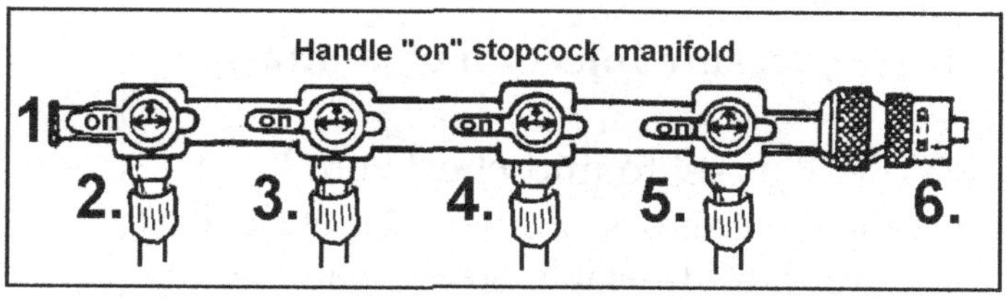

Four-stopcock coronary arteriogram manifold

ANSWER c. Waste bag receives discarded blood. **BE ABLE TO MATCH ALL ANSWERS:**

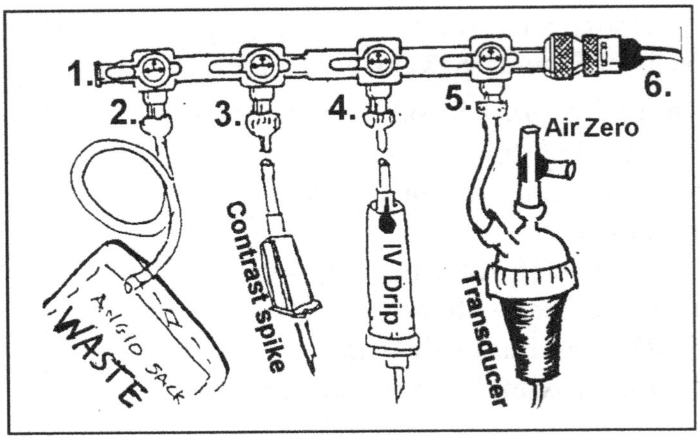

Four Stopcock Manifold setup

1. **SYRINGE:** A contrast injection syringe is attached to this female LL connector. A flush or 3-ring control syringe is used.
2. **WASTE BAG:** This empty IV sack is termed "waste." It receives the discarded blood and flush and prevents the cath team's exposure to blood born contaminants.
3. **DYE:** A dripless spike is used for dye to prevent air bubbles
4. **FLUSH:** A macro drip spike is used for heparinized flush (saline). This may also be connected to position #3. If pressurized flush is used, it requires a special high pressure IV.
5. **TRANSDUCER:** Baim and Grossman recommends use of a micro-transducer here for high fidelity recording. Any movement or tipping of this transducer on-the-table will affect the zero level. For this reason an extension tube is often use to take the transducer off the table (not shown), but it may reduce the frequency response of the system.
6. **CATHETER:** A rotating adapter here allows torquing of the catheter without having to twist the manifold.
7. **AIR ZERO:** A fluid filled IV tube is run from the transducer, off-the-table and set at the height of the patient's "mid-chest-level" for an accurate zero. The Stopcock position shown gives an air zero.

See: Baim and Grossman, chapter on "Percutaneous Approach." **Keywords:** four stopcock manifold setup → waste bag

103. This 3 way coronary stopcock manifold has a built in pressure transducer. What is the tube at #3?

a. Is set up for a waste bag

b. Is set to mid-chest zero level

c. Measures pressure from a second catheter

d. Is for pressure injection of contrast

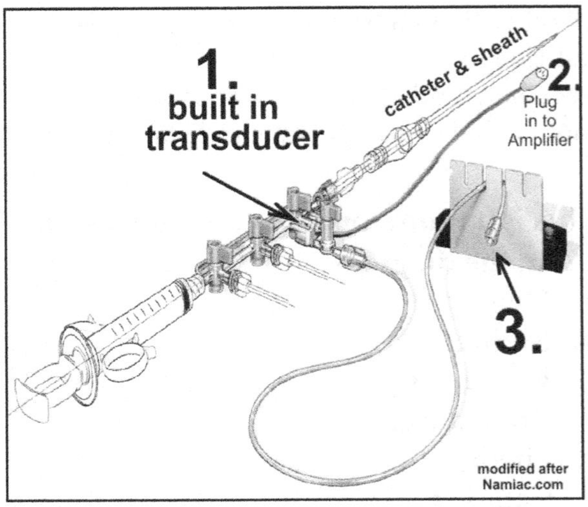

Pressure manifold with built in transducer

ANSWER. B. Is set to mid-chest zero level for off-the-table zeroes. Zero level is at tip of the long tube, off-the-table, so the manifold does not need to be at heart level while recording, the operator can flush bubbles from the transducer himself, and open to zero at any time.

The tube is filled with saline, and the tip (#3) is moved up or down and set to the patient's mid-chest zero level. When the one-way transducer stopcock at #1 is opened, the transducer is given the mechanical (mid-chest) zero level for zero calibration. This also eliminates the problem of recording pressures through long pressure tubes which often resonate with artifacts. Having shorter conducting tubing between catheter tip and transducer improves the fidelity of pressure measurement. **See:** http://www.navilystmedical.com/downloads/eNAVB170_CathBrochure_0512.pdf

104. This 3 way coronary stopcock manifold has a built in pressure transducer. What is shown at #5?

a. To zero line
b. To waste bag
c. To contrast bottle
d. To saline flush bag
e. To transducer connection

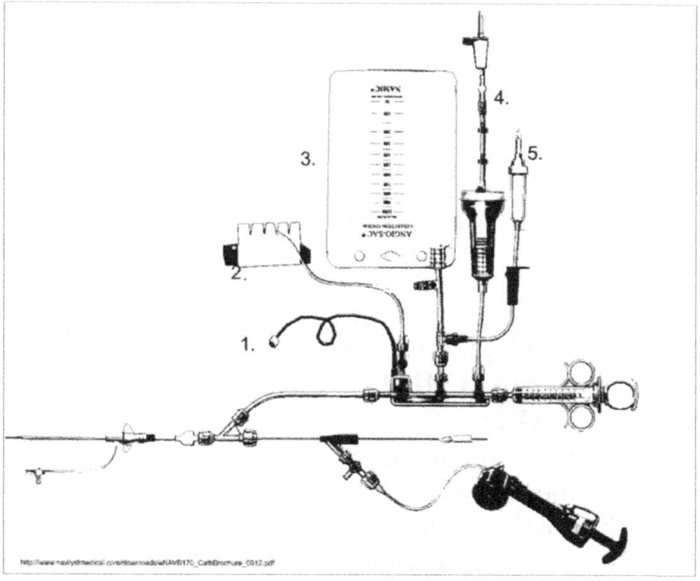

Pressure manifold with built in transducer

ANSWER d. To saline flush bag. When you draw back on the 3-ring syringe you get heparinzed flush for flushing catheters and syringes. Be able to identify all connections in this drawing.

1. Electrical connection to transducer
2. Mid-chest zero set off-table
3. Waste bag for blood and discarded fluids via 2 way T-valve.
4. Contrast line with measuring gauge and no-air limiter. NAMIC® Squeeze™ Contrast Controller
5. Saline line, connected to Waste and 3-ring syringe. Drawing back pulls saline into syringe via 2 way T-valve.
6. Injection syringe
7. Inflation device
8. Guidewire
9. Y-connector or Touhy-Borst
10. Guiding or diagnostic catheter
11. Sheath

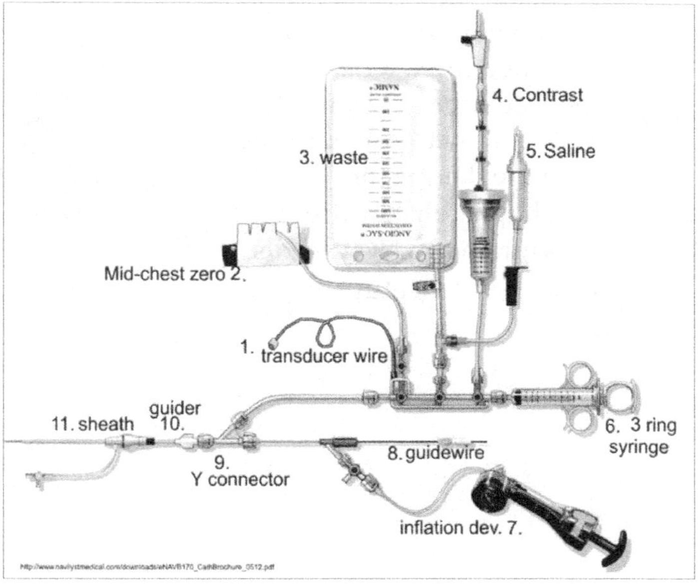

Coronary manifold using NAMIC® devices

See: http://www.navilystmedical.com/downloads/eNAVB170_CathBrochure_0512.pdf

105. What should be attached to the tail of the Swan-Ganz thermodilution catheter labeled #2 (distal) in the diagram?

a. **Cool injectate & temp. sensor**
b. **PA pressure monitoring**
c. **Balloon inflation port (2.5 cc syringe)**
d. **CO computer cable**

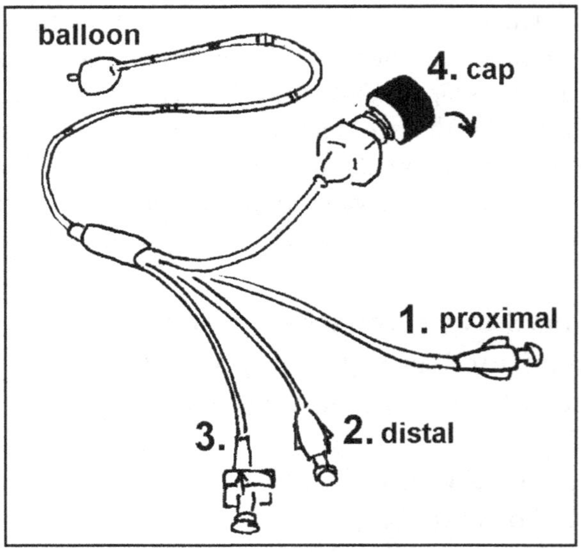

Swan Ganz catheter tails

ANSWER b. PA pressure monitoring. **MATCHED ANSWERS ARE:**

1. Blue proximal female connector for iced injectate
2. Yellow distal female connector for wedge pressure monitoring
3. Female connector with built in plastic one way stopcock for balloon inflation port
4. Threaded three wire connector for CO computer cable conducts power to and from the thermistor.

See: Daily, chapter on "Cardiac Output Measurements."**Keywords:** TDCO Swan catheter setup

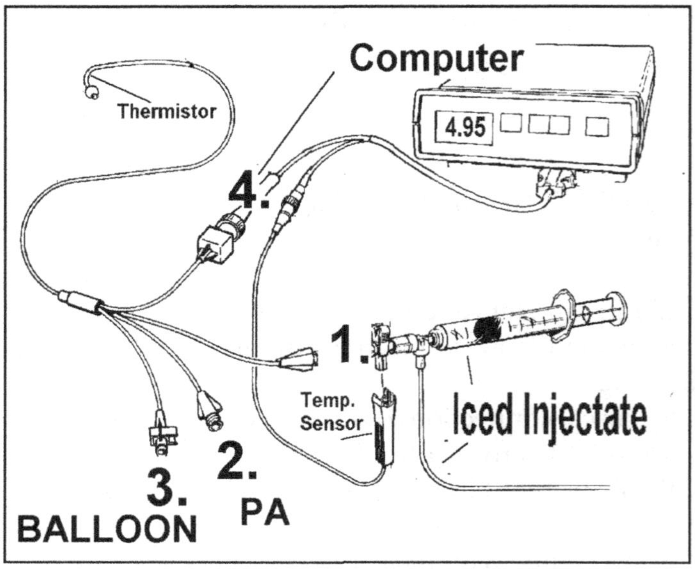

Swan-Ganz Thermodilution setup

106. **This is a manifold setup to monitor Swan-Ganz and arterial pressures following surgery. The stopcocks are the "handle-OFF" type. With the way these stopcocks are turned you can:**

a. Flush the RA catheter

b. Fill the flush syringe

c. Monitor PA pressure

d. Monitor RA and arterial pressure

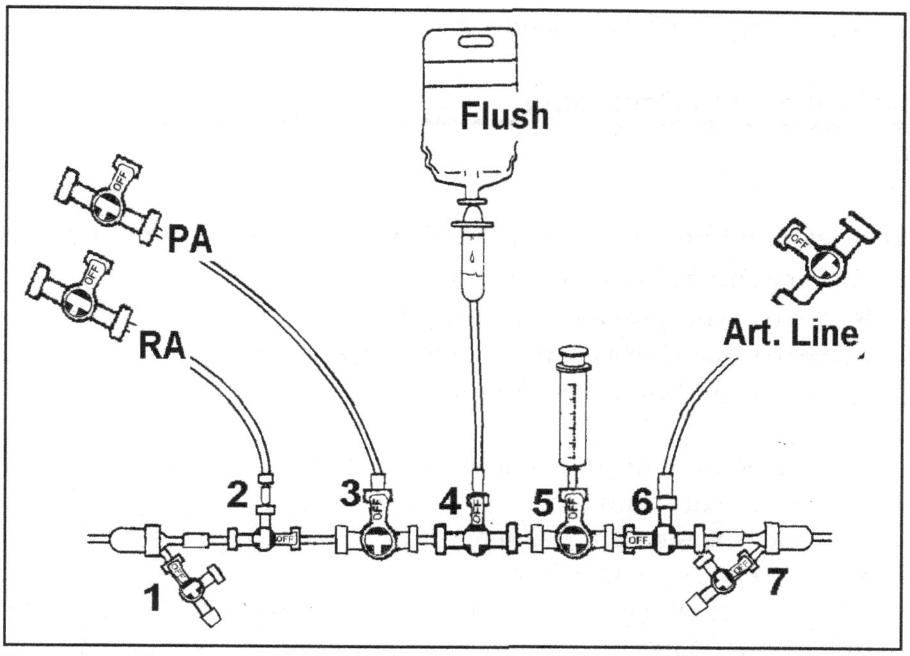

Two transducer manifold for critical care pressure monitoring

ANSWER d. Monitor RA and arterial pressure. Remember wherever the handle of a "handle-off" stopcock is turned, that port is turned OFF. RA pressure enters stopcock #2 and turns left into the left pressure transducer. Arterial pressure turns right at stopcock #6 and enters the right pressure transducer. **STOPCOCKS SHOWN ARE:**

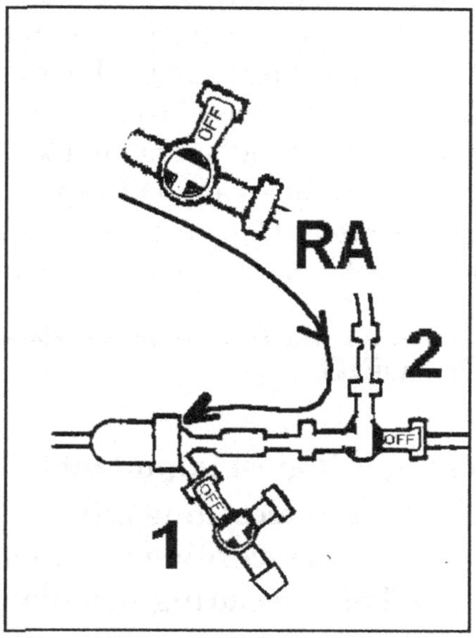

Monitoring RA pressure

1. **Zeroing stopcock closed**, so transducer will not leak. Normally pointed up, not down as shown in this diagram, as it makes it easier to flush out air bubbles. Be sure the top of the air or zero stopcock is set to the patient's mid-chest zero level.
2. **Conducts RA pressure to transducer**, or may be turned to flush the RA line.
3. **Currently turned off.** Can be turned to measure PA pressure of flush PA line.
4. **Flush stopcock turned off.** Can be turned to fill flush syringe or drip into right heart lines.
5. **Flush syringe** used for filling transducers, lines, and flushing catheters.
6. **Conducts arterial pressure to transducer on right**. It can be turned to flush art. line.
7. **Zeroing stopcock closed**, so transducer will not leak. Normally pointed up, not down as shown in this diagram, as it makes it easier to flush out air bubbles. Be sure the top of the air or zero stopcock is set to the patient's mid-chest zero level.

See: Daily, Chapter on "Hemodynamic Monitoring during Critical Care Transport."

Keywords: large stopcock manifold

Calibration and Recording

Set up

107. Bubbles must be carefully flushed from pressure transducers because they:

a. Reduce the dynamic response
b. Reduce compliance of the system
c. Increase the high frequency response
d. Cause air embolism problems

ANSWER a. Reduce the dynamic response. Depending on their amount and location, air bubbles in pressure lines can:

- Reduce the resonant frequency
- Cause excessive damping
- Increase compliance of system that may in turn increase resonance
- Effect the zero level (if large and in the pressure line)

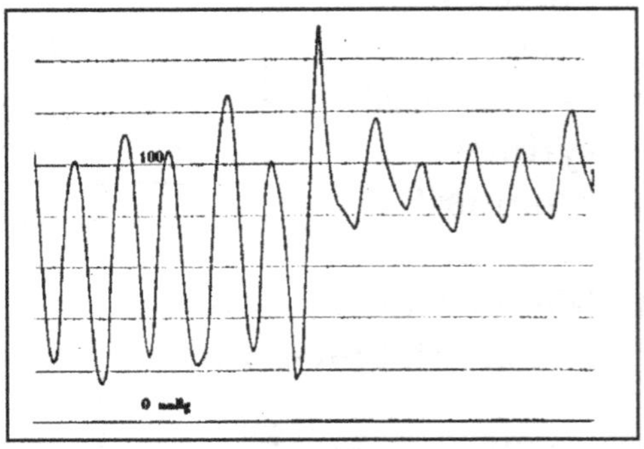

Excessive Damping

In short, bubbles are bad! They compress with each systole making the system much more compliant and resonant. Contrast in the line and small lumen catheters may also have a damping effect.

You must flush all the bubbles out of the transducer. Careful inspect the transducer dome and tubing for adherent bubbles. It helps to snap the transducer with your finger to dislodge bubbles as you flush.

See: Ahrens, Hemodynamic Waveform Analysis, chapter on "Technical Considerations..."
Keywords: Bubbles reduce dynamic response by causing damping

ZEROING

108. When is it most important to"zero" a transducer to atmospheric pressure?

a. Prior to recording arterial pressures
b. Prior to recording ventricular pressures
c. When measuring simultaneous pressures in mitral stenosis
d. When measuring pressure pullbacks across a valve

Answer: c. When measuring simultaneous pressures in Mitral stenosis accurate zeroes on each transducer are critical. The decision to go to surgery may be based upon the diastolic pressure gradient between LA &. LV. Air pressure is 0 mmHg gauge pressure, so the transducers must be open to air while the calibration button is pressed. The transducers must also be at mid-chest level . This assures a common baseline.

109. For a pressure transducer to be accurately zeroed and calibrated it must be:
- **a. Bubble free**
- **b. Open to air**
- **c. Closed on both ends**
- **d. Open to the catheter**

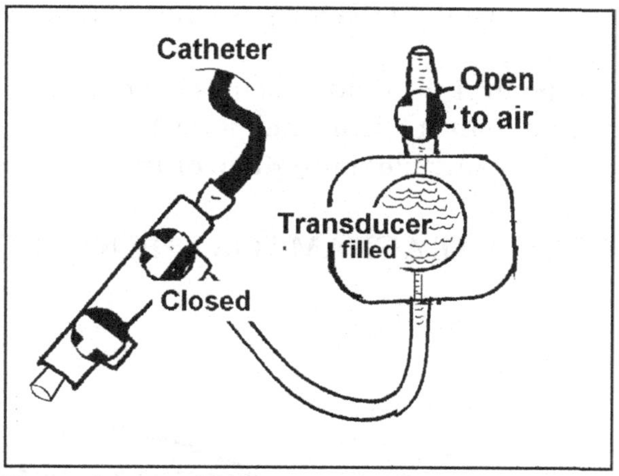

Transducer calibration - Air zero

ANSWER b. Open to air. The zero reference point must be set with one stopcock open to air at the mid-chest reference level. If a zero is set while the transducer has any residual pressure trapped within it, the zero will be incorrectly set to that pressure. Then pressure measurements will all have that static zero error.

Bubbles in a transducer are a NO-NO, but they chiefly affect the dynamic response - damping and resonance. However, large bubbles in the *pressure line* can affect the zero level by displacing the saline column with air.

See: Kern, chapter on "Hemodynamics."
Keywords: accurate zeroes require air zero

110. Disposable transducers are often set up and used "off" the sterile field on a rack near the patient's side. This patient's mid-chest level has been measured and the disposable transducer flushed. For an accurate zero, what part of this transducer system should be leveled to the patient's mid-chest level?
- **a. Top of upper stopcock (a)**
- **b. Middle of transducer (c)**
- **c. Sidearm port of lower stopcock (d)**
- **d. Proximal manifold stopcock (e)**

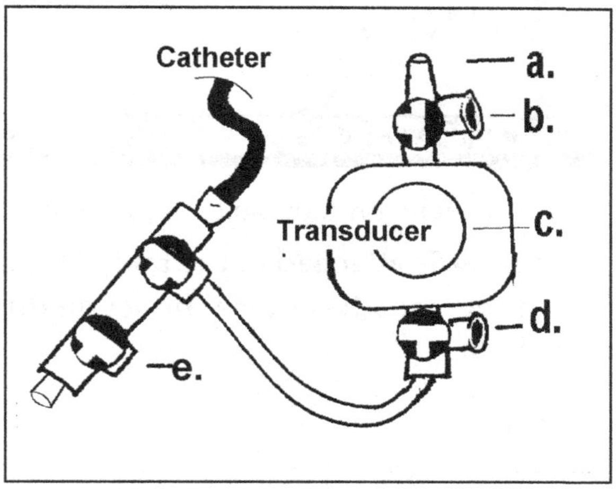

Disposable pressure tube & transducer

ANSWER a. top of upper stopcock. Wherever the top of the fluid column opens to air must be set to the mid-chest level. This is termed "mechanical zero." This becomes the zero reference point at the middle of the patients chest - traditionally the center of the LV.

Fluid transducer zero is not at the center of the transducer, as you might think. When you open the transducer to air, there is

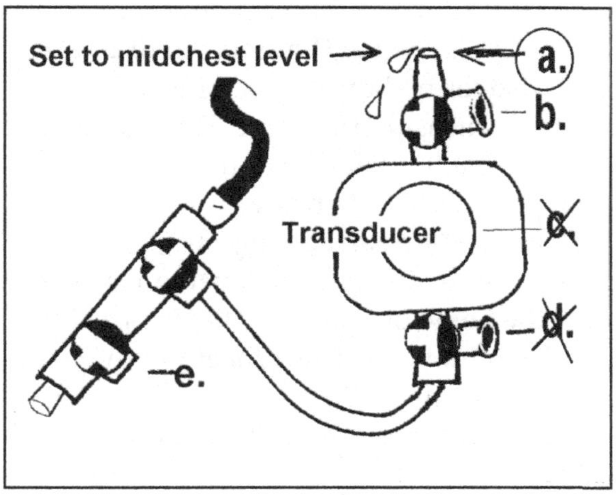

Disposable pressure tube & transducer

always a small column of fluid on top of the transducer (2-3 cm between the transducer element and the top of the stopcock). This small column of saline must be there to "top off" the transducer to eliminate bubbles. Since its presence can't be eliminated, it must be nulled out electronically so the recorder reads zero mmHg at this level. Even though the transducer is on the manifold (Namic) it is the reference stopcock (a) that is set to the zero pressure level.

Wherever the fluid system is open to air becomes the reference point. It should be adjusted to the patients mid-chest level.

See: Company literature **Keywords:** mid-chest zero level = top of stopcock

USE THIS DIAGRAM FOR THE NEXT QUESTION.

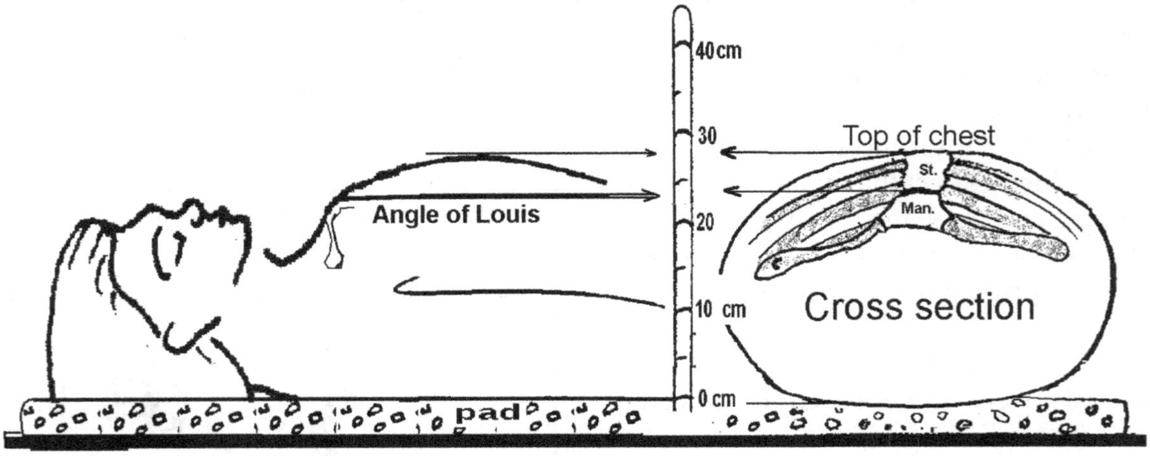

Patient on cath table. Note: top of chest = 27 cm., Sternal angle =23 cm.

111. **-A cm ruler is attached to the table IV pole for setting the transducer zero. Where should the transducer level be set on this pole for an accurate zero reference level?**

a. 11.5 cm
b. 18.5 cm
c. 23 cm
d. 27 cm

ANSWER a. 11.5 cm. This is ½ the chest thickness. Baim suggests measuring the chest thickness with a chest calipers between the back and the sternal-manubrium junction (angle of Louis). Since this patients chest is 23 cm thick at the angle of Louis, the mid-chest level would be ½ of this or 11.5 cm down from the angle of Louis - not at the stomach or thickest chest. Also termed the sternal angle, this is where you measure the chest. Then go down half way. The transducer should be adjusted to that point as shown below.

Baim and Grossman suggests using a yard-stick with an attached level to visualize where the angle of Louis hits the measuring tape. Then move the transducer down ½ of the chest thickness.

Other authors suggest finding the mid

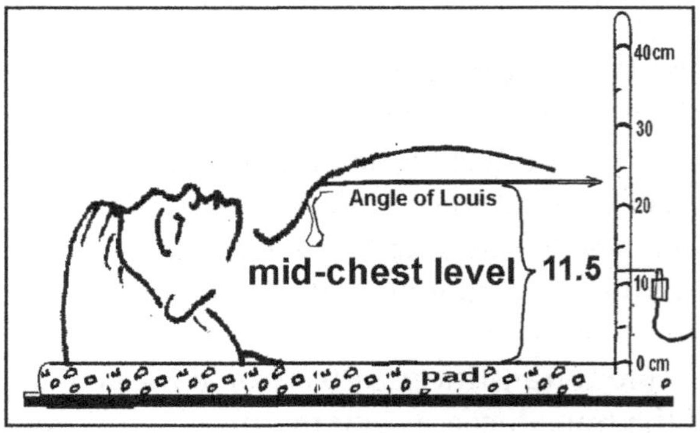

Patient's chest on cath table showing an IV reference pole for setting mid-chest level.

axillary line at the 4th intercostal space (V6 position), marking this on the patient with a pen, and then setting the transducer height to that point with a level.

Darovic strongly recommends using the midchest level, with the zeroing stopcock attached to the transducer. He says,

> *"All circulatory pressure measurements are referenced to the midchest position (one-half of the patient's anteroposterioir diameter) below the sternal angle.... Once the midchest point is identified, it should be marked with an ink pen or felt-tipped marker so that all clinicians have the same external reference."*

See: Darovic, chapter on "Fluid-filled Monitoring Systems" Baim and Grossman, chapter on "Pressure Measurement." **Keywords:** mid-chest level zero @ ½/ AP diameter @ angle Louis

112. A patient with a Swan-Ganz catheter is short of breath. He needs to sit up in bed as shown to breathe. Where should the mechanical zero level be set?

a. Same level as used when reclining
b. Angle of Louis
c. Level of carotid bulb
d. Mid-axillary line - 4th intercostal space

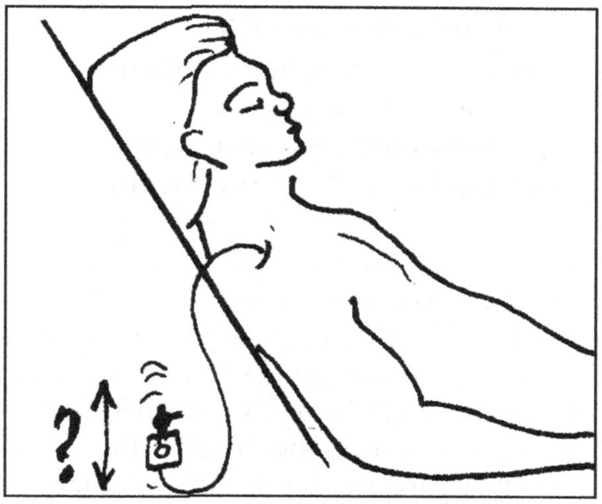

Where Zero level with patient sitting up?

ANSWER d. Mid-axillary line - 4th intercostal space. This approximates the mid-chest level point in all types of patient positions (unless they turn on their side). This mid-chest zero point is termed the "phlebostatic axis." This is an imaginary horizontal reference plane of zero pressure, through the LV. Positioning and balancing the transducer in this "phlebo-static" plane provides a mechanical zero reference.

To avoid having to reset the transducer level every time the patient changes his sitting position some hospitals tape the transducer directly to the chest at this "phlebostatic" point, marked here with a circle.

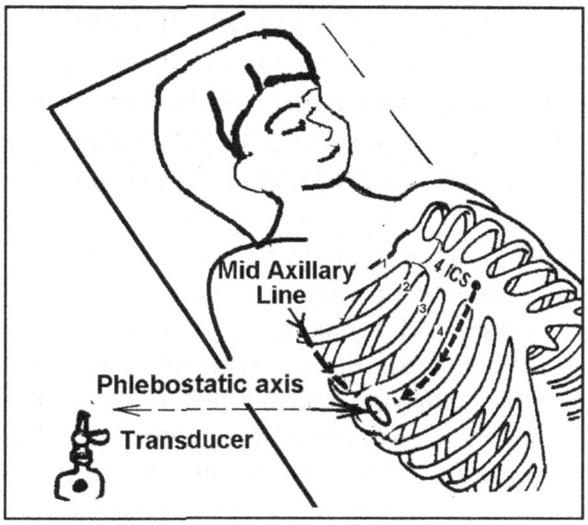

Setting Phlebostatic axis (Transducer Zero), Mid-axillary line 4th intercostal space

See: Ahrens, chapter on "Technical Considerations..." **Keywords:** mid-chest position when sitting up

CALIBRATION

113. You have calibrated a modern pressure recorder which balances and calibrates with one button. The Dr. is waiting for you to record the PA pressure. While the PA is displayed on the screen you accidentally push the calibration button again. A calibration stairs appears on the PA pressure as shown. Your next step should be to:

a. Continue recording PA
b. Press the balance button again
c. Ask for air zeroes again
d. Ask for a mercury calibration
e. Ask the Dr. to flush the PA line

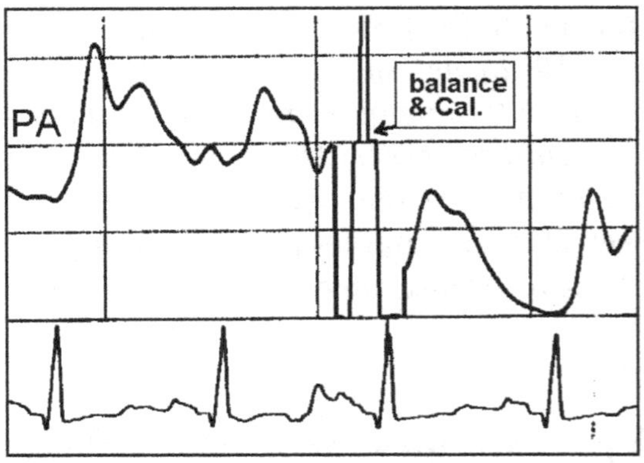

PA x 50

ANSWER c. Ask for air zeroes again. Then rebalance the transducer. Zeroing, balancing, and calibration must be done prior to recording with the transducer open to air. Here, it was done while a pressure was applied to the transducer. This will incorrectly reset the baseline zero level. Note how much lower the PA is after the calibration. The calibration steps must be done in the correct order - described above. You cannot balance or calibrate unless the transducer is open to air. **" Inaccurate data is worse than no data."**
See: Darovic, chapter on "Fluid-filled Monitoring Systems" and Quinton Co. Literature
Keywords: Calibration requires air zero.

114. Pressure transducer zero level may drift throughout a case. Temperature drift should be corrected periodically by:

a. Opening to air and pressing the zero or balance button
b. Pressing the calibration button and adjusting gain
c. Repeating the mercury calibration and adjusting the gain
d. Rechecking the mid-chest transducer level

ANSWER a. Opening to air and pressing zero or balance button. The baseline or zero level is very sensitive to changes in the transducer position and temperature. The zero needs to be checked and re-balanced frequently by this method. This cooling effect is why you should wait a minute after flushing a transducer before calibrating it. Darovic says,

> *"The monitoring system should be rezeroed periodically during use because transducer drift from the zero reference point occurs over time. The main factors causing transducer drift are (91) temperature effects on the transducer: temperature changes of 10 degrees C usually change the monitored pressure by about 1 mmHg, and (2) the effects of transducer domes that contain diaphragms."*

Although most zeroing is now done automatically with a single zero or balance button it is important to understand the 4 steps in calibrating a transducer described below.
See: Darovic, chapter on "Fluid-filled Monitoring Systems." Co. Literature **Keywords:**

Flushing transducer causes Temp. change - rezero

115. The only truly accurate calibration standard for a pressure amplifier and transducer is to use:

- **a. The factory assigned calibration factor**
- **b. The electrical 100 mmHg calibration frequently**
- **c. A mercury manometer to check the calibration factor**
- **d. A sine wave pressure simulator at different frequencies and amplitudes**

ANSWER c. A mercury manometer to check the calibration factor. The factory provided factor may be accurate enough for coronary cases, but should not be relied upon in critical valve gradient measurements. Accurate mercury calibration used to be documented with recorder tracings on EVERY hemodynamic case. Now, transducers are pre-calibrated and seldom checked. But, Hg is the only absolute calibration standard. Kern says,

> "*Most transducers come with a specific gauge factor. This is a number assigned from the factory to a specific transducer that allows the operator to preset the amplifier as a rapid means of calibration. While this may put the amplifier gain 'in the ballpark,' it should not be a substitute for direct manometric calibration.*"

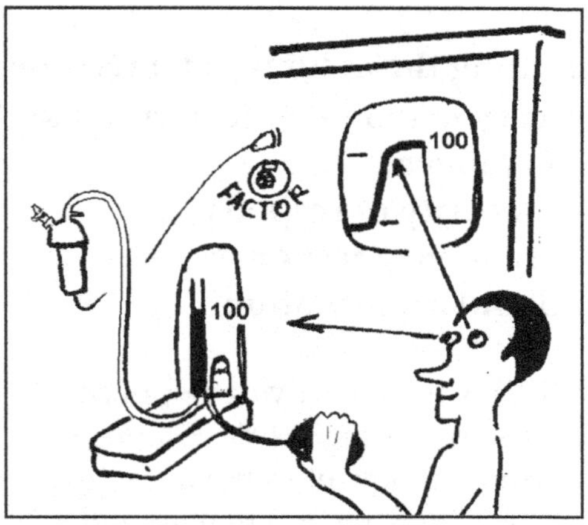

Checking transducer with mercury

See: Daily, chapter on "Principles and Hazards of Monitoring Equipment." **Keywords:** Mercury calibration

116. Setting the calibration factor of a pressure transducer determines:

- **a. The zero level of the transducer in mm Hg.**
- **b. The Wheatstone bridge balance**
- **c. The linearity of the calibration in mmHg/sec**
- **d. The gain of the machine in mmHg/mm deflection**

ANSWER d. The gain of the machine in mmHg/mm deflection gain or sensitivity. Gain is the ratio of output / input. A normal gain on range x 100 is 1:1, where each 1 mm deflection on the recorder results from 1 mmHg pressure. This must be calibrated on the high end with mercury so that 100 mmHg gives 100 mm deflection. As the range number increases, the "gain" decreases and the recorder becomes less sensitive. The range or X number (E.g. X 100) is termed the "full scale" setting or "range." It is the highest pressure you can normally record, and is written on the top line of the monitor grid. E.g., on X 50 the highest pressure you can record is 50 mmHg. Pressures higher than 50 mmHg will be off the top of the monitor scale.

When the correct calibration factor is set into the machine, the electrical calibration signal becomes accurate so it can be used to set the gain thereafter. But only a correct calibration factor determined by a mercury manometer will make the electrical calibration stairs and gain accurate. Although many hospitals use disposable transducers interchangeably, and trust the companies assurance of a fixed calibration factor, you should do mercury calibrations on every valve case, and any time you change transducer brands. Darovic says,

> *"Both disposable and reusable pressure transducers are industry tested and standardized to a fixed sensitivity. Although disposable transducers are usually reliable, reusable transducers, over time, may lose pressure sensitivity and accuracy, usually because of damage of the pressure-sensitive diaphragm or cable. Therefore, calibration checks using a mercury manometer should be periodically done by introducing a known pressure signal from a mercury manometer and by observing the transducer output signal on the digital display and oscilloscope."*

See: Kern, chapter on "Hemodynamics." **Keywords:** gain, sensitivity, range

117. **Checking the accuracy of a recorder's output at several pressure points with a mercury manometer (e.g. 20, 50 & 100 mmHg) determines the:**

a. **Zero level**
b. **Linearity of response**
c. **Frequency response**
d. **Standard deviation**

ANSWER b. Linearity of response. A linear response is a straight line response or proportional output in the useable range.

Linearity is related to gain and is often checked by pumping in 20, 50, then 100 mmHg with a mercury manometer. If the deflections are all "proportional" the gain is "linear" over that range. A linear response to 20, 50 and 100 mmHg on x 100 is shown by plotting measured against actual pressure, as shown. A straight line results if the system is linear.

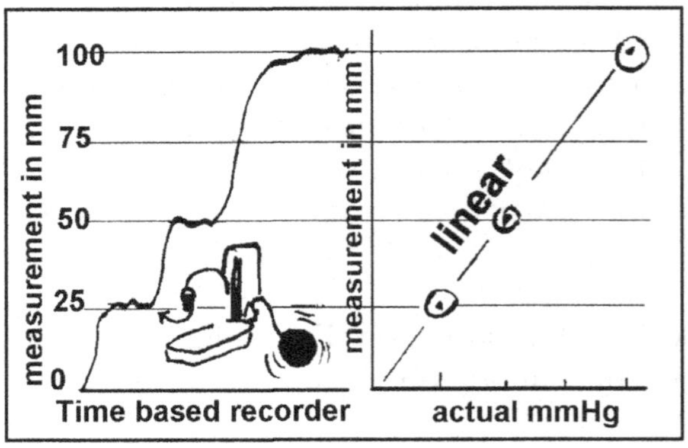

Linear recorder response

At very high pressures > 400 mmHg most transducers become nonlinear. An example of non-linearity might be as follows: 300 mmHg reads 300 mm, but 400 mmHg reads 480 mm. If these higher points are plotted a non-linear curve results instead of the expected straight line. **See:** Kern, chapter on "Hemodynamics." **Keywords:** linearity

RECORDING

118. **When recording right and left heart cath phasic pressures, recorder settings are normally set to paper speed _____ and a time line setting of _____ lines/sec.**

a. **25 mm/sec, 1 line/sec**
b. **25 mm/sec, 5 lines/sec**
c. **50 mm/sec, 10 lines/sec**
d. **50 mm/sec, 25 lines/sec**

ANSWER a. 25 mm/sec, 1/sec. Consider paper speed first. 25 mm/sec is normal for pressures and ECGs. Recordings as fast as 100-200 mm/sec may be used in EP and valve studies. Mean pressures are usually recorded at slower 10 mm/sec speed. You don't want too many time lines on the paper to make pressure analysis difficult. But you need enough lines to make time measurements and accurately correlate the ECG.

Now consider time lines. One vertical time line/sec is normal for pressure recording on speed 25. At faster speeds faster time lines may be helpful. E.g., On valve cases the gradients should be recorded at fast speed for accurate planimetry. Some recorders display a special grid for ECGs with standard ECG lines of 0.04 sec time lines, 1 mm apart so it looks like ECG paper.

See: Kern, chapter on "Hemodynamics" **Keywords:** normal paper speed = 25 mm/sec, time lines = 1/sec.

119. A blood pressure of 160/85 should be recorded on full scale RANGE setting of:

a. **Range x 50**
b. **Range x 100**
c. **Range x 200**
d. **Range x 400**

ANSWER c. RANGE x 200. The range or full scale sensitivity should exceed the highest pressure you want to record. If a pressure of 180 were recorded on range 100, the top 80 mm would be off the top of the chart, and unusable.

Recording on range x 400 will display all the pressure smaller. Since on x 400 the pressure tracing is only ½ the size of x 200, it makes pressures harder to read accurately.

See: Kern, chapter on "Hemodynamics"
Keywords: setting range

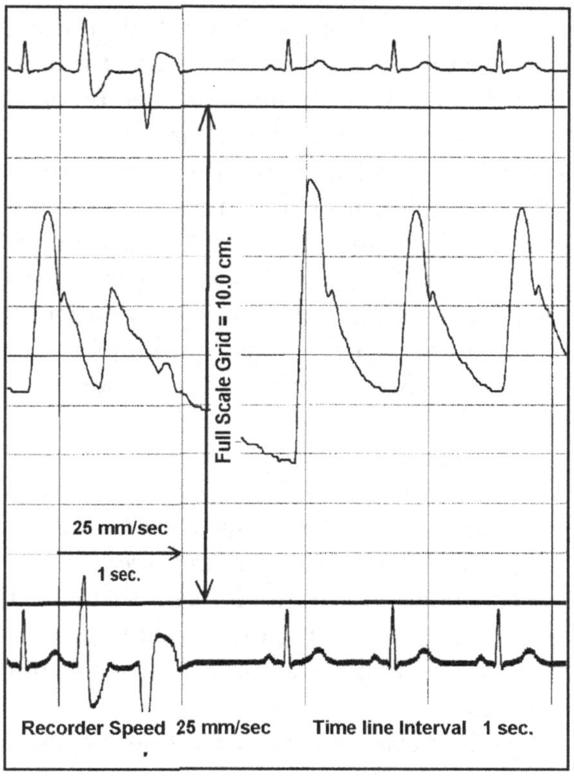

Normal paper speed and time line settings

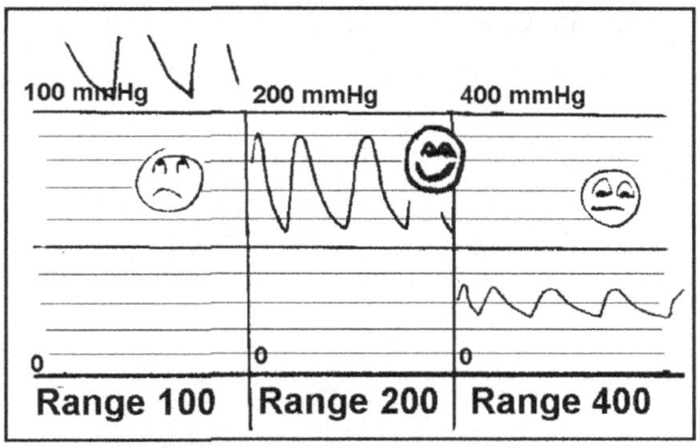

BP of 180/120 recorded on 3 ranges

120. You are recording simultaneous pressures on an aortic stenosis case. The cardiologist doubts the accuracy of your pressure gradient. How can the calibration accuracy of simultaneous pressure recordings be quickly checked?

a. Open all transducers to air and re-zero
b. Replace and accurately recalibrate all transducers
c. Compare arterial pressure to auscultation BP
d. Reverse transducers to see if the gradient remains the same

ANSWER d. Reverse transducers to see if the gradient remains the same. When the pressure tubes are disconnected from both transducers and transducers switched, pressures and gradients should be the same. If one transducer is inaccurate, the gradient will be changed **or even reversed** as shown in the below tracing. It is very embarrassing for the recording tech when this happens!!

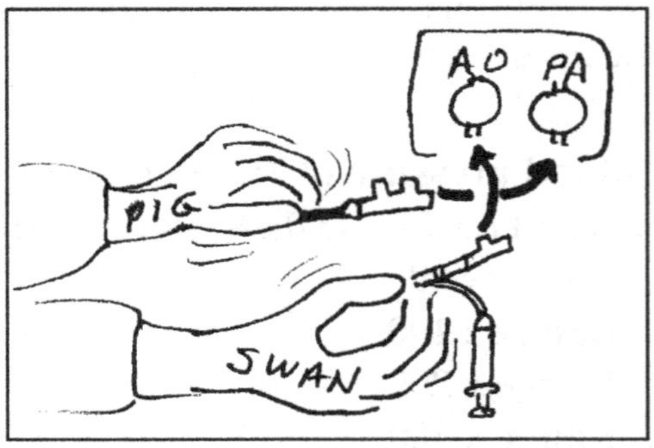

Reversing pressures checks gradient

For example, after recording an initial LV-AO simultaneous gradient, it is noted that the gradient is smaller during the pullback. Reversing the transducers should not change the gradient, if they are equally calibrated. This simultaneous recording shows an AO root systolic higher than LV systolic. This can only happen when the transducers are not equally calibrated . Baim and Grossman say,

"If the unexpected gradient persists, switch catheter attachments between the two involved manifolds. An artifactual gradient reverses direction, whereas a true gradient persists after this maneuver."

A second method is to hook AO pressure to both transducers to see if it reads the same pressure. When in doubt about the accuracy of simultaneous pressures:

- Switch transducers - this should cause no change in pressures.
- Record AO on both transducers - this should cause no change in pressures.

See: Baim, chapter on "Pressure Measurement."
Keywords: Check simultaneous pressures by reversing transducers

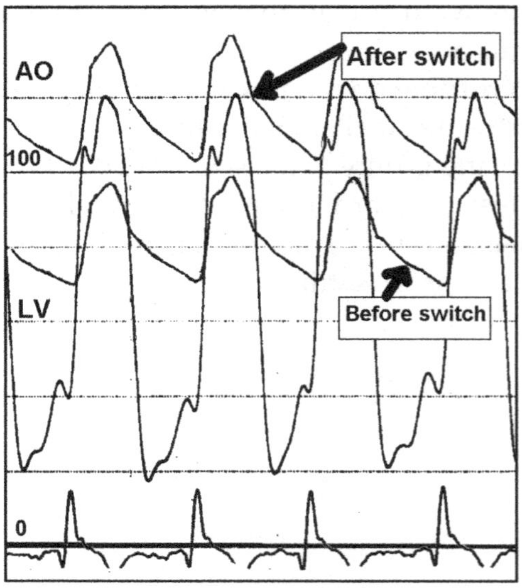

Transducers not EQU-sensitive !

Recording Errors

121. Convert a 27 cm. (270 mm) H_2O CVP pressure to mmHg. (Note that the specific gravity of Hg = 13.6.)
a. 2.5 mmHg
b. 5 mmHg
c. 10 mmHg
d. 15 mmHg
e. 20 mmHg

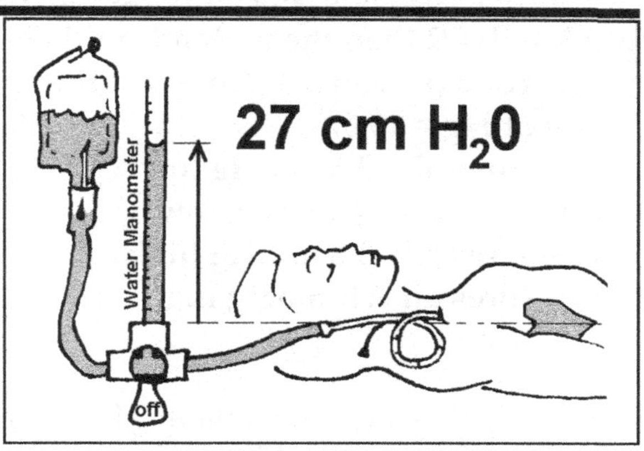

CVP pressure taken with water manometer

ANSWER e. 20 mmHg. CVP measurements are taken with a water manometer and measured in cm H_2O. Since the specific gravity of Hg is 13.6, one mm of Hg = 13.6 mm H_2O. Thus, to convert 270 mm H_2O into mmHg divide it by 13.6 as shown below. Note that the units cancel.

27 cm H_2O = 270 mm H_2O x (1 mmHg/13.6 mm H_2O) = 20 mmHg

Every inch of water is approximately equal to 2 mmHg. Thus for every inch a transducer is set off the mid-chest line, the pressure will be off by 2 mmHg.
See: Quaal, chapter on "Bioinstrumentation of hemodynamic monitoring." **Keywords:** convert CVP water readings into mmHg. divide 13.6

122. The patient is sitting up in bed. A transducer accidentally set below the patient's phlebo-static axis (LA) position will result in a measured pressure that is:
a. Too high
b. Too low
c. Overdamped
d. Underdamped

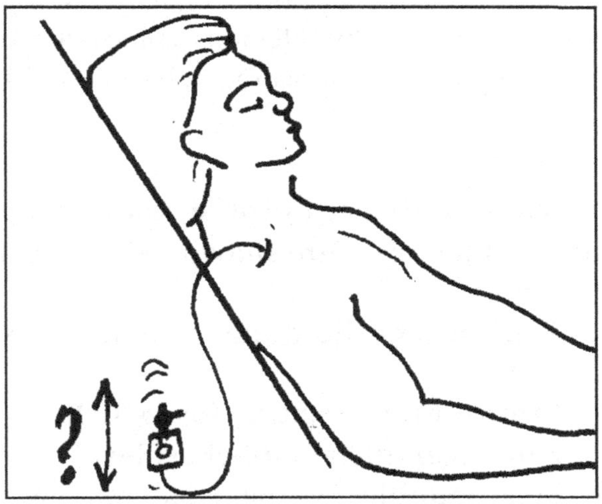

Transducer too low = too high pressure

ANSWER: a. Too high. The real pressure gains energy as it drops down to the transducer. There is a head of pressure above the transducer pressing on it. All measured pressures will be too high by a fixed mmHg. Every inch too low will result in a pressure that is 2 mmHg high. Conversely, a transducer placed above the true zero position will furnish a measure pressure lower than the actual pressure. These small pressure changes caused by improper zeroing may lead to significant errors in diagnosis and perhaps, inappropriate therapy. See: Ragosta, chapter on Normal Waveforms. Keywords: low transducer = high pressures

123. How does placement of a strain gauge 10 cm (100 mm) HIGHER than the patient's mid-chest affect the recorded pressures? (Note that the specific gravity of Hg = 13.6.)

a. Pressures all 13.6 mmHg low
b. Pressures all 7.4 mmHg low
c. Pressures all 13.6 mmHg high
d. Pressures all 7.4 mmHg high

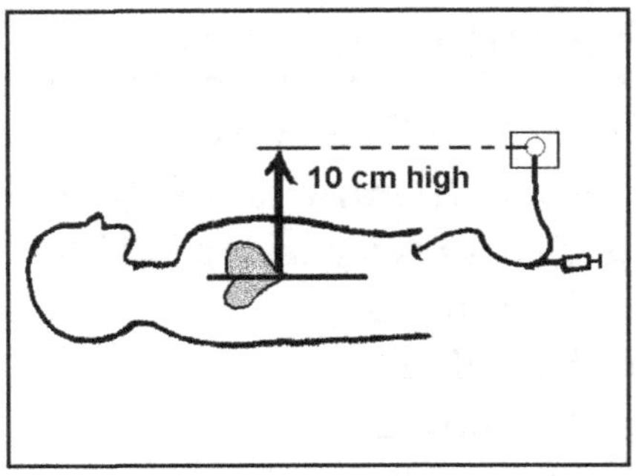

Transducer error - 10 cm high.

ANSWER b. Pressures all 7.4 mmHg low. Try it sometime. Remove the transducer from its holder while it is measuring pressure. As you raise the transducer the pressures all decrease, as shown is the diagram at right. The signal loses "head" as the pressure transducer is raised. This is a zeroing error.

Since the specific gravity of Hg is 13.6, one mm of Hg = 13.6 mm H_2O. Thus, to convert 100 mm H_2O into mmHg divide it by 1.36 as shown below.

10 cm H_2O = 100 mm H_2O x (1 mmHg/13.6 mm H_2O) = 7.4 mmHg.

Note that the units cancel. This is close to the 27 mm example above. Every inch a transducer is set off the mid-chest line, the pressure will be off by approximately 2 mmHg.

See: Kern, chapter on "Hemodynamics" **Keywords:** transducer 10 cm too high lowers measured pressure by 7.4 mmHg

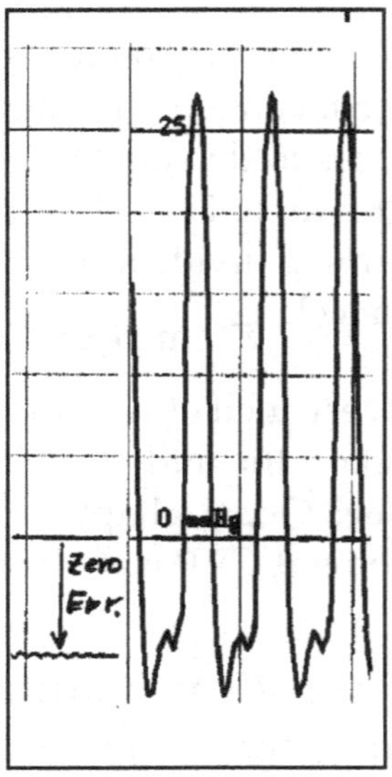

High Transducer

124. Which recording error could result in the incorrect RV pressure shown, with elevated diastole?

a. Transducer calibration factor (check with Hg)
b. Incorrect range setting (use x 100)
c. Zero level (not at mid-chest level)
d. Small bubbles in line (flush system)

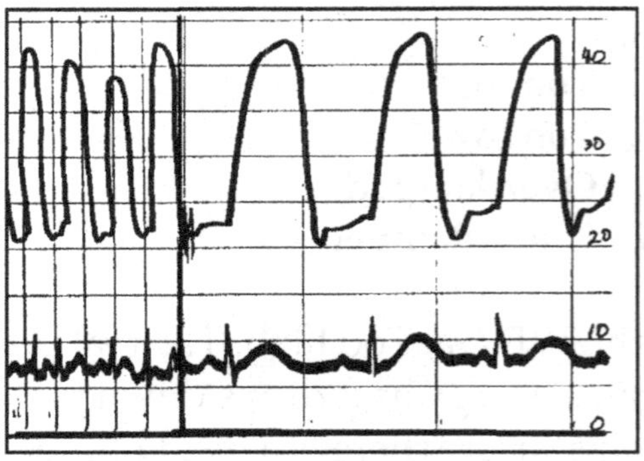

RV Pressure recording error x 50

ANSWER c. Zero level (not at mid-chest level). This diastolic RV reading is excessive. Ventricular diastole readings should normally be near the baseline (0-5 mmHg). Neither is the calibration signal on the baseline. Zero errors shift the entire pressure up or down on the pressure grid by a constant amount. This happens by not setting the transducer to the mid-chest level and/or incorrectly balancing the transducer. This is the opposite error from the previous question, whose transducer was set too high. **See:** Baim and Grossman's chapter on "Pressure Recording." **Keywords:** zero level error (not at mid-chest level)

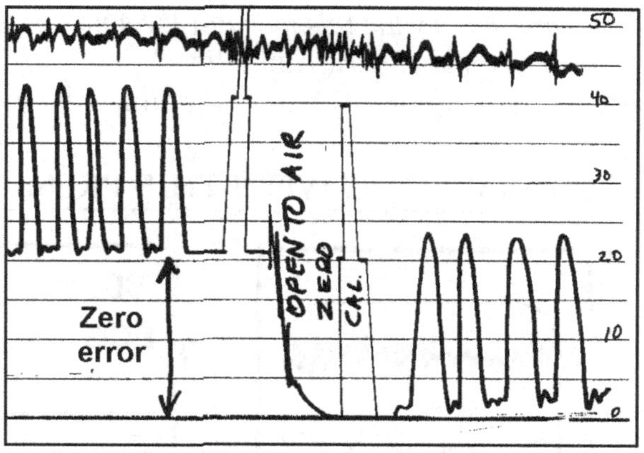

RV Pressure recording error x 40

125. A pressure transducer has been electrically calibrated but only reads 180 mm when 200 mmHg of physical pressure is applied with a BP cuff as shown. For accuracy what needs to be rechecked?

a. Bubbles in transducer

b. Calibration factor error

c. Zero drift error

d. Transducer mid-chest level set too high

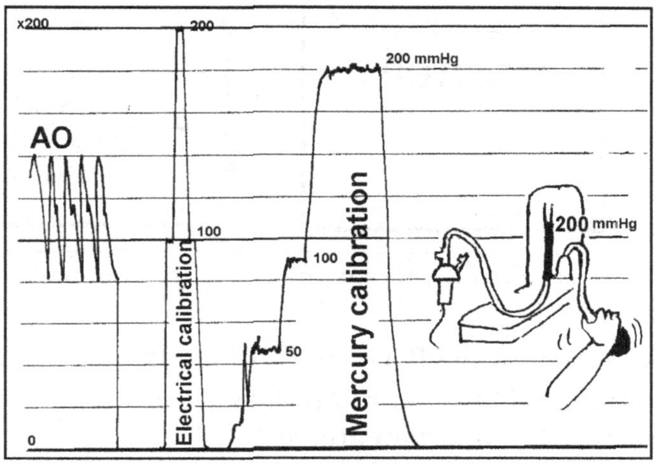

Incorrect reading with mercury calibration

ANSWER. b. Cal factor error. This is what happens when the calibration factor is set incorrectly. Everything calibrates fine electrically. The truth comes out when you calibrate the transducer with mercury. That is why when you get a new brand or model of transducer you should check them with a mercury BP gauge before use. The Calibration factor may need changing.

Note that the AO initially reads 140/80 but, after the adjusting the factor, you find that the correct AO reading is 155/89 mmHg. Kern says,

> "*Most transducers come with a specific gauge factor. This is a number assigned from the factory to a specific transducer that allows the operator to preset the amplifier as a rapid means of*

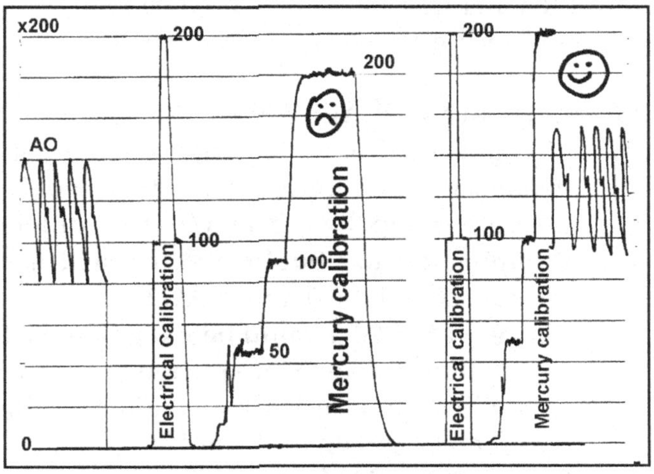

Incorrect reading with mercury calibration

calibration. While this may put the amplifier gain "in the ballpark," it should not be a substitute for direct manometric calibration."

See: Kern, chapter on "Hemodynamics" **Keywords:** calibration factor error errors

WHAT IS WRONG WITH THIS PRESSURE MONITOR?

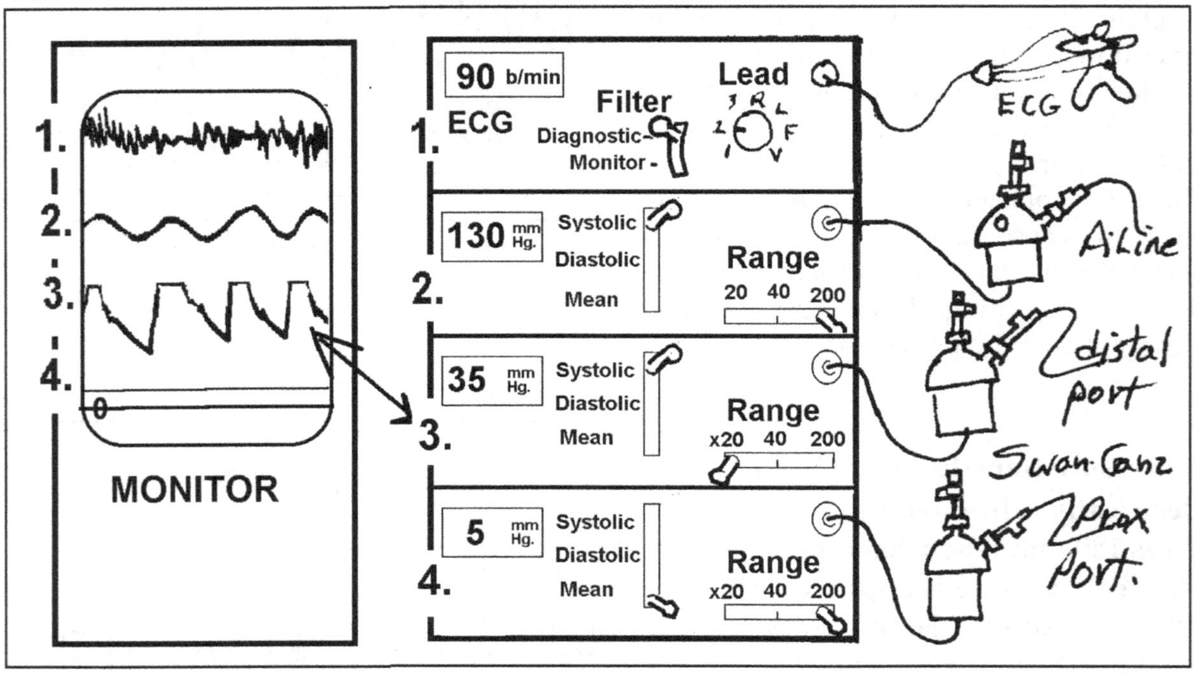

Errors in ECG & pressure monitors (arterial line and Swan-Ganz catheter)

126. A patient in the ICU has an ECG, an arterial line, and a Swan-Ganz catheter with two ports being monitored. What problem is evident on channel #3 (distal Swan port) in the diagram above ?

a. Range set to x 20 (should be x 40)

b. Range set to x 200 (should be x 20)

c. Damping due to bubble in line (flush the system)

d. Filter set to "diagnostic" (reset to "monitor")

ANSWER a. Range set to x 20 (should be x 40). Systolic PA pressure exceeds the amplifier range and is being clipped off by the monitor.

BE ABLE TO MATCH ALL ANSWERS:

#1. ECG noisy: filter set to "diagnostic" (reset to "**monitor**"): This will filter higher frequencies and reduce artifact. However, it is better to eliminate the artifact at the source: re-prep the skin and/or try a different ECG vector lead.

#2. Damping due to a bubble in the line (flush the system): Note the bubble in the transducer and the damped AO tracing.

#3. Range set to x 20 (should be x 40): Systolic PA is 35 mmHg. It is being"clipped" off the monitor display. Since the range is only x 20, twenty mmHg is the highest pressure it can record. Changing the sensitivity to x 40 range will allow you to record pressures up to 40 mmHg.

#4. Range set to x 200 (should be x 20): No pressure waves seen because the amplifier

gain is not sensitive enough. Reset range to x 20 to amplify the RA pressure and make it more readable. Normally X 200 is used only for left heart pressures.
See: Personal Experience **Keywords:** problems with pressure monitoring

127. Computer-read pressures may report a falsely elevated LV-AO peak-to-peak pullback gradient as shown. This may be caused by a recording system with:
a. Contrast in the catheter
b. Catheters with small french size
c. Long pressure tubes
d. Leak in transducer

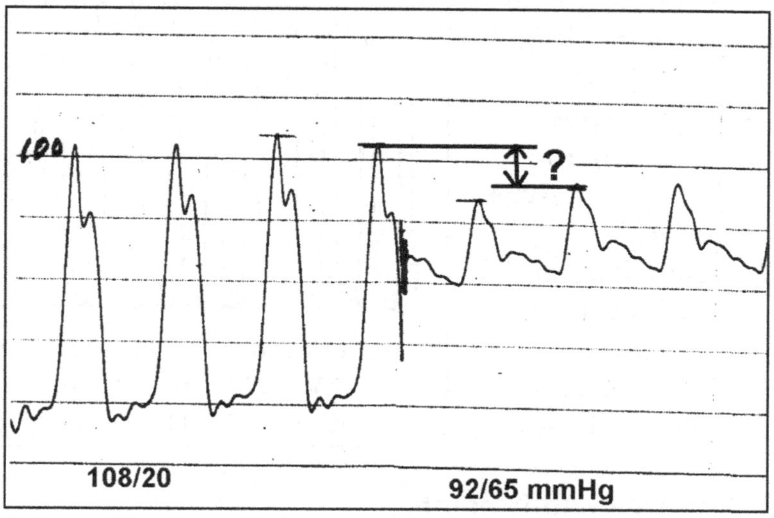

False pullback gradient

ANSWER c. long pressure tubes or an air bubble in the line. Pressure tubes often cause underdamped (resonant) systems. If pressure tubes must be used they should be limited to 2-3 feet in length. Computers may erroneously measure systole from the highest pressure point, even if it is just a spike. The monitoring tech must be able to "read through" the artifact to estimate where the true pressure is and correct the computer markers. I rounded the resonance artifact off (dotted lines). Some hemodynamic computers have filters for filtering these artifacts. This reduces the gradient to zero. This is the problem with resonant systems - you are never sure where systole is. Best correct the resonance first so you do not have to manipulate the data. **You are smarter than computers.**

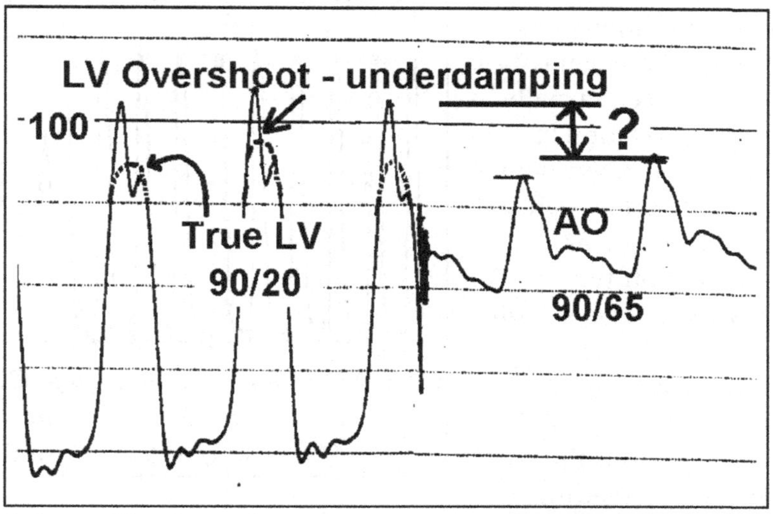

False pullback gradient due to LV resonant spike

See: Baim and Grossman's chapter on "Pressure recording." **Keywords:** long pressure tubes causing false pullback gradient

128. **Note that a computerized recording system has incorrectly read this pressure. What marker adjustment should be made before having the computer re-analyze the tracing?**

a. Delete PVC and post-PVC beats
b. Edit aortic systolic points
c. Edit LV diastolic points
d. Edit LV systolic points

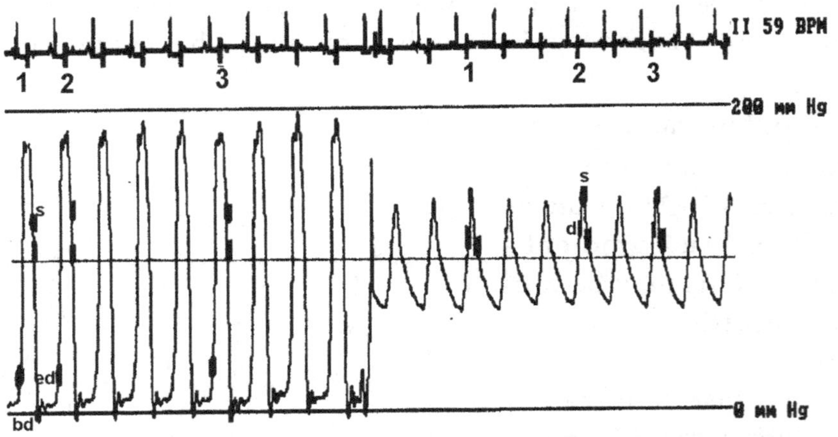

LV→ AO x 200 - COMPUTER PRINTOUT -
LV: 131, 2, 29 mmHg
AO: 139/117,93 mmHg

ANSWER d. Edit LV systolic points. Note that the computer numbers show no gradient between LV and AO. Yet, visually there is a 50 mmHg peak-to-peak gradient.

Incorrect ECG R wave timing was throwing off the pressure analysis. Note that the systolic markers were on the downslope of the LV curve. Besides the LV systole low reading, the diastolic AO reading was too high. This resulted in no systolic gradient. You should realign the ECG triggering. If you can't get the computer accurately triggered from the ECG "R" wave, the makers must be moved manually. This second diagram shows that the ECG is now correctly triggering from the R wave. Both pressures now read correctly. with a systolic gradient of 48 mmHg. You must control the computer, and not let it control you.

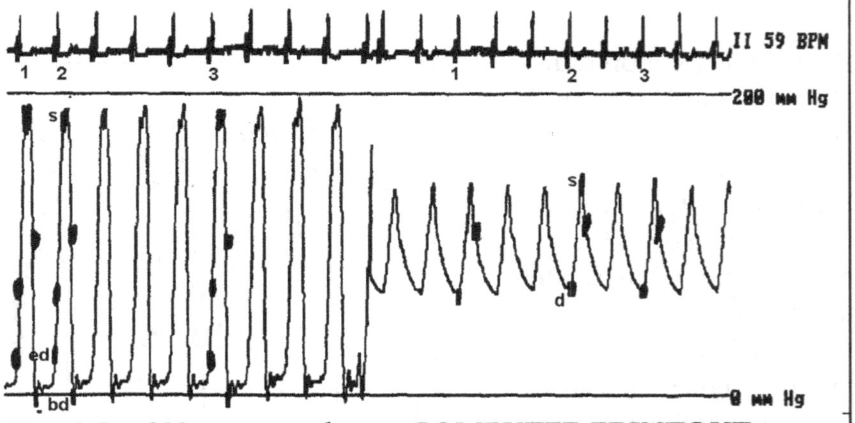

LV→ AO x 200 - reanalyzes- COMPUTER PRINTOUT
LV: 187, 0, 26 mmHg
AO: 139/65,93 mmHg

See: Co. literature and personal experience **Keywords:** ECG and systolic markers off

USE THIS PRESSURE TRACING FOR THE NEXT QUESTION:

129. WHAT ABNORMALITY IS SHOWN ON THIS ECG AND AORTIC PRESSURE RECORDING?

a. **PVCs, unifocal**
b. **Couplets, multifocal PVCs**
c. **Ventricular bigeminy**
d. **Junctional escape beats**

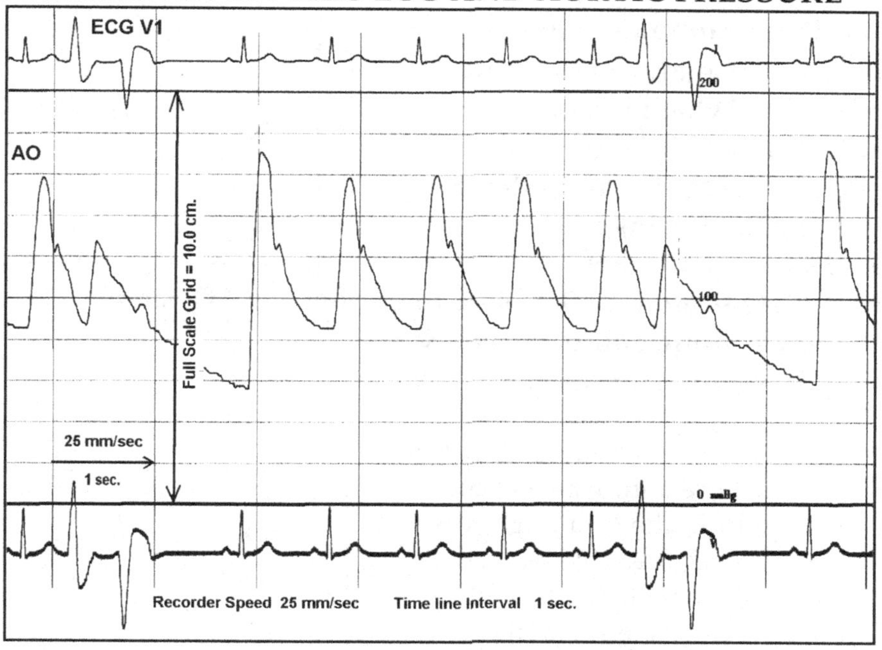

AO Sample x 200, paper speed 25, 1 sec. time lines

ANSWER b. Couplets, multifocal. Couplets are pairs of PVCs. Note how each PVC beat results in a lower arterial pressure. This is because premature beats have reduced filling periods and preload. In this example the first PVC originates from the LV (positive in lead V1), the second PVC of each couplet from the RV (negative in V1). PVCs from different foci are termed multi-formed or multifocal. Each second premature beat (RV-PVC) barely opens the aortic valve. Its arterial pulse only shows a slight bump on the down-slope of the first PVC pulse. **See**: Marriott's Practical Electrocardiography, chapter on "Premature Beats." **Keywords:** PVCs, couplets effect on arterial pulse

130. -What normally happens to the arterial pressure after a PVC? After the compensatory pause, the next sinus beat usually results in a:

a. **Lower systolic and diastolic**
b. **Lower systolic and higher diastolic**
c. **Higher systolic and diastolic**
d. **Higher systolic and lower diastolic**

ANSWER d. Higher systolic and lower diastolic, make for a higher pulse pressure in the post-PVC beat. The sinus beat following a PVC has good atrial kick, unlike the PVCs, and the better preload yields a better stroke volume. Note the dramatic effect of the PVCs above. Often patients don't feel the PVC beat at all, because its ejection is so small. They may only feel the large post-PVC beat. See: Marriott's Practical Electrocardiography, chapter on "Premature Beats." Keywords: post-PVC = larger SV due to atrial kick

THE REAL TIME ARTERIAL PRESSURE RECORDING ABOVE, RESULTED IN THE COMPUTER PRINTOUT BELOW. <u>What's wrong with it?</u>

131. A cath lab computer has incorrectly analyzed this aortic pressure. What marker adjustment should be made before having the computer re-analyze the tracing?

a. Delete beat 2 & 9
b. Delete beats 1, 2, 3, 8, 9, & 10
c. Edit systolic points beats 2 & 9
d. Edit systolic points 1, 2, 8 & 9

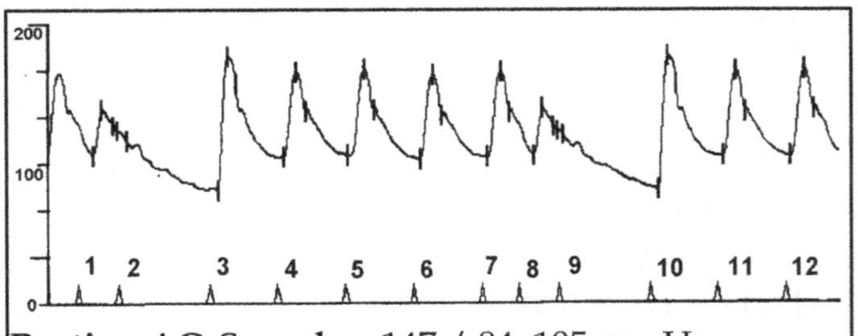

Resting AO Sample: 147 / 84, 105 mmHg

ANSWER b. Delete beats 1, 2, 3, 8, 9, & 10. Each premature beat in the couplet reduces the resulting pressure (PVC beats 1, 2, 8, & 10). Note, that beats 3 &10 are high due to a long filling time associated with the compensatory pause. You have to delete all the abnormal beats. Then when the computer reanalyzes it, the higher correct normal pressure results. Don't analyze PVC or post PVC beats.

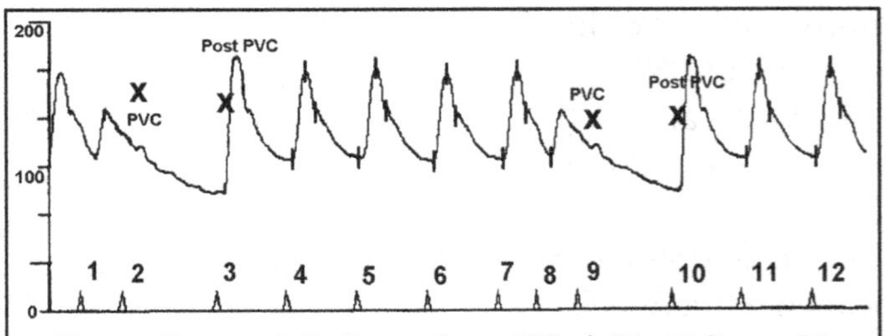

Reanalyzes AO Sample: 158 / 85, 112 mmHg

Note how the markers have been removed from the aortic pressures in beats 1, 2, 3, 8, 9, & 10. You do this by selecting and deleting the PVC and post PVC beats. The re-analyzed pressure correctly reads the 6 normal beats shown at 158/85,112. Computers are only as good as their operator. (GIGO means: garbage in = garbage out.)

See: Co. literature **Keywords:** reading pressures, editing out PVC, couplet beats

132. Pressure from a Swan-Ganz catheter is shown in the diagram. What should be done for a more accurate PA pressure?

a. Insert the catheter further
b. Pull the catheter back
c. Tell the patient to take a deep breath and hold it
d. Have the patient let out a normal breath and hold it with his mouth open

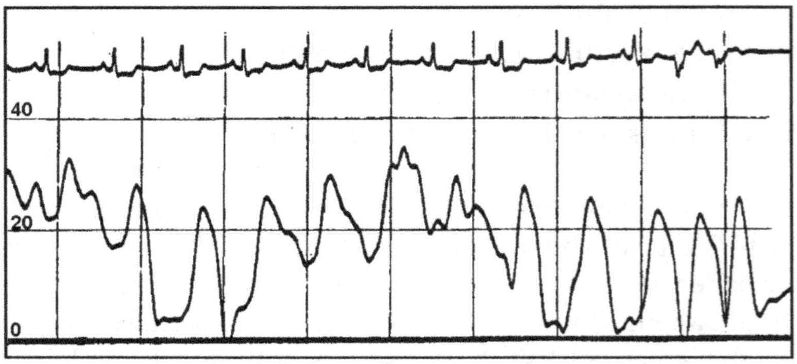

Right heart pressure x 40 via Swan-Ganz (after Daily fig. 5.19)

ANSWER a. Insert the catheter further. This is a mixed RV & PA tracing. The catheter tip is moving back and forth across the pulmonic valve. This often causes frequent PVCs. Breathing maneuvers, inflating the balloon, and inserting the catheter all help the catheter cross the valve into the distal PA for a more stable position.

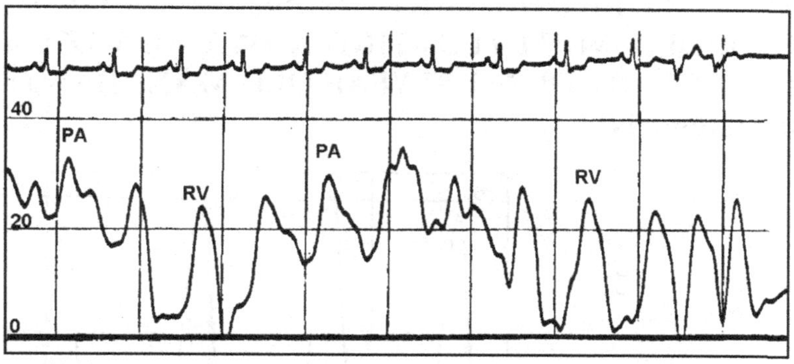

Right heart pressure x 40 via Swan-Ganz (after Daily fig. 5.19)

See: Kern, chapter on "Hemodynamics" **Keywords:** mixed RV & PA pressure

133. After recording the wedge pressure you check the zero and record a calibration. With the transducer open to air you see that the zero level has drifted up as shown. You should:

a. **Re-zero the transducer. Continue with the case.**
b. **Record the incorrect zero level. The 10 mm error can be subtracted after the case.**
c. **Inform the Dr. of the zero drift error, and that the wedge recording should be repeated after you re-balance.**
d. **Inform the cardiologist of an equipment malfunction. Ask for time to re-calibrate the transducers with mercury.**

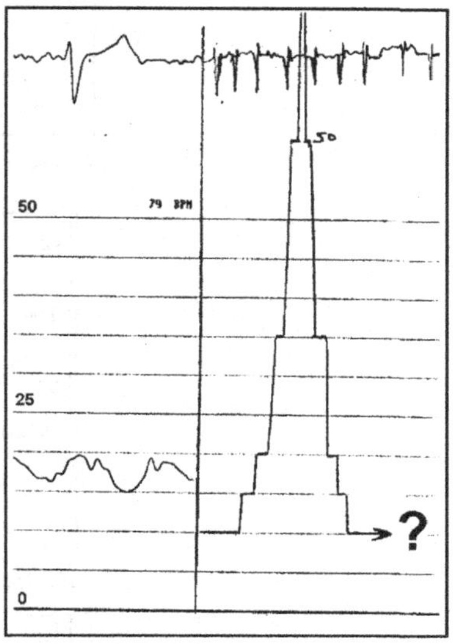

PAW with Cal. stairs steps of 25, 50, 100, & 200 mmHg

ANSWER c. Inform the cardiologist of the zero drift error. After rebalancing the transducer, the PAWP recording should be repeated. The erroneous wedge pressure reads 18 mmHg. while it really is only 8 mmHg. This error can be very significant - perhaps resulting in a false diagnosis of mitral stenosis - perhaps unnecessarily sending the patient to surgery.

Accurate zeroes must be established prior to recording. If the Dr. wants accurate data he will comply with your request. Zero drift is most common when the transducer is moved or flushed (cooled) or balanced without being open to air zero.

See: Kern, chapter on "Hemodynamics" **Keywords:** zero drift, rebalance

THE THREE RIGHT HEART PRESSURES RECORDED BELOW ARE WERE RECORDED WHILE FLOATING A SWAN-GANZ CATHETER INTO THE RIGHT HEART OF AN 83 YEAR OLD MAN. He was found to have moderate aortic stenosis.

1.

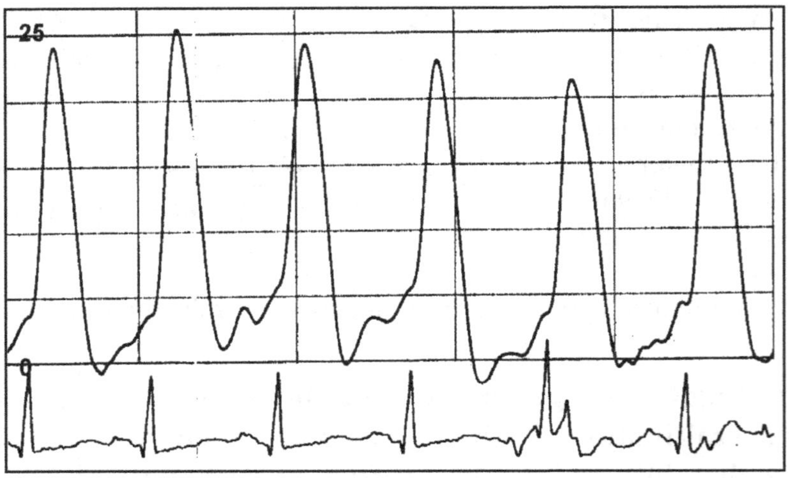

Pressure #1, RV X 50

2.

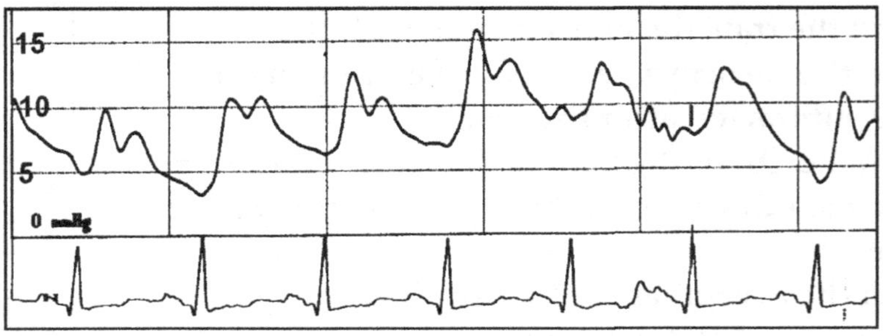

Pressure #2, PA X 50

3.

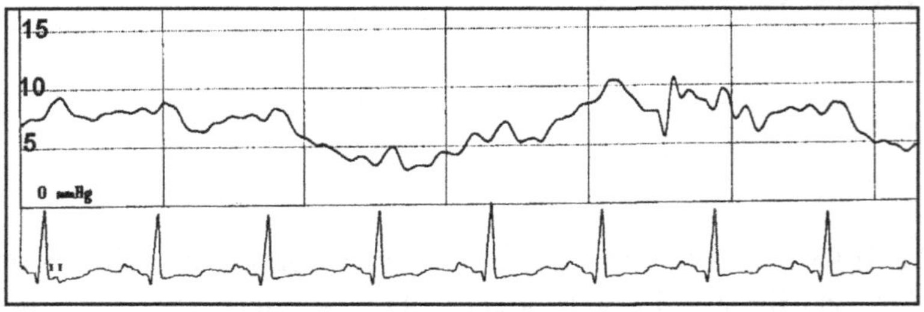

Pressure #3, PAW X 50

134. **What error has probably occurred in the PA pressure tracing #2 above?**

a. **Balloon rupture causing loss of PA pressure**
b. **Catheter kinked in PA**
c. **Mixed wedge & PA pressure**
d. **Recorder range set too high**

ANSWER c. Mixed wedge & PA pressure. #2 above is too low for PA. The reduced systolic PA pressure resembles pulmonary valve stenosis. But the physician thought this unlikely since it is usually found only in children. This PA pressure was taken with the balloon inflated in the main PA. The balloon itself may cause a gradient in a small PA or where the catheter tip has already migrated into a branch of the PA. The resulting PA pressure will appear to be a mixture of main PA and PAW.

Pullback pressures at the right (with balloon deflated of course) show no systolic gradient.

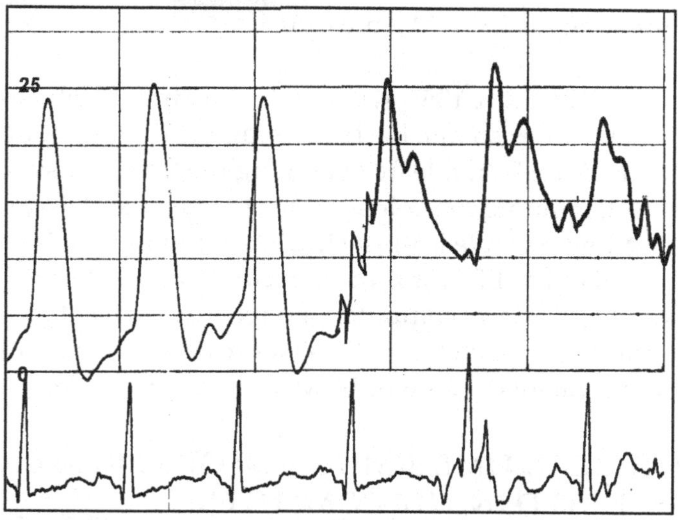

No pulmonary valve gradient seen on pullback

See: Personal experience **Keywords**: False pulmonary stenosis, mixed PA and PAW pressure.

USE THIS DIAGRAM FOR THE NEXT 3 QUESTIONS BELOW:

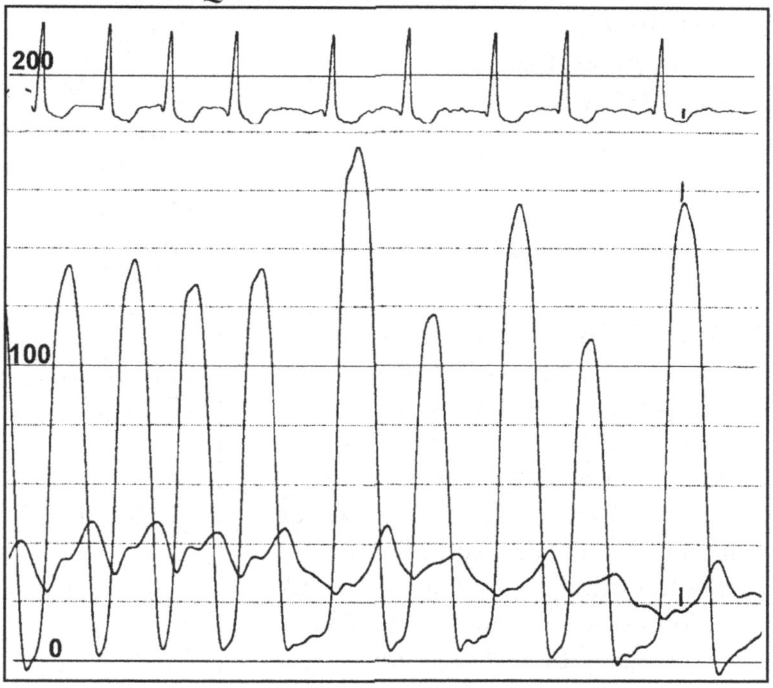

Simultaneous pressures recorded X 200

135. What two simultaneous pressures are probably recorded here?
a. RV, RA
b. LV, PAW
c. LV, AO
d. AO, PA

136. From the 9 beats shown, measure the average ventricular pressure (as a computer would).
a. 120/ 0, 10 mmHg
b. 135/ 1, 9 mmHg
c. 145/ 10, 72 mmHg
d. 155/ 5, 10 mmHg

ANSWERS FOR THE DIAGRAM ABOVE APPEAR TOGETHER BELOW:

135. ANSWER: b. LV, PAW. The LV is evident from the high pressures and the waveform shown. The smaller tracing peaks at the end of diastole with the "v" wave. Small "c" waves are seen. No "a" waves are present due to the presence of atrial fibrillation.

See: Baim and Grossman, chapter on "Pressure Measurements" **Keywords:** Identify simultaneous LV-PAW pressures.

136. ANSWER b. 135/ 1, 9 mmHg. In atrial fibrillation many beats must be averaged since the rate varies so much. The average of the 9 systolic LV beats is 135 mmHg. But an estimate can be made by averaging the first four systolic beats at 136 mmHg

- Beginning diastole varies between -3 and +4 mmHg averaging 1 mmHg.
- End diastole is most clearly seen in the last 5 beats where the rate slows averaging 8-10 mmHg LV-EDP. It is more accurate to measure LV-EDP on X 50 where diastole is expanded. Many computerized recorders must be set to atrial fibrillation mode or they will continue to search for ECG "a" waves. **See:** Baim and Grossman, chapter on "Pressure Measurements" **Keywords:** Measure LV pressure

THE REAL TIME SIMULTANEOUS PRESSURE RECORDING ABOVE, RESULTED IN THE COMPUTER PRINTOUT BELOW. <u>What's wrong with it?</u>

137. What pressure point was incorrectly marked and measured by the computer?

a. Systolic LV
b. Begin diast. LV
c. PAW "a" waves
d. PAW mean

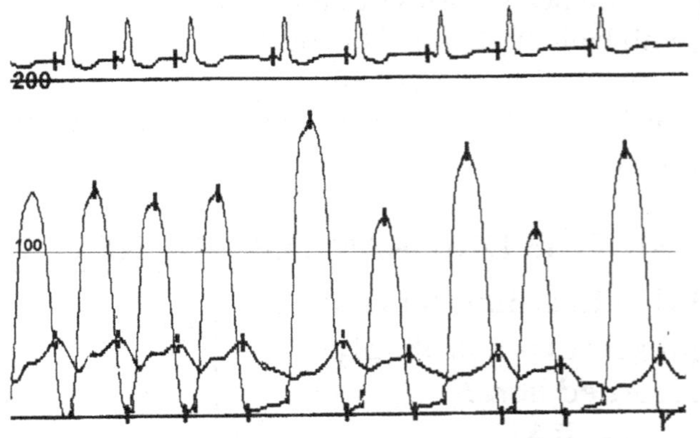

LV & PAW x 200 Computer marked waves
LV: 138/2,11 mmHg
PAW: 38,34,32 mmHg.

ANSWER c. PAW "a" waves. In atrial fibrillation the "a" waves are not present. The computer is misreading the "v" waves as "a" waves.

The small positive waves in early systole are "c" waves. The "v" waves are the largest waves seen here. They coincide with the down-slope of the LV relaxation phase, although this PAW is delayed slightly by transmission through the lungs. The "v" waves vary from 35 to 45 and average 40 mmHg, not 34 as the computer reports. The mean PAW pressure varies from 38 to 24 and averages 32 mmHg over the entire tracing. PAW should read PAW = - , 40 , 32 mmHg (a, v, m). If your Dr. insists on reading "a" waves, where there are none, at least read them where the "a" waves *should be*, prior to systole.

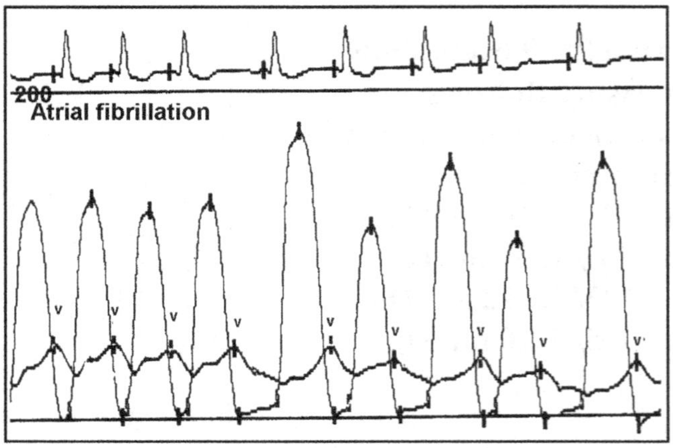

Corrected computer markers in Atrial fibrillation

See: Ahrens, chapter on "Normal Arterial Waveforms" **Keywords:** measure RV

138. "Waveform damping" on pressure waves may be associated with which of the conditions listed below? (Check 4 below.)

a. A drop in systolic pressure
b. Air bubbles in the pressure tube
c. A more pronounced dicrotic notch
d. Total or partial occlusion of a vessel
e. Contrast media in the pressure tubing
f. Vibrations in recorded pressure

ANSWERS: a, b, d, & e. A more pronounced dicrotic notch - would NOT occur, because in damping all sharp components of the waveform are damped or smoothed out. The dicrotic notch may be slurred or excessively smoothed in damped tracings. Kern says, "Wide, rounded waves indicate overdamping (i.e., Not sensitive enough), usually produced by a problem in the fluid path to the transducer..." Vibrations are associated with underdamped or resonant systems. See: Kern chapter on "Hemodynamic Data" Keywords: damping = smoothed pressure waveform

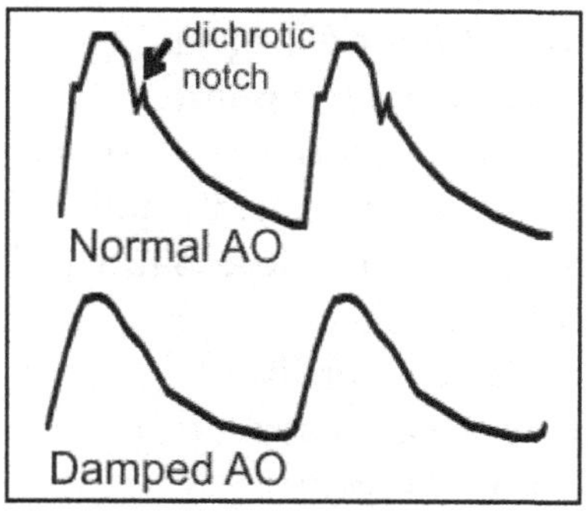

Arterial Pressure

Frequency Response (Beyond scope of registry exam)

139. What fluid filled catheter would give the highest frequency response characteristics?

a. 8 French, 100 cm nylon multiple side hole catheter
b. 6 French, 110 cm polyethylene pig-tail catheter with 3 foot pressure tube
c. 5 French 120 cm. Swan Ganz catheter
d. 5.5 French 100 cm single end-hole coronary catheter

ANSWER a. 8 French, 100 cm nylon catheters multiple side hole. For the best frequency response, you want the resonant frequency to be as high as possible, preferably over 20 Hz. Things that allow the system to respond faster are: shorter tube (cath length), larger diameter tube (cath ID), more rigid tubing (nylon more stiff than Polyurethane or PVC), and less viscous fluid in the catheter (contrast damps and slows the vibration). Catheters with sideholes also respond better than single end hole catheters. Because of their length pressure tubes are usually the worst offender for reducing frequency response. The formula to calculate resonant natural frequency of a fluid filled tubing is:

$$\textit{Natural frequency} = K \times \textit{radius} \sqrt{\frac{\textit{Stiffness}}{\textit{density} \times L}}$$

Because a high frequency response is important, use large diameter, short, stiff catheters and pressure tubes filled with a low density fluid (like saline). K is a constant.
See: Baim and Grossman, chapter on "Pressure Measurements."

140. Pressure tubes connect the fluid filled catheter to the pressure transducer. Which tube below will have the lowest (poorest) frequency response?

a. 50 cm. long soft, small diameter pressure tube
b. 50 cm. long stiff large diameter pressure tube
c. 100 cm. long soft small diameter pressure tube
d. 100 cm. long stiff large diameter pressure tube

ANSWER c. 100 cm. long soft small diameter pressure tube. Pressure tubes should be as short, stiff, and large as practical. So the **poorest** frequency response will occur in the long, soft, and small pressure tubes. **See:** Baim and Grossman's chapter on "Pressure recording." **Keywords:** Pressure tube dynamic response

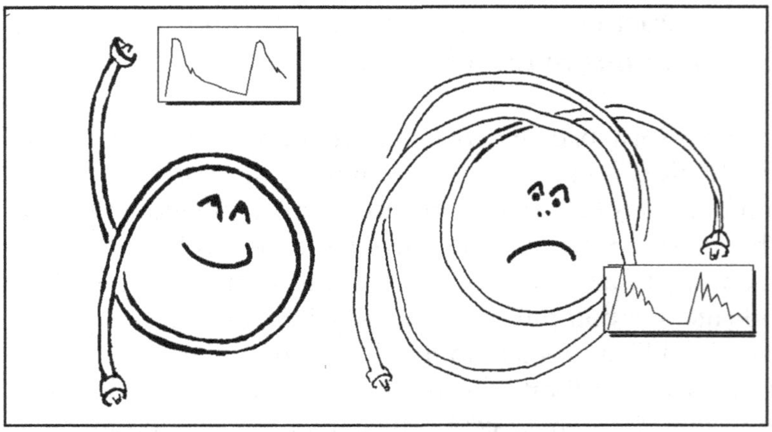

Dynamic response of short and long pressure tubes

141. When a generated square wave is recorded at fast speed through a fluid-filled catheter and pressure transducer system, DAMPING can be measured by:

a. Maximum vertical % overshoot (a)
b. Ratio of overshoot to undershoot (a/b)
c. Horizontal RR interval (c)
d. Horizontal distance between resonant peaks (d)

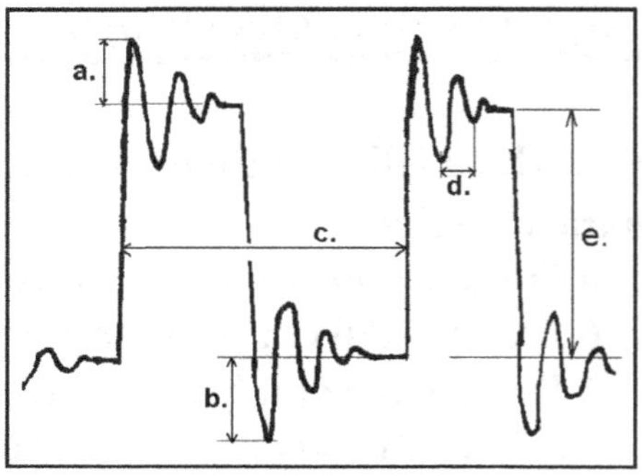

Evaluate system damping

ANSWER a. Maximum vertical % overshoot evaluates system damping. The distance a is the amount of overshoot. Damped systems do not overshoot at all. Only a small amount of overshoot is desirable - around 10% is allowable.

THE MEASUREMENTS SHOWN ARE USED TO MEASURE:

1. **Overshoot** is present in underdamped systems. Note that this is a vertical measurement. The most important measurement is the **ratio** of overshoot to the true height of the square wave or a/e ratio. It can also be estimated from the ratio of successive peaks of the resonant frequency. This example is 25% overshoot.
2. **Undershoot** occurs in LV pressure curves in early diastole, when the pressure wave goes below zero. In a square wave the amount of overshoot equals the amount of undershoot.

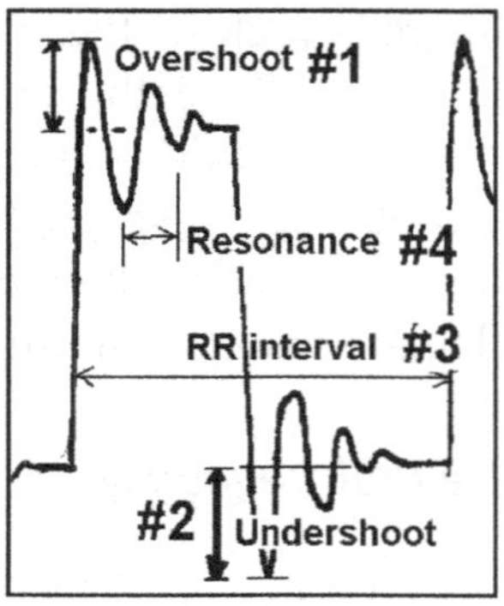

Estimate system damping

3. **RR interval** is used to calculate the fundamental frequency of the patient. The faster the heart rate, the higher the frequency response needs to be. A HR of 60 (where RR = 1 sec) requires a frequency response over 10 Hz. A HR of 120 (where RR = 0.5 sec) requires a frequency response over 20 Hz.
4. **The distance between resonant peaks is the period of the resonant frequency.** It can be used to estimate the frequency response of the fluid filled system, but not the damping. This frequency should exceed 10 x the patients fundamental frequency. Or stated another way, more than 10 resonant cycles need to fit into one RR interval.

THE NEXT 2 QUESTIONS REFER TO THIS DIAGRAM:

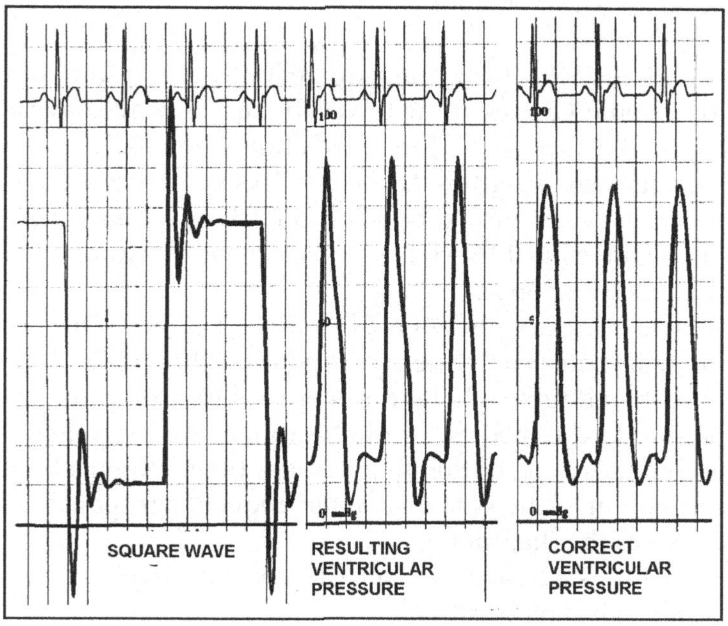

Speed 50 mm/sec, Time Lines 0.2 sec, Range X 100

142. **Evaluate the damping amplitude ratio from the square wave response shown.**
- a. **0 % overshoot, over-damped**
- b. **10 % overshoot, critically damped**
- c. **25 % overshoot, under-damped**
- d. **50 % overshoot, extremely under-damped**

143. **Evaluate the system frequency response (natural frequency of vibration) from the square wave response shown above.**
- a. **6 Hz, inadequate for the heart rate shown**
- b. **12 Hz, barely adequate for the heart rate shown**
- c. **16 Hz, adequate for the heart rate shown**
- d. **24 Hz, exceeds requirements for this heart rate**

BOTH ANSWERS FOR THE DIAGRAM ABOVE APPEAR TOGETHER BELOW:

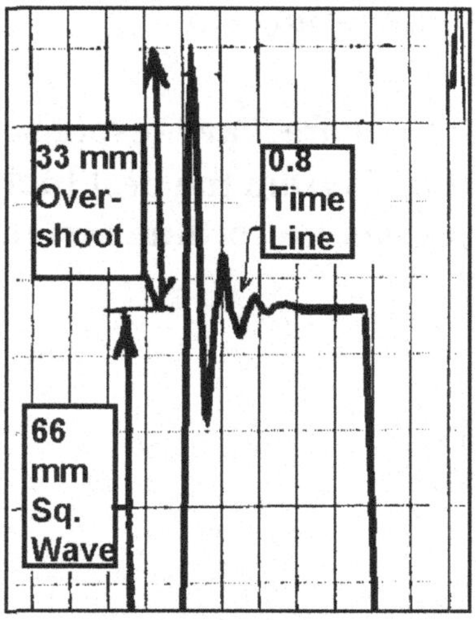

50 % Overshoot (under-damping)

142. ANSWER d. 50 % overshoot, under-damped. Overshoot is 33 mmHg above the 66 mmHg square wave. Note that like the square wave overshoots the plateau, the middle under-damped LV signals overshoot the true systole. The ventricular waveform becomes elongated and "spikey" compared to the correct ventricular pressure on the right. The pressure overshoots the true systolic by 50% and undershoots the beginning diastolic pressures by 50%. When contrast was injected into the pressure line the system shows a better dynamic response, shown at the

right.

Square wave generators or fast flush devices can be used to measure both the damping and frequency response. From this damping amplitude ratio a "damping coefficient" can be calculated and plotted against frequency response (resonant frequency) to assess both dynamic aspects. See Daily or Ahrens. But, this is usually too difficult for all but research purposes. I recommend simply measuring the % overshoot and reducing it to around 10% with the recorder high frequency filter (critical or optimal damping). For adequate frequency response, make sure more than 10 resonant cycles can fit into one RR interval. All of this can be done by inspection of the graph. No calculations are necessary.

See: Baim and Grossman's chapter on "Pressure recording." **Keywords:** under-damping measured by overshoot

143. ANSWER a. 6 Hz, inadequate for the heart rate shown. The resonant cycles at the top of the square wave have a wave length of .8 time lines. Since each time line is 0.2 sec, the resonant wavelength is 0.8 x 0.2 = .16 sec. (Ahrens says the vibration cycles should be less than 0.8 sec.) Changing 0.16 sec into Hz gives 1/0.16 = 6 Hz. This is generally too slow a frequency response.

The heart rate shown is 91 /min or 1.52 Hz. This fast heart rate will require a frequency response of 10 x 1.52 = 15.2 Hz, more than double what our system is currently producing. All the standard remedies should be applied to the system: flush out bubbles and shorten the pressure tube. When a bubble was flushed out of the system a better frequency response results as shown in the diagram.

See: Ahrens, Hemodynamic Waveform Analysis, chapter on "Technical Considerations..."

Keywords: resonant frequency response

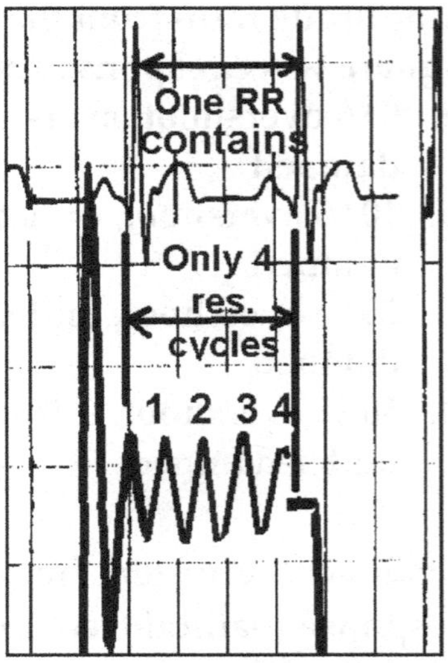

Inadequate frequency response

THE NEXT TWO QUESTIONS REFER TO THIS DIAGRAM. This diagram shows how different catheter lengths and fluid viscosities react to a square wave pressure input.

144. Which square wave response in the diagram is from the best high fidelity LV pressure recording system?

a. #1
b. #2
c. #3
d. #4
e. #5

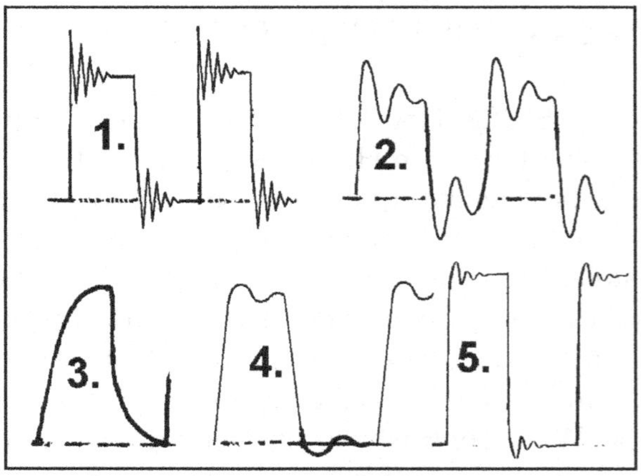

Various degrees of damping & resonance

145. **The type of dynamic square wave response shown at #3 in the diagram above is ______ damped with an ________ frequency response.**

a. **Over-, inadequate**
b. **Critically-, adequate**
c. **Under-, Adequate**
d. **Under-, inadequate**
e. **Critically-, inadequate**

BOTH ANSWERS APPEAR TOGETHER BELOW:

144. ANSWER e. = #5 is the BEST response - the squarest looking wave. It has only 5-10% overshoot and the vibrations are high frequency (>10 Hz/cycle). This is termed "critically damped with adequate frequency response." Most fluid filled recording systems overshoot in systole and undershoot in early diastole often going below zero, and creating false readings and "squiggly" tracings. Your job is to get the highest fidelity pressure tracings possible, with adequate frequency response and adequate damping. This response takes care to achieve. Use short rigid tubes and add contrast to the line for damping. LV pressure is always the hardest to accurately record because of its higher frequency components.
See: Kern, chapter on "Hemodynamics" **Keywords:** optimal damping and frequency response

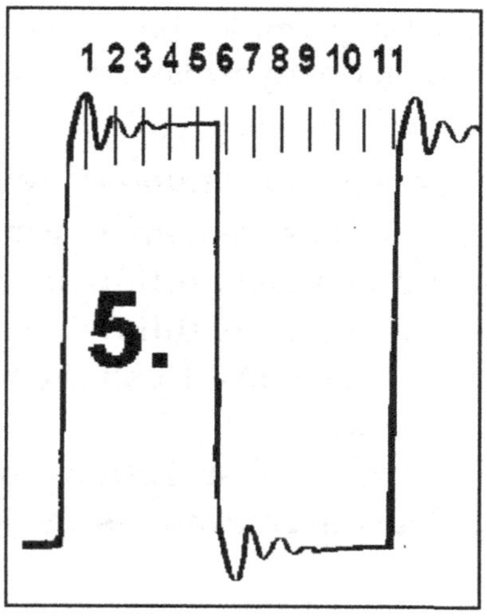

>10 resonant cycles/ RR

145. ANSWER a. = #3 is over damped with INADEQUATE frequency response. Tracings recorded through such a system will be very damped. Systolic readings will all be too low, diastolic too high. Usually caused by bubbles in the system.

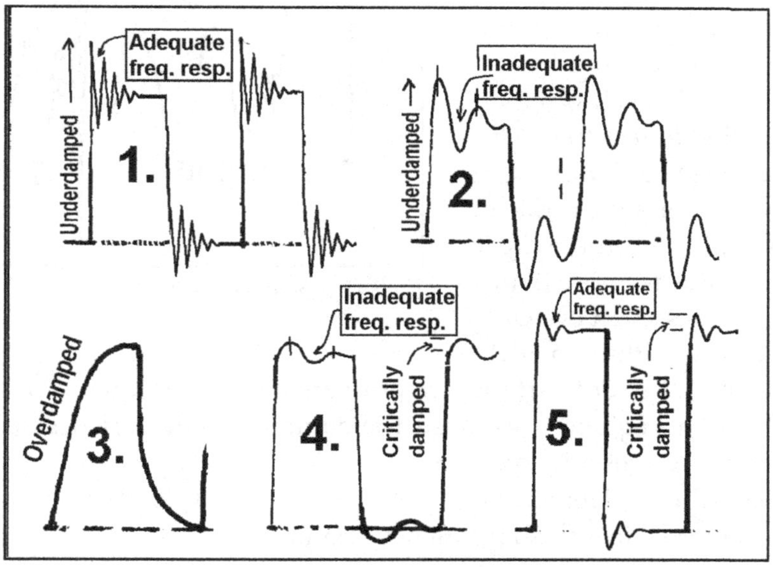

Various degrees of damping and frequency response seen in system response to square wave.

BE ABLE TO MATCH ALL ANSWERS:

#1. Underdamped with adequate frequency response (resonance freq. high enough). Reduce the pressure amplifier filter cutoff.

#2. Underdamped with inadequate frequency response (resonance freq. too low) Check for bubbles in line and reduce the pressure amplifier filter cutoff.

#3. Over damped with inadequate frequency response (resonance freq. too low). Check for bubbles in the line or other damping problems.

#4. Critically damped with inadequate frequency response (resonance freq. too low) Reduce length of pressure tubing and check for air bubbles.

#5. Critically damped with adequate frequency response (resonant freq. high enough). Damping evidenced by % overshoot is around 10% - not over damped. High frequency resonance indicates it can respond adequately to the high frequency components of the LV. (Must be >10 times LVS fundamental freq.) Looks Good!

See: Daily, chapter on "Principles and Hazards of Monitoring Equipment." **Keywords:** adequacy of dynamic response, damping and frequency response

146. How can a continuous flow device in a fluid filled pressure line be used to check the system's frequency response?

a. **Immediately following a fast flush high frequency resonance should occur**
b. **Immediately following a fast flush no resonance should occur**
c. **During a fast flush the transducer pressure should equal the pressure bag pressure**
d. **During a fast flush the pressure should rise to a square peak and level off**
e. **During continuous slow flow, the transducer pressure equal bag pressure**

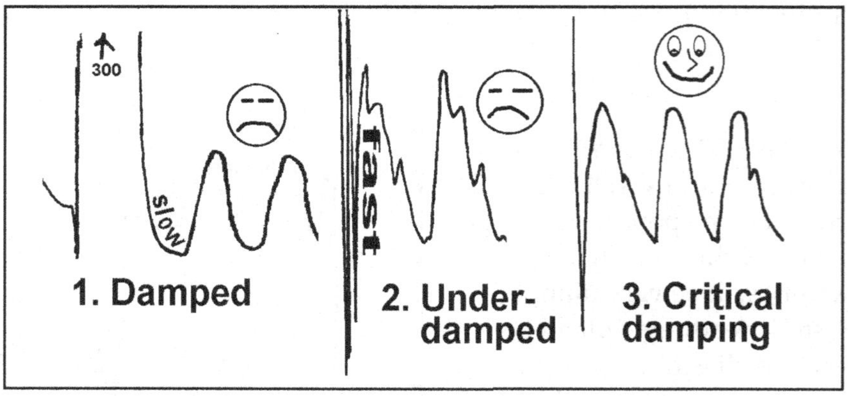

Fast flush responses

ANSWER a.
Immediately following a fast flush high frequency resonance should occur. Resonance should exceed 12 cycles/sec (period of less than .08 sec/cycle or 2 ECG boxes) for a heart rate of 80/min. Another way to state this is; more than 10 of the resonant cycles must fit within one RR interval. Faster heart rates require greater high frequency response (over 20 Hz.). Besides the high frequency response, the damping characteristics need to be evaluated to prevent excessive pressure overshoot.

See: Ahrens, Hemodynamic Waveform Analysis, chapter on "Technical Considerations..." **Keywords:** fast flush frequency response

147. What is the fundamental frequency of an LV pressure curve with a heart rate of 80/min shown?

a. **0.45 Hz.**
b. **0.75 Hz.**
c. **1.33 Hz.**
d. **1.83 Hz.**

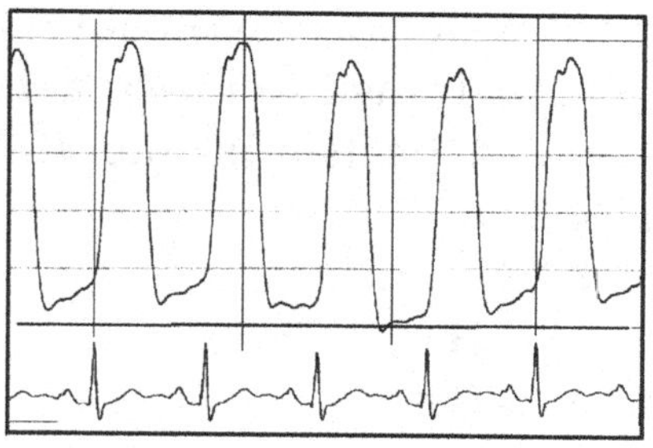

ANSWER c. 1.33 Hz. (Hz. = Hertz = cycles/sec)
Remember the simple formula: frequency = 1 / period

(where the heart's period is the RR interval) Fundamental frequency = 1 / RR interval

Measure the RR interval of one heartbeat, in seconds, and take its reciprocal to get fundamental frequency. E.g.: Fundamental frequency = 1 / RR so Ff. = 1/.75 = 1.33 Hz. You must set up the equation so the units cancel resulting in the units you want. Convert the heart rate from cycles/min into cycles/sec by dividing by 60 sec/min:

Ff. = cycles /sec = (80 cycles/min) / (60 sec/min) = 1.33 cycles/sec.

Note how "minutes" cancel out.

See: Baim and Grossman, chapter on "Pressure Measurements"**Keywords:** fundamental frequency

148. What is the relationship between gain (transducer output/input) over a range of frequencies?

a. **Filtration**
b. **Damping**
c. **Scale factor**
d. **Linearity**
e. **Frequency response**

Answer: e. Frequency response is usually a graph relating output amplitude of a pressure signal to the frequency of the input signal. Modern pressure transducers can respond to frequencies between zero and several hundred 100 Hz. But, the fluid filled catheter system typically reduces the upper useable range to around 20 Hz. Above 20 Hz the output amplitude cannot keep up with input, and may not respond at all above 50 Hz. There is often a peak in these curves near the high limit, showing where resonance occurs in the system. Frequency response curves are commonly used to rate all manner of amplifiers, most notably the performance of stereo audio systems. See: Baim and Grossman, chapter on "Pressure Measurements"**Keywords:** fundamental frequency, Keywords: Frequency response curve

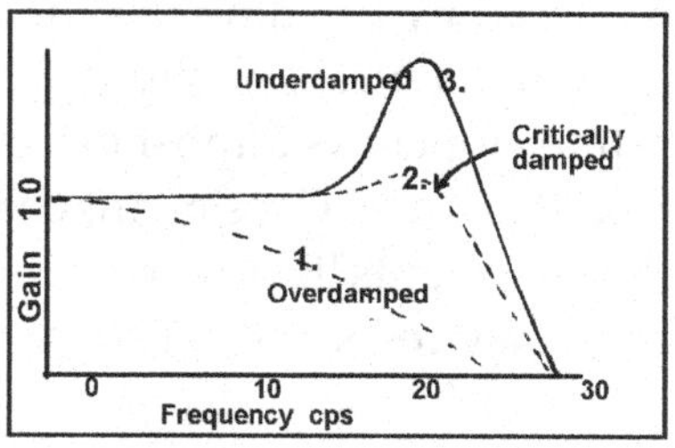

Frequency response curve

149. What is the minimum allowable upper frequency response of a catheter/transducer system to adequately record an LV pressure recorded at a heart rate of 80 beats/min? (i.e. 10th harmonic of the fundamental frequency.)

a. **4.5 Hz.**
b. **8.0 Hz.**
c. **13.3 Hz.**
d. **18.3 Hz.**
e. **80 Hz.**

ANSWER c. 13.3 Hz. The allowable upper frequency limit is considered to be ten times the fundamental frequency of the patients heart rate. We found the fundamental frequency above to be 1.33 Hz. Ten times this is 13.3 Hz. Since the upper usable frequency range is near the resonant frequency, we want the system to vibrate faster than 13.3 times/sec. Ideal response exceeds 20 times the fundamental frequency. Note that the resonance on the last example would be 20 cycles/sec. the peak of the frequency response curve.

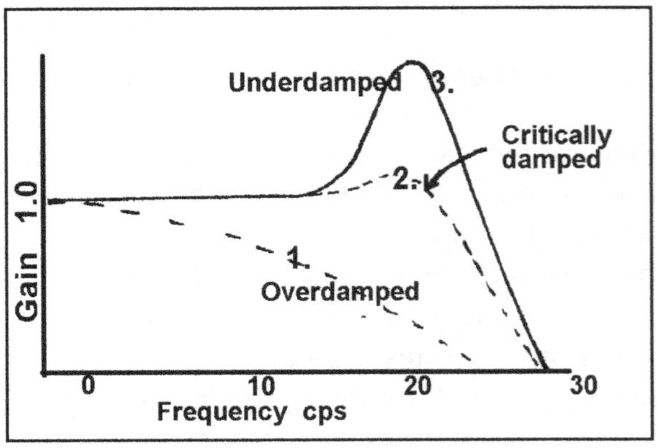

Frequency response curve

In addition to the frequency response discussed (measured on the time axis), damping is the other critical factor (measured on the vertical axis). Once the best upper limit of resonance is achieved, then the ringing system should be damped to reduce the amount of overshoot to 10%. This is called critical damping for a fluid filled system. Optimum damping prevents wild catheter resonance and excessive overshoot. Damping may be increased by flushing the catheter and pressure line with contrast or slightly turning one of the in-line stopcocks almost off.

See: Baim and Grossman, chapter on "Pressure Measurements"**Keywords:** desired upper frequency response = 10 x fundamental

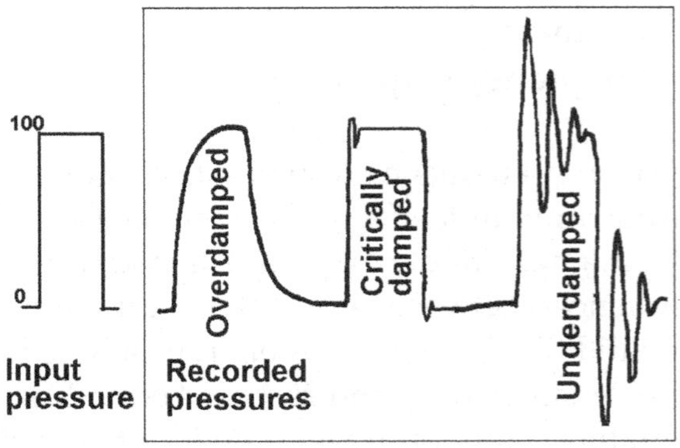

Frequency response to Square wave input

150. What is the minimum allowable high frequency response needed in a catheter transducer system to accurately record the LV pressure shown to the 10th harmonic?

a. 20 Hz.
b. 100 Hz.
c. 200 Hz.
d. 1000 Hz.

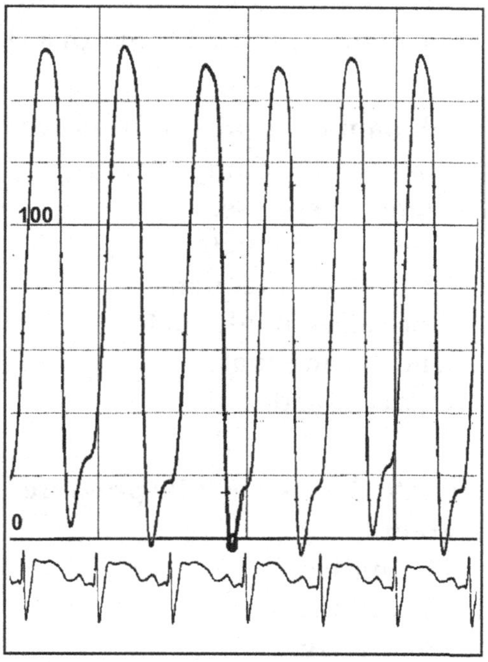

LV X 200, 1 second time lines

ANSWER a. 20 Hz. This tracing has two LV cycles per second for a heart rate of 120 / min. The fundamental frequency is thus 2/sec (frequency = 1 / period or f = 1/ RR interval). The 10th harmonic of 2 Hz is:
2 Hz x 10 = 20 Hz. Simply find the fundamental frequency (which is the heart rate in Hz) and multiply it by 10. Baim and Grossman say,

> "*the essential physiologic information is contained within the first 10 harmonic of the pressure wave's Fourier series. At a heart rate of 120 beats per minute, the fundamental frequency is 2 cycles per second and the tenth harmonic is 20 cycles per second. Thus a pressure measurement system with a frequency response range that is flat to 20 cycles per second should be adequate....*"

See: Baim and Grossman's, chapter on "Pressure recording." Keywords: 10th harmonic

151. When measuring pressures at cath, placing the transducer at the mid-chest position closely correlates with the height of the _____.

a. LV
b. Mid-LA
c. Neck veins
d. Pericardial zero pressure

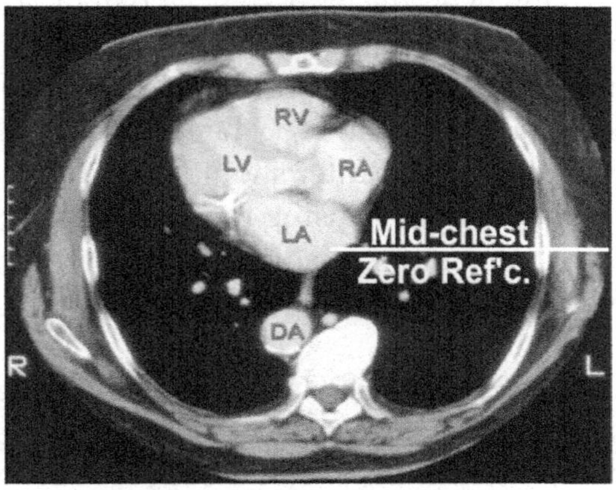

CT showing mid-chest zero reference

ANSWER b. Mid-LA. Ragosta says, Ragosta says, "A major advantage of the midchest position is that is has been shown to correlate with the position of the left atrium by MRI studies.... Frequently, busy catheterization laboratories might position the transducer at the same level for all patients or from a measured, fixed distance from either the table or from the top of the patients chest, without taking into consideration the variations in patient position or body habitus. This practice will lead to marked inaccuracies...." See: Ragosta, chapter on Normal Waveforms.

BOTH QUESTIONS BELOW REFER TO THIS DIAGRAM:
This LV was recorded through a fluid filled transducer/catheter system.

152. **The dynamic response of this system appears ______ damped with ________ frequency response.**
a. **Over-, inadequate**
b. **Critically-, adequate**
c. **Critically-, inadequate**
d. **Under-, adequate**
e. **Under-, inadequate**

153. **Estimate the LV systolic pressure in this diagram.**
a. **115 mmHg**
b. **125 mmHg**
c. **135 mmHg**
d. **145 mmHg**

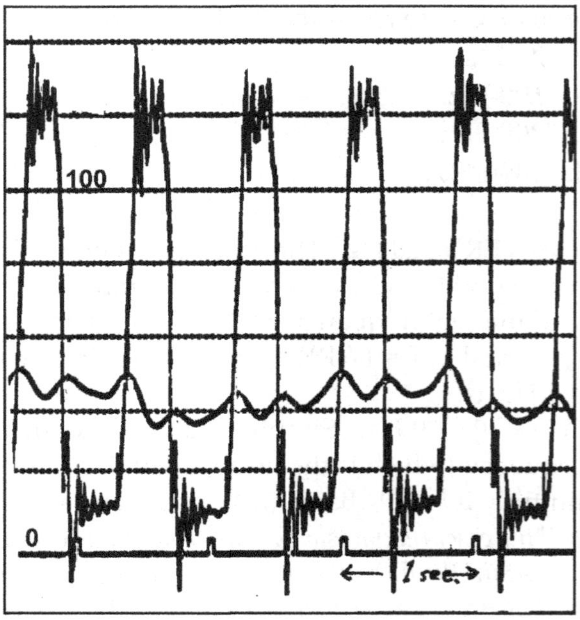

Simultaneous LV and PAW pressure x 200

BOTH ANSWERS APPEAR TOGETHER BELOW:

152. ANSWER d. Underdamped with adequate frequency response. The resonance is very rapid. (over 10 cycles can be fit into one RR interval.) This makes the frequency response adequate. Each resonant cycle is 1 mm in duration and the RR interval is 12 mm. Here 12 resonant cycles can be included within one RR cycle. This indicates adequate high frequency response (> 10 cycles/RR).

However, the excessive overshoot on the resonance indicates inadequate damping. To increase damping, contrast should be flushed into the fluid system and/or the recorder's high frequency cutoff filter should be reduced to 6-10 Hz. Both of these will reduce the overshoot by increasing the damping.

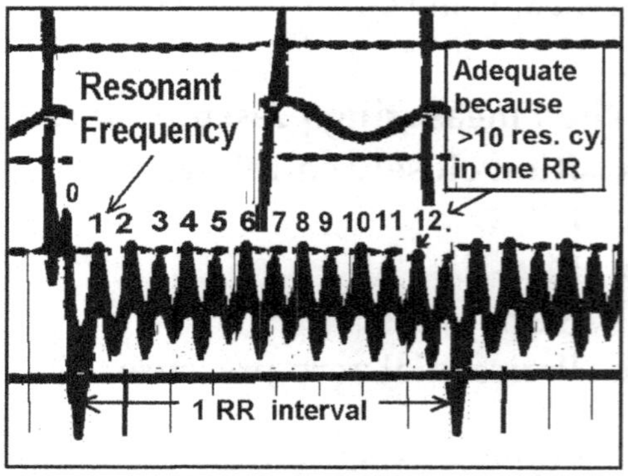

Analysis of a resonant LV signal

See: Baim and Grossman's chapter on "Pressure recording."
Keywords: frequency response

153. ANSWER b. 125 mmHg. The catheter resonance artifact overshoots the systolic pressure by at least 10 mmHg. Under-damping like this resonates around the true pressure. If the resonance is not filtered or damped out, the operator must "read through" the noise. Peak artifact is 140 mmHg and the minimum peaks are around 110 mmHg, making the average between them approximately 125 mmHg. A computerized recorder will over-

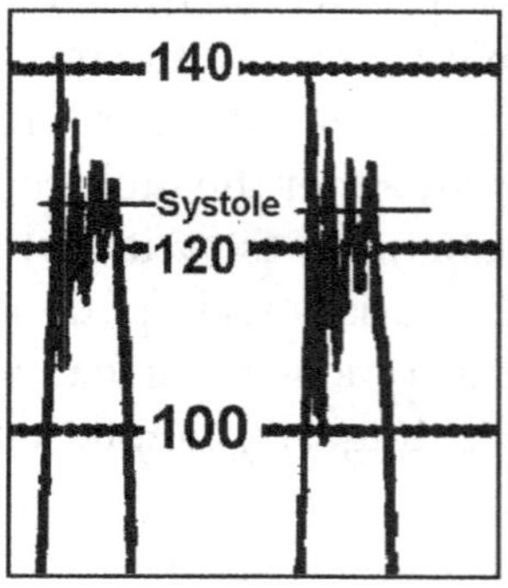

LV systole x 200

read these pressures. **A competent hemodynamic tech must take the time to appropriately move the computer generated markers or filter out the overshoot. Make the computer read the correct systolic pressure**. Diastolic pressures must be corrected in a similar manner. Note that atrial tracings seldom show artifact. But, there is a 30 mmHg diastolic gradient here due to MS.
See: Baim and Grossman, chapter on "Pressure Measurements" **Keywords:** averaging systolic LV resonance

154. During simultaneous LV-FA pressure recording the arterial tracing is 10 mmHg higher than the LV systolic. A sheath pressure higher than the LV systolic pressure indicates:
- **a. AS**
- **b. HOCM**
- **c. Normal response**
- **d. Coarctation of AO**
- **e. Constrictive pericarditis**

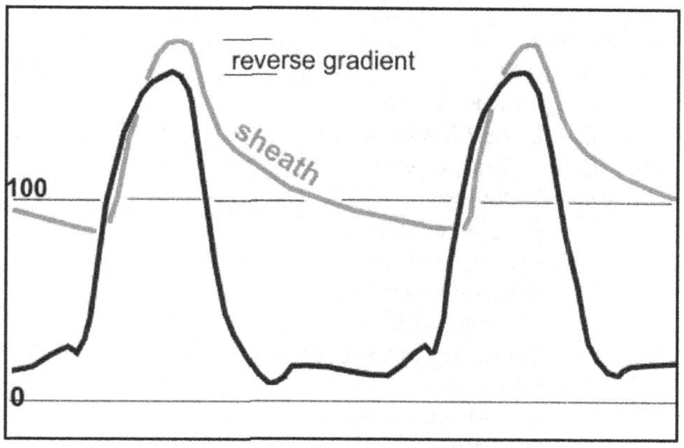

Reverse gradient

Answer: c. Normal response - due to resonant frequencies in the periphery. Ragosta says, "The effect of reflected waves is particularly notable in peripheral arterial waveforms (brachial, femoral, and radial) Peak systolic pressure exceeds central aortic pressure by 10-20 mmHg due to peripheral amplification from reflected waves. The contour of the waveform changes further from the aortic valve, with a steeper upstroke, narrower systolic portion (spiked appearance), and markedly diminished or absent dicrotic notch."
See: Ragosta, chapter on "Normal Waveforms" Keywords: resonance in distal AO=higher AO

REFERENCES:

Baim, D. S. and Grossman W., *Cardiac Catheterization, Angiography, and Intervention*, 6th Ed., Lea and Febiger, 2006
Braunwald, et. al. Ed., *Heart Disease, a Textbook of CV Medicine*, 8th Ed., Saunders, 2008
Kern, M. J., Ed., *The Cardiac Catheterization Handbook*, 3rd Ed., Mosby-Year Book, 2003
Ahrens, T. S., and Taylor, L.A., *Hemodynamic Waveform Analysis*, 1st Ed., W.B. Saunders Co., 1992
Daily, E. K., and Schroeder, J. S., *Techniques in Bedside Hemodynamic Monitoring*, 4th Ed., C. V. Mosby Company, 1989
Darovic, G.O., *Hemodynamic Monitoring: Invasive and Noninvasive Clinical Application*, WB Saunders, 1995
Quall, S.J., *Comprehensive Intra-aortic Balloon Pumping*, CV Mosby Co., 1984
Ragosta, Michael, Textbook of Clinical Hemodynamics, Saunders, 1st Edition, 2008
Wagner G.S., *Marriott's Practical Electrocardiography*, Williams and Wilkins, 1994

OUTLINE: Pressure Recording Systems

1. System Electronics
   a. Transducers
   b. Wheatstone bridge
   c. Carrier amplifier & signal
      i. Modulation/demodulation

2. Plumbing
   a. Stopcocks
      i. handle on/off
      ii. 2 way/ 3 way/ 4 way
   b. Quick flush device
      i. Y device
      ii. Pressure bag
   c. Transducer setup
      i. Arterial line setup
      ii. IV/Swan setup
      iii. Coronary manifold
         (1) Ports
         (2) Flush syringe
         (3) Waste
         (4) Dye
         (5) Pressurized Flush
         (6) Catheter connector
         (7) Transducer/zero
         (8) 2 transducer ICU manifold
      iv. Swan Ganz setup
         (1) Tails
         (2) Ports
         (3) Thermistor

3. Calibration and Pressure Recording
   a. Air Zero
      i. Position at mid-chest level
      ii. Phlebostatic axis
         (1) Mid-axillary, 4th IS
   b. Balance
      i. Balancing Wheatstone bridge
   c. Calibration
      i. Setting Electrical Gain
      ii. Calibration Stairs
   d. Mercury Calibration
      i. Gauge Factor
      ii. Linearity
   e. Dynamic Response
      i. Square wave test
   f. Drift (temperature)

4. Recording
   a. Paper Speeds
   b. Time Lines
   c. Ranges / Full scale
      i. Sensitivity
   d. Reversing transducers

5. Recording Errors
   a. Conversions
      i. cm H_2O (Convert CVP readings)
      ii. mmHg (zero errors)
   b. Transducer/Calibration Factor errors
   c. Arrhythmia
      i. PVC's
      ii. Atrial Fibrillation

6. Monitor controls
   a. Trouble shooting
      i. Range
      ii. Filters
      iii. ECG noise
      iv. Tube/connection errors
         (1) Air bubbles
         (2) Loose stopcocks
      v. Damping/overshoot

7. Editing Pressure Recordings
   a. Markers
   b. ECG Trigger
      i. PVCs
      ii. Atrial Fibrillation
   c. Mixed Pressures
      i. Wedge pressure/PA
      ii. LV/AO
   d. Calibration Stairs errors
      i. Off zero line
   e. Reading Pressures

8. Frequency Response
   a. Fundamental Frequency = 1/RR interval
   b. Heart Rate
   c. Allowable upper frequency limit = 10 x ff
   d. Frequency Response Curve
   e. Natural Frequency of Vibration
      i. Reduced with long pressure tubes
   f. Damping
      i. Overshoot = underdamping
      ii. Critical Damping = 10% overshoot
   g. Testing with fast flush device
   h. Testing with square wave response

PRESSURE PATHOLOGY I

INDEX E4:

General Pressure Pathology

BOTH OF THESE QUESTIONS REFER TO THE DIAGRAM BELOW:

155. The wide arterial pulse waveform labeled #2 in the diagram is termed:
- a. Pulsus alternans
- b. Pulsus bigeminus
- c. Pulsus bisferiens
- d. Pulsus tardus
- e. Corrigan's pulse

156. The arterial pulse labeled #3 in the diagram may be diagnostic of:
- a. Heart failure, myocardial depression
- b. Bigeminy (Alternating sinus, PVC beats)
- c. HOCM
- d. Aortic Stenosis (AS)
- e. Aortic Insufficiency (AI)

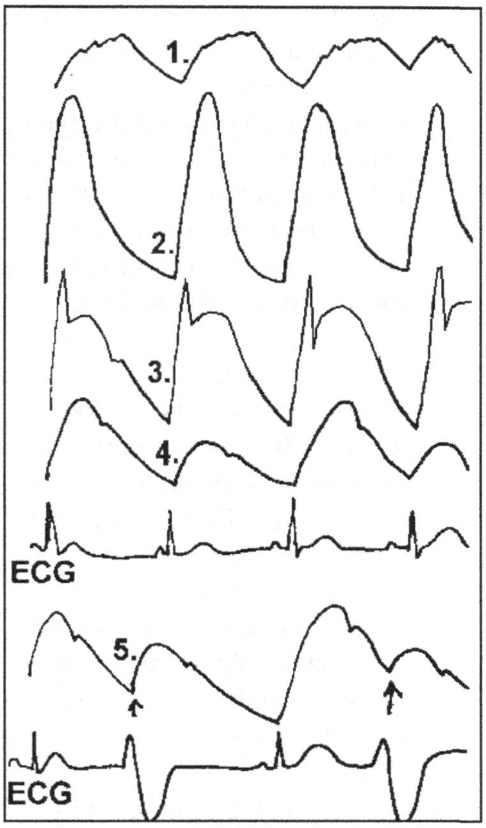

Abnormal aortic pulse tracings

BOTH ANSWERS LISTED TOGETHER BELOW:
155. ANSWER e. Corrigan's pulse. In aortic insufficiency the blood leaks backwards out of the AO into the LV. This loss of aortic blood rapidly drops the arterial pressure.

BE ABLE TO CORRECTLY MATCH ALL ANSWERS BELOW:

1. Pulsus tardus:
   Aortic stenosis slows the upstroke (making it tardy - "Tardus"). The upstroke may have a "shudder" coincident with the ejection murmur and an anacrotic notch (notch on the upstroke wave).
2. Corrigan's pulse:
   Corrigan's pulse is seen in Aortic regurgitation. It is termed Water-hammer because it feels bounding. It shows a rapid upstroke (percussion wave) followed by a rapid collapse (regurgitation) early in diastole. No dicrotic notch is seen, because the aortic valve does not close completely.
3. Pulsus Bisferiens:
   Pulsus bisferiens is a double humped arterial pulse. Both percussion and tidal waves are distinct. It is similar to a dicrotic pulse, which has a large dicrotic notch and pulse following it, except both of the bisferiens pulses are in systole.
4. Pulsus alternans:
   Pulsus alternans is an alternating systolic BP, even though the heart rate is regular. Beats alternate like this: 120/80, 115/75, 120/80, 115/75... Often seen in failing ventricles.
5. Pulsus bigeminus:
   Pulsus bigeminus is caused by ventricular bigeminy. It is distinguishable from pulsus alternans only when compared to the bigeminal ECG.

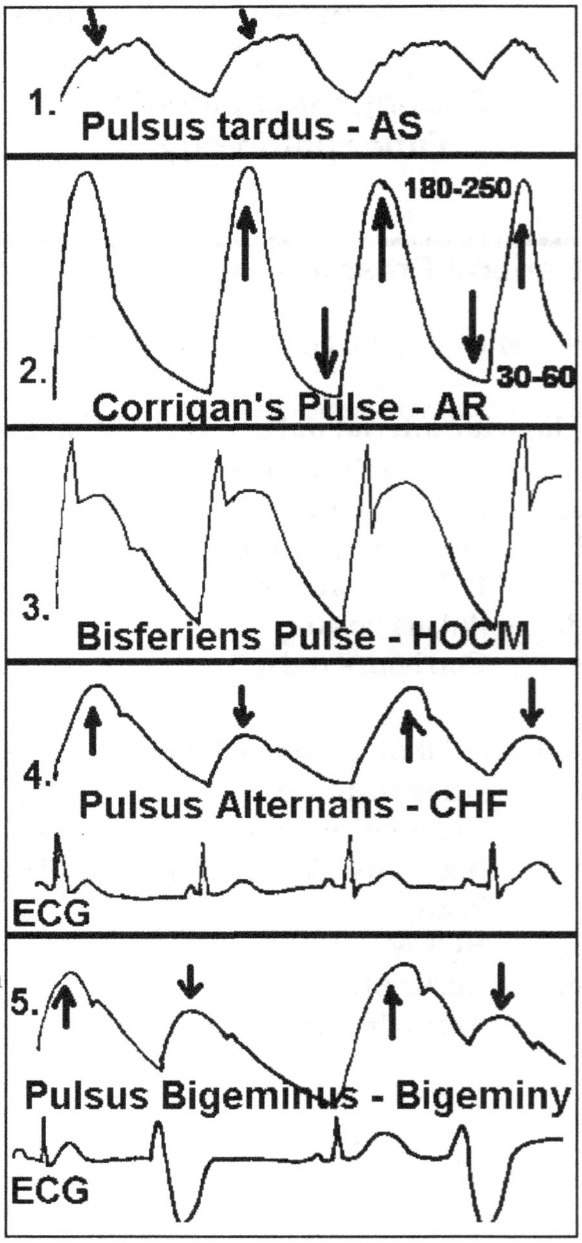

Abnormal aortic pulse tracings

Pulse contours may be palpated in the carotid artery, recorded externally with phonocardiography transducers or recorded through an intravascular catheter connected to a pressure transducer. The wave-form may be diagnostic of the pathology.
See: Braunwald, chapter on "Physical Examination." Keywords: Arterial pulse waves, AS=tardus, AI=Corrigan's, Alternans=CHF, Bigeminus=bigeminy

156. ANSWER c. HOCM or IHSS . BE ABLE TO MATCH ALL ANSWERS:

1. AS: In severe AS the aortic ejection is obstructed and the peak pressures is reduced and delayed.
2. AI/AR: In leaking aortic valves the blood leaks backwards out of the AO into the LV. This loss of aortic blood rapidly drops the arterial diastolic pressure. The systolic may increase to compensate for the reduced cardiac output.
3. HOCM/IHSS: Bisferiens pulse is associated with HOCM/IHSS and AR. In HOCM The LV outflow tract pinches itself off mid-systole. This makes a characteristic notch at the top of the pulse wave. This "bifid" pulse of AR is due to rapid early systolic ejection followed by a reflected wave. It may be seen in any rapid ejection - low resistance system. This arterial configuration is also termed "spike and dome."
4. Heart failure, myocardial depression:
   In alternating pulse, the heart is so weak that it seems to rest every 2nd beat. It is an ominous sign, not specific to any disease - just a severely depressed myocardium.
5. Bigeminy (Alternating sinus, PVC beats):
   Bigeminal pulse is caused by a bigeminal ECG. Every other beat is a PVC followed by a compensatory pause. This pause allows more complete ventricular diastolic filling with every other beat. More preload makes for more complete contraction, and higher systolic BP with the following sinus beats.

See: Braunwald, chapter on "Physical Examination." Keywords: Arterial Pulse waves associated pathology, AS=tardus, AI=Corrigan's, Alternans=CHF, Bigeminus=bigeminy

157. Other words describing a "billowing" heart valve pathology as shown at #1 are:

1. Prolapsed
2. Insufficient
3. Floppy
4. Stenotic

a. 1, 2
b. 1, 3
c. 2, 3
d. 3, 4

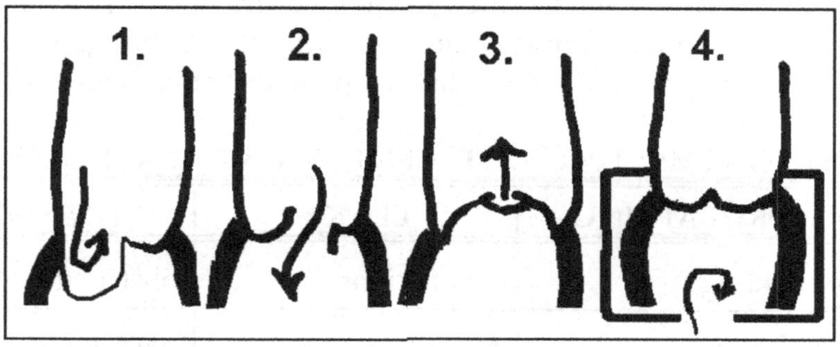

Heart Pathology in heart valves

ANSWER b. 1, 3. Prolapsed and Floppy, also myxomatous, redundant, systolic click, Barlow valve, or buckling. Under pressure a prolapsing valve bulges backward. Mitral regurgitation results. The mitral valve is the most frequently regurgitant

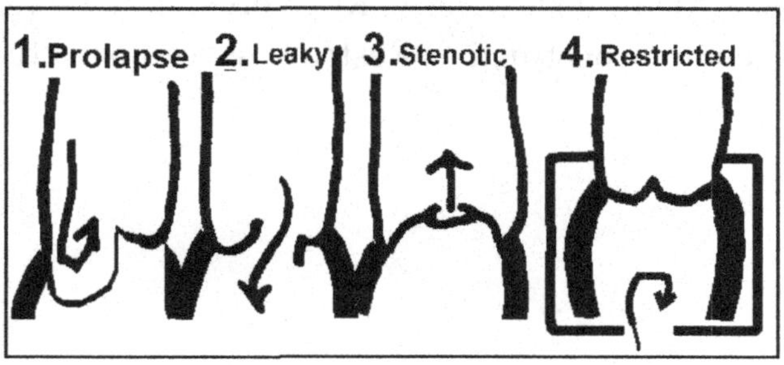

Types of valve pathology

BE ABLE TO MATCH ALL VALVE PATHOLOGIES SHOWN:

1. **A prolapsing** valve does not hold its position when closed. High distal pressure and an enlarged valve causes it to balloon back into the proximal chamber. The AV valves are most prone to prolapse when chordae and papillary muscles are damaged. Occasionally, a prolapsing valve may balloon or buckle so much that it leaks.
2. **A regurgitating valve** leaks. It is not "competent" to do its job of allowing flow in only one direction - it "insufficiently" coapts or closes. Leaky heart valves cause volume overload and dilatation of the proximal chamber. They also cause loss of pressure and cardiac output to the distal chamber.
3. **A Stenotic valve** has a blockage or narrowing that obstructs blood flow. Stenosis restricts blood flow and pinches off the forward cardiac output. (In coronary arteries we sometimes call these obstructions "lesions.") Significant stenosis always causes a pressure gradient due to its high resistance to flow. It results in pressure overload and eventual hypertrophy of the proximal chamber. Regurgitation and stenosis are distinctly different valvular problems, with completely different physiologic consequences. However, calcified valves often exhibits both regurgitation and stenosis. Here, there is a regurgitant jet and a stenotic gradient.
4. **Restrictive defects** form a barrier around the ventricle that limits diastolic filling and venous return. Restriction does not affect the valve leaflets. It is a "diastolic disorder." E.g., in constrictive pericarditis a tight pericardium limits (constricts) ventricular expansion in diastole. The tight pericardium allows a small initial rapid fill, then cannot expand further. Since the venous return is so restricted, the stroke volume and CO are reduced. Restriction is listed in this chapter only because it has distinct hemodynamic consequences. Although this is not a valve problem, I list it here because it is a distinct hemodynamic class of diseases.

SYNONYMS FOR DIFFERENT VALVE PATHOLOGIES:

PROLAPSING	LEAKY	STENOTIC	RESTRICTIVE
buckling	insufficient	obstructive	encased
billowing	regurgitant	narrowing	constricted
floppy	incompetent	blockage	filling limited
redundant	flowing backwards	lesion, gradient	diastolic disorder

See: Medical Dictionary. **Keywords:** Leaky = regurgitant = insufficient = incompetent, Stenotic = obstructive, Restrictive = constrictive

CORONARY ARTERIOGRAPHY MONITORING

158. These pressure waveforms are taken through Judkins coronary catheters being manipulated in the aortic root. Identify the pressure pattern seen at #2 on the diagram.

a. Ventricularization
b. Reduced pressure damping
c. LV (retrograde across valve)
d. High frequency damping (incomplete damping) as from contrast in the catheter.

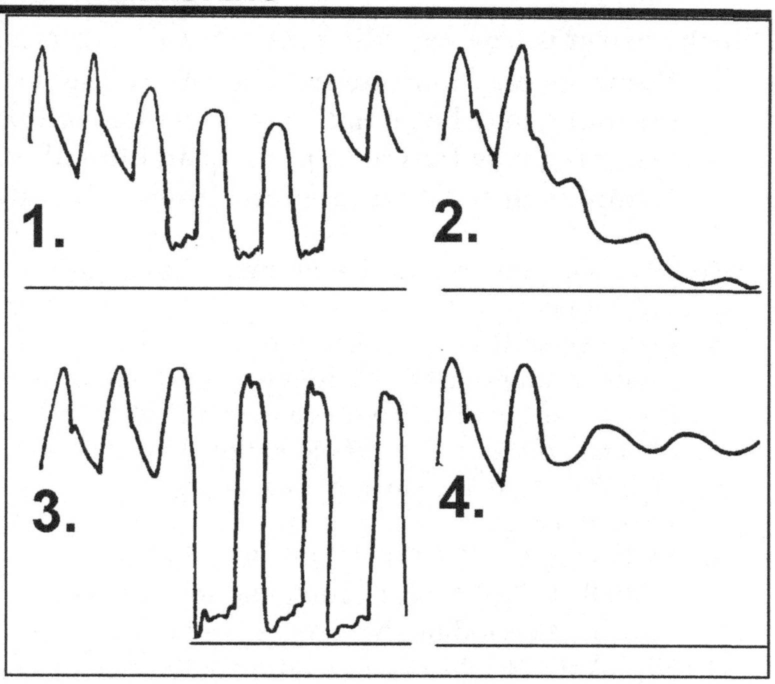

Types of coronary catheter DAMPING

ANSWER b. Reduced pressure damping.

BE ABLE TO CORRECTLY MATCH ANSWERS BELOW:

1. **Ventricularization**: Arterial pressure mimics LV with exception of a lower systolic and higher diastolic. (Associated with left main stenosis)
2. **Reduced pressure damping**: Pressure falls off as the tip is occluded and does not transmit pressure to the transducer
3. **LV** (retrograde across valve): Catheter advanced across Aortic valve into LV. While this is NOT a form of damping, it commonly occurs while attempting to cannulate the coronary ostium. Dangerous ventricular arrhythmias can result if it goes unnoticed.
4. **Reduced high frequency response** (contrast): phasic pressure is smoothed out as the catheter lumen size is reduced due to clot, partial occlusion, or viscous fluid such as contrast or blood in the lumen. These damped waveforms looks as if you had activated the "mean" switch on the recorder.

See: Baim, chapter on "Coronary Arteriography" **Keywords:** Types of Coronary artery damping

159. Which answer is true regarding coronary artery pressure DAMPING?

a. **Damping may indicate significant LAD stenosis**
b. **Damping may be an indicator of cardiac failure**
c. **Damping may lead to tipping up an intimal plaque**
d. **Damping may lead to clot formation in the catheter tip**

ANSWER c. Damping may lead to lifting or tipping up an intimal plaque.

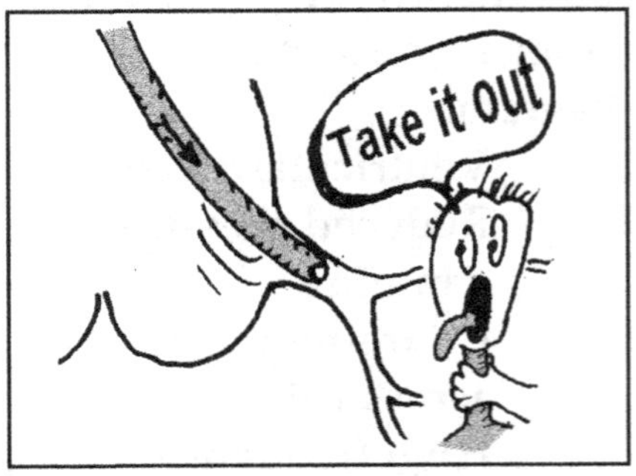

Damping = Possible Ischemia

a. NO: It may indicate left-main coronary ostial stenosis, but not LAD. Damping cuts off blood flow to the heart: When the catheter occludes the coronary orifice it cuts off blood flow to that area. This may lead to ischemia, injury, arrhythmia, etc.

b. NO: DAMPING IS NOT AN INDICATOR OF CARDIAC FAILURE. It is an indicator that your catheter is occluding the coronary ostia.

c. YES: DAMPING MAY cause lifting or tipping up a plaque or dissect the intima in an ostial lesion: Damping means you are occluding the coronary orifice especially in main-stem left lesions. If the orifice is tight anyway and has a atherosclerotic lesion, the catheter tip contact may dissect or tip up a plaque leading to coronary occlusion. Remember left main lesions are dangerous. Damping should be carefully monitored and acted upon. Judkins says,

> "*Careful, continuous catheter tip pressure monitoring is mandatory for procedural safety. Constant, vigilant monitoring will ensure instantaneous recognition of damping. Fluid injection should not be made if there is damping of the catheter tip pressure.* ***If there is any damping or slowed washout on test contrast injection, the catheter should be withdrawn and repositioned.*** *Electrocardiographic changes lag hopelessly behind regional myocardial ischemia produced by catheter malposition....A physician or appropriately trained member of the technical staff should be assigned to monitor pressure and the electrocardiogram throughout the procedure*".

d. NO: DAMPING DOES NOT LEAD TO CLOTS FORMING IN THE CATHETER TIP: Clotting seldom happens in coronary catheters which are large bore and flushed frequently with contrast and heparinized saline. Contrast itself is an anticoagulant. However, long-term small-bore catheters and IVs which are not frequently flushed may clot. A catheter clot may result in pressure damping. Other dangers of damping include the induction of arrhythmia, coronary spasm, and cardiac ischemia.

KNOW THE BAD EFFECTS OF DAMPING.

See: Baim, chapter on "Coronary Arteriography" and Judkins, chapter on "Coronary Arteriography and Left Ventriculography: Judkins Technique." **Keywords:** problems with damping (spasm, tip plaque, cuts off blood)

160. A cardiologist is manipulating a PTCA guider catheter into this patient's right coronary ostia. As the monitoring tech, what would you say to the Dr. regarding the pressure shown?

a. "Damping"
b. "Phasic pressure"
c. "Gradient"
d. "Give me zeros"
e. "Arrhythmia"

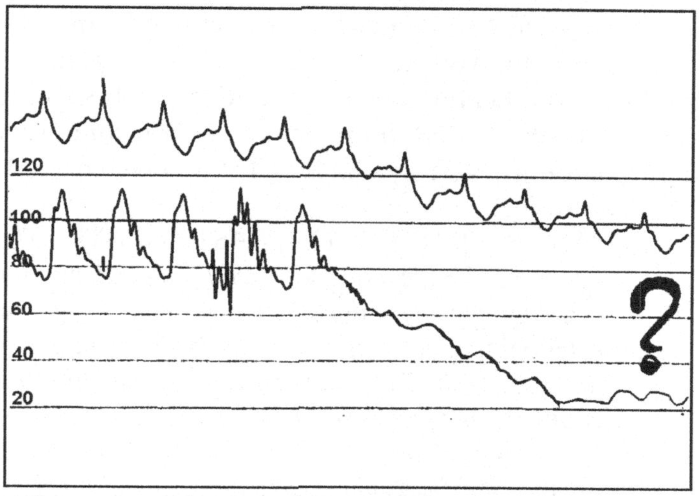

AO pressure during insertion into coronary artery

ANSWER a. "Damping." Pepine says, that in PTCA

> *"Care should be taken to observe arterial pressure from the tip of the guide catheter to be sure that 'damping' does not occur. If either 'damping' or 'ventricularization' occurs, the balloon should be advanced quickly across the stenosis and the guiding catheter withdrawn immediately to a more proximal or ostial position to reestablish adequate coronary flow."*

If damping continues, sideholes may be cut in the guider catheter to allow perfusion into the coronary. **See:** Pepine, chapter on "Coronary Angiography" **Keywords:** identify damping

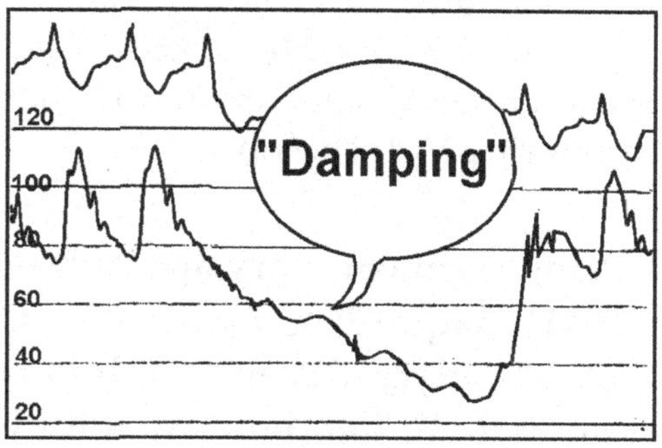

Coronary artery damping restored

161. You are called in to assist with coronary arteriography on an acute MI patient. You are one of only 3 staff in the lab. Your job is to both monitor and circulate on the case. Noting the ECG and the aortic pressure changes shown in the diagram you should notify the Dr. and:

a. Begin CPR
b. Administer precordial thump
c. Charge the defibrillator
d. Prepare the pacemaker
e. Administer Lidocaine

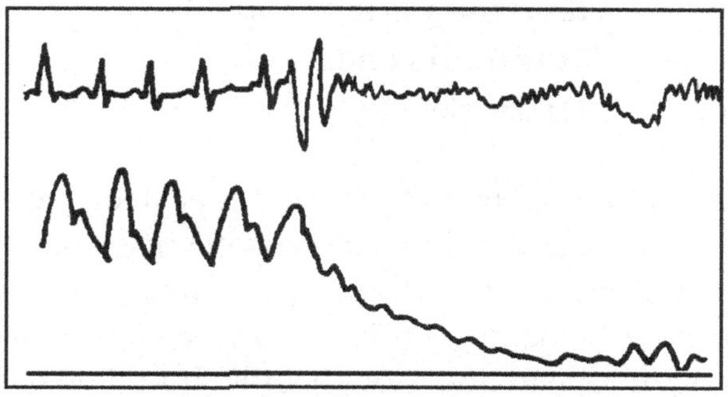
Monitoring ECG and coronaries

ANSWER c. Charge the defibrillator. This is ventricular fibrillation. It is invariably lethal if not immediately treated. In this form of cardiac arrest the heart ineffectively quivers and pumps NO blood. Note the BP on the diagram falls to zero. The patient will only remain conscious for 10 seconds. Brain damage will result within 4 minutes.

The Dr. will normally instruct the patient to COUGH REPEATEDLY to prolong his conscious state. You should prepare the emergency treatment, which is immediate defibrillation. Let the patient go "out", then shock him.

The precordial thump is now only recommended in VF/VT when a monitor and defibrillator are NOT available. CPR will be required if defibrillation is unsuccessful. Braunwald says,

> "*RADIOGRAPHIC CONTRAST AGENTS. These agents may produce a number of adverse hemodynamic, electrophysiological, and renal effects consequent to coronary arteriography. The monomeric ionic contrast agents that have been used in coronary arteriography for many years are high-osmolar methylglucamine and sodium salts of diatrizoic acid. These substances dissociate into cations and iodine-containing anions, resulting in aqueous solutions of 1940 mOsmol/kg, as compared with the osmolality of human plasma of 300 mOsmol/kg. The Hypertonicity of these compounds produces sinus bradycardia, heart block, Q-T interval and QRS prolongation, ST-segment depression, giant T-wave inversion, decreased left ventricular contractility, decreased systolic pressure, and increased left ventricular end-diastolic pressure.... If the contrast agents are injected into a damped coronary catheter with ventricular pressure tracing or given too rapidly in too great a volume (e.g., more than approximately 5 ml for opacification of the right coronary artery), ventricular tachycardia or fibrillation may ensue.*"

See: Braunwald, chapter on "Coronary Arteriography", ACLS manual **Keywords:** monitoring V. Tach./fib

162. During right coronary angiography with Hypaque 76% a patient's ECG shows bradycardia and a fall in the BP as shown. Initial therapy should be to:

a. Have the patient cough
b. Have the patient Valsalva
c. Thump his chest
d. Defibrillate

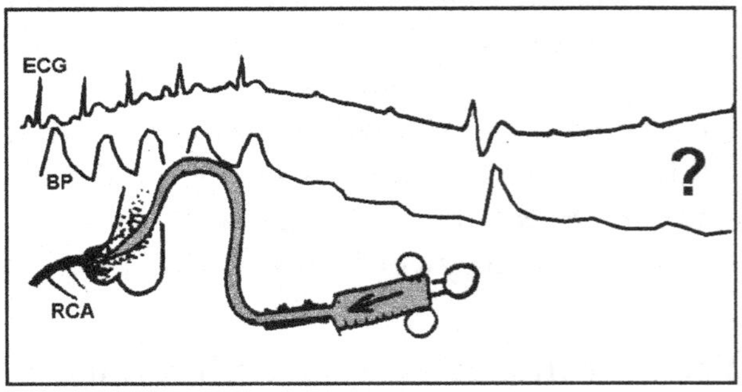

Bradycardia during RCA angiography

ANSWER a. Have the patient repeatedly cough. It is a form of self induced CPR. This patient has developed a complete heart block with inadequate blood flow. Whenever there is cessation of blood flow, have the patient cough repeatedly. Patients that would otherwise have gone "out" may be kept conscious for several minutes by having them cough repeatedly. Cough CPR should be taught to all patients undergoing coronary arteriography.

In addition to the CPR effect, coughing compresses the heart enough to squeeze toxic dye from the coronary arteries. After a few coughs, usually bradycardia and then sinus rhythm resume . Remember, that the right coronary artery feeds the SA and AV nodes. If the contrast makes these nodes ischemic, bradycardia and/or heart block may develop. Consider inserting a prophylactic temporary pacemaker or using low-osmolar contrast agents.

See: ACLS manual. **Keywords:** Cough

163. **You are monitoring the ECG and pressures during left coronary artery angio. injections with Hypaque 76%. With these ST segments and pressure changes you should tell the catheterizing physician:**

a. "Damping."
b. "Ventricularization."
c. "Asystole"
d. Nothing.

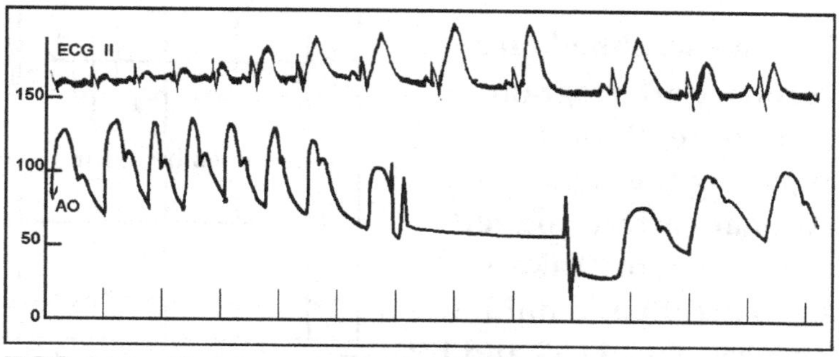

ECG & Aortic pressure during left coronary angiography via Judkins catheter

ANSWER d. Nothing. It is a typical left coronary injection. With LCA injection the ST segments elevate markedly in the inferior leads . The flat pressure line occurs because the pressure stopcock is closed during injection. Mild transient hypotension and bradycardia are also typical of coronary injection. Most experienced practitioners expect these transient ECG and pressure changes with high-osmolar contrast. So don't get too excited unless the BP doesn't come back within 15-20 seconds. These changes can be minimized by using the more expensive low-osmolar or non-ionic contrast materials.
See: Baim, chapter on "Coronary Arteriography" **Keywords:** RCA injection → ST depression, bradycardia, mild hypotension

164. **During ______ coronary angiography with Renografin-60 you may note the ECG and pressure changes shown.**

a. Left coronary artery
b. Right coronary artery
c. Coronary sinus
d. Native internal mammary artery

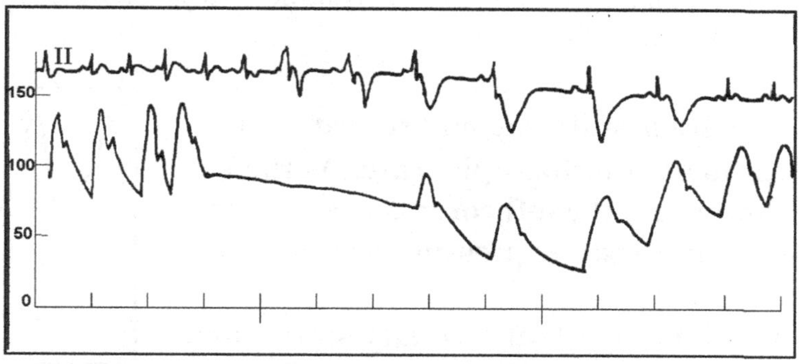

Lead II, ECG & pressure changes during coronary angio.

ANSWER b. Right coronary artery. With RCA injection the ST segments depress markedly in the inferior leads . Mild transient hypotension and bradycardia are typical of coronary angiographic injection. Remember the SA and AV nodes usually arise from the RCA. so watch for continued bradycardia or AV block. Note that the pressure seems to be returning towards normal. Most experienced practitioners expect these transient ECG and pressure changes. So don't get too excited unless the BP doesn't come back within 15-20 seconds. These changes can be minimized with low-osmolal or non-ionic contrast materials. Similar changes may occur with balloon inflation in the RCA.
See: Baim, chapter on "Coronary Arteriography" **Keywords:** LCA injection → ST elevation, bradycardia, mild hypotension

165. You are scrubbed on a coronary arteriogram procedure. Prior to injecting the right coronary artery you tell the patient to "Take a deep breath and hold it." The patient's ECG and BP are shown. Continue by:

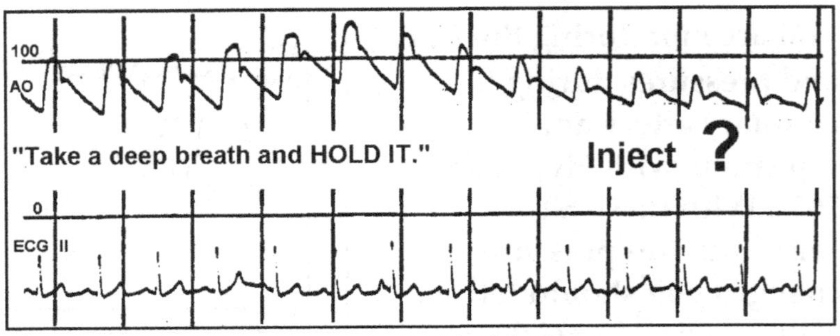

Patient takes a deep breath and holds it

- a. **Injecting 5-8 cc of contrast**
- b. **Removing the catheter from the coronary orifice**
- c. **Telling the patient to take another deep breath and let it all the way out**
- d. **Telling the patient to not bear down, but keep his mouth open**

ANSWER d. Tell the patient to not bear down, but keep his mouth open. Physicians may ask the patient to inhale prior to coronary injection to move the diaphragm off the screen to improve the angio image. A drop in pressure like this is a result of a Valsalva maneuver by the patient. While holding a full breath it is common for patients to bear down producing a Valsalva response. This can interfere with normal coronary flow. To keep the pressure up when the breath is taken in, have the patient keep his mouth open and try to slowly continue taking air in.
See: Kern, chapter on "Hemodynamics" **Keywords:** Identify and prevent Valsalva during coronary injection

166. You are monitoring and recording a coronary arteriography case. As the Dr. cannulates the left coronary ostia this drop in diastolic pressure occurs. This is termed:

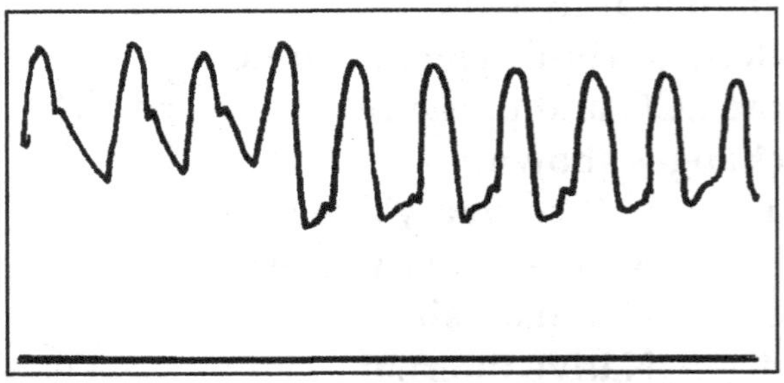
Drop in diastole with coronary cannulation

- a. **Inadvertent coronary sinus entry**
- b. **Inadvertent LV entry**
- c. **Phasic coronary pressure**
- d. **Ventricularization**

ANSWER d. Ventricularization. The normal triangular arterial waveform begins to look like LV - hence the term "ventricularization."Anytime the diastolic pressure falls below the normal AO diastolic level, it may be "ventricularization" and the Dr. should be alerted. "Ventricularization" may be associated with main-stem stenosis and may lead to asystole or bradycardia.

Ventricularization resembles left ventricular pressure, but not exactly . The "ventricularized" systole is usually lower than LV systole - especially if the catheter is in the RCA (RV capillary pressure is lower). Here the catheter is wedged into the coronary orifice, occludes the coronary artery and cuts off blood flow. Even though ventricularization is a dramatic waveform no perfusion is getting down the coronary artery.

In addition to a lower systole the "ventricularized" pressure has a higher diastole than LV and it slopes up, unlike arterial diastole that slopes down. In ventricularization end diastolic atrial kick waves are often seen. Ventricularization is associated with an orifice lesion. **See:** Baim, chapter on "Coronary Arteriography." **Keywords:** coronary wedge = diastolic damping = ventricularization

167. This pressure tracing is a pullback of a pigtail catheter from LV to AO. The low AO diastolic pressure seen on the diagram shows a probable ____ pressure.

- **a. Ventricularization**
- **b. Coronary sinus wedge**
- **c. Aortic insufficiency**
- **d. Mixed LV & AO**

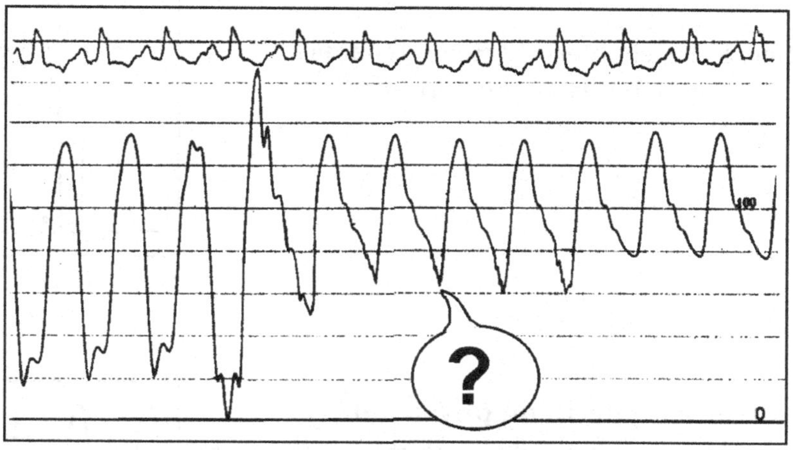

LV to AO pullback

ANSWER d. Mixed LV & AO . When a catheter with many sideholes like a pigtail, is slowly pulled across a valve, it's sideholes may straddle the valve creating a mixed pressure, somewhat like AO and somewhat like LV. These catheters should be briskly pulled back far enough to completely cross the valve. Kern says "This artifact can be easily recognized by the unusual diastolic waveform with a late diastolic shoulder and rapid dip differentiating it from a wide pulse pressure of valvular insufficiency."

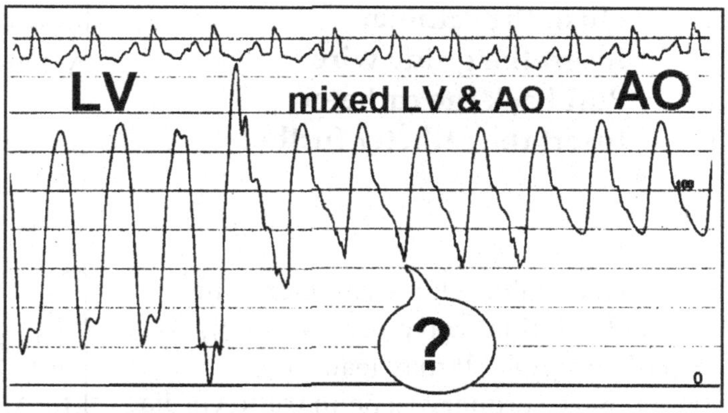

Pigtail LV to mixed LV/AO to AO pullback

This second LV tracing shows a bizarre diastolic decline. This is very rare for LV (LV diastole should always be slowly rising). But note the normal diastolic LV immediately preceding the pullback. Again, this is related to a multiple side-hole catheter positioned across the aortic valve.

See: Kern, chapter on "Hemodynamics."
Keywords: pullback pressure with mixed LV-AO

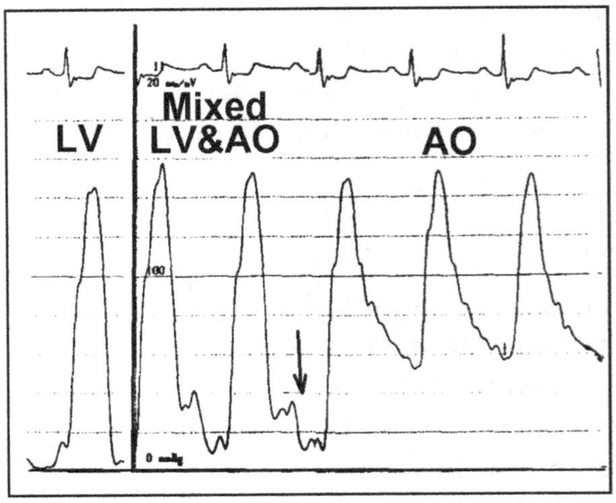

LV, Mixed LV/AO → AO x 200

168. As the catheterizing physician manipulates a guider catheter in the left coronary artery the catheter pressure drops and changes as shown. After you notify the physician of this waveform he should immediately:

a. Flush the catheter
b. Insert the guide wire
c. Pull back the catheter
d. Insert the catheter further

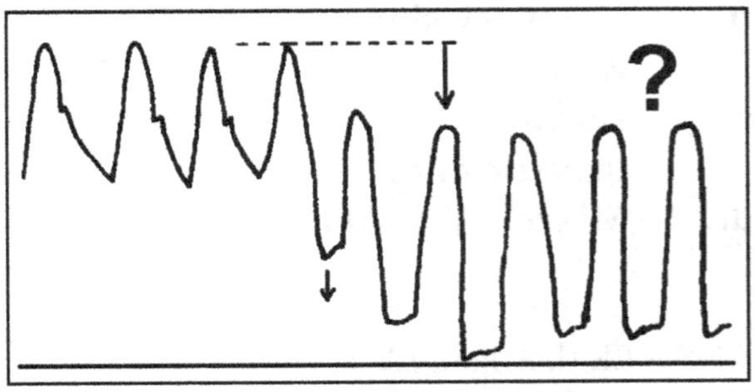

AO pressure during left coronary angio.

ANSWER c. Pull back the catheter. This ventricularization waveform is a dangerous form of damping. It may lead to arrhythmias, coronary ischemia, and cardiac arrest. It is due to occlusion of the coronary orifice and is especially common in main stem left stenosis. Since left main stem disease is so DANGEROUS, the catheter should be drawn back and replaced with one of a smaller tip diameter. If ventricularization continues "Hit and Run" angiographic shots may be necessary. Kern says,

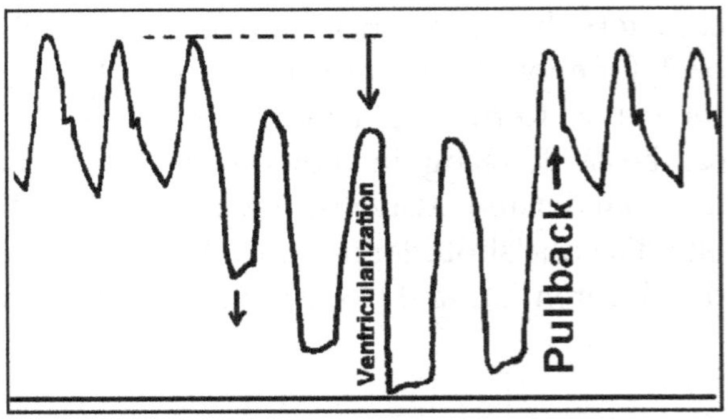

Pullback from "ventricularization" to AO

> *"It is critically important to identify and understand these coronary catheter waveforms. The significance of such an altered waveform during coronary angiography must be appreciated early in the angiographers career to avoid the catastrophic outcome after diagnostic angiography that has been associated with some patients with left main coronary*

stenosis.... This pattern commonly called ventricularized, is very commonly seen in patients with left main stenosis.... Appropriate precautions in patients with suspected left main disease involve performing a non-selective aortic cusp flush, a brief 'hit-and-run' injection in a shallow RAO or AP projection. Minimizing the number of contrast injections is important."

See: Kern, Hemodynamic Rounds, chapter on "Interpretation of Cardiac Pathophysiology From Pressure Waveform Analysis: Coronary Hemodynamics: 1. Coronary Catheter Pressures." **Keywords:** On seeing damping, pull back catheter

169. During coronary arteriography a "ventricularization" pressure waveform is most associated with:

a. Post stenotic dilatation of AO
b. VSD or coronary AV fistula
c. Main stem left coronary lesions
d. Blood clot in the catheter

ANSWER c. Main stem left coronary lesions. These are also termed "widowmaker lesions." A ventricularized pressure pattern is commonly seen during left coronary arteriography in patients with left main stenosis. Although this pattern should not be tolerated for long, angiography may be quickly performed by the "hit and run" technique.
See: Kern, chapter on "Hemodynamics"
Keywords: ventricularization = main stem left lesions

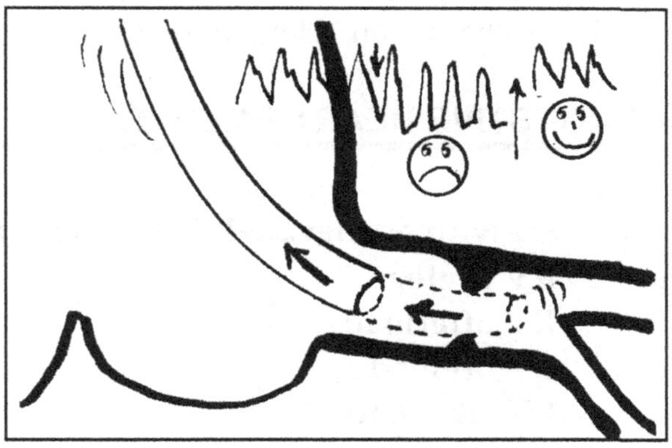
Ventricularization in widowmaker lesion

170. What is demonstrated in the last half of this tracing recorded during a bilateral heart cath and coronary case?

a. Catheter advanced across aortic valve (elevated LV EDP)
b. Catheter pulled back from distal to proximal AO (coarctation)
c. Catheter advanced from PA into RV (pulmonary hypertension)
d. Catheter in stenosed coronary ostium (ventricularization)

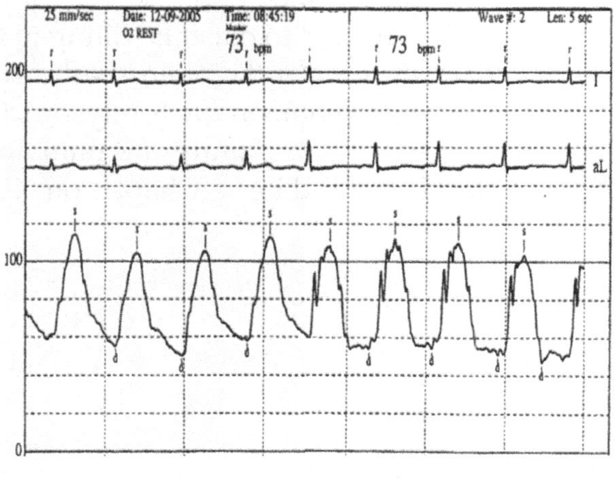

Answer: d. Catheter in stenosed coronary ostium (ventricularization) (E.g., Main left coronary lesion). The arterial pressure changes to a rapid upstroke and downstroke, like the LV. Note the atrial kick waves at d on the ventricularized tracing. Ventricularization pressure is essentially a coronary wedge pressure, reflecting the pressure in the LV capillary bed. Ventricularization is dangerous because is suggests an aorto-ostial coronary

stenosis which has an extremely high cath risk - "widow-maker".
See: Kern, chapter on "Hemodynamic Data" Keywords: ID Ventricularization

171. You are advancing a JL4 catheter into the LCA when the coronary pressure suddenly drops from 120/70 to 90/10 mmHg. This suggests:

a. **Ventricularization**
b. **Coronary artery spasm**
c. **Coronary artery rupture**
d. **Loss of atrial synchrony (AF)**

Answer: a. This is ventricularization in a left main ostial stenosis. The pulse pressure in AO is 50 mmHg, while in this ventricularized trace it is 80 mmHg. Ventriculized tracings usually show a flat or rising diastole with an "a" wave. Besides the ventricular shaped waveform, the ventricularized systolic pressure often drops, as a form of damping. Ventricularization is dangerous because is suggests a aorto-ostial coronary stenosis which has an extremely high cath risk - "widow-maker". If a severe ostial lesion is demonstrated on angio, physicians usually put in an IABP and rush the patient to surgery.
See: Kern, chapter on "Hemodynamic Data" Keywords: Ventricularization

CONGESTIVE HEART FAILURE

172. A patient with an elevated PAW pressure has elevated:

a. **RV preload**
b. **RV afterload**
c. **LV preload**
d. **LV afterload**

ANSWER c. LV preload. LV-EDP and PAW are the two most common indicators of LV preload. Elevated PAW pressure indicates that LA and LV-EDP have increased. These are strictly related to diastolic filling of the ventricle and Starling's law. According to Starling's Law, the greater the preload - the greater the force of contraction. It is a sign that the heart is trying to compensate for dysfunction. Elevated LV preload is often associated with congestive heart failure and pulmonary edema.
See: Berne and Levy, Chapter on "Cardiac Pump." **Keywords:** Preload, LV function.

173. This patient's LV pressure indicates probable congestive heart failure because of the:

- **a. Low dP/dT**
- **b. Elevated LV-EDP**
- **c. Large atrial kick "a" waves**
- **d. Reduces LV systolic pressure**
- **e. Diastolic flutter waves**
- **f. Square root sign**

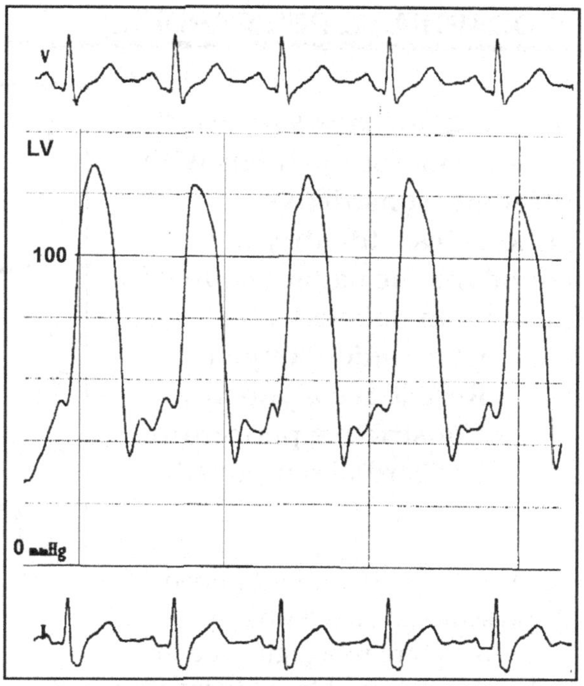

LV Pressure x 200

ANSWER b. Elevated LV-EDP. The hallmark of heart failure is elevated preload as seen in PAWP and LVEDP. Here, the end diastolic LV pressure averages 50 mmHg - where normal is under 12 mmHg. The LV-EDP is measured at the end of diastole immediately prior to LV contraction, between the atrial kick and the LV upstroke. This point also lines up with the ECG "r" wave as shown.

The heart attempts to compensate for poor a damaged heart by filling it more. Then, according to Starling's law the force of contraction should increase. But, in CHF this elevated pulmonary pressure results in pulmonary edema. This patient will be short of breath and have fluid in his lungs. **See:** Berne and Levy, Chapter on "Cardiac Pump." **Keywords:**

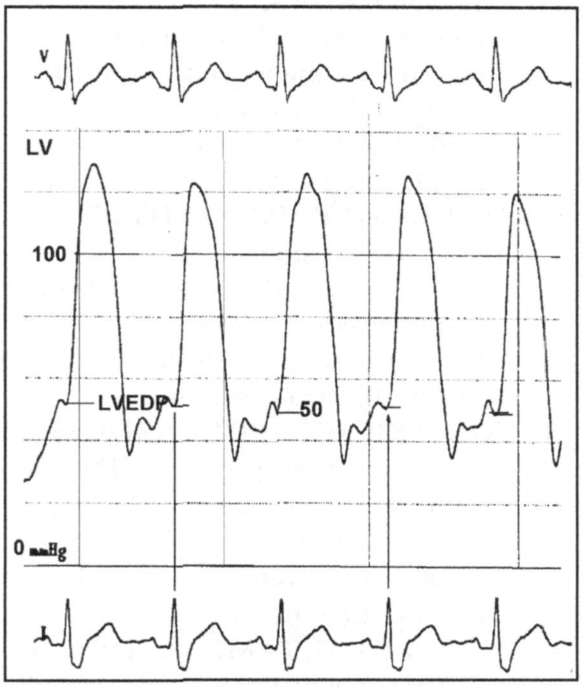

LV pressure x 200

MYOCARDIAL & PERICARDIAL

174. This diagram shows pressure curves from four patients with different constrictive pathologies. Identify the hemodynamic pattern shown in the diagram labeled #1.

a. CHF underdamped
b. Restrictive myopathy
c. Constrictive pericarditis
d. Pericardial tamponade

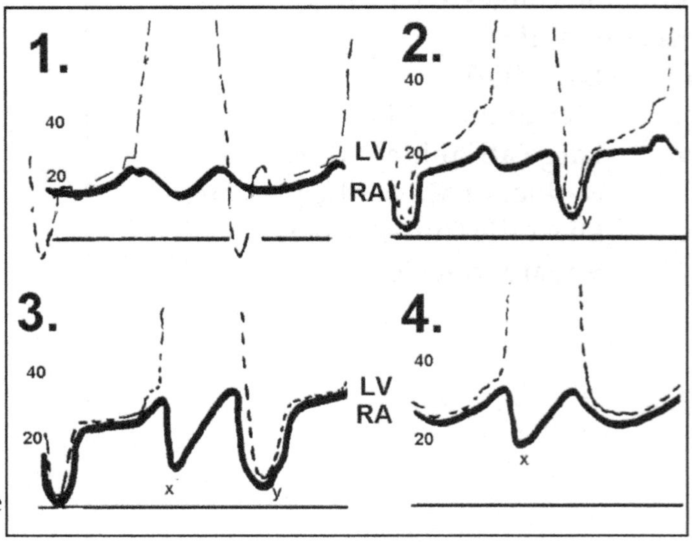

Simultaneous LV & RA pressures patterns x50

ANSWER a. CHF underdamped. The LV pressure labeled #1 has a "pseudo-square root sign" due to underdamped fluid transducer system. LV-EDP is elevated due to fluid congestion backing up into the lungs.

BE ABLE TO CORRECTLY MATCH ALL ANSWERS BELOW:

1. **CHF UNDERDAMPED:**
   Elevated LV-EDP and wedge pressure due to CHF. Underdamped ventricular pressure resonance causes pressure readings overshoot in systole and undershoot the early diastole (often resembling a square root sign). LV should never go below zero. This ringing can be due to a bubble in a long pressure line. See previous chapter on pressure measurements.
2. **RESTRICTIVE MYOPATHY (CM):**
   Elevated venous pressures. RA, RV, and LV show square root sign (rapid "y" descent). Rt. and Lt. sided diastolic pressures do NOT equilibrate. Pulmonary Hypertension is present. Here a stiff hypertrophied LV fills rapidly in diastole, then the pressure plateaus. This square root sign √ pattern is also described as a "dip and plateau pattern."
3. **CONSTRICTIVE PERICARDITIS (CP):**
   Elevated venous pressures. Prominent "x" and "y" descent making an "M" or "W" pattern. The prominent "y" wave dip termed a "square root sign" (√‾) is seen on the diastolic portion of the RA, RV and LV pressures. (seen in LA and PAWP also). There is an elevated diastolic plateau on these pressures. Rt.. and Lt. sided diastolic pressures equilibrate so that RA pressure = RV-EDP = LA = LV-EDP
4. **PERICARDIAL TAMPONADE (PT) :**
   Elevated venous pressures. Diastolic RA and RV collapse. Prominent "x" descent but NO "y" descent seen on atrial pressures (no square root sign √‾). Brachial pulses may disappear or reduce with inspiration (Pulsus Paradoxus).

See: Braunwald, chapter on "Pericardial Disease." . **Keywords:** Constrictive pressure patterns: Pericardial Tamponade, Restrictive Cardiomyopathy, Constrictive Pericarditis, CHF Underdamped.

175. **This patient has equal end diastolic pressures on both sides of the heart (25 mmHg). These simultaneous ventricular pressures show a pattern of:**

a. **Constrictive Pericarditis**
b. **Common ventricle with probable L-R VSD**
c. **Mitral stenosis with secondary pulmonary hypertension**
d. **Left sided CHF with cor pulmonale**

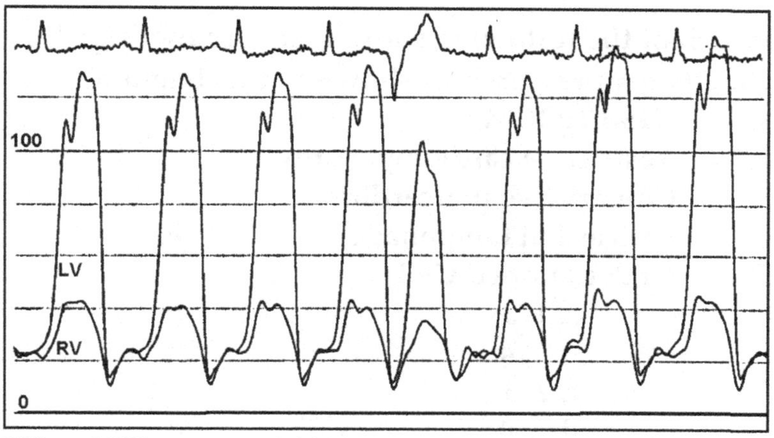

RV and LV pressure X200

ANSWER a. . Constrictive pericarditis.
These ventricular pressures show the square root pattern and diastolic equalization seen in constrictive pericarditis.

- LV EDP is 25 - high.
- RV EDP is 25 - high

Note the square wave pattern with the diastolic "dip and plateau" (Square root sign √) characteristic of constrictive pericarditis. In constrictive pericarditis the diastolic plateau is at approximately the same pressure level in all heart chambers (RA, RV, LA, & LV). In these constrictive patterns there is a deep Y wave. Remember, the letter Y looks like a suction cup, (suction cup effect) and occurs during early rapid ventricular filling phase.

TIN CAN ANALOGY: Imagine the 4 chambers of the heart as 4 water balloons. Imagine trying to fill these balloons in a closed tin can. They would fill only to the limit of the can size. Also, all 4 balloons would be at the same pressure when filling because fluid transmits pressure perfectly and in all directions. This analogy helps explain why all four cardiac chamber diastolic pressures are equal.

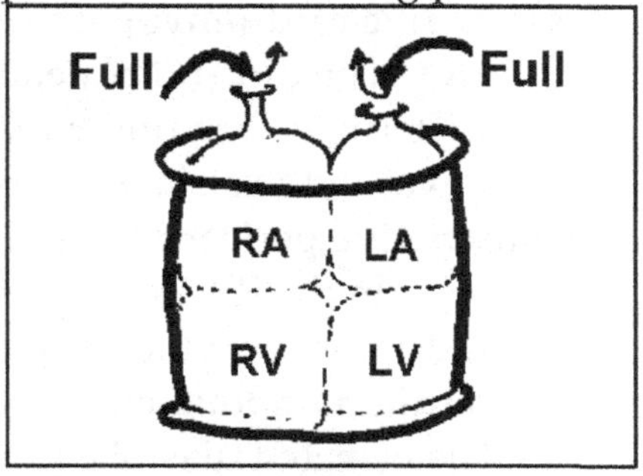

Tin Can compression analogy

Note these pullback pressures show the diastolic phase of all right heart pressures equals the LV diastolic. The LV gram and cardiac echo also help you distinguish between the two restrictive patterns.

See: Baim, chapter on "Profiles in Constrictive Pericarditis." **Keywords:** constrictive pattern, pressure equalization, RA=RV=LV diastole

176. Which of the following show a "square root sign" √‾ in the LV, RV, RA and usually LA pressures, as shown in the diagram?

1. **IHSS/HOCM**
2. **Restrictive cardiomyopathy**
3. **Constrictive pericarditis**
4. **Pericardial tamponade**
5. **Underdamped CHF**

   a. 1, 3
   b. 1, 4
   c. 2, 3
   d. 3, 4

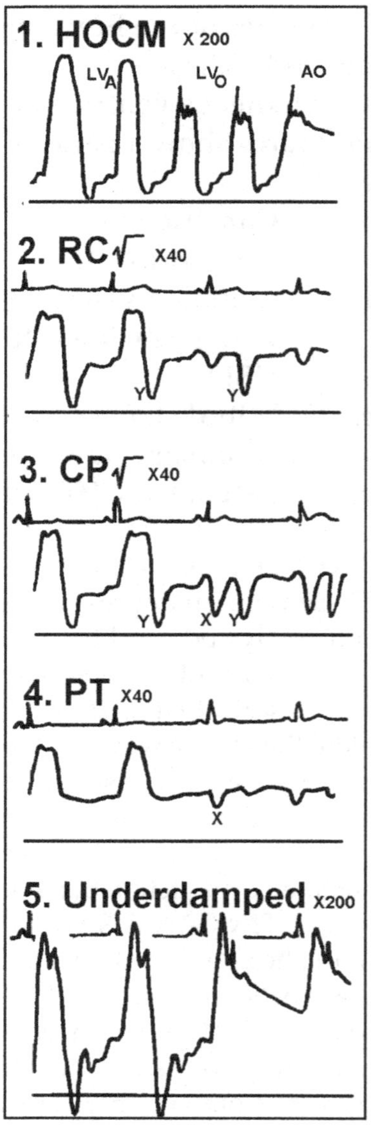

Pullback Pressures

ANSWER c. 2 & 3. Restrictive cardiomyopathy (RC) and Constrictive pericarditis (CP). Square root sign begins with the atrial "y" wave and the "beginning diastolic" ventricular wave. It is the sudden drop in pressure when the AV valve opens and the ventricles fill by the "suction cup effect." In CP this is the only filling the ventricle gets. The rapid diastolic dip ("y wave") is followed by a plateau in which it can't fill further because of its tight "tin can" "constrictive" pericardium. **BE ABLE TO CORRECTLY MATCH ALL ANSWERS BELOW:**

1. **IHSS/HOCM** Pullback pressure x2OO. LV-apex ➔ LV ➔ outflow tract ➔ AO, shows systolic gradient between LV-apex and LV-outflow tract. Small normal "y" waves are seen - No plateau.
2. **Restrictive cardiomyopathy:** pullback from RV to RA on x4O. The dip and plateau waves (√‾) are seen which are termed "beginning diastolic" in the RV and "y" waves in the atria. (Suction cup effect)
3. **Constrictive pericarditis:** pullback from RV to RA on x4O. In the RA pressure two dips are seen - the "x" and "y" wave which make a "W" pattern.
4. **Pericardial tamponade**: Shows pullback from RV to RA. The elevated diastolic level is seen with normal or small atrial waves. (NO √‾)
5. **Undamped transducer:** pullback from LV to AO on x200. Note the peaked pressures which overshoot the true systolic. Also, note the negative beginning diastolic pattern which undershoot diastole. The beginning diastolic wave should not be

below zero. This is an artifact which mimics(√‾) termed a "false of pseudo-square root sign."

One way to remember which diseases have √‾ and which have = is:

- Only the two diseases which include the term "-strictive" show the square root sign
- The two diseases that include the term "pericard-" show pressure equalization
- The pathologic term that includes both "-strictive and pericard-"

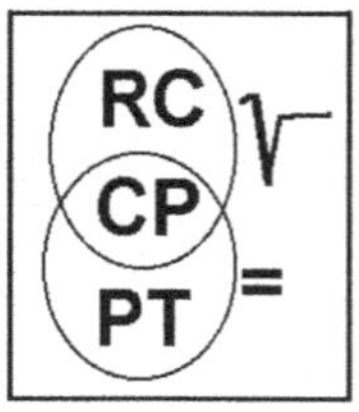

pericard-"√‾", -strictive "="

(constrictive pericarditis) has both square root sign and pressure equalization
See: Baim, chapter on "Profiles in Constrictive ... Restrictive ... Tamponade." **Keywords:** square root sign seen in RC & CP

177. A patient's intra-cardiac pressures all show a deep "y" wave and a diastolic plateau (square root sign). His pressure readings in the box indicate probable:

a. Mitral regurgitation
b. Constrictive pericarditis
c. Pericardial tamponade
d. Idiopathic hypertrophic subaortic stenosis

HEMODYNAMIC FINDINGS
RV = 36/15,25 mmHg
RA = 26,28,20
LV = 95/10,25
LA = 27,22,20
(Square Root sign in all)

ANSWER b. Constrictive pericarditis. Constrictive disease intracardiac pressures all show elevation of the diastolic plateau. But only constrictive pericarditis causes the equalization of diastolic pressures and square root sign (√) as described by a deep "Y" wave. Note how all the end diastolic pressure readings are very close (circled). Distinguish between the hemodynamics of the 3 major constrictive diseases: Restrictive cardiomyopathy, constrictive pericarditis, and pericardial tamponade (RC, CP, & PT).
See: Baim, chapter on "Profiles in Constrictive Disease." **Keywords:** ID pressures of constrictive pericarditis

HEMODYNAMIC FINDINGS
RV = 36/15/25 mmHg
RA = 26/28/20 mmHg
LV = 95/10/25 mmHg
LA = 27/22/20 mmHg
(Square Root sign in all)

178. Despite many pressure similarities tamponade and constriction may be distinguished by their differing RA pressure waveforms. Cardiac tamponade shows a:

a. Large X descent (small or absent Y)
b. Large Y descent (small or absent X)
c. Large A wave (small or absent V)
d. Large V wave (small or absent A)

ANSWER a. Large X descent (small Y). Ward says: " Despite many pressure similar hemodynamic features, tamponade and constriction may be distinguished by the different CVP waveforms... ***In tamponade, the venous pressure waveform appears more monophasic and is dominated by the systolic x pressure descent, while the diastolic y pressure descent is attenuated or absent*** because early diastolic flow from the RA to RV is impaired by the surrounding compressive pericardial fluid collection. " See tracings in next question. This is not termed square root sign, because it is a dip in the X wave and there is no diastolic plateau. Square root involves a dip (Y or suction cup wave) and plateau during diastole, and is associated with constrictive disease.
See: Ward, chapter on "Pericardial constriction and cardiac Tamponade"

179. In what stage of pericardial tamponade are all the intracardiac diastolic pressures elevated and equal (RA = RV-ED = PAW = LV-EDP) as shown?

- a. **Normal hemodynamics**
- b. **Early stage #1**
- c. **Intermediate stage #2**
- d. **End stage #3**

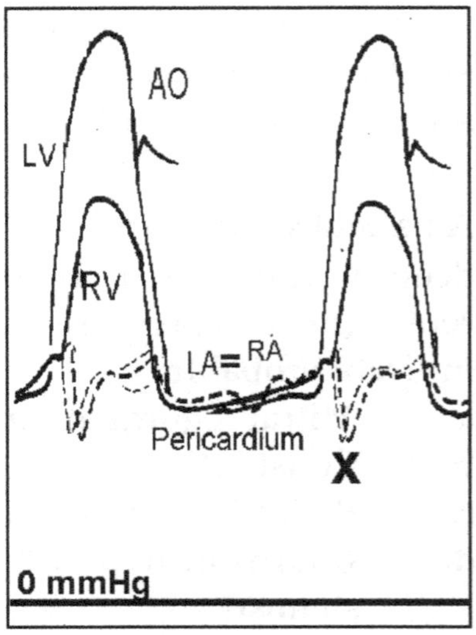

ANSWER d. End stage #3. This final stage of tamponade can be terminal if pericardial pressure is not relieved quickly by pericardiocentesis. In this end stage, ventricular collapse occurs. RA, RV, LA & LV pressures equalize at a very high pressure, systolic BP falls, and pulsus paradoxus is evident. All intracardiac filling pressures are compressed within the overfilled pericardial sack. Note in the diagram below how pericardial pressure normally starts below zero. Then as the pericardium fills and pericardial pressure rises it pushes all the intracardiac diastolic pressures up with it. Impaired filling then reduces systolic function. Note how systole falls with rising diastolic pressures. When intrapericardial pressure rises above the RA systolic pressure, inversion and collapse of the RA free wall occurs. **See:** Kern, Hemodynamic Rounds **See:** Kern, Hemodynamic Rounds on "Pericardial Compressive Hemodynamics, Part I." **Keywords:** ID stages of pericardial tamponade

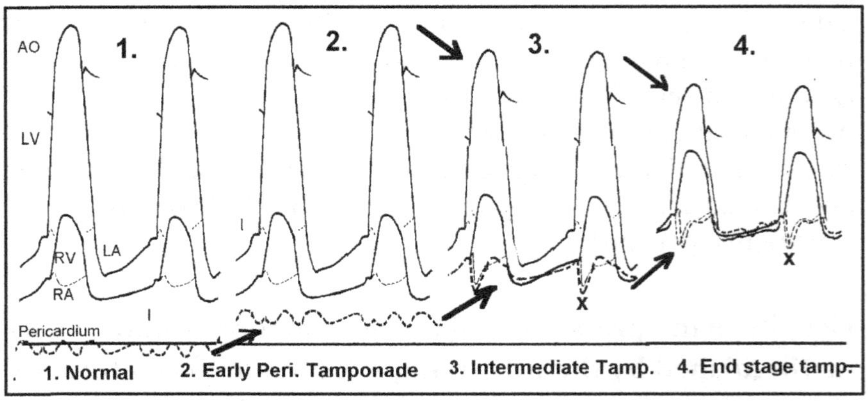

LV, AO, LA, RV, and RA pressures x200 Stages of pericardial tamponade

180. Kussmaul's sign, showing increased venous pressures, is associated with:

- a. **Atrial septal defect**
- b. **Third degree block**
- c. **Pulmonary embolus**
- d. **Pericardial tamponade**
- e. **Constrictive pericarditis**

Answer: e. Constrictive pericarditis. Kussmaul's Sign is a paradoxical rise in the height of jugular venous pulse during inspiration (normal response is drop in venous pressure with inspiration), which occurs frequently in patients with chronic constrictive pericarditis and sometimes in congestive heart failure. See: Braunwald chapter on "Physical assessment"

181. Your physician asks you to record simultaneous RV and LV pressures on the same scale. Why?

a. Screen for ventricular dextrocardia
b. Screen for valvular stenosis or regurgitation
c. Screen for restrictive or constrictive pathology
d. Screen for right or left sided heart failure
e. Screen for right or left sided ventricular hypertrophy

Answer: c. Screen for restrictive or constrictive pathology. Ragosta says, "Combination Left Ventricular and Right Ventricular Pressures: This maneuver is performed to screen for the presence of restrictive or constrictive physiology and should be a part of all complete, hemodynamic evaluations." This relates to ventricular concordance and discordance with respiration. See: Ragosta, chapter on "Normal Waveforms" Keywords: simultaneous RV-LV screens for restrictive or constrictive pathology

182. This simultaneous LV - RV pressure tracing demonstrates diastolic pressure equalization with:

a. Spike and dome pattern and constrictive pericarditis
b. Spike and dome pattern and pericardial tamponade
c. Square root sign of constrictive pericarditis
d. Square root sign of pericardial tamponade

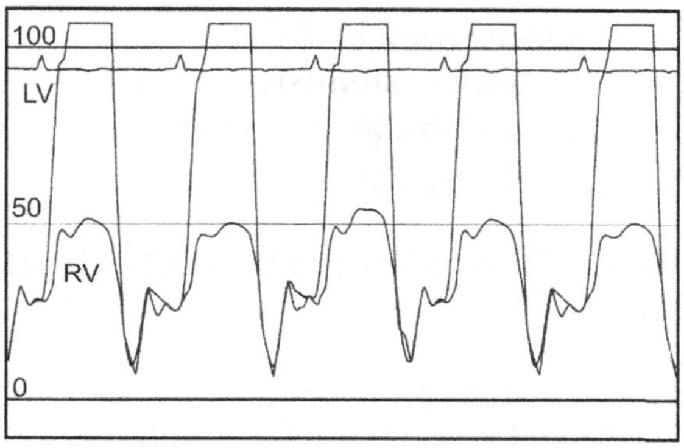

LV & RV After Ragosta Cardiac Catheterization Text

Answer: c. Square root sign (Dip and plateau) of constrictive pericarditis. The ventricular rapid filling phase is exaggerated making a deep "y" wave, followed by a diastolic plateau where the two ventricular pressures equalize. This dip and plateau pattern looks like a square root sign in math $\sqrt{\ }$. They equalize because of the rigid pericardium which allows filling of both chambers up to the same maximum point (like a balloon in a can). Remember the 2 diseases with square root sign end in "-strictive". See: Ragosta, chapter on "Classic Hemodynamic Waveforms" Keywords: CP = square root sign + diastolic equalization

CONGENITAL PATHOLOGY

BOTH QUESTIONS BELOW REFER TO THIS DIAGRAM :

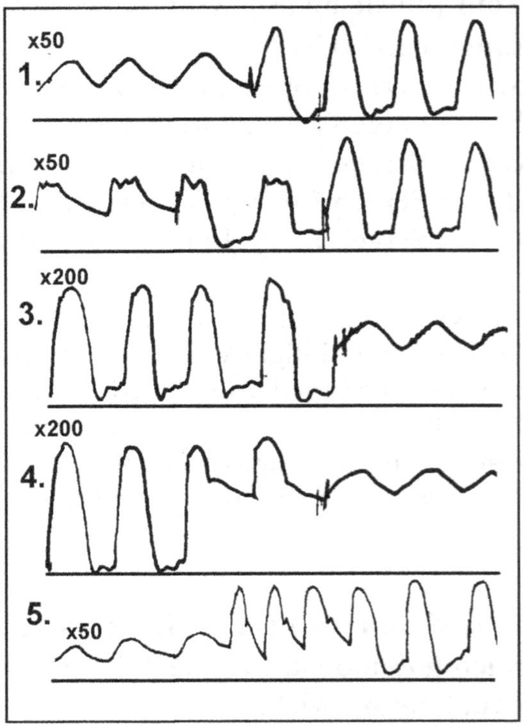

Congenital Obstruction - Pullback Pressures

183. Identify the abnormal pullback pressure labeled #2 in the diagram.
- **a. Infundibular stenosis**
- **b. Coarctation of PA**
- **c. Pulmonary stenosis**
- **d. Tricuspid stenosis**

184. What congenital defect is diagnosed by the pullback labeled #4.
- **a. Coarctation of the PA**
- **b. Coarctation of AO**
- **c. Pulmonic stenosis**
- **d. Infundibular stenosis**
- **e. Aortic stenosis**

BOTH ANSWERS ARE LISTED TOGETHER BELOW:

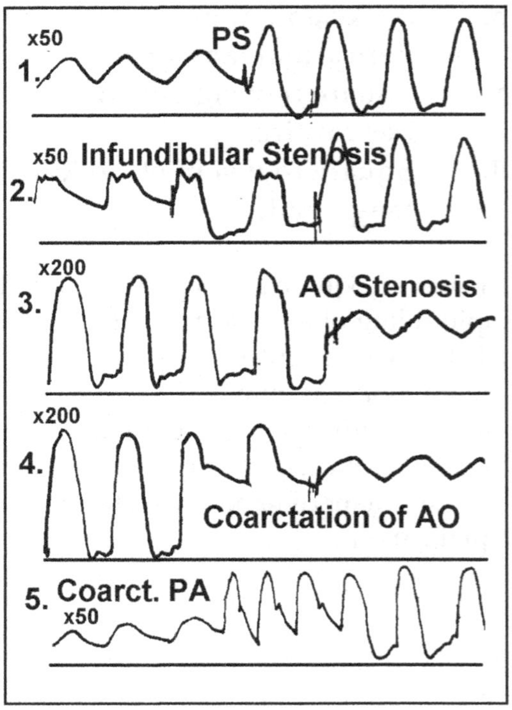

Pullbacks in Congenital Obstruction

183. ANSWER #2 = a. Infundibular stenosis. The PA and chopped-off LV systolic pressure match. RV systolic inflow pressure is increased over the middle RV outflow track. This is a type of HOCM/IHSS in the RV. **See:** Kern, chapter on "Hemodynamics." **Keywords:** ID Pullback tracings, RV outflow infundibular stenosis

184. ANSWER #4=b. Coarctation of AO. In mild coarctation there is only a systolic pressure gradient. BE ABLE TO MATCH ALL ANSWERS:

1. PULMONIC STENOSIS: Pullback from PA to RV on x 50. Systolic gradient across the pulmonic valve. slow upstroke of PA pressure. Simultaneous pressures indicated on diagram at right.

2. INFUNDIBULAR STENOSIS: Pullback from PA-RV outflow-RV inflow on x 50. It shows Subvalvular (infundibular) stenosis. The RV outflow systolic peak appears "chopped off." This is a "dynamic gradient" within the RV outflow tract

(infundibulum) similar to IHSS/HOCM on the left side.

3. AORTIC STENOSIS: Pullback from LV to AO on x 200. Systolic gradient is noted across the aortic valve. Simultaneous pressures indicated on diagram above.

4. COARCTATION OF AO: Pullback from LV-Ascending AO - Descending AO on x 200. Systolic gradient within the aorta, across the coarctation. Aortic systolic pressures differ. Diastole is the same. In the early milder stages of coarctation only a systolic gradient is noted. The descending aortic tracing appears damped with a slow upstroke.

5. COARCTATION of PA: Pullback from branch PA - Main PA -RV on X 50. Severe gradient noted between the two PA tracings. Late in severe coarctation the gradient both occurs in both systole and diastole.

See: Baim, Chapter on "Cardiac Catheterization in Infants and Children"

185. These are right heart catheter pullback pressure tracings. What abnormality is labeled at #2?

a. Pulmonary arteriolar gradient

b. Pulmonary valvular gradient (PS)

c. Intra-RV gradient (Infundibular stenosis)

d. Tricuspid valvular gradient (TS)

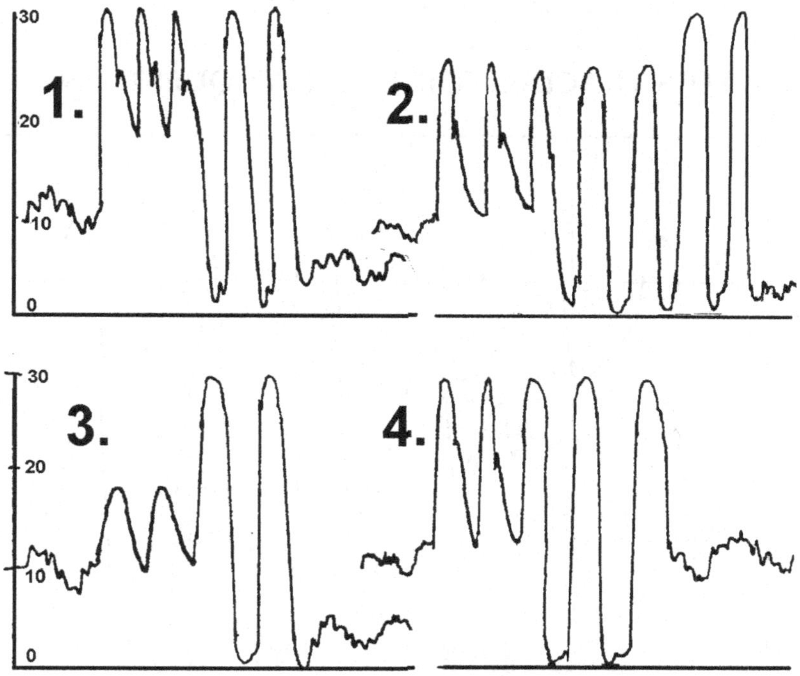

Swan-Ganz Right Heart catheter pullback

ANSWER c. Intra-RV gradient (Infundibular stenosis) .

BE ABLE TO MATCH ALL ANSWERS:

1. Pulmonary Arteriolar gradient:

Compare the initial PAW to the PA pressure that follows. The PAW mean should equal the PA end-diastolic pressure or not be more than 6 mmHg lower. Here there is a 10 mmHg. gradient indicative of possible stenosis between the PA and the pulmonary arterioles/capillaries. This can happen in pulmonary hypertension and various lung diseases. With increased CO this gradient occurs normally.

2. Infundibular stenosis (intra-RV gradient):

Compare the RV outflow with RV inflow pressures. They should be the same. An intra-cavity systolic gradient due to infundibular stenosis exists. (analogous to HOCM/IHSS)

3. Pulmonary Valve stenosis (Pulmonary valvular gradient):

Compare the PA systolic to the RV systolic pressure. **They should be equal**. A systolic gradient exists due to a tight pulmonic valve. (analogous to AS)

4. Tricuspid valve stenosis (Tricuspid valvular gradient):

Compare RV diastolic with RA mean pressure. They should be the same. A tricuspid valve gradient exists. (comparable to MS)

NORMAL RT. HEART PULLBACK should look like this with equalization of PAW ≈ PA-edp, PA syst. = RV syst., RV-edp = RA mean.

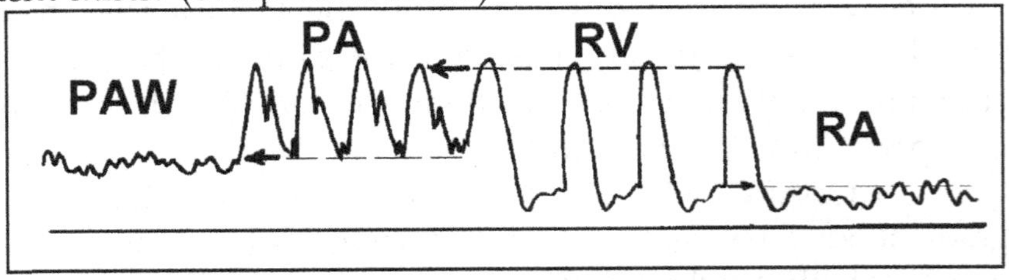

Normal rt... Ht. pullback: PAW-PA-RVO-RV-RA

See: Baim, chapter on "Profiles in Valvular Ht. Disease." **Keywords:** Right heart pullback, arteriolar stenosis, pulmonary stenosis, infundibular stenosis. tricuspid stenosis

USE THIS TRACING FOR THE NEXT QUESTION:

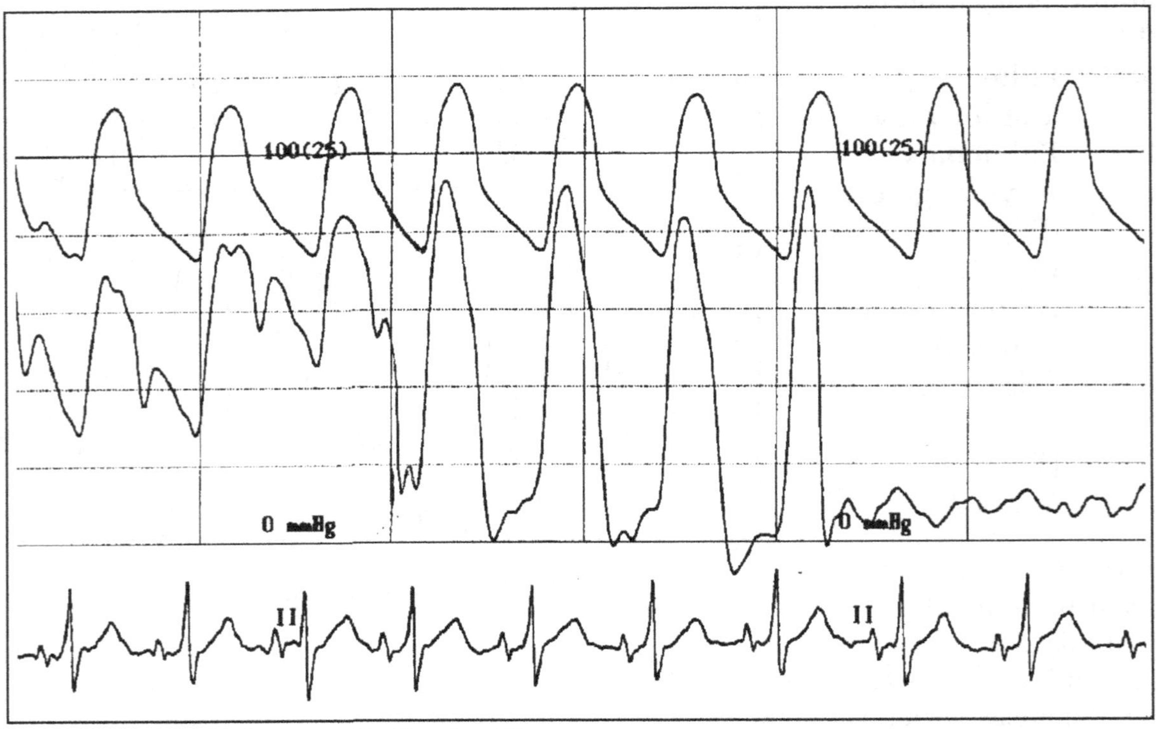

AO x 200 with Right heart Pullback x 50.

186. **The pressure tracings above are AO on x 200 and a right heart pullback on x 50. These pressures are consistent with a diagnosis of:**

a. **Normal valve function**

b. **Pulmonary valve regurgitation**

c. **Tricuspid valve regurgitation**

d. **Aortic regurgitation**

ANSWER a. Normal valve function. Pressures are all within the normal range. They read as:

AO 117/74, 93 mmHg
PA 18/8,13
RV 23, 0, 2
RA 3,3,2

There appears to be a slight pulmonary stenosis gradient. But this is only because we do not have enough PA to get a steady end expiratory reading.
See: Kern, chapter on "Hemodynamics." Keywords: normal right heart pullback

THE NEXT TWO TRACINGS ARE FROM THE SAME CYANOTIC CHILD.

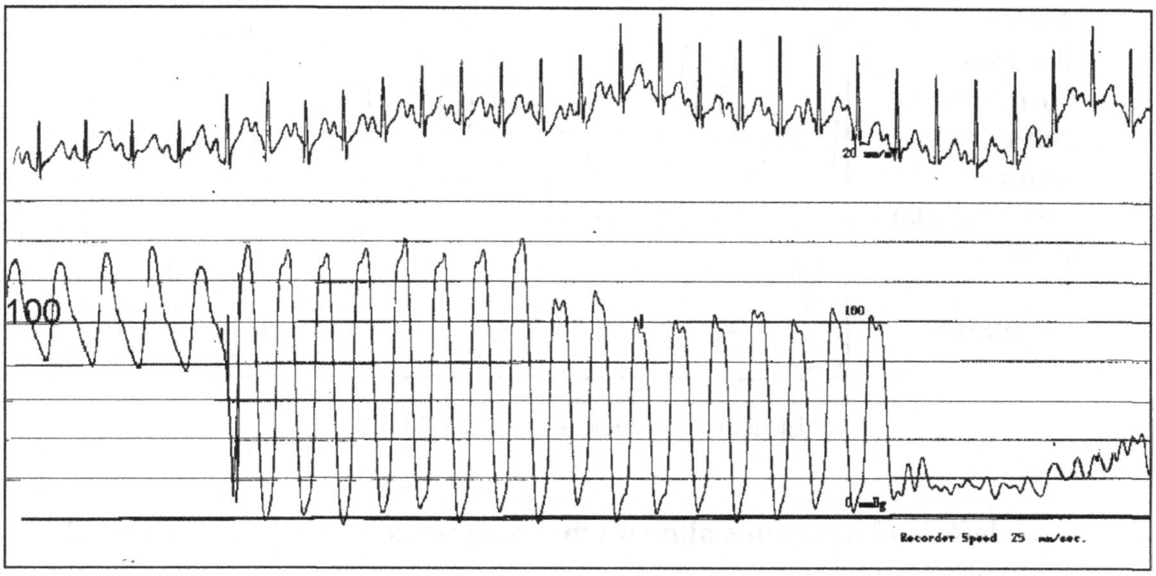

AO - LV - RV - RA x 200

187. A right heart catheter was pulled back from the AO. This pullback passes through a/an:

a. PDA
b. ASD
c. VSD
d. Coarctation of AO

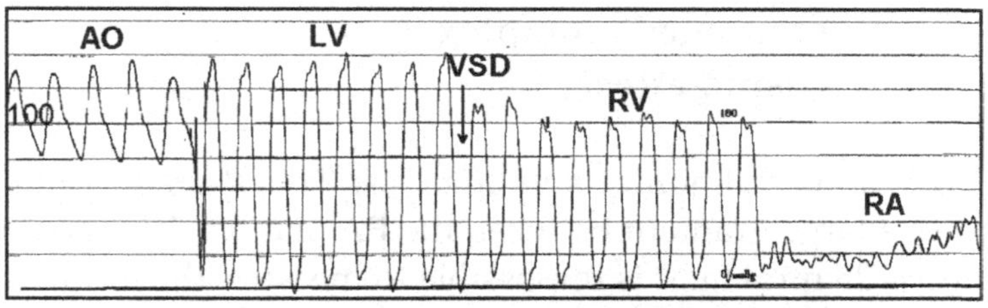

Catheter pullback from AO →LV→VSD→RV→RA.

ANSWER c. VSD. Catheter pressures pass from AO →LV→VSD→RV→RA. Note the 30 mmHg pressure gradient across the ventricular septal defect. This usually indicates a relatively small defect or very high shunt flow. Large VSDs, just like normal valves, show no gradient. Initial catheter position is shown in this drawing.
See: Kern, Hemodynamic Rounds on."Adult Congenital

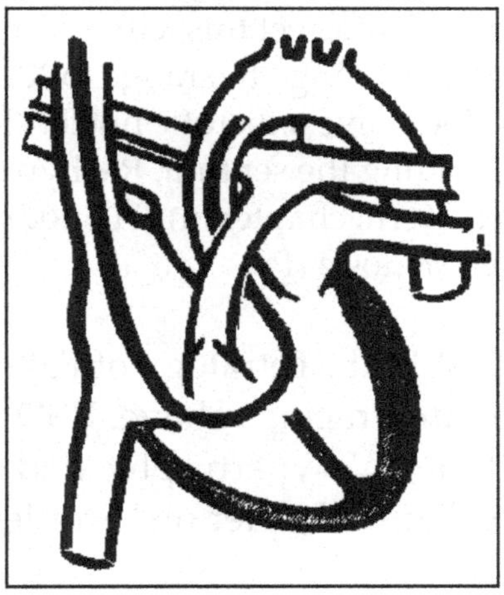

AO →LV→VSD→RV→RA

Anomalies." Keywords: VSD

188. **A pediatric Swan Ganz catheter was pulled back from the lungs in the same cyanotic child shown above. The pressure recording below suggests a diagnosis of:**

a. **Aortic stenosis**
b. **Pulmonic valve stenosis**
c. **Infundibular stenosis**
d. **PA coarctation**

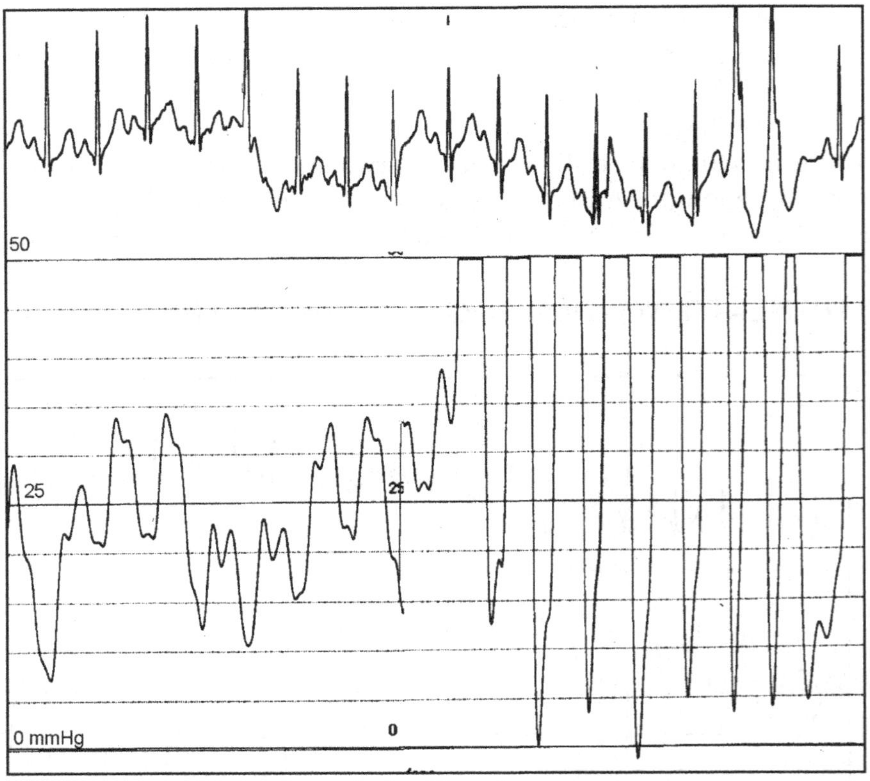

Right heart pullback recorded x 50 scale

189. **With these defects (2 questions above) what diagnosis is likely in this child?**

a. **Transposition of great vessels**
b. **Tetralogy of Fallot**
c. **Eisenminger's complex**
d. **Tricuspid atresia**

ANSWER b. Pulmonic valve stenosis. This PA→RV pullback shows a large gradient between the PA and RV. The gradient exceeds 25 mmHg. It is impossible to measure the gradient exactly because the RV systolic pressure is off the scale, at the top of the paper. To correct this, either extend the grid to the top of the paper, or change the range to X 100. The PA waveform is distorted but does have a dicrotic notch. Tetralogy of Fallot has: VSD, AO over-riding the septum, RV hypertrophy, and pulmonary stenosis. See: Kern, chapter on "Hemodynamics." Keywords: Pulmonary valve stenosis (PS)

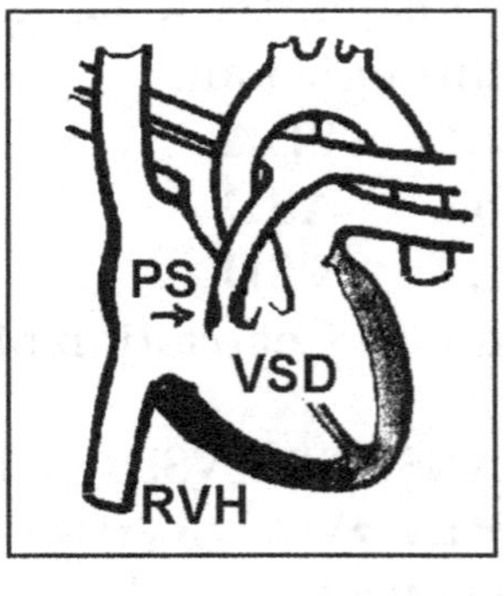

ANSWER b. Tetralogy of Fallot. Two of the criteria for TET are shown in the pressure tracings above: VSD and pulmonary stenosis. The other criteria for TET include RV hypertrophy and overriding aorta can best be diagnosed with echo. See: Baim, chapter on "Profiles in Congenital Heart Disease." Keywords: Tetralogy of Fallot (TET)

USE THIS TRACING FOR THE NEXT 2 QUESTIONS:

190. **A pediatric Swan Ganz catheter was pulled back from the lungs. The pressure recording below suggests a diagnosis of:**

a. **Aortic stenosis**
b. **Pulmonic valve stenosis**
c. **Infundibular stenosis**
d. **PA coarctation**

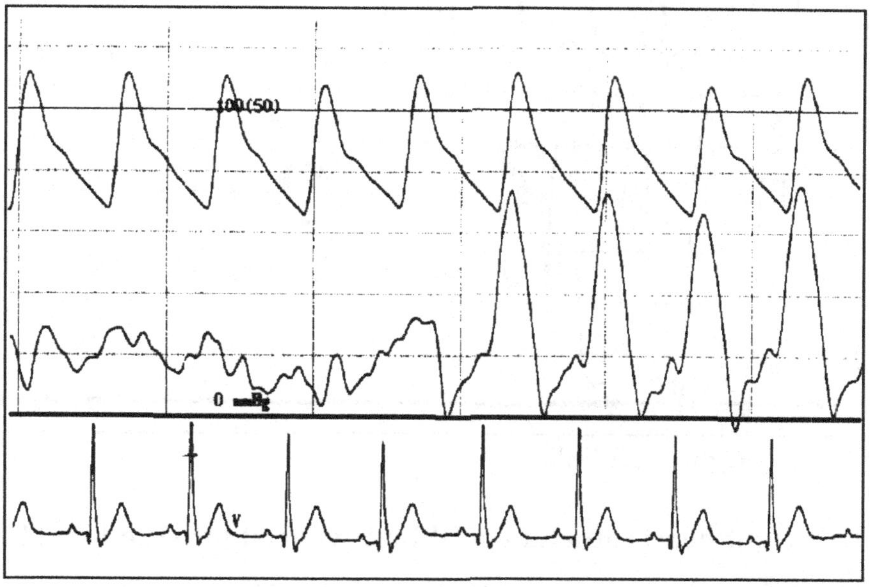

AO (x 200 scale) with MPA→RV pullback recorded (X 100 scale)

ANSWER b. Pulmonic valve stenosis.

The pullback shows a 25 mmHg peak-to-peak systolic gradient between Main PA and RV, indicating pulmonary valvular stenosis. Although PA tracings in PS are often severely distorted, a distinct PA dicrotic notch is evident. These simultaneous tracings are recorded at different scale settings - AO on x 200 and PA-RV on x 100.

See: Kern, chapter on "Hemodynamics." Keywords: Pulmonary valve stenosis (PS)

191. **How would you read the RV pressure above? (Note the 2 different sensitivities/scales)**

a. **15/ 2/ 10 mmHg**
b. **30/ 0/ 20 mmHg**
c. **35/ 0, 10 mmHg**
d. **80/ 0, 20 mmHg**

ANSWER c. 35/0, 10 mmHg. or 35/0 /10 mmHg.

These simultaneous tracings are recorded at different scale settings - AO on x 200 and PA-RV on x 100. For the right heart channel, this makes each line 10 mmHg.

AO = 110/68, 85 mmHg
MPA=15/7, 10 mmHg
RV =35/0, 10

See: Kern, chapter on "Hemodynamics." Keywords: Pulmonary valve stenosis (PS)

USE THIS PULLBACK TRACING FOR THE NEXT QUESTION.

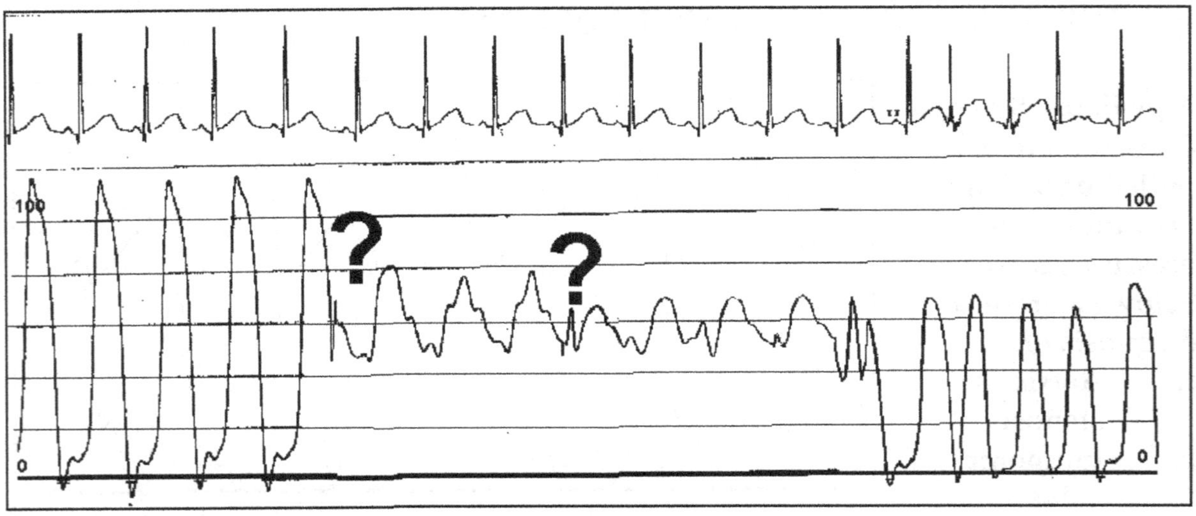

LV-AO - Right heart Pullback x200

192. This right heart catheter could be advanced into the LV. The above pull back suggest:

a. AS and PDA

b. AS and VSD

c. PDA and VSD

d. Coarctation of AO

ANSWER a. AS and PDA. This pullback goes from LV➔AO➔PDA➔PA➔RV. There is an initial drop in pressure across the AO valve indicating AS. In the center of the tracing the AO tracing slightly drops the systolic pressure, while the diastole remains the same. This is characteristic of most PDA and coarctation pullbacks. The location of the catheter prior to pullback is shown in the drawing. Note how it crosses the PDA in the center of the tracing. There is no gradient from PA to RV. See: Kern, Hemodynamic Rounds on."Adult Congenital Anomalies." Keywords: AS and PDA pullback

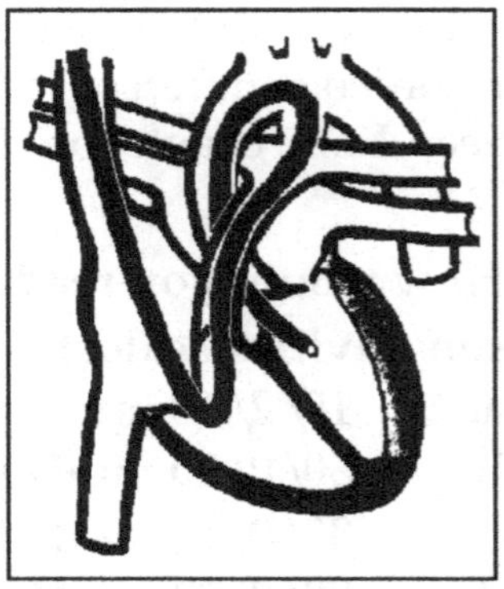

LV➔AO➔PDA➔PA➔ RV pullback

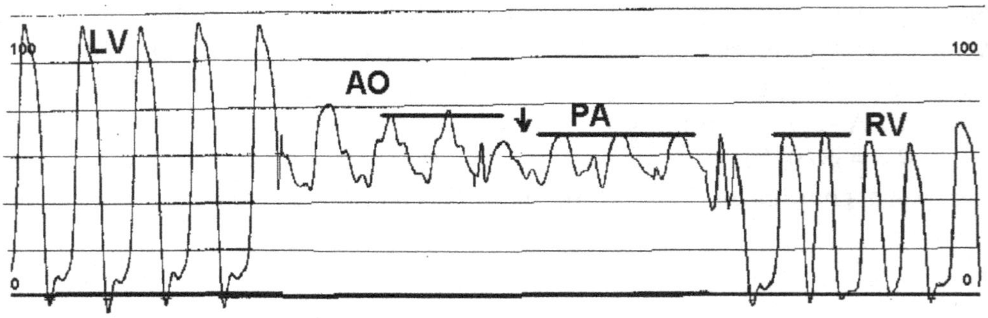

Catheter pullback in child with combined AS and PDA

OTHER PRESSURES

193. During transseptal cardiac catheterization you are monitoring Brockenbrough needle pressure on X40. The cardiologist advances the needle and you note the waveform shown at #3. The most likely position of the needle tip is ___.

a. Aorta
b. LA
c. Pericardium
d. Myocardial wall

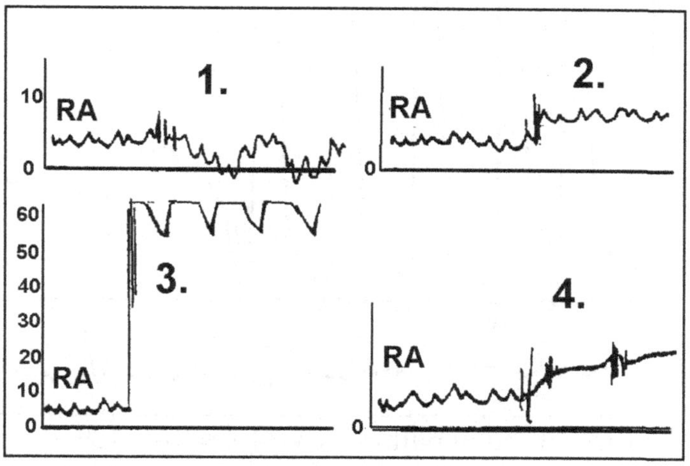

Brockenbrough needle monitored Pressure

ANSWER a. Aorta. This is an OOPS! Note that part of the arterial waveform is visible at the top of the screen. BE ABLE TO MATCH THE OTHER WAVE-FORMS SHOWN with the needle tip position below.

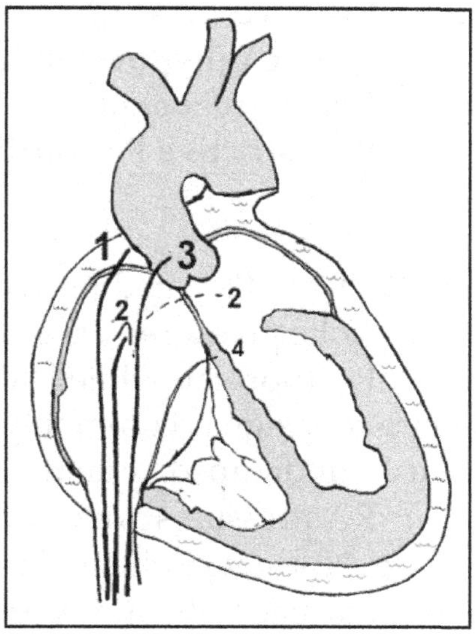

1. PERICARDIUM. As the needle crosses into the pericardium the pressure drops suddenly because of negative pleural pressure. This can lead to the potential complication of tamponade. When the small needle tip is withdrawn it usually heals over. Do not advance the catheter. That just widens the hole, and tamponade is more likely.
2. LA: GOOD! That is what you want. LA pressure is 5-12 mmHg. with "a" and "v" waves. This can be checked by drawing a small blood sample (it should be bright red) or by a contrast test injection through the needle.
3. AORTA: Aortic pressure is off the screen. Pressure monitoring is essential to see inadvertent aortic puncture. When the small needle tip is withdrawn it usually heals over. Do not advance the catheter if the needle is in the aorta. That just widens the hole, and tamponade is likely. If bleeding does occur the Brockenbrough catheter can be used to plug the puncture site while the patient is taken to surgery. Pericardial centesis in the lab may be lifesaving.
4. MYOCARDIUM: THIS pressure appears damped because it is intra-myocardial, within atrial or aortic tissue. Small test injections (done by hand) may stain the myocardium, mark it, and make it more visible. With this, if the needle is found to be in the free it should be withdrawn. Advance only if it is within the in the interatrial septum or LA.

See: Baim , Chapter on "Percutaneous Approach" Keywords: Transseptal complication → AO puncture & tamponade

USE THIS TRACING FOR THE NEXT QUESTION:

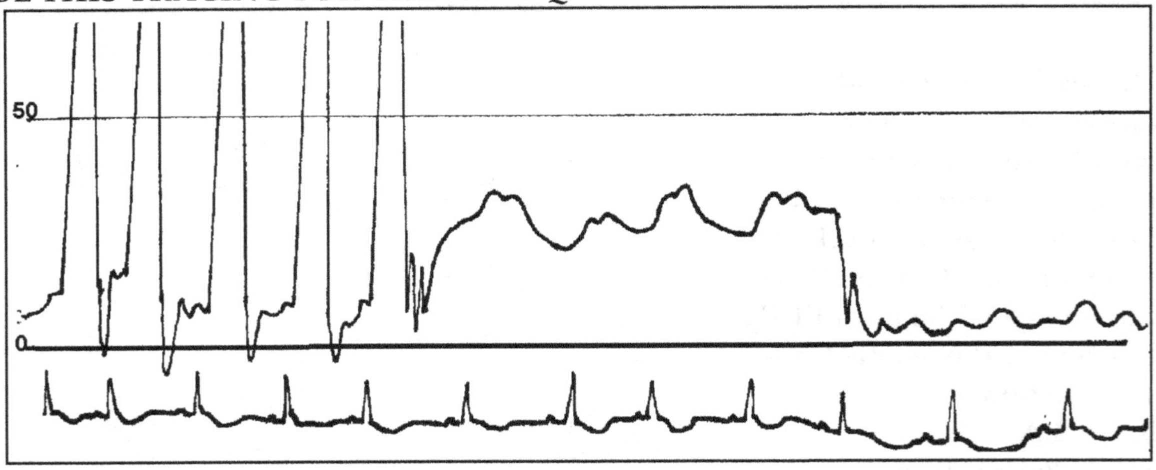

Brockenbrough pullback LV→LA→RA x 100

194. The recording above was made as a Brockenbrough transseptal catheter was pulled back. What is abnormal about it?

- a. **Elevated LV-EDP (CHF)**
- b. **Elevated LA (MS)**
- c. **Low RA (hypovolemia)**
- d. **Square root sign (Constrictive Pericarditis)**

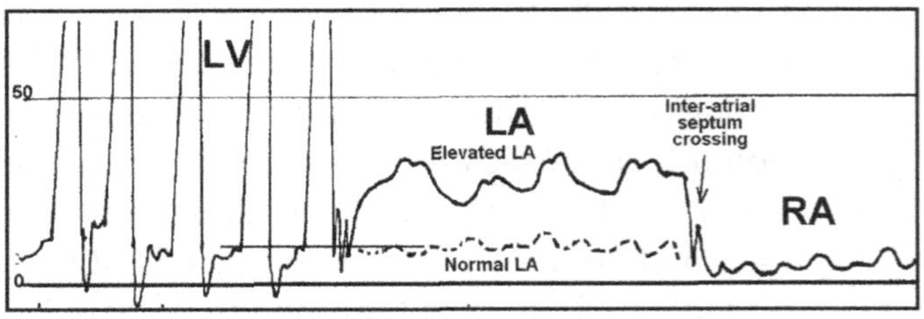

Pullback of antegrade Brockenbrough catheter

ANSWER b. Elevated LA (MS). LV diastolic pressures are around 10 mmHg (normal) while LA pressure is elevated at around 25 mmHg. False square root sign is commonly seen in LV tracings recorded from an undamped system (LV should never go below zero). RA pressures are low and normal at around 5 mmHg. Normal LA is similar to PAW = 5-13 mmHg. See: Verel, Cardiac Cath and Angiography, 1973, chapter on "Measuring Pressure" Keywords: transseptal pullback with MS

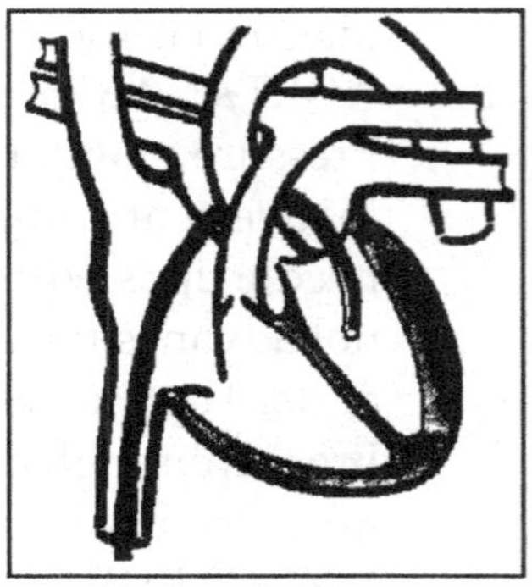

pullback LV→LA→RA

REFERENCES:

Ahrens, T. S., and Taylor, L.A., *Hemodynamic Waveform Analysis,* 1st Ed., W.B. Saunders Co., 1992

Baim, D. S. and Grossman W., *Cardiac Catheterization, Angiography, and Intervention,* 7th Ed., Lea and Febiger, 2004

Braunwald, et. al. Ed., *Heart Disease, a Textbook of CV Medicine,* 8th Ed., Saunders, 2008

Berne R. M. and Levy, M. N., *Cardiovascular Physiology,* 6th Ed., Mosby Year Book, 1992

Daily, E. K., and Schroeder, J. S., *Techniques in Bedside Hemodynamic Monitoring,* 4th Ed., C. V. Mosby Company, 1989

Darovic, G.O., *Hemodynamic Monitoring: Invasive and Noninvasive Clinical Application,* WB Saunders, 1995

Kern, M.J., *Hemodynamic Rounds: interpretation of cardiac pathophysiology from pressure waveform analysis,* St. Louis, Wiley-Liss, 1993

Kern, M. J., Ed., *The Cardiac Catheterization Handbook,* 4th Ed., Mosby-Year Book, 2003

Pepine, J. C., and Hill, J. A., et. al., *Diagnostic and Therapeutic Cardiac Catheterization,* 2nd Ed., Williams and Wilkins, 1994

Ragosta, Michael, Textbook of Clinical Hemodynamics, Saunders, 1st Edition, 2008

Taylor, E. J. Ed., *Dorland's Medical Dictionary,* 27th ed., W. B. Saunders Co.,1988

Verel D. and Grainger R., *Cardiac Catheterization and Angiography, an Introductory Manual,* 2nd Ed., Churchill Livingstone, 1973

Ward, Johnathan B, *Atlas of Cardiovascular Monitoring,* Churchill Livingstone, 1998

OUTLINE: Pressure Pathology

1. IDENTIFY ARTERIAL PULSE contours & pathologies
- a. Pulsus alternans = CHF
- b. Pulsus bigeminus = PVCs
- c. Pulsus bisferiens = HOCM
- d. Pulsus tardus = AS
- e. Corrigan's pulse = AI

2. IDENTIFY VALVE PATHOLOGIES
- a. Prolapsed, floppy
- b. Insufficient, incompetent
- c. Leaky, insufficient
- d. Stenotic, obstructive

3. CORONARY ARTERIOGRAPHY
- a. Identify damping waveforms
- 1. Ventricularization
  - Main stem lesion danger
  - Widowmaker
  - c. Reduced pressure damping
  - d. LV (retrograde across valve-not ventricularization)
  - e. High frequency damping (incomplete damping)
  - f. mixed LV-AO
- b. BAD EFFECTS OF DAMPING
  - 1. cuts off blood flow - ischemia
  - 2. may tip up a plaque or dissect
  - 3. spasm
  - 4. Main stem lesion danger
  - Ventricularization
  - pull back catheter

- c. EFFECTS OF HIGH-OSMOLAR CONTRAST ON CORONARIES
  - 1. bradycardia
  - 2. hypotension
  - 3. asystole/arrhythmia
    - Bradycardia - SA,
    - AV node with
    - RCA
    - Cough CPR
  - 4. RCA injection = ST depr. in II
  - 5. LCA injection = ST elevation LII
  - 6. Normal recovery post injection

- d. CONGESTIVE HEART FAILURE PRESSURES
  - 1. Low dP/dT
  - 2. elevated LV-edp & wedge

3 CONSTRICTIVE - RESTRICTIVE PRESSURES
- 1. Square root sign
  - CM - restrictive myopathy
  - CP - Constrictive pericarditis
  - Tin-can analogy
- 2. Distinguish from
  - PT - Pericardial tamponade
  - Under damped
  - CHF - Congestive heart failure
- 3 SIMULTANEOUS PRESSURE RECORDINGS - WHY?
  - RV-LV, Restrictive/constrictive
  - LA (wedge)- LV, MS
  - AO-LV, AS, HOCM

4. MYOCARDIAL & PERICARDIAL
- 1. Restrictive cardiomyopathy
- 2. Constrictive Pericarditis
  - Tin can analogy
- 3. Pericardial Tamponade
- 4. HOCM
- 5. Kussmaul's sign

5. CONGENITAL PATHOLOGY
- 1. Coarctation of the PA
- 2. Coarctation of AO
- 3. Pulmonic Stenosis
  - pulmonary arteriolar gradient
  - infundibular stenosis
- 4. Aortic Stenosis
  - HOCM
- 5. Mitral stenosis
  - cor-triatriatum
  - LA myxoma
- 6. Tricuspid stenosis
- 7. Shunts
  - ASD, PDA, VSD
  - Tetralogy Fallot

6. OTHER PATHOLOGY
transseptal stick pressures
- 1. Aorta
- 2. LA
- 3. Pericardium
- 4. Myocardial wall
- 5. LV-LA-RA pullback

VALVULAR & Practice Tracings

INDEX E5:

1. Valvular Stenosis and Regurgitation

ABNORMAL VALVULAR PRESSURES

General

195. **In the simultaneous pressure tracing diagram shown, identify the chamber/vessel labeled at #1 and what valvular disease it represents.**

a. **AO, HOCM**
b. **AO, AS**
c. **AO, AR**
d. **PAW, MS**
e. **PAW, MR**

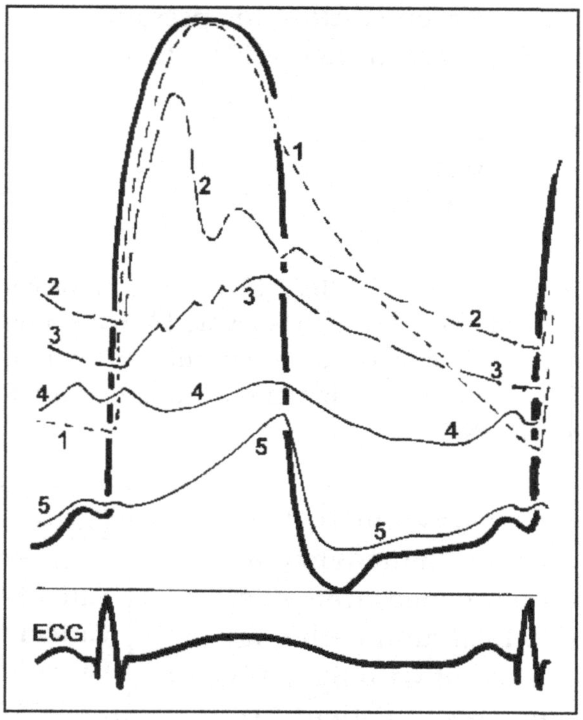

Normal LV pressure tracing simultaneous Abnormal Aorta and LA (PAW) tracings.

BE ABLE TO CORRECTLY MATCH ALL ANSWERS BELOW:

1. AO, AR:

AO, AR. Note that no gradient exists (no stenosis). But the diastolic AO pressure is very low. This continues to fall as blood leaks from the AO into the LV and in severe AR may fall to the LV-edp.

2. AO, HOCM:

AO, HOCM (Previously called IHSS). Although this is not a "valvular" disease, it is similar to AS in many respects. LV-AO gradient occurs because the LV outflow track is itself a dynamic stenosis. It obstructs flow during systole. There may be an initial (tidal wave) and then a sudden release - only to obstruct again as the LV walls come closer together. (See: bisferiens pulse). Pullback tracings identify two levels of pressure within the LV - one above and one below the obstruction. No gradient exists between the subvalvular LV chamber (not shown) and the AO. Gradient exists between the apical LV tracing and the AO (shown).

3. AO, AS:

AO, AS. Note the classic pulsus tardus with slow AO upstroke. A gradient exists between the LV & AO throughout systole, that is usually greatest in mid-systole. The diamond shaped murmur peaks in systole just like the gradient.

4. PAW, MS:

PAW, MS. Note the PAW-LV gradient throughout diastole.

5. PAW, MR:

PAW, MR. Note that no gradient exists (No gradient, no stenosis). But the v wave late in systole indicates the LA is flooded with blood from the leaky mitral valve The LV pressure tracing is shown in dotted lines. Remember how normal simultaneous tracings overlap (See - Wiggers diagram). Normal AO-LV tracings should match in systole. Normal LV-PAW tracings should match in diastole.

See: Braunwald, chapter on "Physical Examination." Keywords: valvular defects, simultaneous pressures, HOCM, AS, AR, MS, MR

196. This box summarizes Jack Black's hemodynamic pressure measurements. All of his pressure readings are normal EXCEPT:

a. PAW

b. PA

c. RV

d. RA

PATIENT # 196 CARDIAC PRESSURES			
	LV	= 140/0,10	mmHg.
	AO	= 150/80,100	mmHg
a.	PAW	= 12,10,8	mmHg
b.	PA	= 25/10,17	mmHg
c.	RV	= 25/2,6	mmHg
d.	RA	= 10,22,12	mmHg

Jack Black's pressure readings at rest

ANSWER d. RA 10,22,12 mmHg. Normal RA pressure is 6, 5, 3 mmHg. The chief abnormality here is the elevated V wave possibly indicative of tricuspid regurgitation. You should be able to scan a computer printout of pressure levels and identify abnormalities. **See:** Braunwald, chapter on "Valvular Heart Disease." **Keywords:** ID abnormal pressure levels - RA

197. This box summarizes 4 patients' hemodynamic pressure measurements. What valvular pathology is consistent with the left heart pressures of Patient #1?

a. Aortic Stenosis

b. Mitral Stenosis

c. Aortic Regurgitation

d. Mitral Regurgitation

Pressures	PAW	LV	AO
Patient #1	**5, 25, 12**	**120/0, 4**	**120/80, 95**
Patient #2	**10, 8, 7**	**136/2, 7**	**140/46, 75**
Patient #3	**15, 17, 13**	**112/3, 6**	**110/72, 88**
Patient #4	**12, 10, 7**	**163/7, 12**	**110/70, 87**

Pressures of 4 different patients with valvular Ht. Dis.

ANSWER d. Mitral Regurgitation. Note patient #1's elevated V waves of 25 mmHg indicative of Mitral Regurgitation where PAW = 5, 25, 12 mmHg (a, v, m).

BE ABLE TO CORRECTLY MATCH ALL ANSWERS BELOW:

Patient #1 = MR, elevated PAW V wave

Patient #2 = AR, low AO diastolic

Patient #3 = MS, PAW - LV diastolic gradient

Patient #4 = AS, LV-AO systolic gradient

See: Braunwald, chapter on "Valvular Heart Disease." Keywords: ID MR by pressure readings

USE THIS SIMULTANEOUS PRESSURE FOR THE NEXT QUESTION:

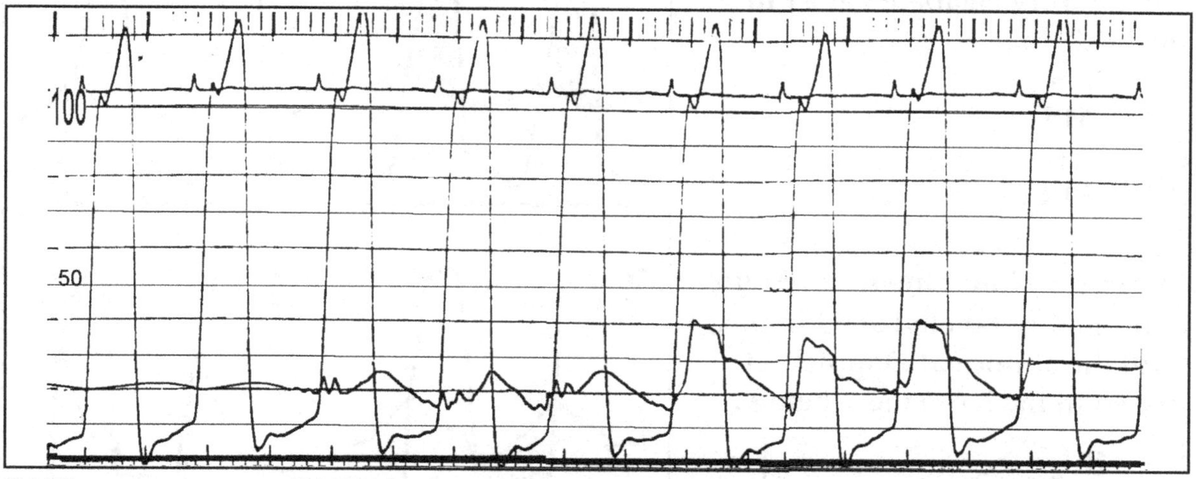

PAW mean, PAW phasic → PA phasic, PA mean x 100

198. **The pressures above are recorded simultaneously and on the same range to rule out a diagnosis of:**

- **a. MR (large v waves in PA)**
- **b. MS (end-diastolic gradient)**
- **c. PS (systolic gradient)**
- **d. PR (end-diastolic gradient)**

ANSWER b. Check for MS (end diastolic gradient across mitral valve). Since the PA diastolic pressure is a good reflection of the mean wedge pressure or LA, it can be used to detect a Mitral Stenosis end diastolic gradient between LA and LV during diastole. Since the PA is normally only a few mmHg higher than the wedge pressure, it is difficult to accurately assess small gradients. But simultaneous LV and PA *gives an idea as to the mitral gradient.* If the end diastolic PA-LV gradient is less than 4 mmHg, MS can be ruled out. PAW and LV still need to be recorded simultaneously on expanded range (x 50).

There is a significant 10 mmHg gradient across the mitral valve (LV diastole = 10, PAW mean = 20). Use of the PA diastole and mean allows visual estimation of the mean mitral valve gradient.

See: Braunwald, chapter on "Valvular Heart Disease. **Keywords:** PA-EDP, LV-EDP gradient

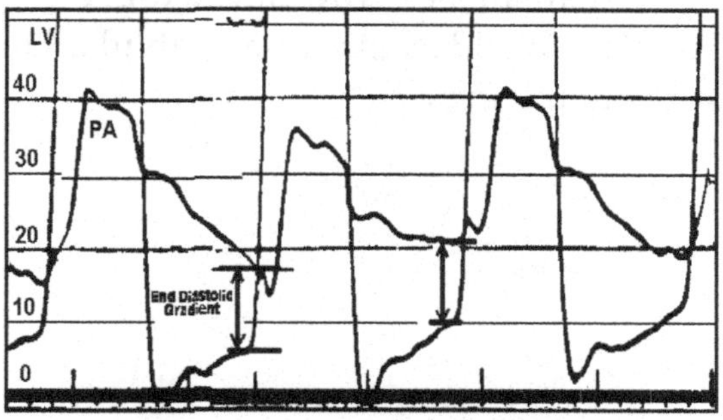

Simultaneous PA-LV - gradient of MS

THE NEXT 2 QUESTIONS REFER TO THIS DIAGRAM:

199. What simultaneous pressure abnormality is labeled at #1 in the box?

a. AS
b. MS
c. AR
d. MR

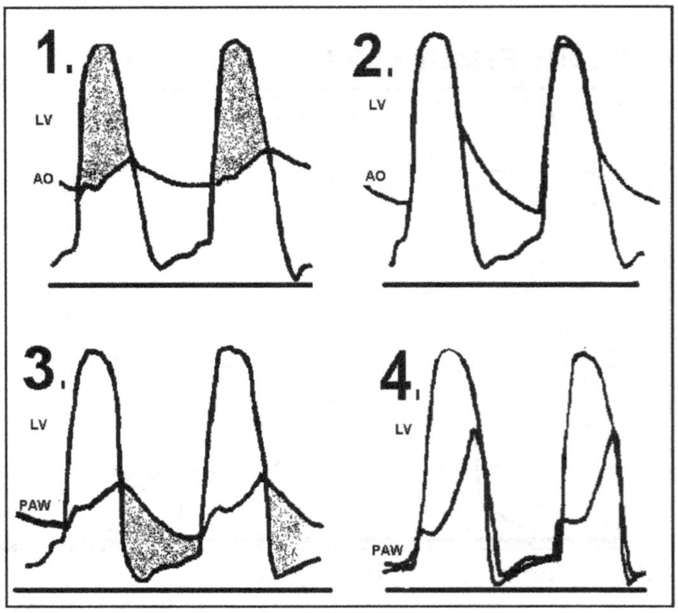

Valvular heart diseases x 200

200. Match the simultaneous pressure abnormality labeled at #2 in box, with the abnormal Doppler jet drawn in the RAO view below.

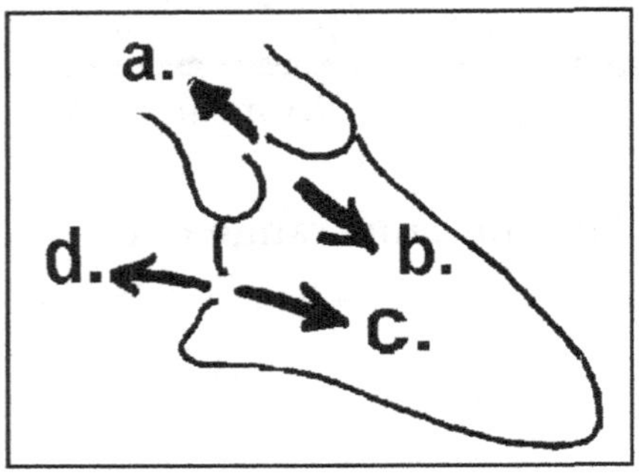

Turbulent high velocity jets

BOTH ANSWERS FOR THE DIAGRAM ABOVE APPEAR TOGETHER BELOW:

199. ANSWER a. AS = Aortic Stenosis. Systolic gradient between LV and AO.

BE ABLE TO CORRECTLY MATCH ALL ANSWERS BELOW:

Patient #1 = AS, LV-AO systolic gradient
Patient #2 = AR, low AO diastolic
Patient #3 = MS, LA-LV diastolic gradient
Patient #4 = MR, elevated LA"V" wave

See: Braunwald, chapter on "Valvular Heart Disease." **Keywords:** ID AS by simultaneous pressure tracings

200. ANSWER #2 = AR = b. Aortic regurgitant reverse high velocity turbulent jet. These jets are best seen in 2D color flow Doppler imaging, but can also be visualized with angiographic injections into the chamber upstream to the jet.

See: Braunwald, chapter on "Valvular Heart Disease."
Keywords: Match AR with its Doppler jet

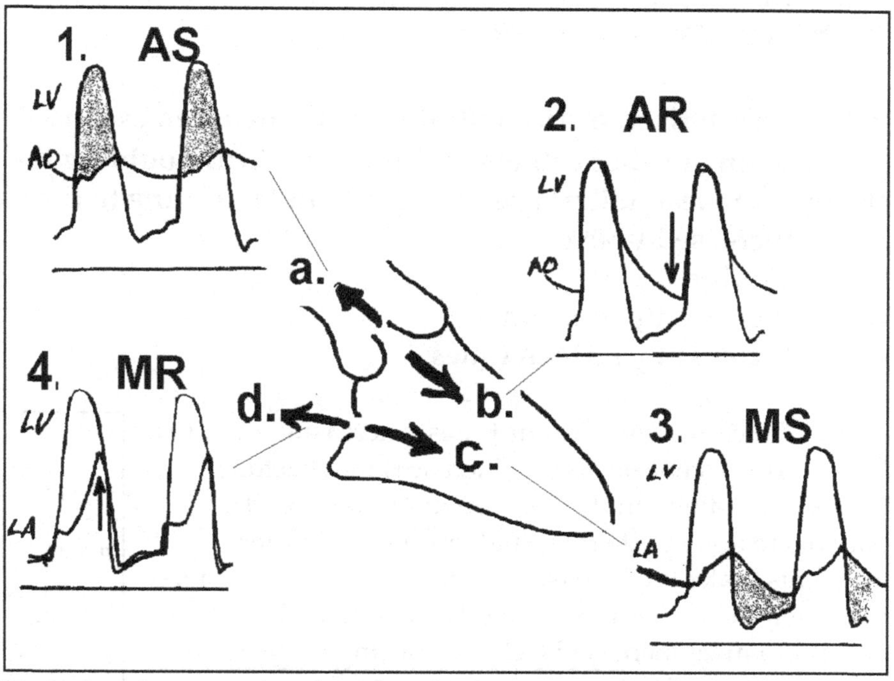

Turbulent jets associated with valvular stenosis and regurgitation.

MITRAL STENOSIS

201. In MS characteristic PAW pressures show:

a. Rapid "x"descent
b. Rapid "y" descent
c. Slowed "x"descent
d. Slowed "y" descent

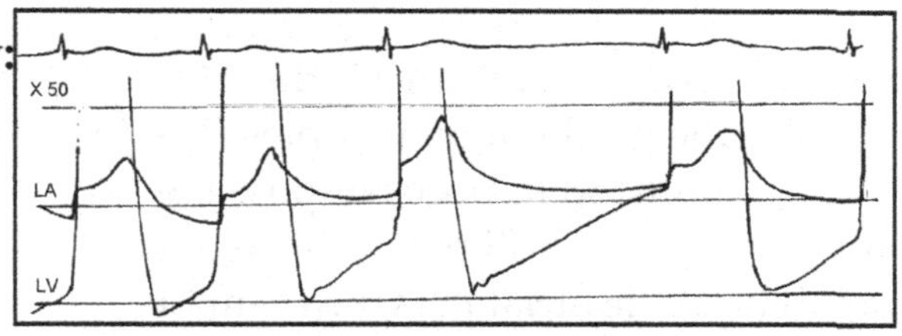

Mitral Stenosis: Simultaneous LA & LVX 50

ANSWER d. Slowed "y" descent. The reduced slope of the "y" descent maintains the diastolic gradient. Remember the "y" wave indicates the rapid filling of the ventricle - rapid filling suction cup. In MS the ventricle cannot fill rapidly so the atrial pressure remains high during diastole. Although the ventricle tries to suck in atrial blood, and the atria hypertrophy and rise in pressure to push it in faster, the tight valve gets in the way and obstructs filling. This slowed "y" descent shown is so characteristic, the pressure ½ time measurement is used to evaluate MS severity. And the Doppler pressure half time is one of the common measurements taken in suspected MS.

In sinus rhythm the "a" wave may be elevated to provide better atrial kick and filling across the tight mitral valve. However, atrial fibrillation often develops in which case there is no "a" wave, but the end diastolic LA pressure is still elevated above the LV-EDP. This is termed the "end diastolic gradient of MS." LV diastole is usually normal or low to encourage filling. This pressure is recorded on X50 - an expanded scale to better see the diastolic events (gradients). Note the irregular heart rate due to atrial fibrillation.

See: Kern, Hemodynamic Rounds "Mitral Valve Gradients" **Keywords:** MS, pressures, LA → "a wave" normal . LV-EDP

202. Patients with fixed orifice mitral stenosis are often exercised or given inotropic drugs during cardiac catheterization. How will doubling the cardiac output change the mean mitral pressure gradient (according to the valve area formula)?

a. **Increase by 50%**
b. **Double**
c. **Increase by four times**
d. **Increase by sixteen times**

ANSWER c. Increase by four times. Increasing the CO or flow across a stenosis always increases the diastolic pressure gradient. In the lab, you may exercise MS patients to accentuate marginal gradients. Larger gradients make the measurement more accurate. Since most stenotic valves have a fixed orifice size, they cannot expand to meet increased CO. According to the Hakki valve area equation:

$$ValveArea = CO / \sqrt{MeanGradient}$$

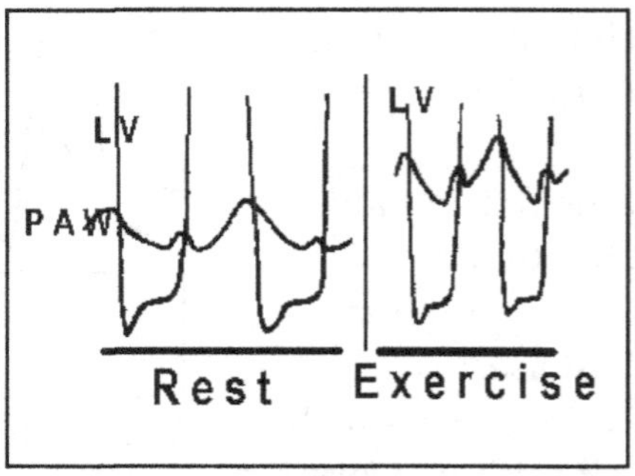

MS: LA-LV in rest & Ex. x 50

or rearranged:

$$CO = [ValveArea]\sqrt{MeanGradient}$$

So, with a fixed valve area if the CO doubles the gradient quadruples (2 = √4). This relationship imposes impossible limitations on an MS patient's exercise capability. The atrial pressure cannot increase that dramatically. Since the pressure cannot easily quadruple, the CO cannot easily double. Even small increases in CO may lead to dramatic increases in PA and PAW pressure resulting in pulmonary edema. E.g. Grossman's CO - gradient graphs show that with a fixed valve size of 0.5 square cm., it is almost impossible for the CO to rise above 5.0 L/min.

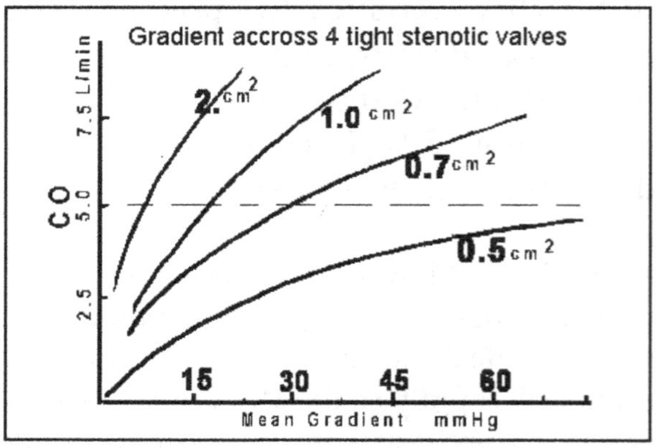

Relation between CO & MS gradient

See: Braunwald, chapter on "Valvular Heart Disease." **Keywords:** MS; ↑ CO = ↑↑ mean diastolic gradient

203. **A patient has pure chronic mitral stenosis, a stiff LV, and atrial fibrillation. Besides an elevated PAWP it is common for the PAWP in such patients to show :**

a. Large "a" waves
b. Large "v" waves
c. A rapid "x" descent
d. A rapid "y" descent

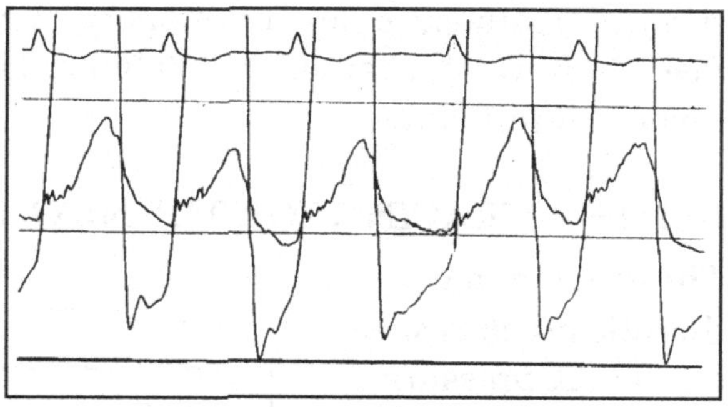

Pure Mitral Stenosis with V waves x 40

ANSWER b. Large "v" waves. Although large "v" waves re usually associated with MR, not MS, this is an exception. Kern says,

> *" the presence of large V waves in mitral stenosis is common, often reflecting a low compliance (stiff) chamber, and does not necessarily indicate clinically significant mitral regurgitation."*

Increased mean LA pressure is necessary to get blood through the tight valve. But, without "a" waves to increase the pressure, the "v" waves must do it. V waves are not specific to MR. The y descent slows in mitral stenosis, preventing atrial pressure from equalizing with ventricular diastolic pressure. This creates the end-diastolic gradient of MS.

See: Kern, Hemodynamic Rounds on "Mitral Valve Gradients" **Keywords:** V waves in MS common

MITRAL REGURGITATION

204. **-Elevated central venous pressure and large right atrial systolic "V" waves as shown at # 1 on the diagram usually indicate:**

a. Mild tricuspid regurgitation (TR)
b. Severe tricuspid regurgitation (TR)
c. Mild pulmonary regurgitation (PR)
d. Severed pulmonary regurgitation (PR)

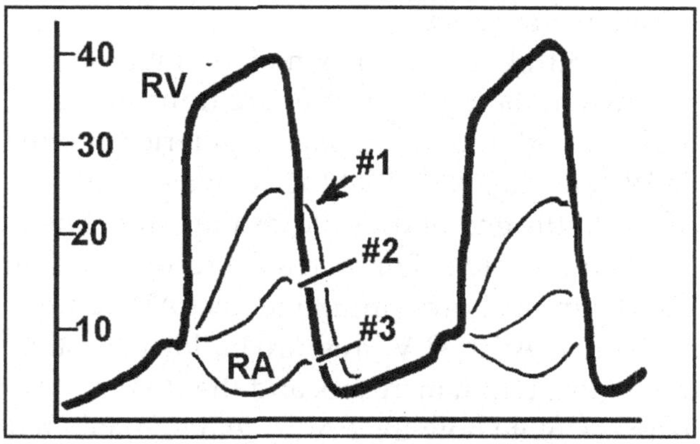

"V" waves RV & RA x 50

ANSWER b. Severe tricuspid regurgitation (TR). RA and RV-EDP are slightly elevated. The RA tracing shows absence of "x" descent and elevated "v" wave in systole." Pressures in the RV may increase.

CORRECTLY MATCHED ANSWERS ARE:

1. Severe TR - ventricularization - large "v wave" to 30 mmHg
2. Mild TR - small "v wave" to 18 mmHg.
3. Normal RA pressure "v wave" to 8 mmHg.

The most common cause of TR is dilation of the tricuspid annulus as a complication of RV failure. The valve ring is stretched so much that the leaflets fail to coapt correctly. Compensatory dilation of the RV develops. TR usually requires no surgical treatment unless pulmonary hypertension develops.

See: Braunwald, chapter on "Valvular Heart Disease." **Keywords:** RA "v" wave, severe TR pressures

USE THIS TRACING FOR THE NEXT QUESTION:

205. The exaggerated dicrotic notches seen on the PA pressure shown are due to:

a. Pulmonic valve stenosis
b. Severe mitral insufficiency
c. Hypertrophic and stiff LV
d. Hypertrophic and stiff RV

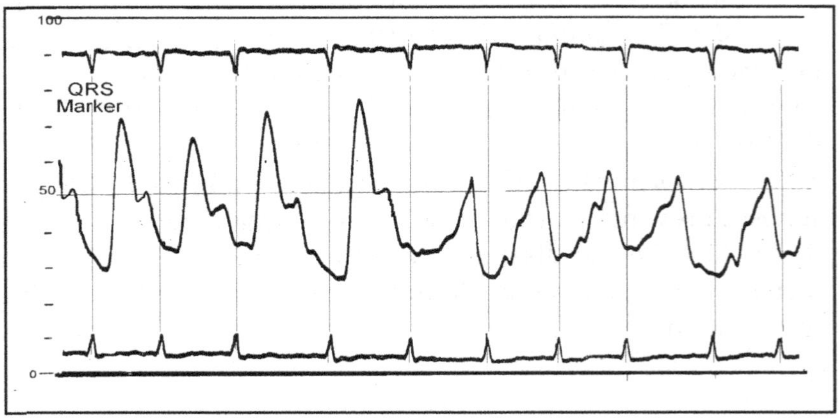

PA→PAW with Swan Ganz inflation x 100 -
After Daily and Schroeder, Chapter on PA catheter monitoring

ANSWER b. Severe mitral insufficiency.
Severe mitral insufficiency may become so severe that the LA "v" waves are transmitted back through the pulmonary capillaries into the PAWP tracing. Note that the "v" wave peak comes at the end of diastole, as the same time as the dicrotic notch. For increased recognition this 2nd diagram shows simultaneous PAW & PA pressures. As the LV pressure builds in systole the regurgitation increases and the PAW "v" increase. Note how the PA "v" waves match with the dicrotic notch.

See: Braunwald, chapter on "Valvular Heart Disease." **Keywords:** RA "v" wave, severe TR pressures reflected into PA

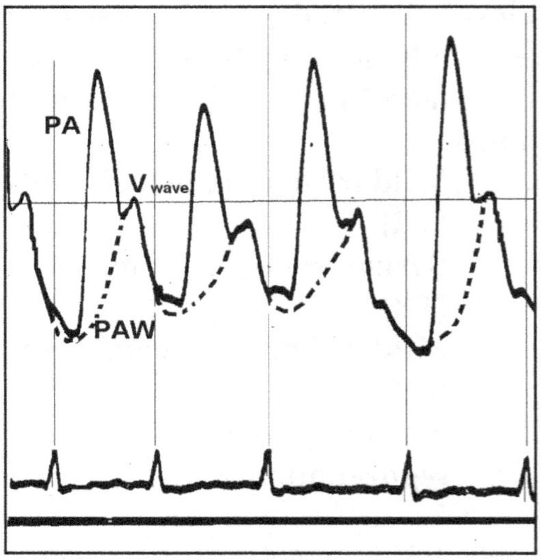

MR "v" waves reflect into PA.
LV, PAW-PA pullback x 100
after Daily & Schroder

206. Mitral regurgitation is virtually certain when atrial "v" waves:

- **a. Are over 40 mmHg**
- **b. Exceed the height of the "a" wave**
- **c. Exceed 3 time the atrial mean pressure**
- **d. Occur throughout systole and extend into diastole**

ANSWER c. Exceed 3 time the atrial mean pressure. Baim says that,

> *" V waves greater than twice the mean left atrial (or pulmonary artery wedge) pressure are suggestive of severe mitral regurgitation, and when the height of the v wave is three times the mean pulmonary capillary wedge or left atrial pressure a diagnosis of severe mitral regurgitation is virtually certain. I hasten to point out, however, that the absence of a prominent v wave by no means rules out severe mitral regurgitation."*

The size of the v wave is very dependent on left atrial compliance.
See: Baim, chapter on "Profiles in Valvular Heart Disease." Keywords: MR, Stage with largest PVR

207. Elevated PAW "v" waves may be associated with which of the following conditions? (Check4 below.)

- **a. Ventricular septal defect**
- **b. Atrial fibrillation**
- **c. Dilated and failing LV**
- **d. Enlarged compliant LA**
- **e. Mitral regurgitation**
- **f. Mitral stenosis**

ANSWERS: a, b, c, & e. Large "V" waves are found in MANY other conditions besides mitral regurgitation (MR). That is the point of this question. Large V waves don't always mean MR is present. Neither does the absence of V waves rule out significant MR. In MR the V waves only appear with a small stiff LA is unable to accept the pressure. Significant V waves may be present in:

- **Yes: VENTRICULAR SEPTAL DEFECT: High flow states with increased CO and atrial filling such as acute VSD from MI.**
- **Yes: ATRIAL FIBRILLATION: Large V waves are common in atrial fibrillation**
- **Yes: DILATED AND FAILING LV: LV failure the LV fails to pump blood effectively out of the LA. LA blood thus accumulates in the veins increasing the V waves.**
- **NO: ENLARGED COMPLIANT LA: In longstanding MR the LA wall is usually very dilated and floppy. And the LA may be huge. These compliant Left atrial chambers can absorb large regurgitant flows with no significant increase in pressure. The result is that even with significant mitral regurgitation, these patients PAW "v" waves may appear normal.**
- **Yes: MITRAL REGURGITATION: Seen in acute MR where the LA compliance is normal. Being relatively small and stiff, it can only absorb significant regurgitation by increasing diastolic pressure (v wave).**

See: Baim, chapter on "Profiles in Valvular Heart Disease." **Keywords:** conditions with large V waves = lots besides MR

THE NEXT THREE TRACINGS ARE FROM THE SAME PATIENT.

208. Joe Smith has acutely ruptured chordae tendineae. The characteristic pressures of acute MR are shown in this pressure tracing . Identify all of the abnormalities associated with acute MR. (Check 4 below.)

a. **Large V waves**
b. **Arterial hypotension**
c. **Elevated LV-EDP**
d. **Early diastolic filling gradient**
e. **Systolic ejection gradient**
f. Reduced LV ejection fraction

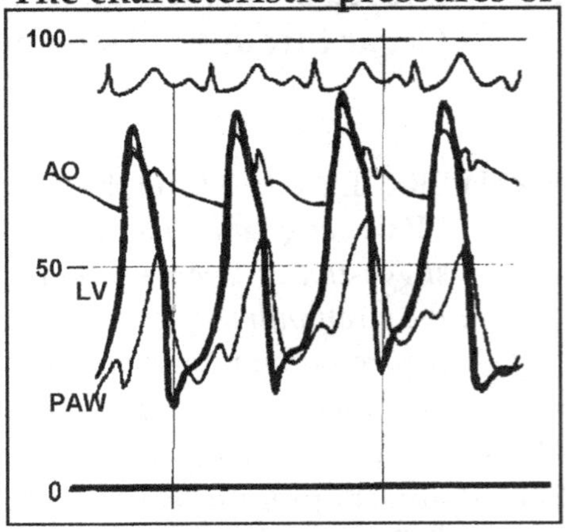

Joe Smith: Simultaneous AO, LV, LA X 100

ANSWERS: a, b, c, & d. No LV-AO gradient of AS is present. However, mitral flow gradients may occur in early diastole because of the increased diastolic flow, in compensation for the MR. The hemodynamic signs of severe acute MR in a normal sized LA seen on this tracing are:

- **Yes:** Large V waves are not always diagnostic of MR
- **Yes:** Arterial hypotension (poor perfusion pressure due to low forward CO)
- **Yes:** Elevated LV-EDP often over 40 mmHg (CHF)
- **Yes:** Early diastolic filling gradient. A diastolic flow gradient and murmur are often present due to initial high total flow across the valve.
- **Yes:** Total left ventricular minute flow (LVMF) may be large in order to compensate for the regurgitation.
- **No:** No LV-AO systolic gradient of AS is present.
- No. LV EF will increase to compensate for MR.

See: Baim, chapter on"Valvular Heart Disease" **Keywords:** conditions with large v waves are many besides mitral regurgitation

209. Joe Smith (above) received therapy for his acute MR. This second recording shows improvement due to probable:

a. **Nitroprusside therapy**
b. **Balloon valvuloplasty**
c. **Mitral valve replacement**
d. **Aortic counterpulsation**

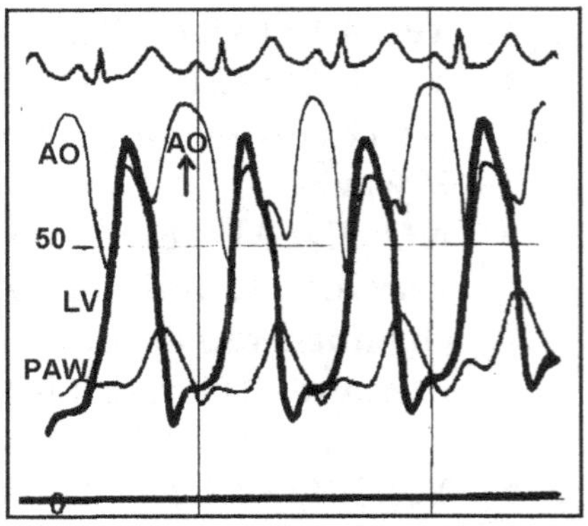

Joe Smith: post- therapy for MR: Simultaneous AO, LV, LA pressures X 100

ANSWER d. Aortic counterpulsation (IABP). Compared to the previous tracing, note the increased diastolic AO pressure and reduced PAW "v" waves.. Balloon pumping is used in MR to reduce afterload. It helps "pull" blood out of the ventricle so less is available to leak back. Nitrates drugs may also be used to reduce afterload. **See:** Baim, chapter on "Profiles in Valvular

Heart Disease." **Keywords:** conditions with large V waves are many besides MR

210. This same patient above had a left heart cath and LVgram that showed 3+ MR. This pullback tracing shows:

a. More severe V waves

b. Improved LV-EDP

c. Bisferiens pulse

d. IABP diastolic augmentation

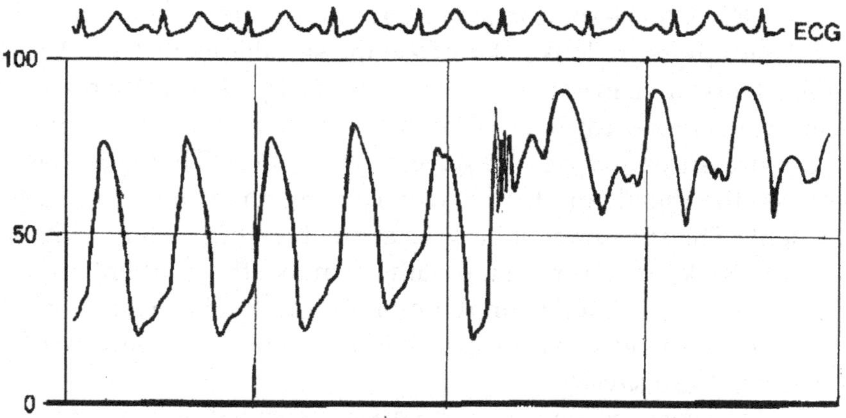

Joe Smith: LV➔AO pullback x 100

ANSWER d. IABP diastolic augmentation. The IABP was operating on 1:1 mode during this LV➔AO pullback, as the pigtail catheter was pulled-back across the active counter-pulsating balloon. Note diastolic augmentation of the BP with inflation of the balloon. A properly sized inflated balloon allows room for a catheter to pass alongside. IABP reduces the LV afterload, by reducing the LV systolic pressure. This decreases the leak backwards because additional stroke volume is pulled forward out of the ventricle with each systolic deflation of the balloon. IABP is an excellent temporary measure to stabilize MR patients awaiting surgery. **See:** Braunwald, chapter on "Valvular Heart Disease" **Keywords:** hemodynamic signs of MR

AORTIC STENOSIS

211. During a bilateral heart cath, you record continuous FA tracings via a 6 F sheath sidearm. The sheath contains a 6 F pigtail catheter that is pulled back from LV-AO while recording the pressures shown . This pullback shows that:

a. Significant valvular aortic stenosis is present

b. HOCM/IHSS gradient is present (no valvular AS)

c. FA sheath is too small, producing a false gradient

d. Pigtail too small, producing damped LV & AO pressures

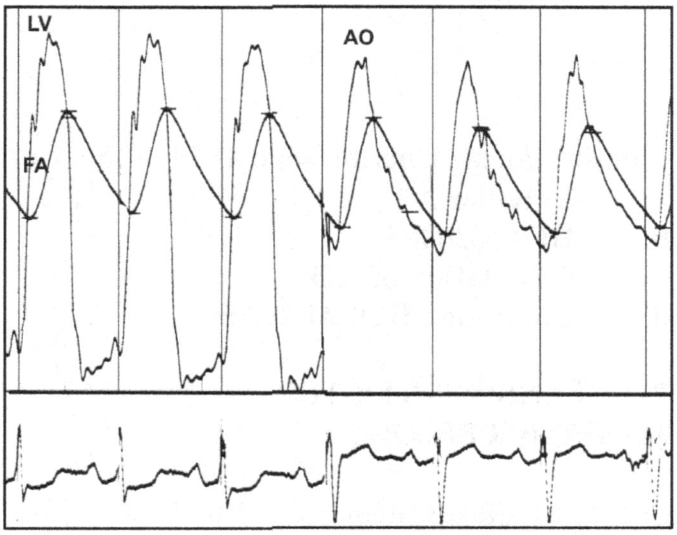

FA sheath pressure with LV➔AO pullback x 200

ANSWER c. FA sheath is to small, producing a false gradient. This example of a damped AO sheath pressure looks like AS on the simultaneous LV-FA tracing. However, on pullback no valve gradient is seen. This damped sheath pressure results from insufficient clearance between catheter OD and sheath ID. The last half of the tracing shows that FA sheath pressures and AO pressure do not match. There may be inadequate clearance between the sheath and the catheter causing an intrinsic gradient that looks like an AS gradient. The sheath must be at least one French size larger than the catheter or this false gradient is likely. To small a sheath can make the gradient appear greater than it really is. A valve area calculated from these pressures will be erroneously low. This could cause you to recommend valve surgery before it is needed. Beware of pressures from sheath sidearms. Kern says,

> "*Whenever using the femoral artery pressure to assess aortic valve gradients, always match pressures in both transducers prior to obtaining aortic-left ventricular gradients. Zero alignment of both systems and simultaneous pressure recordings (both phasic and mean) with a zero position check against transducer drift from baseline after recording will insure accuracy. A discrepancy should be reconciled or transducer changed.*"

Note that iliac disease, coarctation, incorrect transducer calibration or zeroing could produce similar pressure patterns.
See: Kern, chapter on "Hemodynamics." **Keywords:** estimate LV-AO gradient from LV-FA

BOTH QUESTIONS BELOW REFER TO THIS DIAGRAM:

212. Identify the obstruction seen at #1 in this LV-AO pullback tracing.
- a. **Valvular AS**
- b. **HOCM/IHSS**
- c. **Coarctation of AO**
- d. **Combined HOCM & AS**

213. Identify the obstruction seen at #3 in this LV-AO pullback tracing.
- a. **Valvular AS**
- b. **HOCM/IHSS**
- c. **Coarctation of AO**
- d. **Combined HOCM & AS**

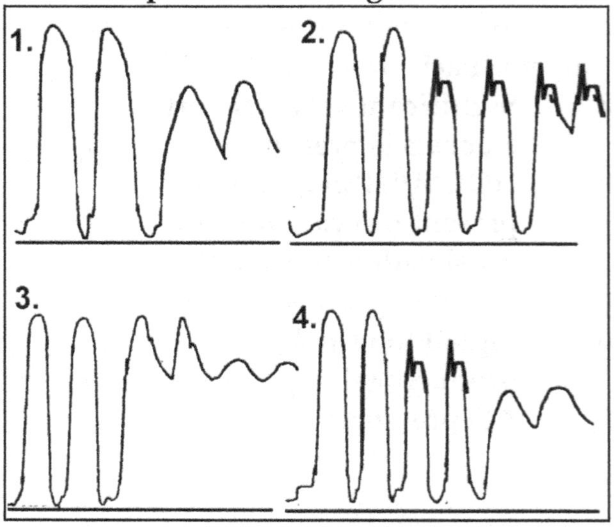

Left heart catheter Pullback pressures x 200

BOTH ANSWERS LISTED TOGETHER BELOW.

212. ANSWER a. Valvular AS. The classic valvular aortic stenosis tracing shows a drop in systolic pressure as the catheter tip crosses the AO valve. The catheter crosses

the valve between the two distinctive pressure tracings of the LV and then the AO. In a normal pullback the LV systolic should equal AO systolic. **See:** Kern, chapter on "Hemodynamics" **Keywords:** Pullback, AS

213. ANSWER c. Coarctation of AO. Note the drop in systolic pressure as the catheter tip crosses the constriction in the aortic arch.. In severe coarctation the diastolic levels may also drop below ascending aortic diastolic pressure. No gradient is seen across the aortic valve only across the arch.

MATCH THE Chambers and pressures shown in this diagram with pathology below.

1. **Valvular AS**
2. **HOCM/IHSS = Subvalvular Stenosis (spike & dome).**
3. **Coarctation AO = Supravalvular**
4. **Combined HOCM & AS.** (These two gradients would not normally be seen combined together in one patient.)

Note how the systolic pressure drops suddenly across each stenosis. HOCM is a subvalvular stenosis within the outflow track of the LV. Valvular AS is in the valve itself. Coarctation of the AO is above the valve (just beyond the aortic arch). **See:** Kern, chapter on "Hemodynamics." **Keywords:** Pullback, AS

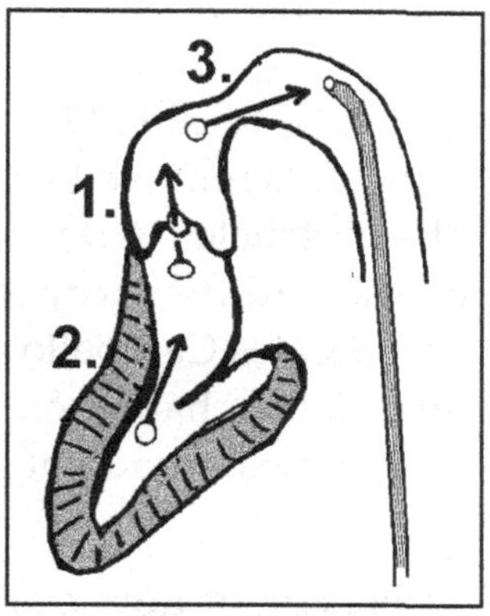

Pullback sites shown

BOTH QUESTIONS BELOW REFER TO THIS DIAGRAM:

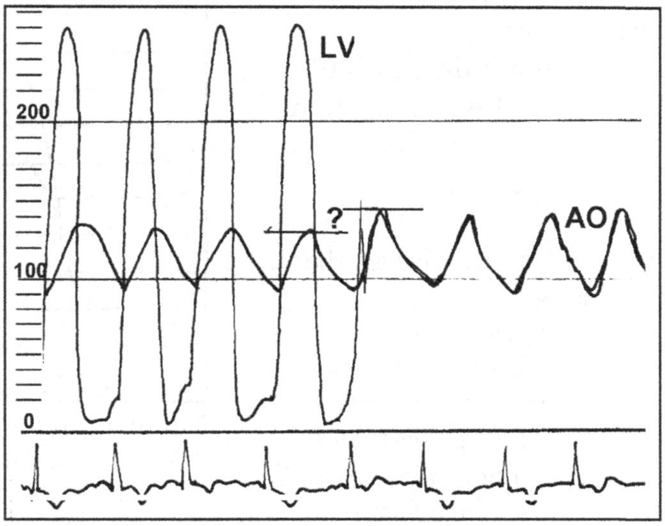

Relief of catheter obstruction in tight AS

214. In critical aortic stenosis a rise in systolic arterial pressure during LV→AO pullback (due to relief of catheter obstruction) is termed:

a. **Hoffman's sign**
b. **Brockenbrough's sign**
c. **Kussmaul's sign**
d. **Carabello's sign**

215. Estimate the true peak-to-peak gradient seen here?

a. **90 mmHg**
b. **115 mmHg**
c. **130 mmHg**
d. **145 mmHg**

BOTH ANSWERS LISTED TOGETHER BELOW.

214. ANSWER d. Carabello's sign (exaggerated here). Baim says,

> "*An interesting hemodynamic finding, describe by Carabello and coworkers, is a rise in arterial blood pressure during left hear catheter pullback in patients*

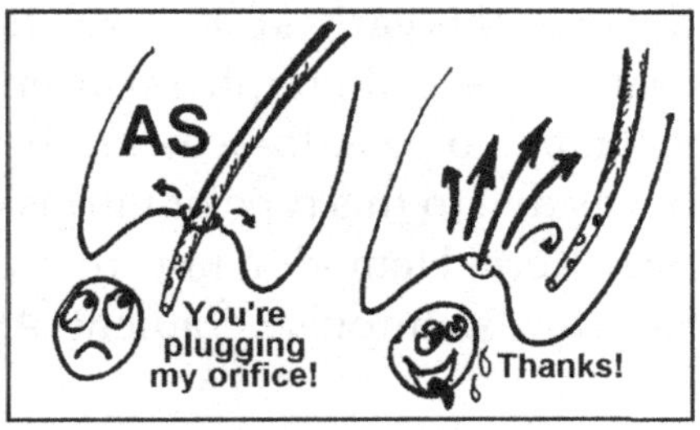

Carabello's Sign is tight AS

with severe aortic stenosis...is an ancillary hemodynamic finding of critical aortic stenosis. The mechanism of this phenomenon is most likely related to partial obstruction of an already narrowed aortic orifice by the retrograde catheter and relief of the obstruction when the catheter is withdrawn."

This slight reduction in AO pressure with a catheter across a tight valve may increase simultaneously recorded pressure gradients by as much as 5 mmHg. **See:** Baim, chapter on "Profiles in Valvular Heart Disease." **Keywords:** AS with

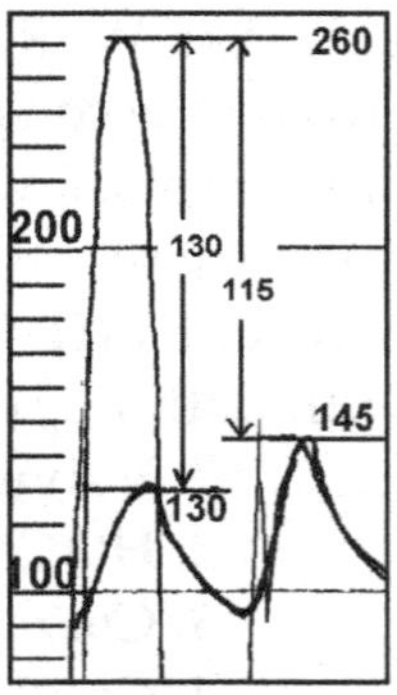

Carabello Sign

215. ANSWER b. 115 mmHg This smaller gradient results when the catheter is removed from the tight aortic valve. LV systole is 260 mmHg. The obstructed AO is 130, while the unobstructed AO is 145 mmHg. The gradient (difference) between 260 and 145 is 260 mmHg. This drawing exaggerates Carabello's sign for demonstration purposes.
See: Baim, chapter on "Profiles in Valvular Heart Disease." **Keywords:** peak to peak gradient in AS angina

216. This type of aortic stenosis gradient showing very little peak to peak gradient is termed a/an:

- **a. Dynamic gradient**
- **b. Tidal wave gradient**
- **c. Impulse gradient**
- **d. Anacrotic notch**

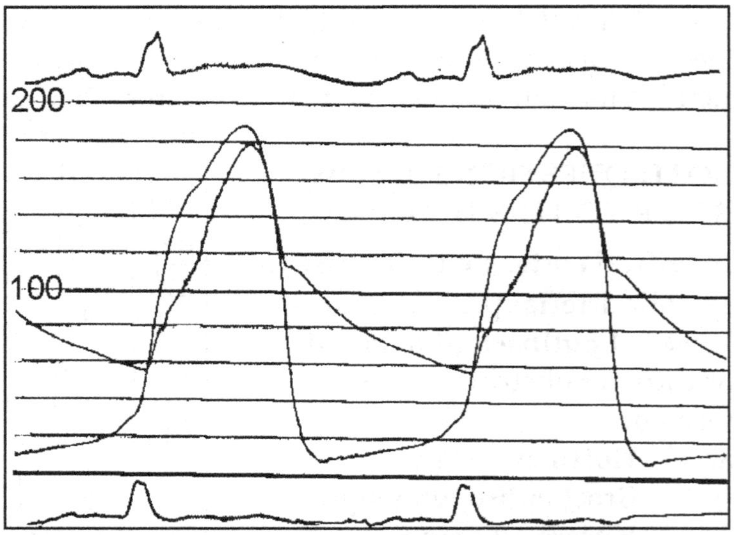

Minimal early systolic aortic valve gradient x 200, After Kern's, Hemodynamic Rounds on Aortic stenosis

ANSWER c. Impulse gradient. Kern says,

"the early systolic gradients of an "impulse type" may be normal in younger patients with vigorous hearts, especially during high flow states such as exercise... The peak to peak gradient is obviously much smaller than the mean or instantaneous gradient."

This type of gradient occurs only in early systole. Impulse gradients are very difficult to detect on pullback because of the minimal peak-to-peak gradient. This is a rare exception where the mean gradient may exceed the peak-to-peak gradient. In femoral artery tracings this early systolic gradient may be confused with the delayed upstroke characteristic of peripheral arterial pressures. We had a case like this where there was virtually no peak-to-peak gradient, but still a mean gradient and a small aortic valve area. It was due to this type of intrinsic gradient.
See: Kern, Hemodynamic rounds, "The Stenotic Aortic Valve."
Keywords: Impulse gradient, AS, normal aortic gradient

HOCM/IHSS

USE THIS TRACING FOR THE NEXT QUESTION:

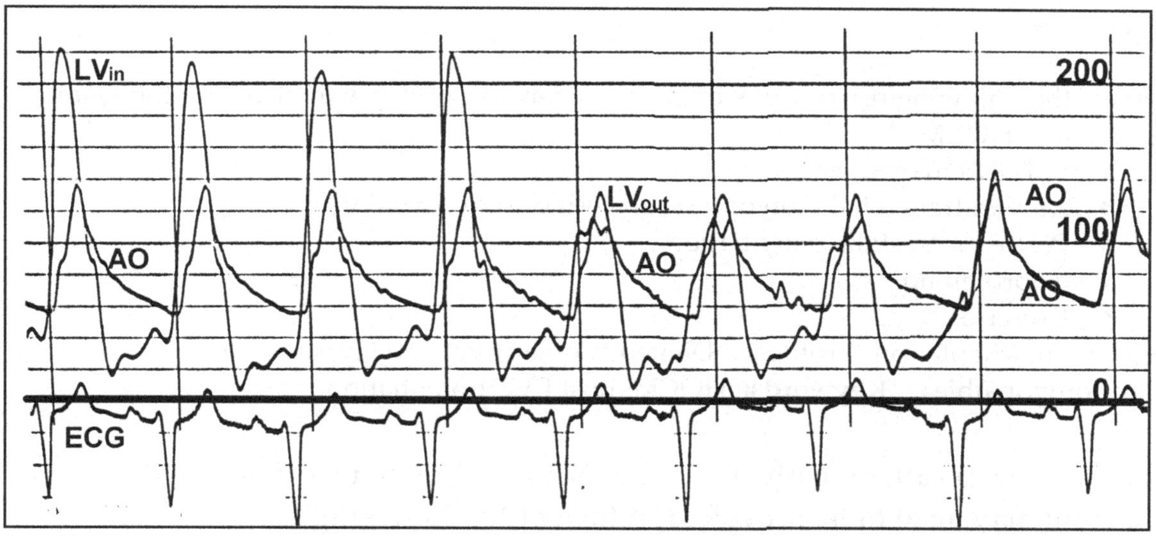

Simultaneous tracings X200. Ao and Pullback out of LV apex

217. These simultaneous pressure tracings were recorded at heart cath. One catheter remains in the AO while the second is pulled back from LV to AO. What pathology is present?

a. **Aortic stenosis**
b. **Coarctation of the aorta**
c. **Infundibular stenosis**
d. **Hypertrophic obstructive cardiomyopathy**

ANSWER d. Hypertrophic obstructive cardiomyopathy. This is HOCM or IHSS. Note the 200 mmHg systolic pressure falls to 140 mmHg systolic mid-tracing. It shows the gradient within the LV chamber outflow track. The Aortic systolic tracing matches with the LV outflow track systolic. No valvular aortic stenosis is present. At the end of the tracing the LV catheter is pulled back to the AO. The two aortic tracings match indicating a good equisensitive transducer calibration.
See: Baim, chapter on "Cardiomyopathy." Keywords: pressure pullback in HOCM, IHSS

218. A dramatic hemodynamic feature of hypertrophic obstructive cardiomyopathy (HOCM/HCM/IHSS) is the:

a. **Elevated LV-EDP with square root sign**
b. **Right ventricular hypertension and heave**
c. **Venous pulsus paradoxus**
d. **Intraventricular systolic pressure gradient**

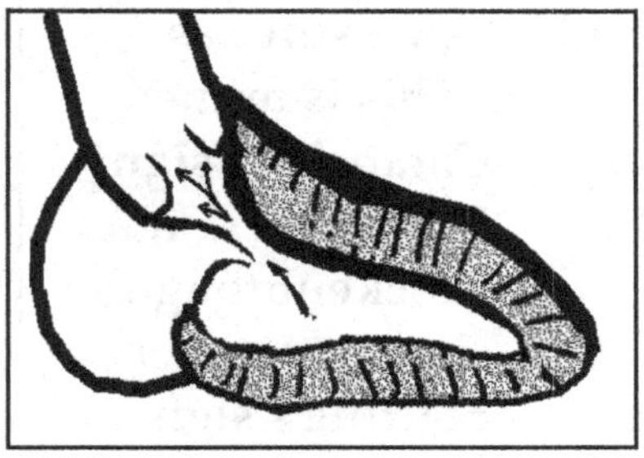

ANSWER d. Intra-ventricular systolic pressure gradient. Baim says,

"*The pressure gradient is present between the body and*

the outflow track of the left ventricle. A key feature of this systolic gradient and most of its associated findings is their variability. Most patients with hypertrophic cardiomyopathy do not have a systolic pressure gradient at rest but may develop one with appropriate provocative maneuvers..."

One of the following provocative maneuvers may be necessary to bring out the systolic gradient of HOCM:

- Valsalva maneuver
- Amyl nitrate inhalation or nitroglycerine administration
- Post-extra systolic potentiation
- Isoproterenol
- Exercise

See: Baim, chapter on "Profiles in Dilated (Congestive) and Hypertrophic Cardiomyopathies." **Keywords:** HOCM, post PVC potentiation

219. During a heart cath on patients with HOCM, an intraventricular pressure gradient may need to be provoked. Which of the following may be used to provoke the gradient? (Check all that apply.)

a. **Isoproterenol**
b. **Nitroglycerine**
c. **Beta blockers**
d. **Valsalva maneuver**
e. **Exercise**

ANSWERS: a, b, d, & e Beta blockers are the mainstay of therapy for HOCM and would NOT be used to provoke it. Drugs such as Inderol slow and relax the heart at both rest and exercise thus reducing the interventricular gradient. The provocative maneuvers described in the previous question may be necessary to bring out and diagnose the gradient. Provocation causes the ventricle to contact harder, thereby increasing the gradient of HOCM. The interventricular gradient of HOCM/IHSS often comes and goes. **See:** Braunwald, chapter on "Cardiomyopathy." **Keywords:** provocative maneuvers in HOCM

220. While monitoring a constrictive pericarditis patient's right heart cath you notice that inspiration is associated with increasing jugular and RA pressures as shown. This is termed:

a. **Carabello's sign**
b. **Kussmaul's sign**
c. **Brockenbrough's sign**
d. **Starling's sign**

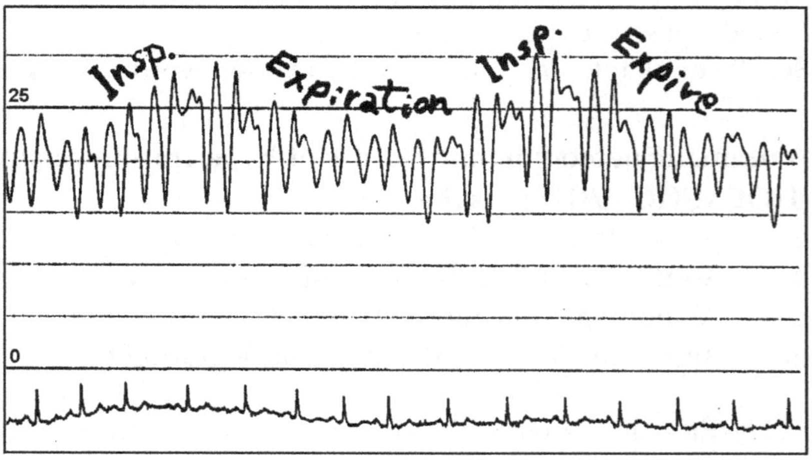

Venous pressure increase with inspiration

ANSWER b. Kussmaul's sign. Normally the venous pressure decreases with inspiration and increases with expiration. It normally follows the diaphragm. This tracing does just the opposite. In constrictive pericarditis we see just the opposite movement. Braunwald says,

> *"systemic venous pressure may actually increase with inspiration i.e., Kussmaul's sign....striking abnormality of constrictive pericarditis is the failure of intrathoracic pressure changes during respiration to be transmitted to the pericardial space and intracardiac chambers. As a consequence, during inspiration, systemic venous and right atrial pressures do not fall and venous flow into the right atrium does not increase, in contrast to the situation in normal subjects and patients with cardiac tamponade."*

See: Braunwald, chapter on "Pericardial Diseases." **Keywords:** Kussmaul's sign

221. A HOCM patient in the cath lab is on a nitroglycerine drip. You notice that with PVCs the LV pressure increases but the BP pressure drops as shown. This is termed:

a. Carabello's sign
b. Kussmaul's sign
c. Brockenbrough's sign
d. Starling's sign

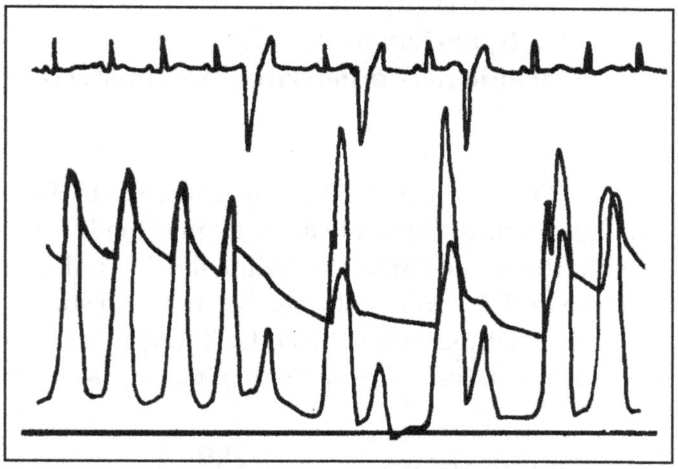

Post PVC beats increase HOCM gradient x 200

ANSWER c. Brockenbrough's sign. PVCs are usually followed by a compensatory pause. This increases the preload and makes the post PVC beat harder. Post PVC beats in normal individuals typically contact to a higher systolic pressure. But in HOCM the opposite happens. In HOCM when the LV beats harder it pinches off the outflow track and increases the gradient as shown.

In HOCM post PVC beats may also show this increased gradient. Since nitroglycerine reduces afterload, preload and the LV size it tends to increase the interventricular obstruction of HOCM. Nitroglycerine, Isuprel, and Valsalva are often used in the cath lab to potentiate this gradient and observe the dynamic interventricular obstruction.

In AS the valve is typically calcified and rigid, this makes the relationship between LV systole and AO systole constant - not dynamic. The AO systolic will be a constant % of the peak LV. Aortic stenosis patients having PVCs will increase both LV and AO pressure in the post-PVC beat, like in normal physiology.

See: Braunwald, chapter on "Valvular Heart Disease." **Keywords:** IHSS, HOCM, Brockenbrough's sign

AORTIC REGURGITATION

222. In which type of aortic regurgitation (AR) may the aortic diastolic pressure fall to the LV-EDP as shown?

- a. **Chronic LV hypertrophied AR (Calcific)**
- b. **Severe acute AR (dissected AO root)**
- c. **Chronic compensated AR (LV hypertension)**
- d. **Chronic decompensated AR (in atrial fibrillation)**

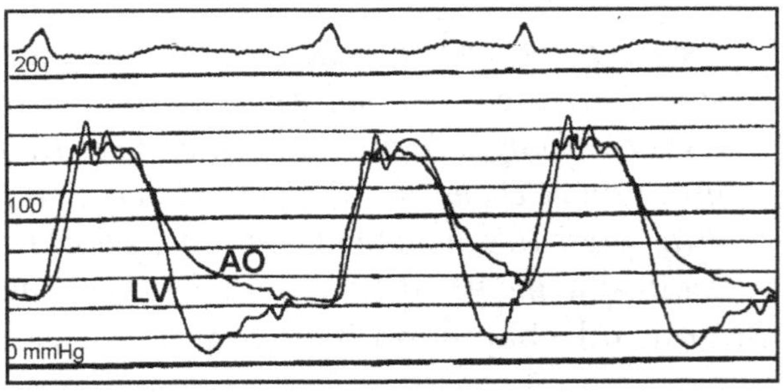

AR with equality of LV-EDP and AO-EDP (After Kern's, Hemodynamic rounds on AR)

ANSWER b. Severe acute AR. In severe acute AR the AO and LV end-diastolic pressures equalize. So much blood leaks back into the LV that much of LV filling is retrograde through the aortic valve. With time this LV will compensate by dilating to accommodate the increased diastolic volume. See next question.
See: Kern, Hemodynamic rounds, "Interpretation of Cardiac Pathology From Pressure Waveform Analysis: Aortic Regurgitation." **Keywords:** AR stages of LV dilation

223. This diagram shows simultaneous LV and AO pressures seen in the various stages of aortic regurgitation (AR). The pressure tracings indicated at #3 indicates:

- a. **Chronic decompensated AR**
- b. **Normal LV**
- c. **Severe acute AR**
- d. **Chronic compensated AR**

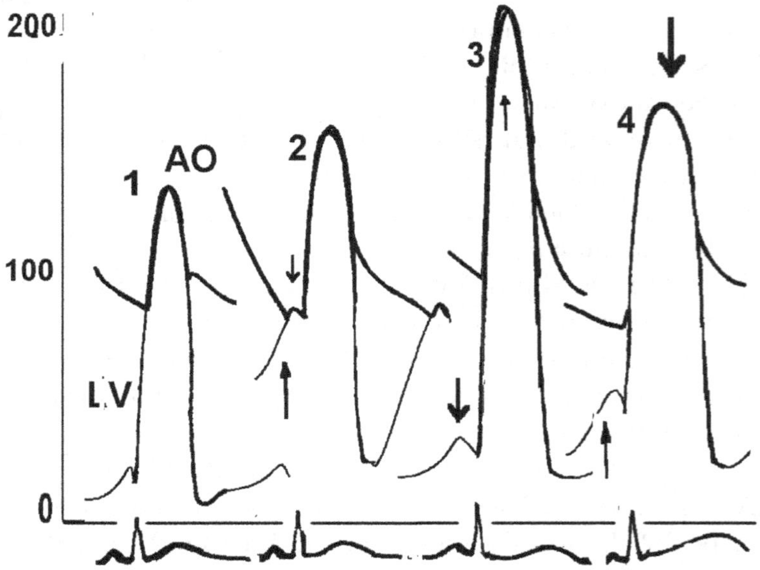

LV-AO pressures seen in stages of AR

ANSWER d. Chronic compensated aortic regurgitation (AR). The most bounding arterial pressures are seen in the chronic compensated phase. The patient may be asymptomatic because the LV dilates and increases in pressure and stroke volume to compensate for the chronic backwards blood leak. The LV-EDP may normalize because of increased CO. Decompensation occurs when the LV is unable to compensate for the leak by dilating and increasing systolic pressure. It finally goes into failure in stage 4.

CORRECTLY MATCHED STAGES OF AORTIC REGURGITATION ARE:
Pressures measured in mmHg are:

Stages of Aortic Regurgitation	Aortic BP in mmHg.	LV edp in mmHg
1. Normal LV	120 /80	10
2. Severe acute AR	130 /70	↑↑ 50
3. Chronic compensated AR	↑ 190 / ↓ 60	12
4. Chronic decompensated AR	↑ 170 / ↓ 60	↑ 25

See: Braunwald, chapter on "Valvular Heart Disease." **Keywords:** AS stages, pressures in each

224. The classic arterial pulse of severe aortic valve regurgitation (AR) shows _____ systolic AO pressure and ____ diastolic AO pressure.

a. **Elevated, elevated**
b. **Elevated, reduced**
c. **Reduced, reduced**
d. **Reduced, elevated**

ANSWER b. Elevated systolic, reduced diastolic pressure. Baim says,

"*The large stroke volume entering the aorta with systole produces an elevated systolic pressure, whereas the regurgitation produces a lowered diastolic pressure.*"

A bounding Corrigan's or Water-hammer pulse is seen in Aortic regurgitation. It shows a rapid upstroke (percussion wave) followed by a rapid collapse (regurgitation) early in diastole. No dicrotic notch is seen, because the aortic valve does not close completely.

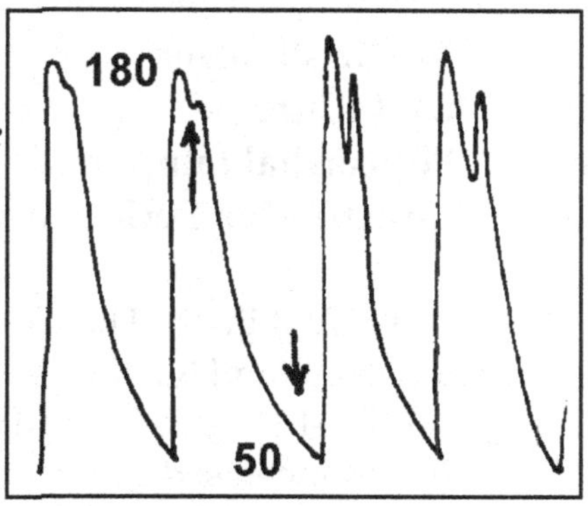

AR: high systolic, low diastolic

However, Older patients with calcific aorta may develop similar pressures, so low AO diastolic pressure is not always diagnostic. The AR pulse may also be bisferiens or notched as shown.

The amount of blood regurgitating may be as much as 60% of the forward stroke volume. With this the heart dilates and hypertrophies to become so large that it may be called "cor bovium" or "cow heart."

See: Braunwald, chapter on "Valvular Heart Disease" **Keywords:** AR, high systolic, low diastolic pressure

225. A common hemodynamic finding in severe AR is:

a. Narrow LV pulse pressure
b. Narrow arterial pulse pressure
c. Systolic FA pressure is higher than LV systolic
d. Diastolic FA pressure is lower than LV beginning diastolic

ANSWER c. Systolic arterial pressure higher than LV systolic, like a reverse gradient due to huge wave reflections. The large LV stroke volumes pumped into the aorta exaggerate the peripheral amplification of systolic arterial pressures. Baim says:

> *Another hemodynamic finding in aortic regurgitation is the amplification of peak systolic pressure in peripheral arteries (especially the femoral and popliteal) so that peak systolic femoral artery pressure may exceed central aortic pressure by 20 to 50 mmHg. This is essentially an exaggeration of a normal phenomenon... but emphasizes the importance of central aortic pressure measurement in aortic regurgitation."*

See: Baim, , chapter on "Profiles in Valvular Heart Disease." **Keywords:** Peripheral artery amplification in AR

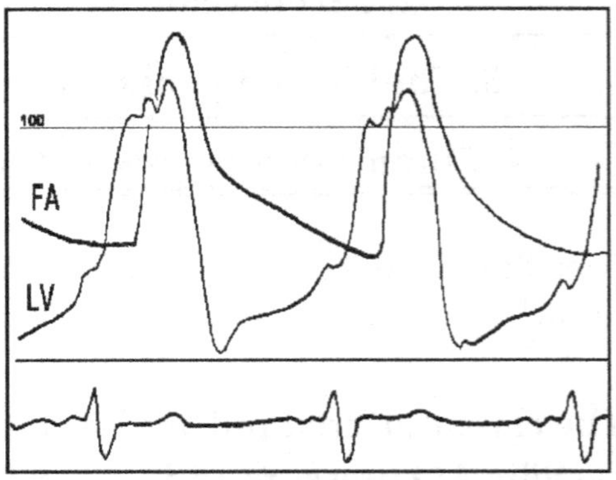

AR Peripheral artery overshoot, **after Kern, chapter on Hemodynamic Data**

PRACTICE PRESSURE TRACINGS

226. This LV→AO pullback shows probable:

a. Aortic stenosis
b. LV failure
c. Pericardial tamponade
d. Constrictive Pericarditis

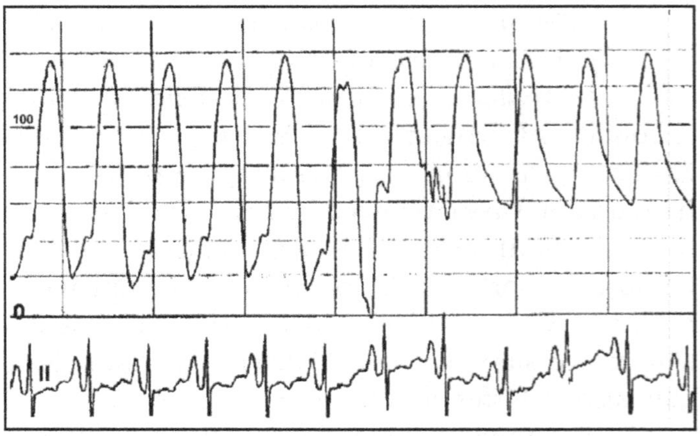

LV→AO pullback x 200

ANSWER b. LV failure. The LV-EDP is elevated at 40 mmHg. Normal wedge and LV-EDP is 5-12 mmHg. This indicates increased preload from left heart failure and probable pulmonary edema. LV failure is usually caused by coronary artery disease, but it could be any of several cardiac diseases. There is no systolic gradient of AS.

See: Braunwald, chapter on " Physical Exam." Keywords :Elevated LV-EDP= LV Failure

227. **This pressure tracing shows a pullback from LV➔AO with a simultaneously recorded PAW. What abnormality is shown?**

a. **AS**
b. **AR**
c. **MS**
d. **MR**

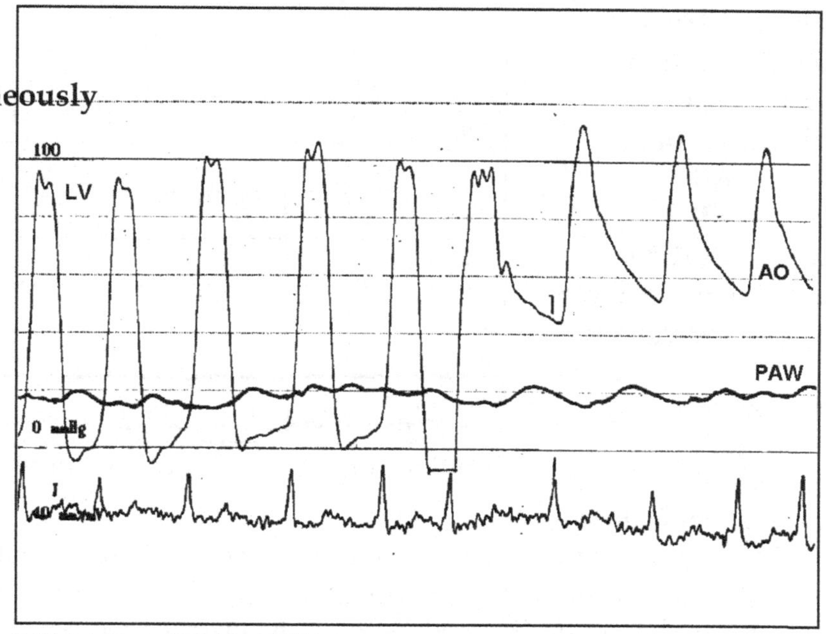

LV➔AO pullback x 200

ANSWER c. MS. The LV➔AO pullback is normal. However, the simultaneous LV and PAW tracing shows a MS diastolic gradient of about 15 mmHg.
See: Kern, chapter on "Hemodynamics."
Keywords: MS gradient

228. **This LV➔AO pullback tracing shows probable:**

a. **AS**
b. **AR**
c. **AS + AR**
d. **HOCM/IHSS**

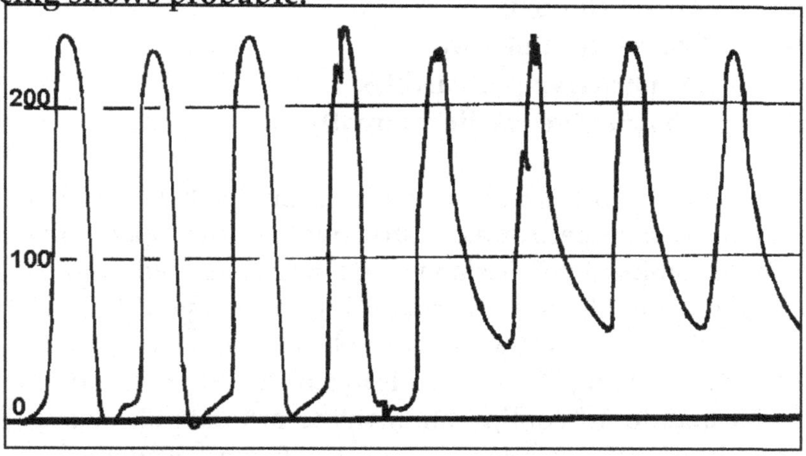

LV➔AO pullback x 200

ANSWER b. Severe acute AR. The wide pulse pressure with low diastole suggests severe aortic regurgitation. Baim says that in AS:

> "*The large stroke volume entering the aorta with systole produces an elevated systolic pressure, whereas the regurgitation produces a lowered diastolic pressure.*"

The LVMF will be increased to compensate for the regurgitation back into the LV. The more leak exists, the lower the aortic diastole. In severe AI the aortic pressure may drop to the level of the LV-EDP. **See:** Braunwald, chapter on "Valvular Heart Disease."
Keywords: AR, high systolic, low diastolic pressure

229. The pullback tracing shown suggests a diagnosis of:

a. AS

b. AR

c. HOCM

d. Constrictive pericarditis

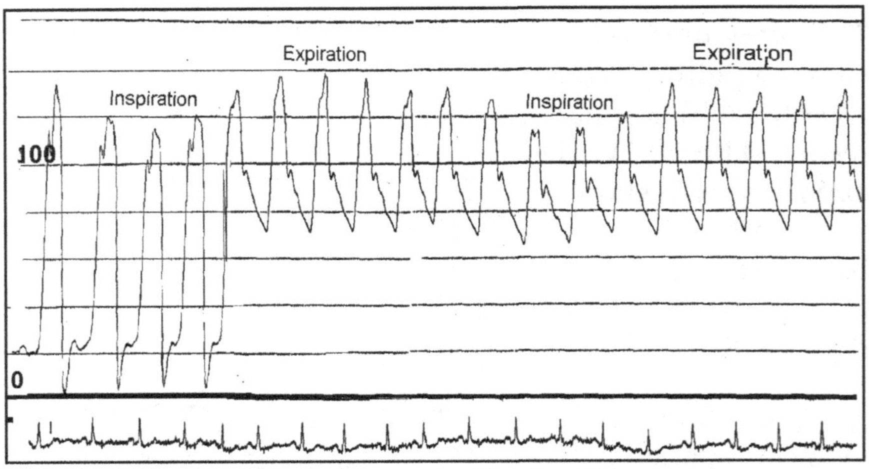

Simultaneous PAW with LV-AO pullback x 200

ANSWER d. Constrictive pericarditis (CP). Two salient features of CP are pulsus paradoxus and square root sign. These are both present. The other hemodynamic feature, Pressure equalization, will require a right heart cath.
See: Kern, chapter on "Hemodynamics." **Keywords:** Constrictive pericarditis

230. Which obstructive pathology below has a rapid initial arterial upstroke and often the "spike and dome" configuration as shown ?

a. Aortic stenosis

b. Coarctation of aorta

c. Constrictive pericarditis

d. Obstructive cardiomyopathy

ANSWER d. Obstructive cardiomyopathy/HOCM/IHSS. In patients with hypertrophic obstructive cardiomyopathy the initial prominent percussion wave is associated with rapid ejection of blood into the aorta during early systole, followed by a rapid decline as the dynamic obstruction pinches off the LV. This pinching off often leads to a bisferiens, notched or "spike and dome" configuration on the arterial pulse wave.
See: Braunwald, chapter on " Physical Exam." **Keywords:** AO Pulse in AS

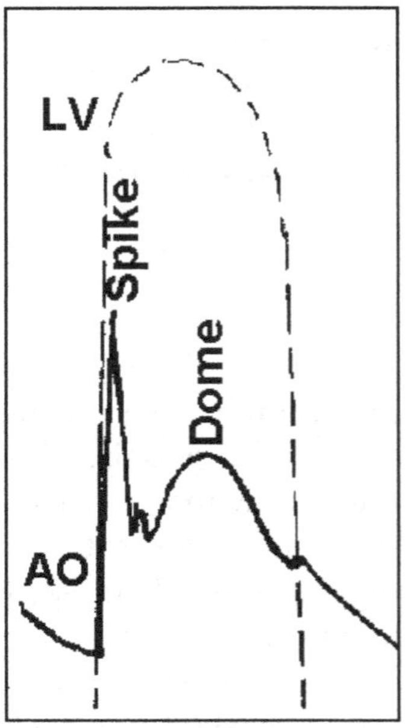

Simultaneous LV-AO

USE THIS SIMULTANEOUS TRACING FOR THE NEXT QUESTION:

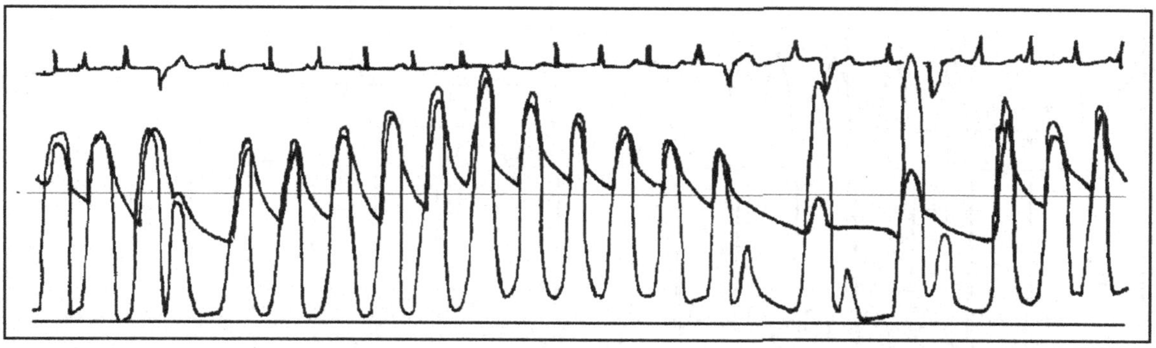

Simultaneous LV-AO x 200 recorded with Valsalva maneuver - after Kern

231. This patient was asked to Valsalva after a few beats of this tracing was recorded. The PVCs following the Valsalva are indicative of:

a. Aortic stenosis
b. Coarctation of aorta
c. Coronary artery disease
d. Hypertrophic obstructive cardiomyopathy

ANSWER d. Hypertrophic obstructive cardiomyopathy/HOCM/IHSS. The 4th beat shows a PVC with normal aortic response - no gradient. But with the Valsalva, where the pressure falls in the center of the tracing, two PVCs are recorded with Brockenbrough's sign. Here a large gradient exists between LV and AO that was not there in the first PVCs. A Valsalva reduced venous return and LV size. This brings the mitral valve and septum closer and the obstruction increases. This easy maneuver tests for HOCM or IHSS.
See: Braunwald, chapter on "Physical Exam." **Keywords:** Valsalva producing HOCM/IHSS

USE THIS TRACING FOR THE NEXT QUESTION:

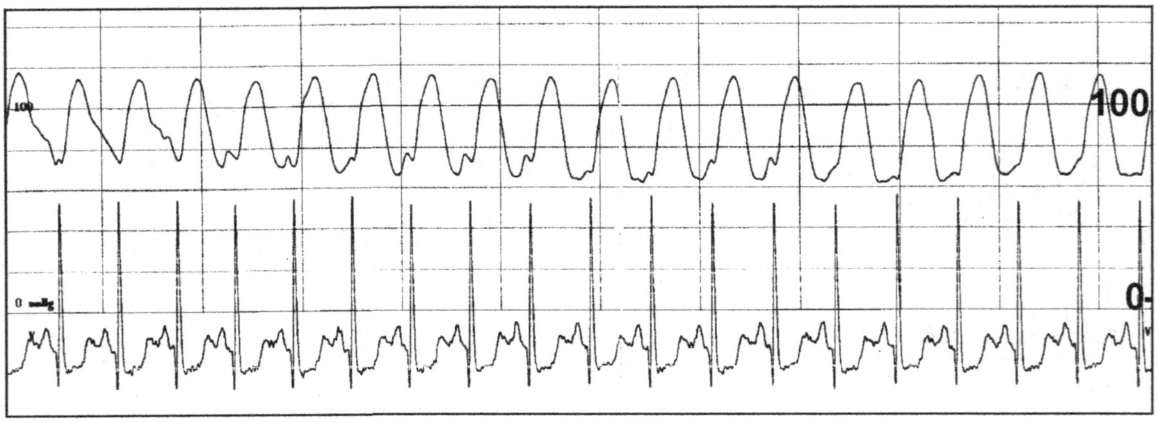

AO x 200 pressure via 6 Fr. JL4 catheter

232. During coronary arteriography you note the pressure changes above that suggest:

a. **Reduced pressure damping**
b. **Ventricularization damping**
c. **Catheter enters LV**
d. **Catheter enters RV via pericardial cushion defect**

ANSWER b. Ventricularization damping. Note the normally triangular aortic waveform changes into a ventricular shaped pattern with rising diastole, termed "ventricularization." It is a form of damping where the coronary orifice is obstructed by the catheter tip. This patient had a tight "widowmaker" orifice LAD lesion. Immediate surgery was recommended based upon arteriography and these pressure patterns, picked up by an astute technologist. Surgery confirmed the significant "widowmaker stenosis."

With ventricularization the systolic pressure usually drops. However, here the abnormality is seen only in diastole. Note the atrial kick waves and rising diastole, characteristic of ventricularization. This is essentially a coronary "wedge" pressure.
See: Braunwald, chapter on " Physical Exam." **Keywords:** Ventricularization damping

THE NEXT 2 QUESTIONS REFER TO THIS DIAGRAM:

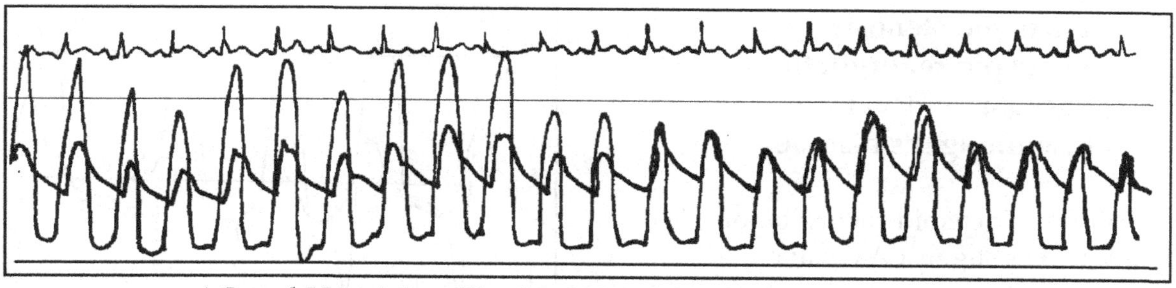

AO and LV→AO pullback x 200 - after Kern.

233. The pressure tracing above shows two simultaneous pressure tracings recorded at heart cath. One catheter remains in the AO while the second is pulled back from LV to AO. The LV→AO pullback suggests:

a. Aortic stenosis
b. Aortic regurgitation
c. Infundibular stenosis
d. HOCM/IHSS

234. The fluctuating aortic systolic pressure in the pullback tracing above suggests:

a. Pulsus alternans & LV failure
b. Pulsus alternans & pericardial tamponade
c. Pulsus paradoxus & LV failure
d. Pulsus paradoxus & pericardial tamponade

BOTH ANSWERS FOR THE DIAGRAM ABOVE APPEAR TOGETHER BELOW:

233. ANSWER d. HOCM or IHSS. This is "Hypertrophic Obstructive Cardiomyopathy" or the old name "Idiopathic Hypertrophic Cardiomyopathy." . Note the 130 mmHg systolic pressure falls to 90 mmHg systolic mid-tracing. The initial tracing shows the systolic gradient within the LV outflow track. At other times, the Aortic systolic tracing matches with the LV outflow track, so no consistent valvular AS is present.
See: Baim , chapter on "Cardiomyopathy." Keywords: pressure pullback in HOCM, IHSS

234. ANSWER d. Pulsus paradoxus & pericardial tamponade. The systolic BP varies between 100 and 75 mmHg. More than a 10 mmHg change indicates pulsus paradoxus and probable pericardial tamponade. Tamponade compresses the ventricular cavities and may set up circumstances for Intra-ventricular gradients as seen in HOCM.
See: Kern, Hemodynamic Rounds on, "Intraventricular Pressure Gradients."Keywords: Pulsus paradoxus and pericardial tamponade

235. This simultaneous pressure tracing recorded at right heart cath suggests probable:

a. **Tricuspid stenosis**
b. **Tricuspid regurgitation**
c. **Valvular endocarditis**
d. **Eisenminger's disease**

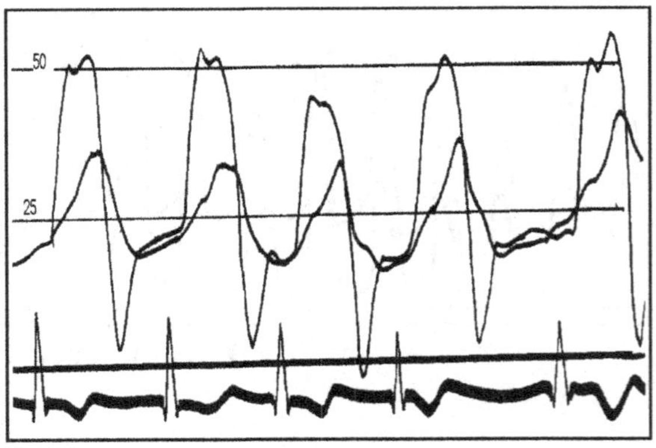

Simultaneous RV & RA x 50

ANSWER b. Tricuspid regurgitation. The large V waves suggest AV valve regurgitation.

There is an early diastolic gradient due to increased forward flow to compensate for the regurgitation. By mid-diastole the RV-RA pressures equalize, thus ruling out tricuspid stenosis. **See**: Kern, Hemodynamic Rounds on, "Tricuspid Valve..." **Keywords:** Valsalva producing HOCM/IHSS

236. The left heart pressures in the box, were recorded at heart cath. What is the most likely diagnosis?

a. **AI**
b. **AS**
c. **MI**
d. **MS**

RECORDED PRESSURES	
PAW=	24 , 20 ,20 mmHg.
LV =	130 / 0 , 4 mmHg.
AO =	130 / 90 , 105 mmHg.

ANSWER d. MS. The LA pressures and PAW are considerably higher than the LV EDP indicating the end diastolic gradient or MITRAL STENOSIS. Note that the AO systole equals the LV systole - a good sign. No AS is present.
See: Kern, chapter on "Hemodynamics." **Keywords:** LA-LV gradient = MS

USE THIS TRACING FOR THE NEXT QUESTION:

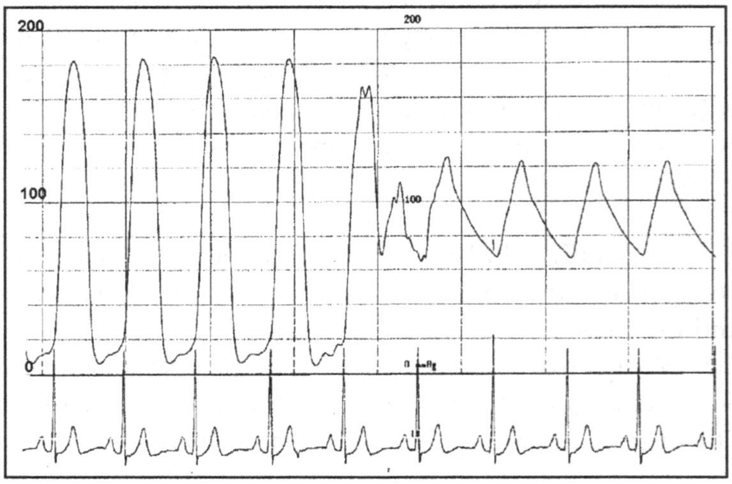

LV➔AO pullback x 200

237. The pullback pressure tracing above is diagnostic of:

a. **Coarctation of the aorta**
b. **Supravalvular aortic stenosis**
c. **Subvalvular aortic stenosis**
d. **Valvular aortic stenosis**

ANSWER d. Valvular aortic stenosis. Pullback pressures drop suddenly from an LV systolic of 183 to an AO systolic of 123 mmHg. This is a significant 60 mmHg gradient diagnostic of aortic stenosis. The aorta shows pulsus tardus slowed upstroke.

It is normal for the transition beats to show irregularity as the catheter crosses the valve. Small gradients are sometimes noted in pullbacks when immediately preceded by LV angiography. Thus it is important to wait several minutes post LV-gram if AS is suspected.

See: Braunwald, chapter on "Valvular Heart Disease." **Keywords:** Pullback showing AS gradient

238. This simultaneous pressure tracing suggests a diagnosis of:

- a. **Pure AS**
- b. **Mixed AS - MR**
- c. **Pure MS**
- d. **Mixed AS - MS**

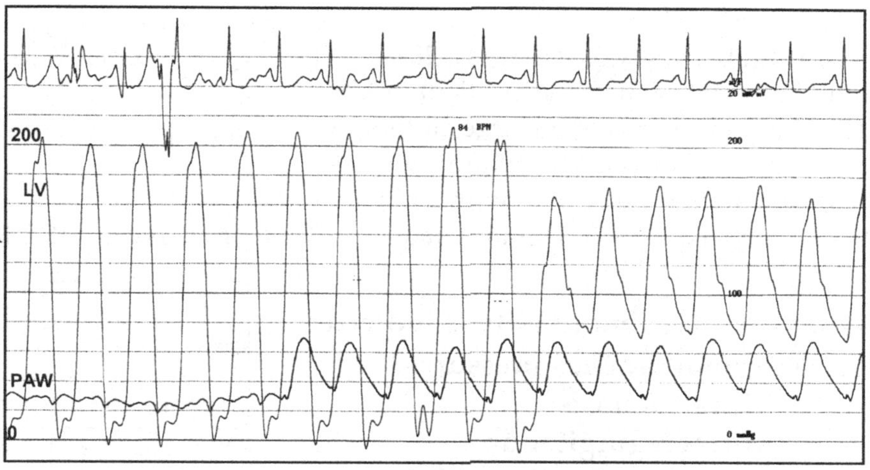

Pullbacks LV-AO, and PAW-PA tracing X 200

ANSWER d. Mixed AS - MS. A systolic gradient occurs between the LV-AO of 40 mmHg indicating aortic stenosis. Diastolic gradient between LV-LA of 10 mmHg indicates MS. When the PAW balloon is deflated, PA pressure end diastolic again shows an MS gradient. **See:** Kern, chapter on "Hemodynamics." **Keywords:** mixed AS-MS

239. As shown in this pressure tracing post-PVC accentuation of an LV-AO gradient indicates:

- a. **Valvular aortic stenosis**
- b. **Supravalvular AS**
- c. **Impulse gradient**
- d. **HOCM/IHSS**

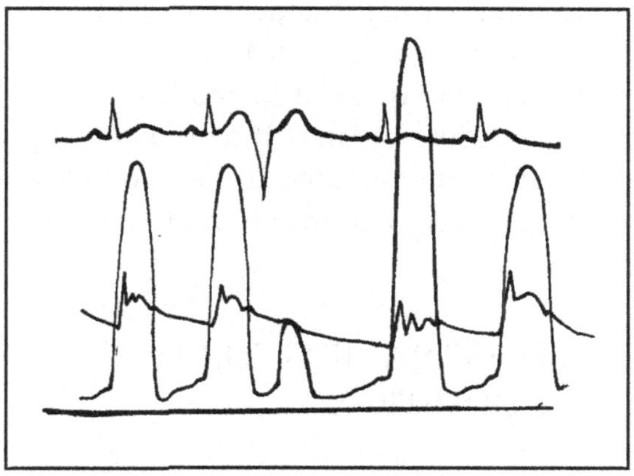

Simultaneous LV AO pressures X200

ANSWER d. Subvalvular obstruction, also termed IHSS or HOCM. After the long compensatory pause of a PVC, the gradient between LV-AO increases. This drop in AO pressures after a PVC is not seen in normal or AS patients, and is termed "Brockenbrough's sign" (The same Dr. that invented the Brockenbrough catheter). **See:** Baim , chapter on "Profiles in hypertrophic cardiomyopathies." **Keywords:** Subvalvular (Obstruction HOCM/IHSS) = Brockenbrough's sign.

240. This patient, who had rheumatic fever as a child, now has a diastolic blowing murmur. The simultaneous pressure tracing shown suggests a diagnosis of:

a. Pure MR
b. Pure MS
c. Pure TS
d. Mixed MS -MR

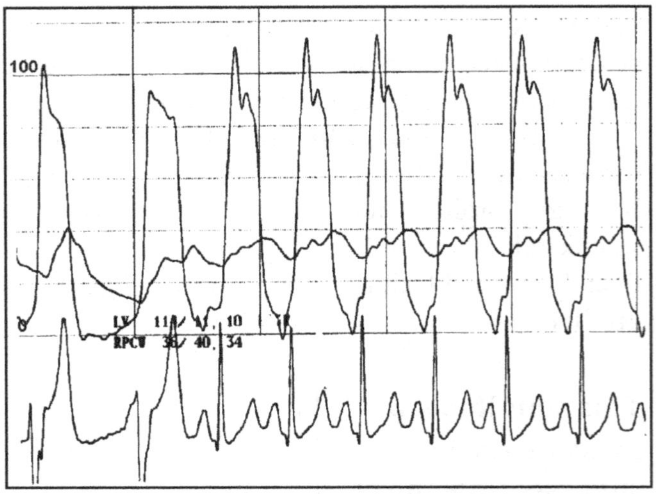

Simultaneous LV & PAW tracing X 200

ANSWER b. Pure MS. There is a 20-30 mmHg LV-PAW diastolic gradient of MS. The V waves are not extra large, although this does not rule out MR. Mitral stenosis is almost always associated with a history of rheumatic fever.
See: Kern, chapter on "Hemodynamics." **Keywords:** mixed AS-MS

241. What valvular abnormality is indicated in these simultaneous pressures?

a. Mitral stenosis
b. Mitral regurgitation
c. Constrictive pericarditis
d. Pericardial tamponade

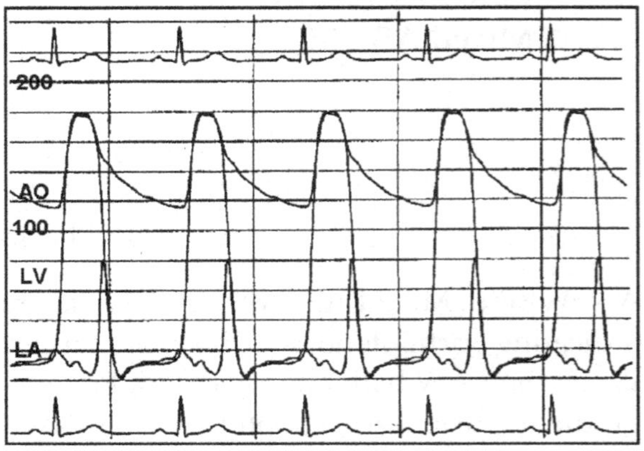

Simultaneous LV, LA, and AO pressures X 200

ANSWER b. Mitral regurgitation. The large V waves of 80 mmHg on the LA pressure indicate Mitral Regurgitation. The V wave is more than 3 times the mean of 25 mmHg. With the "v" waves occurring so late in systole, this may be late systolic mitral valve prolapse. Note the matching diastolic LV & LA pressures indicate no mitral stenosis. This pressure was generated by electronic simulator.
See: Kern, chapter on "Hemodynamics." **Keywords:** ID pressures of MR - V wave

USE THIS TRACING FOR THE NEXT QUESTION.

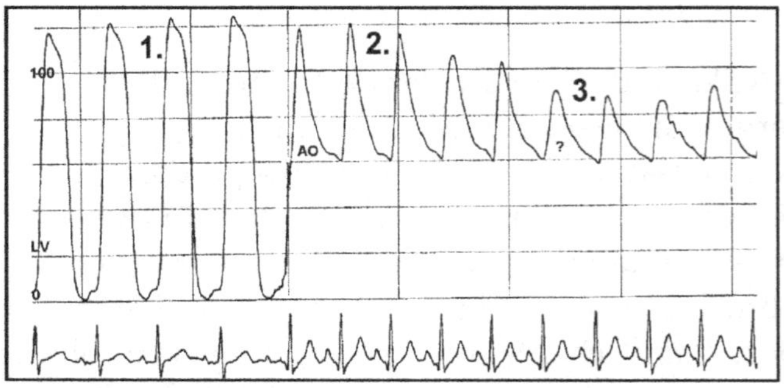

LV→AO pullback x 200

242. This pullback pressure above was recorded as the pigtail catheter was slowly pulled back slowly from LV apex to descending AO. This tracing suggests a diagnosis of:

a. Hypertrophic obstructive cardiomyopathy (HOCM)
b. Aortic stenosis
c. Aortic regurgitation
d. Coarctation of aorta

ANSWER d. Coarctation of aorta. Note the drop in systolic pressure from the ascending to descending AO, as the catheter pulls through the stenotic area. The tracing shows the following 3 pressure areas:

1. LV
2. AO arch: The LV→AO pullback is normal.
3. AO descending: There is a 30 mm systolic gradient between these aortic pressures.

See: Baim chapter on "Congenital Heart Defects." Keywords: Pressure pullback in Coarctation of AO

USE THIS TRACING FOR THE NEXT QUESTION.

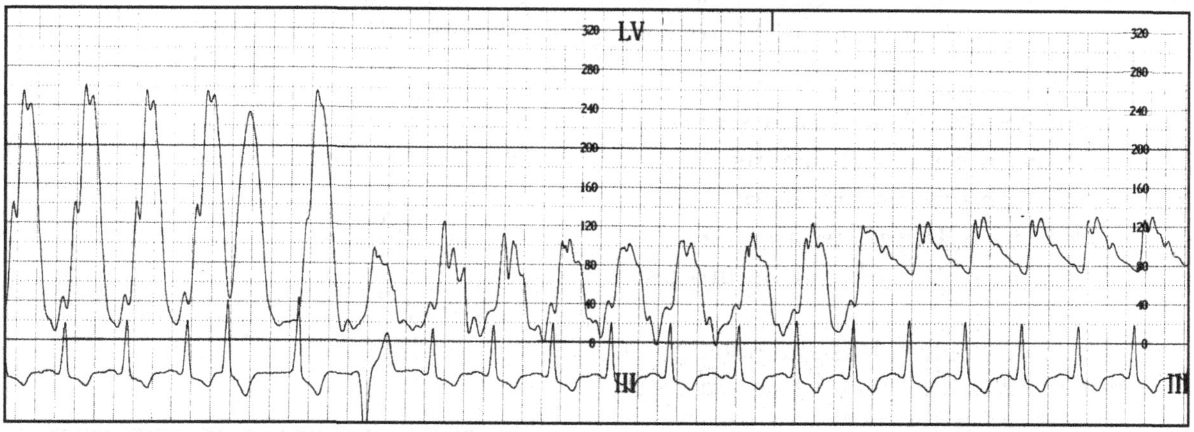

LV→AO pullback x 400

243. This pullback pressure above was recorded as a pigtail catheter was pulled back from the LV apex into the aorta. This suggests a diagnosis of:

a. Coarctation of aorta
b. Patent ductus arteriosus
c. Hypertension induced LV failure
d. Hypertrophic obstructive cardiomyopathy (HOCM)

ANSWER d. Hypertrophic obstructive cardiomyopathy (HOCM) or the old name "Idiopathic Hypertrophic Cardiomyopathy." Note the 260 mmHg LV systolic pressure falls to 100 mmHg systolic mid-tracing. You can tell that the initial chamber is LV by the rapidly rising high pressure levels. The middle tracing strongly resembles the original LV with a lower systole. It is from the LV outflow track. A 120-160 mmHg gradient occurs within the LV outflow track. This is usually due to a thick hypertrophied LV that contracts down on itself, pinching off the outflow and the systolic pressure. The Aortic systolic tracing matches with the LV outflow track showing that no valvular AS is present. See: Baim , chapter on "Cardiomyopathy." Keywords: pressure pullback in HOCM, IHSS

244. This RA tracing suggests a diagnosis of:

a. Mitral regurgitation

b. Constrictive pericarditis

c. Tricuspid stenosis

d. Tricuspid regurgitation

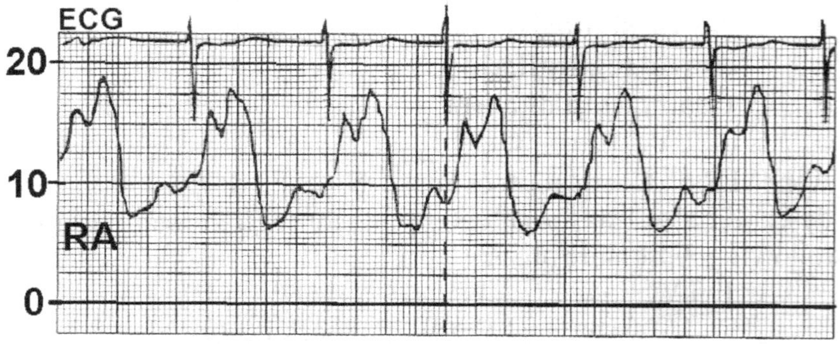

CVP or RA tracing with ECG (after Ward)

ANSWER d. Tricuspid regurgitation. Note the large systolic waves, that look more like RV. Ward say: "A tall regurgitant v wave and a steep y descent in the central venous pressure (CVP) trace are the hallmarks of tricuspid regurgitation. The holosystolic nature of the regurgitation is illustrated by the fusion of c and v waves, which essentially obliterates the normal systolic x descent in CVP. " The systolic (c & v waves) are the large waves following the QRS complex. See" Ward, chapter on "Patterns of Valvular Heart Disease"

245. This tracing suggests a diagnosis of:

a. AS with pulsus alternans

b. AS with pulsus bigeminus

c. HOCM with pulsus alternans

d. HOCM with pulsus bigeminus

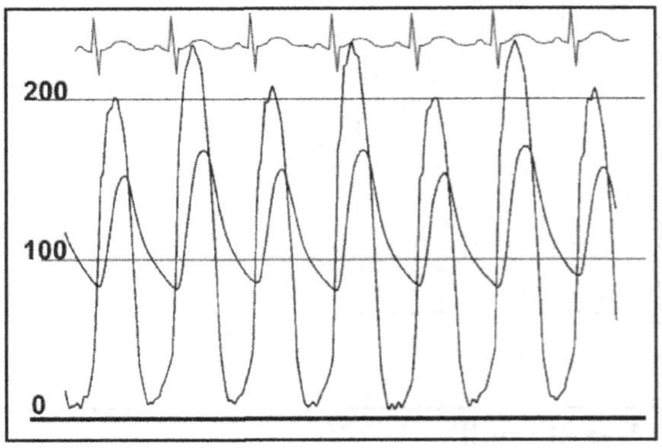

Simultaneous LV AO pressures X200 - after Ragosta

ANSWER a. AS with pulsus alternans. Note the sinus rhythm, the LV-AO gradient, high LV-edp and alternating systolic pressure (alternans). Systolic hypertension. AS with probable failing heart. See: Ragosta, chapter on "Hemodynamic Waveforms". Keywords: AS, pulsus alternans

REFERENCES:

Ahrens, T. S., and Taylor, L.A., *Hemodynamic Waveform Analysis*, 1st Ed., W.B. Saunders Co., 1992

Baim, D. S. and Grossman W., *Cardiac Catheterization, Angiography, and Intervention*, 6th Ed., Lea and Febiger, 2006

Berne R. M. and Levy, M. N., *Cardiovascular Physiology*, 6th Ed., Mosby Year Book, 1992

Braunwald, et. al. Ed., *Heart Disease, a Textbook of CV Medicine*, 8th Ed., Saunders, 2008

Daily, E. K., and Schroeder, J. S., *Techniques in Bedside Hemodynamic Monitoring*, 4th Ed., C. V. Mosby Company, 1989

Darovic, G.O., *Hemodynamic Monitoring: Invasive and Noninvasive Clinical Application*, WB Saunders, 1995

Kern, M. J., Ed., *The Cardiac Catheterization Handbook*, 3rd Ed., Mosby-Year Book, 2003

Kern, M.J., *Hemodynamic Rounds: interpretation of cardiac pathophysiology from pressure waveform analysis*, St. Louis, Wiley-Liss, 1993

Pepine, J. C., and Hill, J. A., et. al., *Diagnostic and Therapeutic Cardiac Catheterization*, 2nd Ed., Williams and Wilkins, 1994

Ragosta, Michael, Cardiac Catheterization, an Atlas and DVD, Saunders, 1st Edition, 2010

Taylor, E. J. Ed., *Dorland's Medical Dictionary*, 27th ed., W. B. Saunders Co.,1988

Verel D. and Grainger R., *Cardiac Catheterization and Angiography, an Introductory Manual*, 2nd Ed., Churchill Livingstone, 1973

Ward, Johnathan B, *Atlas of Cardiovascular Monitoring*, Churchill Livingstone, 1998

Omid Salehian MD, Cardiac Hemodynamic Evaluation: Online Manual, http://faculty.ksu.edu.sa/Hussam%20Al-Faleh/Postgraduate/Hemodynamic%20manuel.pdf

OUTLINE: PRESSURE PATHOLOGY

1. GENERAL PATHOLOGY
   a. Arterial Pulse Patterns
      i. Pulsus alternans
      ii. Pulsus bigeminus
      iii. Pulsus bisferiens
      iv. Pulsus tardus
      v. Corrigan's pulse
   b. Associated Pulse Pathology
      i. Heart failure
      ii. Bigeminy
      iii. HOCM
      iv. Aortic Stenosis (AS)
      v. Aortic Insufficiency (AI)
      vi. Corrigan's pulse
   c. Valvular Pathology synonyms
      i. Prolapsing, buckling, billowing, floppy, redundant
      ii. Leaky, insufficient, regurgitant, incompetent, back-flow
      iii. Stenotic, obstructive, narrowed, blockage, gradient
      iv. Restrictive, encased, constricted, filling limited, diastolic disorder
2. CORONARY ARTERY MONITORING
   a. Ventricularization = mainstem
   b. Reduced pressure damping
   c. Reduced high frequency damping
   d. Valsalva
   e. Mixed LV-AO
   f. Arrhythmia
      i. Asystole
      ii. V Tach.
      iii. V. Fib.
      iv. Therapy for
         (1) precordial thump
         (2) defibrillation
         (3) pacemaker
         (4) Lidocaine
         (5) Remove catheter
   g. Contrast Effects
      i. RCA = ST depression
      ii. LCA = ST elevation
      iii. Bradycardia
      iv. Hypotension
      v. Toxicity
3. HEART FAILURE PATHOLOGY
   a. Starling's Law: preload
   b. CHF = ↑preload = ↑ LVEDP = ↑ PAWP

4. MYOCARDIAL/PERICARDIAL PATHOLOGY
   a. False √ (Y WAVE) LV underdamping
   b. Restrictive Cardiomyopathy √ y
   c. Constrictive Pericarditis = & √ y
   d. Pericardial Tamponade = of diastolic pressures
   e. Stages of PT: early, intermediate, end stage
   f. Pulsus paradoxus

5. VALVE PATHOLOGY
   a. GENERAL VALVE
      i. AS (valvular) = LV-AO systolic gradient
      ii. HOCM = IHSS = subvalvular
      iii. AR, low AO diastolic
      iv. MS, PAW - LV diastolic gradient
      v. MR, elevated PAW V wave
      vi. ID pressure levels and waves
      vii. Associated Doppler jets
      viii. Mixed lesions (AS & MS, AS & AR)
   b. MITRAL STENOSIS
      i. Diastolic Gradient LV-PAWP
      ii. Sloe Y descent
      iii. Exercise
         (1) ↑CO = ↑↑Gradient
      iv. V waves may be seen in stiff LV
   c. MITRAL REGURGITATION
      i. Tricuspid Regurgitation (TR)
      ii. Significant v waves (3 x mean PAW)
      iii. Reflected V waves (in PAWP)
      iv. V waves seen in:
         (1) VSD
         (2) Atrial Fibrillation
         (3) Dilated/failing LV
         (4) Enlarged/compliant LA
         (5) Acute Mitral Regurgitation
      v. Characteristics acute ruptured chordae (↑v, ↑ LVEDP, diastolic filling ↑y, ↑LVMF)
      vi. Therapy for severe/acute MR
         (1) IABP (ID 1:1 & 2:1 counterpulsation)
         (2) Nitrates (↓ afterload)
   d. AORTIC STENOSIS
      i. Valvular
      ii. HOCM = IHSS
      iii. Coarctation (supravalvular Obstr.)
      iv. Combined: sub-valve, valvular, supra-valvular
      v. Carabello's Sign - cath obstruction
      vi. Impulse gradient
      vii. Pullback patterns
         (1) Infundibular stenosis
         (2) Coarctation of PA
         (3) Pulmonary stenosis
         (4) Tricuspid stenosis
         (5) Coarctation of AO
         (6) Aortic Stenosis
         (7) Pulmonary Arteriolar gradient:
      viii. Recording FA via sheath (1 F larger)
      ix. HOCM
         (1) Dynamic intraventricular systolic gradient
         (2) Kussmaul Sign (↑ PAWP insp.)
         (3) Brockenbrough sign (↓ Post-PVC AO beat, ↑gradient)
         (4) Provocative maneuvers:
            (a) Valsalva maneuver
            (b) Amyl nitrate inhalation
            (c) nitroglycerine
            (d) Post-extra systolic potentiation
            (e) Isoproterenol
            (f) Exercise
   e. AORTIC REGURGITATION
      i. Stages
      ii. ↓ AO diastolic (wide pulse pressure)
      iii. Water-hammer pulse = Corrigan's pulse = bounding

6. CONGENITAL PATHOLOGY
   a. Pullback pressure patterns
      i. Coarctation of the PA
      ii. Coarctation of AO
      iii. Pulmonic Stenosis
      iv. Infundibular Stenosis
      v. Aortic Stenosis
      vi. VSD, ASD, PDA
      vii. Tetralogy Fallot
7. OTHER PRESSURE PATHOLOGY
   a. Transseptal Needle patterns
      i. LA
      ii. Pericardium
      iii. AO
      iv. Myocardial wall
   b. Transseptal pullback patterns
      i. MS
   c. Valsalva pattern
      i. Normal phases
      ii. Abnormal
8. PRACTICE TRACINGS

FICK CO and SHUNT CALCULATIONS

INDEX: E6

General Cardiac Output

246. Match the cardiac output abbreviation labeled #3 (LVMF) with its definition below.

a. Amount of blood pumped by the heart adjusted to body size

b. Quantitative angiographic CO

c. Indicator dilution CO using cooled saline

d. Average pulmonary CO measured via oxygen extraction

HEMODYNAMIC ABBREVIATIONS
1. TDCO
2. Fick CO
*3. LVMF
4. CI

ANSWER b. Quantitative angiographic CO is also termed Left Ventricular Minute Flow (LVMF)

MATCH THE OTHER HEMODYNAMIC ABBREVIATIONS

1. TDCO = Indicator dilution CO using cooled saline (Thermodilution CO)
2. Fick CO = Average Pulmonary CO measured via oxygen extraction (Oxygen consumption per AV difference)
* 3. LVMF = Quantitative angiographic CO (Left Ventricular Minute Flow)
4. CI = Amount of blood pumped by the heart adjusted to body size (Cardiac Index)

See: Yang, chapter on "Cardiac Output." Keywords: CO definitions

247. Match the oxygen abbreviation labeled #2 (SaO_2) in the box with its definition below.

a. Arterial blood O_2 saturation

b. Arterial blood O_2 content

c. Partial pressure of arterial O_2

d. Oxygen consumption rate

e. Inspired O_2%

BLOOD GAS ABBREVIATION
1. $\dot{V}O_2$
***2. SaO_2**
3. CaO_2
4. FIO_2
5. PaO_2

ANSWER a. Arterial blood O_2 saturation. In blood

abbreviations the first large capital letter represents the **type** of measurement taken. E.g., Content, Saturation, Partial pressure. The second small letter, represents the location of the blood sample E.g.. arterial, venous, mixed venous, capillary. The last capital letters represent the gas measured e.g. oxygen, CO_2. An initial capital V and F indicate Ventilation or Fraction.

MATCH THE OTHER BLOOD GAS ABBREVIATIONS SHOWN:

1. $\dot{V}O_2$: Oxygen consumption rate in ml/min as used in the Fick CO technique (the dot above the V indicates rate/min)
*2. **SaO_2**: Saturation of arterial Oxygen, as measured by oximetry
3. CaO_2: Content of arterial Oxygen, as calculated from O_2 sat. & Hgb
4. FIO_2: Fraction of inspired Oxygen, normally 21% unless pt. is on O_2.
5. PaO_2: Partial pressure of arterial oxygen, as in arterial blood gas PO_2

See: Underhill, chapter on "Hemostasis" **Keywords**: Blood O_2 abbreviations

248. The units of #1 in the box (Q) in hemodynamic formulae are usually:

a. **Vol. %**
b. **mmHg**
c. **L/min**
d. **ml/min**
e. **gm/dl**

HEMO. PARAMETER

***1. $\dot{Q}$** (also termed Q dot)
2. O_2 Consumption
3. A-V difference
4. P O_2
5. Hemoglobin

ANSWER c. L/min. $\dot{Q}$ (or Q dot) is flow of a quantity of blood in L/min. The dot means per unit time. Q even without the dot, may be used as an abbreviation for CO, as in the Q_p/Q_s or Pulmonary blood flow /Systemic blood flow.

MATCH THE OTHER HEMODYNAMIC PARAMETERS

1. Q (as in Q_p/Q_s)	= **L/min**
2. O_2 Consumption	= **ml/min**
3. A-V difference	= **vol. % or ml/decaliter**
4. P O_2	= **mmHg**
5. Hemoglobin	= **gm/deciliter or gm %**

See: Yang, chapter on "Cardiac Output." **Keywords:** CO units

249. "Indexed" hemodynamic parameters like "Stroke Index," are corrected for the patient's:

a. **Age and sex**
b. **Ideal body weight**
c. **Heart size**
d. **Body surface area**

ANSWER d. Body surface area is what many cardiac parameters are "indexed" to, because it has been found to be the most closely correlated with body size. Cardiac size and output are normally larger in larger people, and are more accurately assessed by "indexing" them. Thus Cardiac Output is divided by BSA to get Cardiac Index. BSA calculation involves plotting the patient's height and weight on a nomogram. Normal adult BSA ranges from

1.5 to 2.0 square meters (M^2). See: Tortora chapter on "Cardiovascular System: Blood Vessels" also, Keywords: BSA

250. Identify all of the physiologic measurements that can be adjusted to a patient's body size (indexed). (Check 3 below.)

a. **EDV**

b. **CO**

c. **Valve area**

d. **Q_p/Q_s**

e. EF

ANSWERS: a, b, & c. Q_p/Q_s and EF are ratios which do NOT vary with body size. Even if each Q_p and Q_s were indexed, BSA would cancel out in the ratio. Ratios of the same units are dimension-less and cannot be indexed e.g., Q_p/Q_s, EF, RF, and hematocrit. Most physiological measurements increase as the size of the person increases. Indexing adjusts the measurement so that it can then be compared to a normal population of people irrespective of body size. For example, cardiac output (CO) adjusted to body size is termed cardiac index (CI). It is simply cardiac output divided by the persons body surface area:

$$CI = CO/BSA$$

BSA is a more accurate index of body size than just weight alone. Any term with the word "index" behind it means it has been adjusted to that patient's BSA.

See: Braunwald, Chapter on "Evaluation of LV Function"

Keywords: CI, index adjusts for body size

251. The normal resting cardiac output varies with age, position, and BSA. Estimate the normal resting cardiac index (CI) for the patient #1 (reclining 7 year old child) in the box.

a. **2.0 L/min/M^2**

b. **2.5 L/min/M^2**

c. **3.5 L/min/M^2**

d. **4.5 L/min/M^2**

Patient # 251

***1. Reclining 7 year old child**

2. Standing 7 year old child

3. Reclining 70 year old adult

4. Standing 70 year old adult

ANSWER d. 4.5 L/min/M^2. Grossman says,

> *"the normal cardiac output appears to vary with age, steadily decreasing from approximately 4.5 L/min/M^2 at age 7 to approximately 2.5 L/min/M^2 at age 70... In addition to age, cardiac output is affected by posture, decreasing approximately 10% when rising from a lying to a sitting position and approximately 20% when rising (or after being tilted) from a lying to a standing position. Also, body temperature, anxiety, environmental heat and humidity, and a host of other factors influence the normal resting cardiac output."*

Normal reclining CI declines with age from 4.5. to 2.5 L/min/m^2. Thus the overall average CI for a reclining middle aged individual is around 3.5 L/min/M^2.

CORRECTLY MATCHED ANSWERS ARE:

1. Reclining 7 year old child = 4.5 L/min/M^2 (children have high metabolic rate)
2. Standing 7 year old child = 3.5 L/min/M^2 (reduced 20% from reclining CI)
3. Reclining 70 year old adult= 2.5 L/min/M^2
4. Standing 70 year old adult = 2.0 L/min/M^2 (reduced 20% from reclining CI)

See: Baim and Grossman, chapter on "Blood Flow measurement." **Keywords**: normal CI declines with age from 4.5 to 2.5 L/min/M^2.

252. Estimate the average predicted resting reclining cardiac output of a large healthy man from data in the box.

a. **3 L/min**
b. **5 L/min**
c. **7 L/min**
d. **9 L/min**

Patient # 252
Age = 70
Wt = 86 Kg
BP = 146/86
HR = 79 /min
BSA = 2.0 M^2

ANSWER b. 5 L/min. From above question we know the average Cardiac Index of a reclining 70 year old patient is 2.5 L/min/M^2. To get Cardiac Output, multiply the BSA times this average CI. CO = CI x BSA = 2.5 x 2 = 5.0 L/min. Of course this is only an average for normal individuals and it varies ± 10%. **See**: Baim and Grossman, chapter on "Blood Flow measurement." **Keywords**: normal resting reclining CO

Blood O_2

253. Normal adult female hemoglobin is:

a. **10 gm % (or gm/dl.)**
b. **13 gm % (or gm/dl.)**
c. **18 gm % (or gm/dl.)**
d. **22 gm % (or gm/dl.)**

ANSWER b. 13 gm % or gm/dl. (deciliter). The normal values for male blood hemoglobin concentration ranges from 14 - 18 gm/100 ml (females normal values are 2 gm/100 lower than men due to menses). This number can be approximated by taking ⅓ of the measured hematocrit. However, this method is not as accurate as measuring Hgb. directly. Eg. Hct. of 45%: Hgb. = Hct/3 = 45/3 = 15. gm. %
See: Tilkian, Clinical Implications of Laboratory Tests "Complete Blood Count **Keywords:** Blood, Hgb. normal

254. Which right heart O_2 saturation is normally the highest?

a. **SVC**
b. **IVC**
c. **CS**
d. **RV**
e. **PA**

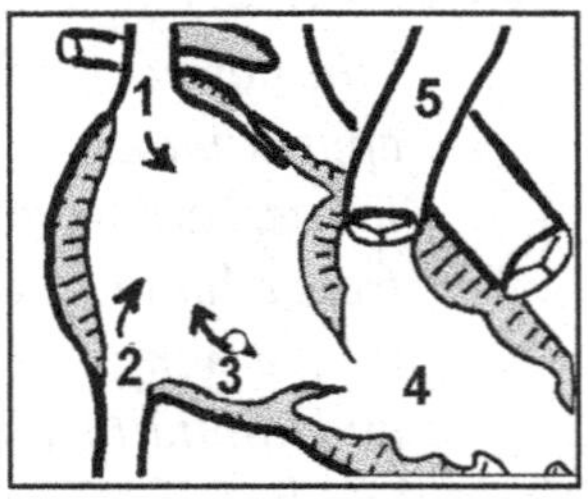

Right heart blood

ANSWER b. IVC blood shown at #2 receives blood from the lower body and abdominal organs that utilize little oxygen. E.g. the kidneys are mainly a pressurized water extractor. While the upper body and the brain are large consumers of O_2. Remember the coronary sinus returns the lowest saturation in the heart - around 40% O_2 saturation. Remember too, the best mixed venous blood is from the

PA. **See:** Todd's Vol. 2 **Keywords**: IVC is highest rt. ht. sat.

O_2 CONTENT

255. The actual amount of O_2 carried in blood (in vol.% or ml/L) is defined as the oxygen ____.

a. **Content**
b. **Capacity**
c. **Saturation**
d. **Dissociation**

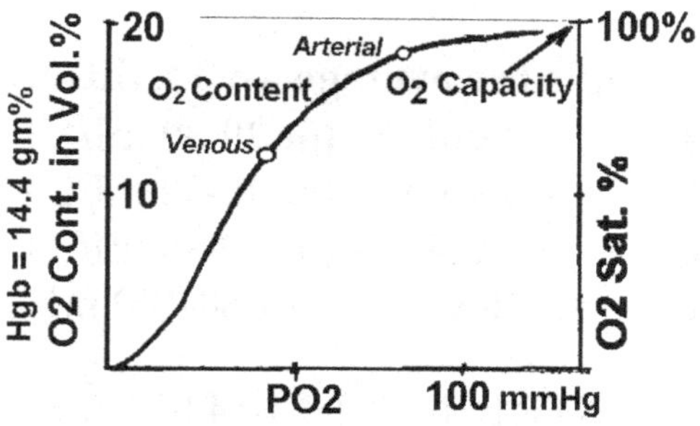

ANSWER a. O_2 content is the amount (cc.) of O_2 contained in a quantity ml of blood. O_2 content is directly proportional to % O_2 Saturation. But O_2 content varies non-linearly with the PO_2 (see O_2 dissociation curve diagram). Note this curve has two vertical axes, one for O_2 content (assuming Hgb of 14.4 gm % or gm/dL) and one for O_2 saturation. The formula for O_2 content is:

Note that some labs use 1.34 or 1.39 instead of 1.36 vol%/gm/dL Hgb as their constant. These definitions are essential background in the calculation of Fick Cardiac Output. **See:** Baim and Grossman, chapter on "Blood Flow and CO" **Keywords:** O_2 content

256. For Fick CO blood O_2 content is usually expressed in units of:

a. **gm O_2/dL**
b. **mm Hg. (PO_2)**
c. **Grams O_2 / Liter of blood**
d. **ml O_2 / 100 ml blood**

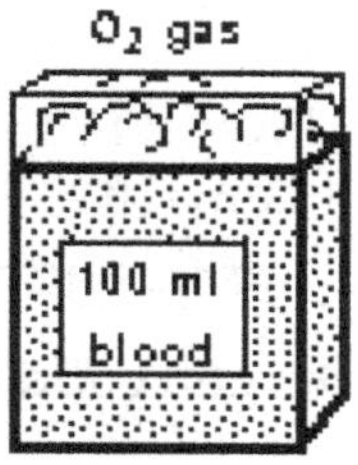

ANSWER d. ml O_2/100 ml blood. This is the unit for volume percent, e.g. the actual amount of oxygen in the blood. As shown, it is the percentage by volume, or the volume of gaseous oxygen that can be extracted from 100 ml of blood. The units of O_2 content and A-V difference are:

Oxygen content in Vol % = ml O_2/100 or ml O_2/ deciliter blood

When it is multiplied by 10 it becomes ml / L of blood. This is the unit needed in the Fick CO calculation to get CO in L/min. That is also why the denominator of the Fick equation is multiplied x 10 - to convert from deciliters to Liters of blood. Some authors use O_2 content units already multiplied by 10. These units are in ml O_2/L of blood.
See: Baim and Grossman, chapter on "Blood Flow Measurement: The Cardiac Output"
Keywords: vol. % = ml O_2/100 ml blood

257. The normal O_2 content of blood in the left heart is:

a. **11-12 vol % (or 110-120 ml/L)**
b. **18-22 vol % (or 180-220 ml/L)**
c. **25-30 vol % (or 250-300 ml/L)**
d. **40-50 vol % (or 400-500 ml/L)**

ANSWER b. 18-22 vol %. The normal O_2 saturation in the left heart is 96%. So using the above formula for O_2 content, O_2 cont. = 0.96 x 1.36 x 15 Hgb = 19.6 vol%
See: Baim and Grossman, chapter on "Blood Flow Measurement: The Cardiac Output"
Keywords: normal left heart O_2 content 19 vol. %

258. What is the average a-v O_2 difference in resting adults?

a. **2-3 vol % (or 20-30 ml/L)**
b. **4-5 vol % (or 40-50 ml/L)**
c. **6-8 vol % (or 60-80 ml/L)**
d. **8-10 vol % (or 80-100 ml/L)**

ANSWER b. 4-5 vol % or 40-50 ml/L). Normal arterial and venous oxygen levels average 96% and 75% O_2 sat. Using the O_2 content formula: venous O_2 content averages 0.75 x 1.36 x 15 = 15.3 vol %.
A-V difference = arterial O_2 content - venous O_2 content = 19.6 - 15.3 = 4.3 vol %. This is the average number found in the denominator of the Fick CO equation. Being in the denominator, as A-V difference widens the CO decreases.
See: Baim and Grossman, chapter on "Blood Flow Measurement: The Cardiac Output"
Keywords: normal a-v difference = 4-5 vol%

259. Calculate the O_2 Volume % of the blood sample shown in the box. (Hint: Hgb = Hct/3)

a. **14.1 vol % (or 141 ml/L)**
b. **16.3 vol % (or 163 ml/L)**
c. **17.9 vol % (or 179 ml/L)**
d. **18.4 vol % (or 184 ml/L)**
e. **21.0 vol% (or 210 ml/L)**

Patient # 259
Hct = 45%
Hgb ?
SaO_2 = 80%
PaO_2 = 50 mmHg

ANSWER b. 16.3 vol % (or 163 ml/L). Use the hematocrit to estimate the Hgb. Hgb = 45/3 = 15 gm/dL. This is a normal Hgb and Hct so the O_2 capacity should be around 20. vol%. 80% of this number is 16. vol %. The formula is:

Oxygen content in Vol % = % Sat x 1.36 x Hgb

Using this formula: O_2 Content = 1.36 x Hgb x % sat./100
= 1.36 x 15 x 0.80 = 16.3 vol % (or 163 ml/L)
See: Baim and Grossman, chapter on "Blood Flow Measurement: The Cardiac Output"
Keywords: O_2 content = 1.36 x Hgb x % sat./100

260. Identify 3 recommended procedures for storing blood gas samples taken at cath that are not analyzed immediately. (Select 3 below.)

a. **De-bubble the syringe**
b. **Pre-flush the syringe with heparin**
c. **Withdraw catheter dead space prior to sampling**
d. **Store at body temperature**
e. **Transfer blood to glass syringe**

ANSWERS: a, b, & c. Storing at body temperature is NOT correct. Icing ABGs is routine. Unless blood samples are capped and iced immediately, the blood gas values will change. At body temperature room air O_2 will be absorbed, CO_2 will diffuse out, and the warm living blood cells will continue to metabolize. Plastic syringes are commonly used. Peterson says,

> "*Every effort should be made to ensure that the blood samples are collected anaerobically and are free from contaminating saline or excess heparin... Any air bubble is expelled, and the syringe is capped. The sample should be analyzed promptly. If this is not possible, the sample must be kept on ice.*"

Initially prepare the syringe dead space with a heparin solution. Use it to wet the syringe with anticoagulant, then expel most of it. Do this prior to sampling to prevent dilution of the sample. Baim states that if the patient is fully heparinized, heparin need not be added to the syringe. After blood is drawn, point the syringe up and eject any air bubbles. Syringes containing dry heparin are available. Use a waste syringe to draw back the catheter dead space, so the sample is not contaminated with flush solution. See: Bain, chapter on "Cardiac Output", **Keywords**: Cap and ice ABGs immediately

261. For Fick CO where should the arterial blood sample be taken?

- **a. Ascending AO**
- **b. Descending AO**
- **c. Pulmonary artery**
- **d. Any systemic artery**

ANSWER d. Any systemic artery. Yang says,

> "*In determining the* ***AVO$_2$*** *difference any systemic artery may be utilized for arterial blood sampling, because the O_2 content of the arterial blood is uniform throughout the body. The mixed venous blood is preferably sampled from the pulmonary artery, where the mixing is adequate.*"

This is true for any arterial blood gas sample: radial, brachial, or femoral - all the same. **See:** Yang, chapter on "Cardiac Output." **Keywords:** arterial sample from any artery

262. From the list below, select the blood analyzers that the O2 content for A-V difference and Fick CO calculation may be measured on. (Select 3 below.)

- **a. Van Slyke apparatus (O_2 content analyzer)**
- **b. Clark polaragraphic (PO_2 electrode)**
- **c. Spectrophotometer (oximeter)**
- **d. Scholander apparatus (% O_2)**
- **e. Finger pulse oximeter (O_2 sat.)**

ANSWERS: a, b, & c. The Scholander is for analyzing air samples for O_2 consumption, but CANNOT be used for blood. Finger oximeters not used for PA blood. Yang says,

> "*The final step in the calculation of CO is the determination of O_2 content in the arterial and venous blood samples. This is generally carried out using one of the following instruments: (1) Van Slyke manometric apparatus, which measures all the O_2 bound Hb and dissolved in plasma) present in the sample (CO_2); (2) the Clark O_2 electrode (generally*

part of an instrument that also measured PCO_2 and pH) and; (3) the spectrophotometer, which measures the hemoglobin saturation (S) in the sample-...."

See: Yang, chapter on "Cardiac Output." **Keywords**: Scholander gas analyzer (cannot analyze blood)

263. Using the data in the box calculate this patient's Hgb. arterial O_2 content.

a. **8.4 vol.% (or 8.4 ml/L)**
b. **10.8 vol.% (or 108 ml/L)**
c. **12.5 vol.% (or 125 ml/L)**
d. **14.7 vol.% (or 147 ml/L)**

Patient # 263 - O_2 DATA ON ANEMIC PATIENT
PaO_2 = 65 mmHg
SaO_2 = 90% by oximetry
Hgb. = 12.0 gm/dL.
O_2 carrying capacity = 1.36 ml O_2/gm %. Hgb.

ANSWER d. 14.7 vol.%. O_2 content = Hgb. x carrying capacity x % sat.

C_aO_2 = 12 x 1.36 x .90 = 14.7 vol.%. | Oxygen content in Vol % = % Sat x 1.36 x Hgb |

Note that the SaO_2 is changed into its decimal equivalent (90% = 0.90). Content of arterial O_2 (C_aO_2) is the actual amount of O_2 combined with Hgb. in arterial blood. Physically dissolved O_2 in the plasma can be calculated from the PO_2 but is not usually calculated because it is insignificant unless the patient is on oxygen. Be able to discriminate between useful and superfluous data in questions. Here ignore the given PaO_2. (Note: PaO_2 = Partial Pressure of arterial blood Oxygen) **See:** Baim and Grossman, chapter on "Cardiac Outputs" **Keywords:** Blood, O_2 Content, Calculation CaO_2

264. Which arterial blood gas parameter will be reduced in an anemic patient?

a. **C_aO_2 (vol %)**
b. **P_aO_2 (mm Hg.)**
c. **S_aO_2 (% Sat.)**
d. **SaCO (arterial carbon monoxide)**

ANSWER a. C_aO_2 (vol %). This stands for: Content - arterial - O_2. In anemia the hemoglobin level is low. This will reduce the O_2 carrying capacity of the blood and with it the O_2 content. However, the O_2 saturation and PO_2 values do **not** decrease in anemia, unless hypoventilation or lung disease are present.

ABBREVIATIONS LISTED ARE:

1. C_aO_2 (vol %) = Content of arterial oxygen
2. P_aO_2 (mm Hg.) = Partial pressure of arterial O_2
3. S_aO_2 (% Sat.) = Saturation of arterial O_2
4. SaCO (arterial carbon monoxide) = Saturation of arterial carbon monoxide

See: Underhill, chapter on "Systemic and Pulmonary Circulations - O_2 transport." **Keywords**: reduced C_aO_2 (vol %) in anemia

O_2 CAPACITY & SATURATION

265. What is the theoretical oxygen carrying capacity of adult hemoglobin?

a. **1.00 ml O_2/ gram Hgb**
b. **1.36 ml O_2/ gram Hgb**
c. **1.96 ml O_2/ gram Hgb**
d. **2.54 ml O_2/ gram Hgb**

ANSWER b. 1.36 ml. The maximum amount which can be carried (at 100% saturation) is termed the "O_2 capacity" in Volume % units.

Most labs use 1.36 ml/mg%. Thus is the constant you multiply times the hemoglobin value to get the theoretical oxygen capacity in volume %.

The formula is: Theoretical oxygen carrying capacity = 1.36 x Hgb

The capacity is then multiplied by % saturation to get oxygen content in vol %. It is used every time you measure a Fick CO with O_2 sats. Various authors use factors ranging from 1.34 to 1.39. Baim and Grossman say,

> "*In several textbooks the constant is given as 1.34, but studies on crystalline human hemoglobin suggest that the correct number may be 1.36. Whatever its correct value, the formula is only an approximation.*"

We will use 1.36 ml/mg% in these questions.
See: Baim and Grossman, chapter on "Blood Flow Measurement: The Cardiac Output"
Keywords: theoretical oxygen carrying capacity of Hgb

266. The normal O_2 capacity of venous and/or arterial blood is:

a. **12 vol% (or 120 ml/L)**
b. **15 vol% (or 150 ml/L)**
c. **20 vol% (or 200 ml/L)**
d. **24 vol% (or 240 ml/L)**

ANSWER c. 20 vol% (or 200 ml/L). Normal Hgb is 15 gm/dL. O_2 capacity = Hgb x 1.36 vol% / gm/dL
O_2 cap. = 15 gm/dL x 1.36 vol% / gm/dL= 20.4 vol%. This is a trick question because the capacity of venous blood is the same as arterial blood. Bubble oxygen through it and it will become fully oxygenated. This 100% saturation point is its theoretic O_2 capacity. The formula is:

Normal oxygen carrying Capacity = 1.36 x Hgb = 1.36 x 15 = 20.4 vol %

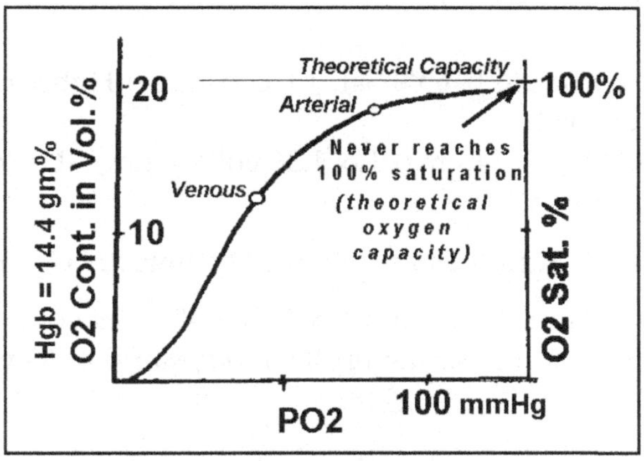

O_2 Dissociation Curve

The top of the curve shown is the "O_2 capacity." This theoretical capacity can be calculated but cannot be reached in the body due to imperfect oxygenation and the normal thebesian and bronchial shunts. In a patient with Hgb of 14.4 gm/dL as shown 100%, O_2 saturation = O_2 Capacity = 20.0 vol% (top of curve).

We use a Hgb of 14.4 gm/dL frequently because it works out to such a nice round vol. % number. Some authors (like Baim) use O_2 content and capacity units already multiplied by 10. These units are in ml O_2/L of blood. If you prefer using these larger units for this example: Capacity = 1.36 x Hgb x 10 = 1.36 x 15 x 10 = 204 ml O_2/L blood
See: Baim and Grossman, chapter on "Blood Flow Measurement: The Cardiac Output".
Keywords: Normal O_2 capacity

267. **O_2 saturation is defined as:**

a. **1.36 x Hgb**
b. **O2 content x 1.36 x Hgb**
c. **O2 content / O2 capacity x 100%**
d. **Ratio of oxygenated to deoxygenated hemoglobin x 100%**

ANSWER c. O2 content / O2 capacity x 100% as measured by VanSlyke or other oxygen analyzer. O2 capacity can be measured on the same blood sample by bubbling O2 through it. The ratio of these O2 contents is the classic O2 saturation.

But, the most common way O2 saturation is measured is with the oximeter, which analyzes the color of the blood. O2 content can then be estimated by multiplying the patients measured O2 sat. x hemoglobin x 1.36 (which is the normal affinity of Hgb for O2). O2 capacity then can be estimated by 1.36 x the patient Hgb. The ratio of these 2 calculations is the standard way saturation is measured in cath labs. See: explanation on above question:
See: Kern, chapter on "Hemodynamics." **Keywords**: Calculate O_2 saturation

268. **From the data given calculate the O_2 saturation.**

a. **54% Sat.**
b. **65% Sat.**
c. **86% Sat.**
d. **92% Sat.**

<u>**Patient # 268**</u>
O_2 content = 12.5 vol%
P O_2 = 70 mmHg
Hgb. = 14.0 gm/dL.
O_2 carrying capacity = 1.36 ml O_2/gm/dL

ANSWER b. 65% Sat. O_2 capacity = Hgb x 1.36 vol% / gm/dL. First determine O_2 Capacity.
O_2 cap. = 14 gm/dL x 1.36 vol% / gm/dL= 19.0 vol%. Substitute this into the % sat. formula.

O_2 Saturation = 100 % x O_2 content / O_2 capacity

O_2 Saturation = 100 % x 12.5 vol% / 19 vol% = 65% Saturation.
See: Kern, chapter on "Hemodynamics." **Keywords**: Calculate O_2 saturation

BOTH QUESTIONS BELOW REFER TO THIS O_2 DISSOCIATION CURVE - GRAPH:

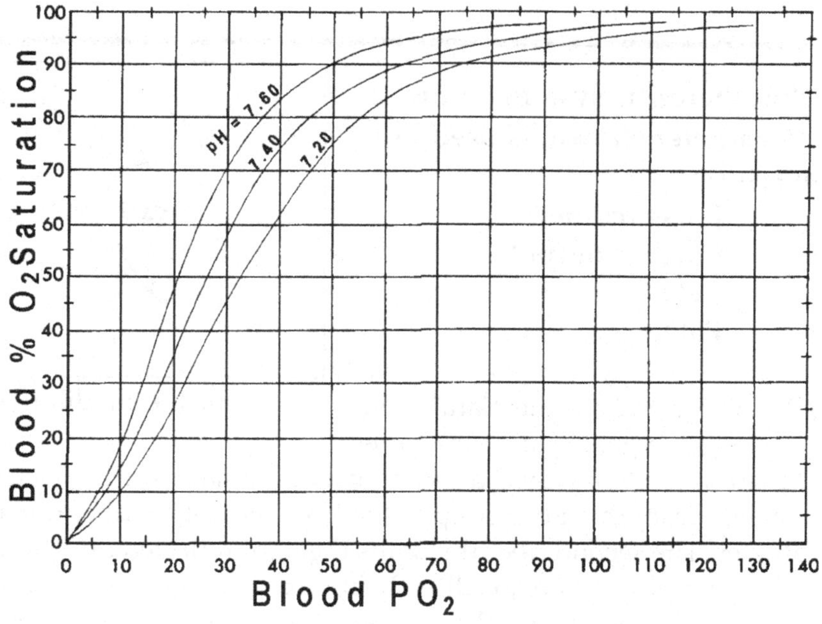

O_2 dissociation curve

269. **From the oxygen-hemoglobin dissociation curves shown, estimate the blood O_2 saturation which has a PO_2 of 30 mmHg and a pH of 7.20.**

a. 45 % sat
b. 55% sat
c. 65% sat
d. 75% sat

270. **If the Hgb = 15 gm/dL, pH = 7.40, PO_2 of AO = 90 mmHg, and PA = 40 mmHg estimate the a-v difference.**

a. 4.3 vol.% (or 43 ml/L)
b. 5.3 vol. % (or 53 ml/L)
c. 6.6 vol. % (or 66 ml/L)
d. 7.5 vol. % (or 75 ml/L)

BOTH ANSWERS FOLLOW CONSECUTIVELY:

269. ANSWER a. 45 % sat. Find the PO_2 of 50 mmHg on the horizontal axis of the graph and follow it up to the 7.20 pH curve. Then follow it over to the % sat scale on the side. Read 45%. Note what a tremendously different % saturation results if the 7.40 or 7.60 pH curves are used. This is an example of why PO_2 should not be used to estimate the oxygen content of venous blood. This curve shifts normally to the left in acidotic venous blood to facilitate O_2 unloading in the tissues. **See**: Underhill, chapter on "Systemic an Pulmonary Circulations - O_2 transport." **Keywords:** Blood, O_2 dissociation curve, PO_2, % O_2 Sat.

270. ANSWER a. 4.3 vol. % (or 43 ml/L). Using the 7.40 oxygen dissociation curve a PO_2 of 90 mmHg yields an O_2 saturation of 96%. 40 mmHg yields 75%. The O_2 saturation difference is .96 - .75 = 0.21 or 21%. This then needs to be changed into volume percent. O_2 content a-v difference = 1.36 x 15 x 0.21 = 4.3 vol %. After being multiplied by 10, this number can be put directly into the Fick CO denominator. However, because of the steepness of this curve is not very accurate for estimation of venous% saturation. **See:** Peterson, chapter on "Methods of Blood Flow" **Keywords:** Estimate a-v difference from O_2 dissociation curve

SvO_2

271. The fiberoptic system on the PA catheter shown, is used to measure:

a. Pulse oximetry
b. Cardiac output
c. SvO_2
d. PaO_2

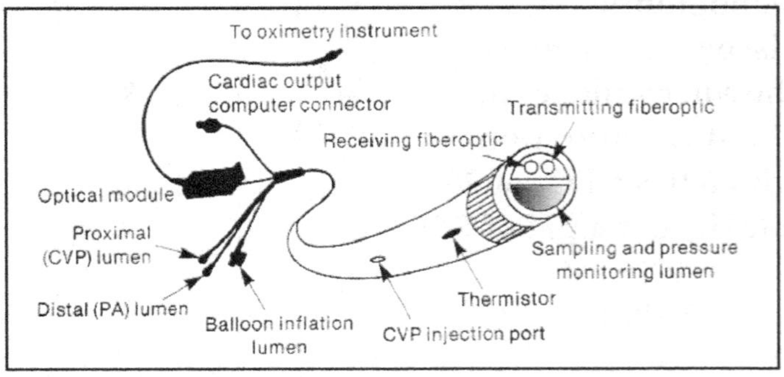

Fiberoptic thermodilution Swan (Oximetrix, Inc)

ANSWER c. SvO_2 is the "Saturation of venous oxygen." This is the same O2 saturation you would draw from a PA catheter during Fick CO, except it is measured instantly from the catheter tip in the PA. One optical fiber transmits light out the tip of the catheter. The second fiber transmits the light reflected off RBCs at the catheter tip back to the computer which reads directly in mixed venous O2 saturation or SvO_2.

The abbreviation PaO_2 means "partial pressure of arterial oxygen" - which is measured on an ABG , not via light oximetry , as saturation is.
See: Darovic, chapter on Continuous Monitoring of "Mixed Venous Oxygen Saturation SvO_2. "

272. SvO2 is an indicator of:

a. The systemic vascular oxygenation
b. Efficiency of oxygen transfer in the lungs
c. The arterial red blood cell saturation
d. Tissue oxygen supply / oxygen demand balance

ANSWER d. Tissue oxygen supply / oxygen demand balance should be 1:1 in a normal resting state. When supply of oxygen is adequate to meet demands the SvO_2 is normal at 75%. If the supply goes down for any reason, or the demand goes up, as on exercise, the SvO_2 will decrease. In extremis venous blood may look BLACK. Darovic says: "SvO2 monitoring is a sensitive indicator of the oxygen supply/demand balance. When the SvO2 values fall to less than 50 percent, the patient should be rapidly assessed for conditions that increase oxygen demand. . . . . . . .tissue hypoxia, now recognized as the common thread throughout all shock syndromes and well known as the most common cause of organ dysfunction, failure, and death. . . . Acute changes in the patient's oxygen supply/demand balance may be simply and safely assessed in the clinical setting by two technologies. First, continuous SvO2 monitoring [via Swan-Ganz fibreoptic catheters] ... Second, pulse oximetry can be used with cardiac index and hemoglobin values to estimate the amount of oxygen delivered to the body cells"
See: Darovic chapter on "Continuous Monitoring of Mixed Venous Oxygen Saturation (SvO_2)"

273. The normal range for SvO_2 is:

a. **50 - 65%**
b. **65 - 77%**
c. **75- 85%**
d. **85 to 95%**

ANSWER b. 65 - 77%. Tilkian says: "Normal saturation of mixed venous blood ranges from 65 to 77% . . . .A fall in SvO_2 below 60% lasting for 5 minutes or longer indicates a compromise in at least one of the determinants of oxygen transport (cardiac output, hemoglobin, or arterial oxygenation) . . . ." Tissue hypoxia may result.
See: Tilkian, chapter on "Hemodynamic Monitoring"

274. Your patient is being monitored with a thermodilution fiberoptic SvO_2 PA catheter. Impending deterioration of the patient is imminent when the:

a. **Wedge pressure elevates above 10 mmHg or >5% over 1 to 2 minutes**
b. **Wedge pressure elevates above 20 mmHg or >10% over 3 to 5 minutes**
c. **SvO_2 drops below 75% or drops >5% over 1 to 2 minutes**
d. **SvO_2 drops below 60% or drops >10% over 3 to 5 minutes**

ANSWER d. SvO_2 drops below 60% or drops >10% over a 3 to 5 minute period. Tilkian says: "Continuous monitoring of SvO_2 with a fiberoptic catheter provides immediate information on changes in cardiopulmonary function and balance between oxygen demand and supply. A decrease of any of the determinants of oxygen supply (cardiac output, hemoglobin, or arterial saturation) is usually associated with a decrease in SvO_2. On the other hand, If the SvO_2 begins to decline (no matter what the value) immediate assessment must be performed to determine the cause. . . . **Sustained reduction in SvO_2 of 10% or greater over a 3 to 5 minute period should prompt the above assessment, as this finding frequently warns of impending deterioration**. ... Brief, minor changes in SvO_2 (5% or less) are clinically insignificant.... "
See: Tilkian, chapter on "Hemodynamic Monitoring"

275. From the list below, identify 3 causes of reduced mixed venous SvO2. (Select 3 below)

a. **Reduced cardiac output**
b. **Reduced hemoglobin levels**
c. **Reduced arterial oxygenation**
d. **Reduced oxygen consumption**
e. **Left to right shunt**

ANSWERS: a, b, & c. Reduced oxygen consumption is NOT associated with reduced SvO_2. To the contrary, reduced oxygen consumption means reduced oxygen extraction, narrowed a-v difference, and elevated SvO_2. Reduced O2 consumption is good, suggesting a restful state. L-R shunt would increase the SvO2.

Tilkian says: "If the SvO_2 begins to decline (no matter what the value) immediate assessment must be performed to determine the cause. . . . increase in oxygen consumption can usually be readily determined as the cause if the patient has just become active, had a seizure, spiked a temperature, developed pain, etc. A decrease of any of the determinants of oxygen supply (cardiac output, hemoglobin, or arterial saturation) is usually associated with a decrease in SvO_2. . . . any change in oxygen consumption is associated with an inverse change in SvO_2 ."
See: Tilkian, chapter on "Hemodynamic Monitoring"

276. In the bedridden patient, what is the most common cause of decrease in SvO_2?

a **Hypoxemia (decreased SaO_2)**
b. **Pain or fever (increased O2 consumption)**
c. **Hypertension (increased afterload)**
d. **Hypoperfusion (decreased TDCO)**

ANSWER: d. Hyoperfusion (decreased TDCO).Tilkian says: "Hypoperfusion is the most common cause of decreased SvO_2. To confirm this, cardiac output determinations should be performed. Cardiac output measurements are made when hemodynamically indicated, rather than at some routine or preset time. Use of continuous SvO_2 monitoring has also reduced the need for routine arterial blood gas sampling." The principal other factor is increasing demand such as pain, fever, increased work of breathing, etc. O2 supply factors don't usually change quickly such as: anemia or reduced SaO_2. When you draw a PA blood sample, realize that really black blood suggests a wide a-v difference and a low CO.
See: Tilkian, chapter on "Hemodynamic Monitoring" Keywords: decreased SvO_2 = Low CO

Oxygen Consumption

277. What is the percentage of oxygen in ambient air?

a. **13.5%**
b. **18%**
c. **21%**
d. **Varies with altitude**

ANSWER c. 21.% or more accurately 20.93%. This number is constant all over the world and at any altitude. The barometric pressure and PO_2 changes, but the percentage of gases in the air does not. The remaining 79% is almost all nitrogen. **See:** Egan, chapter on "Blood gases and acid base." **Keywords**: Ambient air = 21% O_2

278. What is the PO_2 of inspired room air in Colorado Springs (PiO_2) with a barometric pressure of 713 mmHg at body temperature and pressure saturated (BTPS)?

a. **21 mmHg**
b. **80 mmHg**
c. **140 mmHg**
d. **150 mmHg**

ANSWER c. 140 mmHg. To get the effective barometric pressure the water vapor tension (a constant of 47 mmHg at body temp.) must be subtracted. 713 mmHg - 47 mmHg = 666 mmHg. Then, since room air is only 21 % O_2, take 21% of the barometric pressure. 666 x .21 = 140 mmHg. This number is the maximum PO_2 that arterial blood can achieve at 100% saturation. The number is also used as the calibration point for many blood gas machines. Since the barometric pressure varies, this PiO_2 must be calculated each day with the current P_B. At sea level where the barometric pressure is near 760 mmHg, PiO_2 is 150 mmHg.
See: Egan, chapter on "Blood gases and acid base." **Keywords**: Room air PO_2

279. What is the average *(assumed)* oxygen consumption in the normal resting adult male?

a. 100 - 140 ml/min
b. 200 - 300 ml/min
c. 450 - 600 ml/min
d. 800 - 1200 L/min

ANSWER b. 200 - 300 ml/ min. Average normal resting basal O_2 consumption index is 125 ml O_2/BSA in M^2. When this number is multiplied by an average adult male BSA (E.g., 2.0 M^2) it gives the *assumed* normal adult oxygen consumption. Although it is very inaccurate, this is the way O2 consumption is usually calculated for the Fick CO in cath labs.

BSA x 125 ml O_2/BSA/ M^2 = 2.0 M^2 x 125 ml O_2/BSA/ M^2 = 250 ml O_2/min.

Of course, this varies widely with age, sex, sedation level, temperature, and body position. Pepine says, "*oxygen consumption should be estimated only when it cannot be measured....*" .
See: Pepine, chapter on "Blood Flow Measurement" and Yang, chapter on "Cardiac Output." **Keywords:** normal VO_2 = 200-300 ml/ min

280. What is the average oxygen consumption per square meter of BSA in the normal resting adult?

a. 100 ml/min/M^2
b. 125 ml/min/M^2
c. 150 ml/min/M^2
d. 175 ml/min/M^2

ANSWER b. 125 ml/ min/ M^2. Average normal resting basal O_2 consumption index is 125 ml O_2/BSA/ M^2. This when multiplied by the patient's BSA gives the normal adult VO_2 or oxygen consumption. This is the basic number for estimation of O_2 consumption as used by many computer-based Fick methods. For more accuracy estimated O_2 consumption may incorporate the patient's age, heart rate, and condition. Although VO_2 is commonly estimated, this practice is grossly inaccurate. Grossman says, "*assumed values for O_2 consumption are likely to introduce considerable error.*"
See: Baim and Grossman, chapter on "Blood Flow measurement" **Keywords:** normal average VO_2/M^2 = 200-300 ml/ min/ M^2

281. The greatest error in measuring Fick CO is:

- a. **Not measuring O2 consumption and blood samples at the same time**
- b. **Blood oxygen saturation measurement**
- c. **Measuring blood Oxygen content**
- d. **Estimating O2 consumption by formula**

ANSWER d. Estimating O2 consumption by formula. Computers all estimate the O2 consumption based formulas based on patient age, weight and height. The various formulas all give different values for O2 consumption.

Kern says: "Estimates of resting VO2 derived from conventional formulae are inaccurate, especially in severely obese individuals. When accurate hemodynamic assessment is important for clinical decision making, VO2 should be directly measured." Kern recommends using a metabolic cart like that used in cardiopulmonary exercise stress testing. A mask is used to collect expired air.

See: Kern, chapter on "Hemodynamics."

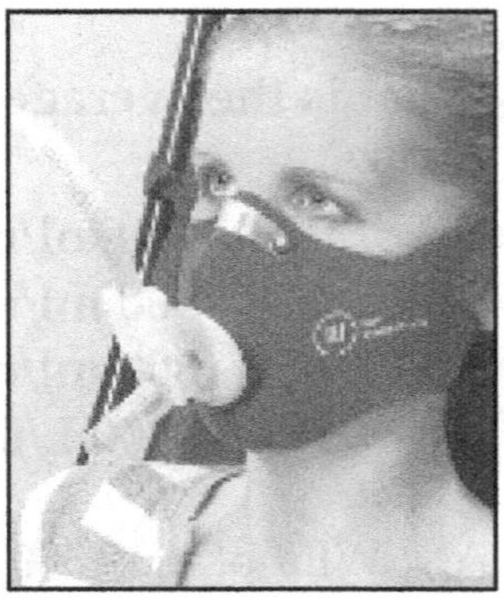

282. Your emphysema (COPD) patient must remain on nasal cannula O_2 throughout the heart cath. How can a measured O_2 consumption and Fick CO be done?

- a. **It cannot be done while he is on oxygen**
- b. **Pinch off the nose gently, leaving the nasal cannula running**
- c. **Include both Hgb and dissolved O_2 in the a-v difference calculation**
- d. **Use the metabolic rate meter hood, with O_2 running**

ANSWER a. It cannot be done on O2. The patient must be off O_2 for 10 - 15 minutes prior to Fick measurement. Kern says,

> *"Mixing the supplemental oxygen with room air makes determination of the oxygen content of the inspired air difficult (if not impossible) to calculate. Therefore, supplemental oxygen therapy should be discontinued at least 10 to 15 minutes before determination of the cardiac output by the Fick technique. If oxygen cannot safely be discontinued, an alternative to the Fick technique should be used."*

See: Kern, chapter on "Hemodynamics." **Keywords**: Fick cannot be done on O_2

283. If a patient's arterial oxygen saturation is still abnormally low (<91%) after breathing pure oxygen via a non-rebreathing mask for 30 minutes, the patient has a/an:

- a. **Anatomic R-L shunt**
- b. **Physiologic R-L shunt**
- c. **Impaired lung diffusion**
- d. **Uneven distribution of inspired air (V/Q abnormality)**

ANSWER a. Anatomic R-L shunt, like an ASD or VSD. Grossman says,

> *"If full arterial blood oxygen saturation cannot be achieved by face-mask administration of*

oxygen (it is best in this regard to use a rebreathing mask that fits snugly), a right-to-left shunt is presumed to be present, and its anatomic site and magnitude should be determined using the methods described...."

Physiologic shunts are due to uneven distribution of air in the lungs that bypass alveoli. This looks like a R-L shunt, resulting in low arterial saturation. But these can be corrected by breathing 100% O_2 for 30 minutes. If the saturation is still abnormally low an anatomic R-L shunt is present. **See**: Baim and Grossman, chapter on "Shunt Detection and Measurement." **Keywords**: low sat (<91%) on pure oxygen = anatomic R-L shunt

Fick CO

284. The Fick principle states that the uptake of a substance by any organ (VO_2) is:

a. The blood flow to that organ divided by the arteriovenous concentration difference of the substance

b. The arteriovenous concentration difference of the substance divided by the blood flow to that organ

c. The product of the arteriovenous concentration difference of the substance and the blood flow to that organ.

d. The difference between the concentration of blood entering the organ (arterial) and the concentration of blood leaving the organ (venous)

ANSWER c. The product of the arteriovenous concentration difference of the substance and the blood flow to that organ. This is the familiar Fick equation slightly rearranged: Oxygen consumption = (a- v difference) x CO.

Pepine says,

> ***"The Fick principle is based on the simple concept of conservation of mass and can be applied to flow through any system in which a substance (indicator) either enters or leaves the flowing stream at a measurable rate."***

Note, in the Fick formula A-V difference in vol. % must be multiplied by 10 to get correct units. See: Pepine, chapter on "Blood Flow Measurement." Keywords: Fick principle

285. What is the "gold standard" cardiac output measurement technique on cardiac patients with relatively low cardiac outputs?

a. Fick CO

b. TDCO

c. LVMF

d. Green Dye

ANSWER a. Fick CO is the classic steady state CO method, although it is time consuming and difficult to perform accurately. Pepine says,

> *"the Fick method is generally regarded as being most accurate when cardiac output is low and arterial-venous oxygen content difference is large.... In animal studies, the Fick cardiac output agrees well with direct measurements of flow. In humans, the Fick output is often considered a "gold standard" for cardiac output measurements, and the accuracy of other*

techniques is determined by comparison with the Fick method... In fact, there is ample opportunity for error,..."

Peterson says, "

It is not easy to measure oxygen consumption, and significant errors may also creep into the measurement of the oxygen contend of arterial and mixed venous blood. It is therefore critically important that persons whose responsibility it is to interpret hemodynamic data thoroughly understand the Fick principle, appreciate the limitation of its application in the cardiac catheterization laboratory, and become familiar with what values to expect on the technician's work sheet. It is unwise simply to look at the bottom line, a practice that may eventually lead to acceptance of an erroneous cardiac output.... The method of Fick has great advantages over other methods of determining cardiac output in that it yields not only the cardiac output but also oxygen consumption and the oxygen content of mixed venous blood and systemic arterial blood, all of which are of great physiologic and clinical significance. Correctly measured, oxygen consumption identifies the metabolic state and arterial oxygen saturation is a measure of ventilation, whereas cardiac performance is directly related to the content of oxygen in mixed venous blood.

See: Peterson, chapter on "Methods of Blood Flow" and Pepine chapter on "Blood Flow Measurement." Keywords: Fick CO most accurate

286. What O_2 saturation values should be used to calculate the a-v difference in the Fick equation from the diagnostic saturation run shown? (No shunt was found.)

Patient # 286	- O_2 Saturations
RA = 71 %	PAW = 96%
RV = 72%	LV = 94 %
PA = 73%	AO = 94 %

a. **0.94 - 0.71**
b. **0.94 - 0.73**
c. **0.96 - 0.72**
d. **0.96 - 0.73**

ANSWER b. 0.94 - 0.73. The best mixed blood samples are downstream from the ventricles. AO and PA are the standard chambers used in the Fick CO. This is true only if no shunts exist. When shunts are present calculate SBF and PBF, not the standard Fick CO. O_2 content is traditionally used in the Fick equation; however, O_2 saturation units may be substituted for vol. % if the 1.36 x Hgb. factors are included as shown.

$$\text{Fick CO} = \frac{O_2 \text{ consumption}}{(O_2 \text{ Sat. a - v dif}) \times 1.36 \times \text{Hgb } 10}$$

See: Baim and Grossman, chapter on "Blood Flow Measurement: The Cardiac Output" Keywords: for Fick CO use best mixed AO-PA samples as a-v difference

287. Which set of O_2 saturations taken at cath indicate the lowest CO? (Assume constant oxygen consumption and Hgb levels.)

a. **Patient A AO = 89% sat PA = 50%**
b. **Patient B AO = 91% sat PA = 60 %**
c. **Patient C AO = 96% sat PA = 70%**

ANSWER a. Patient A AO = 89% sat PA = 50%. The darkest venous blood has the lowest saturation, the widest AV difference, and the lowest CO. More O_2 is extracted in low CO because the blood moves so slowly through the capillary bed. Note in the Fick formula, if the venous blood content drops this widens the av difference which acts to increase the denominator and reduces the Fick CO. Arterial O_2 content varies only with respiratory status, not CO. Note, that this formula and the previous formula are the same. This formula just uses blood samples already converted from O2 Sat. to O2 content. See: Peterson, chapter on "Methods of Blood Flow" Keywords: Blackest venous blood = lowest CO.

$$\downarrow \text{Fick CO} = \frac{O_2 \text{ consumption}}{(a - \downarrow v \text{ dif}) \times 10}$$

Fick CO Calculations

288. Calculate the Fick CO from the data in the box:

a. **4.0 L/min**
b. **5.0 L/min**
c. **6.0 L/min**
d. **10.0 L/min**

Patient # 288
VO_2 = 200 ml/min
Hgb = 15 gm % or gm/dL
AO blood =20 vol %
PA blood = 15 vol %

ANSWER a. 4.0 L/min. Use Fick formula. Fick CO = VO_2 / [(a-v dif.) x 10]

CO = VO_2 / (a - v diff. x 10) = (200 ml/min) / [(20 - 15 vol) % x 10)]
= (200 ml/min) / [(5.0 vol) % x 10)] = (200 ml/min) / [(5.0 vol) % x 10)] = 4 L/min
See: Kern, chapter on "Hemodynamics." Keywords: Calculate Fick CO

BOTH QUESTIONS BELOW REFER TO THIS DIAGRAM.

289. From the data in the box calculate an *assumed* O_2 consumption.

a. **65 ml O_2/min**
b. **125 ml O_2/min**
c. **225 ml O_2/min**
d. **275 ml O_2/min**

Patient # 289
Predicted VO_2 = 125 ml/min/ M^2
BSA = 1.8 M^2
Hgb = 13 gm % or gm/dL
AO blood = 95 % O_2 saturation
PA blood = 65 % O_2 saturation

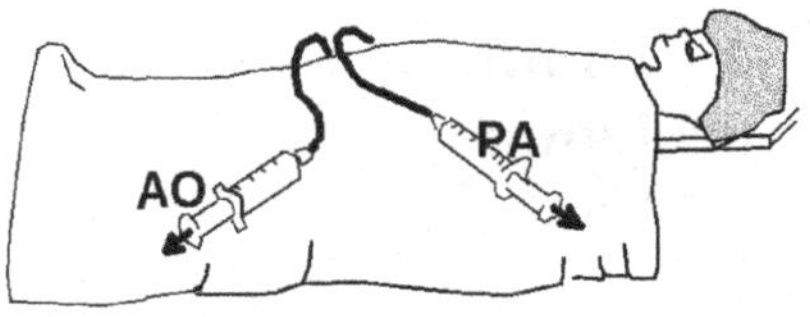

290. Calculate the Fick CO from the data in the box.

a. **4.24 L/min**
b. **5.76 L/min**
c. **6.50 L/min**
d. **7.75 L/min**

BOTH ANSWERS FOLLOW CONSECUTIVELY:

289. ANSWER c. 225 ml O_2. Although this estimation tends to

O_2 consumption = minute ventilation$_{\text{corr. STPD ml/min}}$ x (Room air O_2 %- Expired air O_2%) / 100%

be inaccurate, most labs multiply the average O_2 consumption/BSA (125) times the BSA to get an assumed O_2 consumption = (125 ml / min/ M^2) x BSA. In this example assumed O_2 consumption = 125 x 1.8 = 225 ml O_2 / min. See: Kern, chapter on "Hemodynamics."
Keywords: calculate *assumed* oxygen consumption

290. ANSWER a. 4.24 L/min. An assumed oxygen consumption may be used as the numerator of the Fick equation. This is a common method used by computers in calculating Fick CO.
1. Assume VO_2 = 225 ml O_2/min.
2. Calculate the a-v difference in vol %.
    a-v difference = (AO sat - PA sat) x 1.36 x Hgb
    a-v difference. = (.95 - .65) x 1.36 x 13 = (0.30) x 177 = 5.31 vol % (53.1 ml/L)
3. Calculate Fick CO = O_2 consumption / (a-v difference x 10)
    Fick CO = 225 ml O_2/min / (5.31 x 10) = 4.24 L/min. The diagram shows simultaneous drawing of the Fick blood samples with no O_2 consumption mask on the patient. See: Peterson, chapter on "Methods of Blood Flow" also, Kern, chapter on "Hemodynamics."
Keywords: Estimate a-v difference from O_2 dissociation curve

FOUR QUESTIONS BELOW REFER TO THE DATA IN THIS BOX:

<u>**Patient # 291**</u>
Corrected minute ventilation = 8.5 L/min
Expired air = 18% O_2
AO blood = 20 vol % O_2
PA blood = 15 vol % O_2
Respiratory Quotient = 1.0
Age = 59 Ht. = 60 inches Wt=140 Lbs.
Estimate BSA below

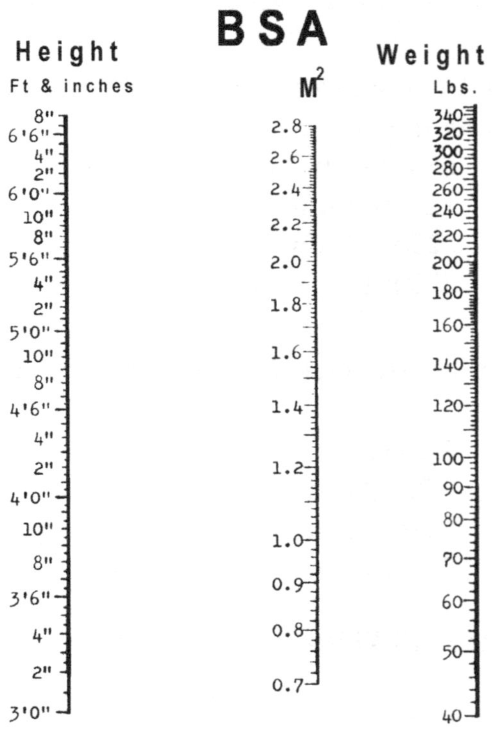

291. **Calculate the O_2 consumption from the data in the box.**
- a. **153 ml/min**
- b. **198 ml/min**
- c. **255 ml/min**
- d. **270 ml/min**

292. **Calculate the Fick CO from data in the box.**
- a. **3.6 L/min**
- b. **4.1 L/min**
- c. **4.8 L/min**
- d. **5.1 L/min**

293. **Estimate the BSA from the nomogram.**
- a. **1.60 M^2**
- b. **1.70 M^2**
- c. **1.80 M^2**
- d. **2.00 M^2**

294. **Calculate the cardiac index (CI) on this patient.**

a. **3.2 L/min**
b. **4.1 L/min**
c. **4.8 L/min**
d. **5.1 L/min**

ALL FOUR ANSWERS FOLLOW CONSECUTIVELY:

291. ANSWER c. 255 ml/min.
$VO_2 = V_E \times (FiO_2 - FeO_2)$ = Ventilation of expired air x (Fraction of inspired O_2 - Fraction of expired O_2) = (8.5 L/min) (.21 - .18) = (8,500 ml/min) x .03 = 255 ml/min:
See: Kern, chapter on "Hemodynamics."

292. ANSWER d. 5.1 L/min. Since we calculated the oxygen consumption above as 255 ml/min, all we need to do for Fick CO is divide by the a-v difference x 10. The a-v difference is AO - PA blood content, already listed in the box. Do not get the O_2 consumption and ventilation data (21% room and 18% expired air O_2) mixed up with the Fick blood gas data (20 vol% and 15 vol% blood O_2). Each must be used in their correct equations.
Fick CO = (255 ml O2/min) / [(20 - 15 vol%) x 10]
Fick CO = 255 / 50 = 5.1 L/min
See: Kern, chapter on "Hemodynamics." Keywords: calculate Fick CO

$$\text{Fick CO} = \frac{O_2 \text{ consumption}}{(\text{a - v dif}) \times 10}$$

293. ANSWER a. 1.60 M^2. Use the nomogram by aligning a ruler between the height of 5.0 feet (60 inches) and the weight 140 Lbs. Read the BSA where the ruler intersects the middle BSA line. It reads 1.60 M^2. BSA can also be calculated on a pocket calculator using the Dubois and Dubois height-weight equation:
$BSA = 71.84\ Wt^{0.425}\ Ht^{0.725}$, where Wt is in kg, and Ht in cm.
See: Yang, chapter on "Cardiac Output" and appendix Keywords: Calculate BSA

294. ANSWER a. 3.2 L/min/M^2. Cardiac index (CI) is the cardiac output (CO) divided by the BSA. See: Kern, chapter on "Hemodynamics."

$$CI = CO / BSA$$

295. **Your patient is receiving 5 L/min of oxygen by nasal cannula. Before taking Fick CO blood samples on a bilateral heart cath:**

a. **Turn the O_2 level down to 1-2 L/min**
b. **Take the patient off oxygen for 1 – 5 min**
c. **Take the patient off oxygen for 10 – 15 min**
d. **Take the patient off oxygen for at least 1 hour**
e. **Have the patient deep breath room air for 1-2 minutes**

O_2 consumption = minute ventilation$_{\text{corr. STPD ml/min}}$ x (Room air O_2 %- Expired air O_2%) / 100%

ANSWER: c. Take the patient off oxygen for 10 – 15 min. Kern says, "Supplemental oxygen is often administered to a patient during diagnostic cardiac catheterization. Mixing the supplemental oxygen with room air makes determination of the oxygen content of the inspired air difficult (if not impossible) to calculate. Supplemental oxygen therapy should be discontinued at least 10 to 15 minutes before determination of CO by the Fick technique. If oxygen cannot be discontinued safely, an alternative to the Fick technique should be used. [i.e., thermodilution]"
See: Kern, chapter on "Hemodynamic Data" Keywords: Fick=off oxygen for10 – 15 min

296. Given the following information, calculate the oxygen consumption. CO = 6.0 L/min, AO sat = 95%, A-VO$_2$ diff = 5.0 vol %, BSA = 1.70 M^2

a. **3.0 L/min**
b. **200 ml/min**
c. **250 ml/min**
d. **300 ml/min**

Answer: d. 250 ml/min. Rearranging the Fick equation: VO$_2$= (A-V dif) (10) (CO) = 5.0 x 10 x 6.0 = 300 ml O$_2$/min. A question like this is used to check your algebra calculation skills. See: Kern, chapter on "Hemodynamic Data" Keywords: Fick CO & O2 consumption

297. Given the following information, calculate the A-VO2 difference. Hgb = 14.8 gm%, O$_2$ binding coefficient = 1.39, Oxygen consumption = 212 ml/min, AO saturation = 95%, PA saturation = 75%.

a. **2.0 vol %**
b. **20.0 vol %**
c. **4.11 vol %**
d. **41.1 vol %**

Answer: c. 4.11 vol %, O$_2$ Content = Hgb x 1.39 x O$_2$ Sat.
AO O$_2$ Content = 14.8 x 1.39 x .95 O$_2$ Sat. = 19.54 vol %
PA O$_2$ Content = 14.8 x 1.39 x .75 O$_2$ Sat. = 15.43vol %
A - V O$_2$ dif = AO O$_2$ Content - PA O$_2$ Content = 19.54 - 15.43 = 4.11 vol % or 41.1 ml/L
See: Kern, chapter on "Hemodynamic Data" Keywords: calculate O2 content in vol%

298. The formula for O$_2$ carrying capacity (content at 100% sat.) in ml O$_2$/L is:

a. **(hemoglobin) X (1.36)**
b. **(hemoglobin) X (1.36) X 10**
c. **(oxygen saturation) X (1.36)**
d. **(oxygen content) X (hemoglobin) X 10**

Answer: b. (hemoglobin) X (1.36) X 10: The O$_2$ capacity is the perfect O$_2$ content if the O$_2$ Sat. were to reach 100%. Normal O$_2$ capacity is 20 m. O$_2$/ 100 ml (This is the unit of vol %). The unit in ml/L is 10 times larger. Thus the 10 in the normal Fick equation. Normal O$_2$ carrying capacity = 200 ml O$_2$/L. Some texts use the Hgb. conversion factor of 1.34 or 1.39 instead of 1.36 as the O$_2$ binding coefficient .

See: Kern, chapter on "Hemodynamic Data" Keywords: O_2 capacity = (hgb.) X (1.36) X 10

299. Calculate the mixed venous oxygen content. Oxygen consumption = 200 ml/min, Hemoglobin = 12.0 gm%, Pulmonary artery saturation = 60%, AO saturation = 95%, BSA = 1.76 , Heart rate = 76 beats/min, O_2 binding coefficient = 1.39.

a. **6.0 vol % or ml/deciliter of blood**
b. **8.5 vol % or ml/deciliter of blood**
c. **9.5 vol % or ml/deciliter of blood**
d. **10.0 vol % or ml/deciliter of blood**

Answer: d. 10.0 vol % The best mixed venous blood is the PA. PA oxygen content formula is O_2 Content = Hgb x 1.39 x PA O_2 Sat. = 12.0 x 1.39 x .60 = 10 vol % See: Kern, chapter on "Hemodynamic Data" Keywords: best mixed venous= PA, convert to vol%

300. Calculate the <u>Fick cardiac output</u>. Oxygen consumption = 200 ml/min, Hemoglobin = 12.0 gm%, Pulmonary artery saturation = 60%, AO saturation = 95%, BSA = 1.76, Heart rate = 76 beats/min.

a. **3.5 L/min**
b. **4.2 L/min**
c. **4.6 L/min**
d. **5.3 L/min**

Answer: a. 3.5 L/min. Fick CO = VO_2 / (A-V dif) x 10 = 200 / (12 x 1.36 x 10) x (.95 - .60) = 200 / 57 = 3.5 L/min. Exam questions may provide irrelevant information, such as BSA and heart rate. Beware of just subtracting O2 saturations, because it is not yet an A-V difference in terms of Vol %. The Hgb and O_2 binding coefficient must be factored in. See: Kern, chapter on "Hemodynamic Data" Keywords: Fick CO

301. Calculate the <u>cardiac index</u>. Oxygen consumption = 250 ml/min, Hemoglobin = 14.0 gm, Pulmonary saturation = 69%, AO saturation = 98%, O_2 binding coefficient = 1.36 O_2/g hgb., BSA = 1.76, Heart rate = 76 beats/min

a. **1.99 L/min/M^2**
b. **2.39 L/min/ M^2**
c. **2.57 L/min/ M^2**
d. **3.01 L/min/ M^2**

Answer: c. 2.57 L/min/ . Fick CO = VO_2 / (A-V dif) x 10 = 250 / (14)(1.36)(10)(.98 - .69) = 250 / 55.2 = 4.53 L/min. Then CI = CO/BSA = 4.53 / 1.76 = 2.57 L/min/M^2
You can subtract the O_2 sats. directly, as shown, only if you convert that sat. difference into volume %, with the Hgb x 1.36 (or 1.39 O_2/g hgb.) O_2 binding coefficient .
See: Kern, chapter on "Hemodynamic Data" Keywords: calculate CI = CO/BSA

Shunts

302. Which 3 methods below can be used for evaluating intracardiac shunts? (Select 3 below)
- **a. Oximetry**
- **b. Angiography**
- **c. Dye dilution curves**
- **d. Intra chamber pressure gradients**
- **e. IVUS**

ANSWERS: a, b, & c. All of the above methods are used to measure CO and shunts EXCEPT pressure gradients and IVUS. These are only used to evaluate a stenosis. Large shunts typically show no gradient and IVUS is for vessel anatomy.
See: Kern, chapter on "Hemodynamics." Keywords: methods to evaluated shunts do not include not measuring gradients

303. When evaluating <u>pulmonary</u> blood flow (#1) on a patient with a shunt, what two blood samples must be collected and analyzed for oxygen content?
- **a. AO - PA**
- **b. AO - RA**
- **c. LA - PA**

<u>Patient # 303</u>
*1. Pulmonary blood flow (PBF)
2. Systemic blood flow (SBF)
3. Fick CO (no shunt)

ANSWER c. LA - PA. The PBF and SBF are only used when shunts are present. To measure Fick blood flow through any system you need the O_2 contents of the blood entering and leaving the system. Think about the capillary system being studied. If you are measuring pulmonary blood flow, sample from the veins and arteries nearest the lung - LA and PA or even pulmonary veins and PA.
BE ABLE TO CORRECTLY MATCH ALL ANSWERS BELOW:
1. Pulmonary blood flow (PBF) uses pulmonary venous - pulmonary arterial or (LA - PA)
2. Systemic blood flow (SBF) uses systemic arterial - systemic venous or (AO - RA)
3. Fick CO (no shunt) uses best mixed arterial and best mixed pulmonary or (AO - PA).

If no shunts are present, the standard Fick CO is measured. Here the average O_2 sat. is the same everywhere in the right heart, so the best mixed values are taken (AO and PA).
Keywords: AV difference in PBF = LA - PA

304. During heart catheterization, cyanotic cardiac shunts show a _______ in O_2 saturation on the _____ side of the heart.
- **a. Step-up, Left**
- **b. Step-up, Right**
- **c. Step-down, Left**
- **d. Step-down, Right**

ANSWER c. Step-down, Left. Cyanotic lesions shunt from Right to Left (R-L). The dark venous blood is shunted into the red arterial blood lowering its O_2 saturation. This causes the O_2 saturation to drop on the left side of the heart, often so severely that blue cyanosis is seen. Where the O_2 sat. drop occurs is the shunt entry point. The magnitude of the step-down determines the size of the shunt.

Large shunts with balanced pressures may show both R-L and L-R shunting. This is termed a "bidirectional shunt." These rare shunts show both saturation step-up on the Rt. side and step-down on the Left side. See sample question later in this chapter.
See: Braunwald, chapter on "Congenital Heart Disease" Keywords: Cyanotic = sat. step-down on Left side

305. In a child with a L-R ASD, the systemic venous sample used in the systemic blood flow calculation may be taken from the:

a. **SVC**
b. **IVC**
c. **RA**
d. **RV**

ANSWER a. SVC. In children the SVC saturation is often used instead of averaging SVC and IVC samples (Flamm equation) to estimate systemic venous O_2 sat. It is usually only a few percentage away from the Flamm average. An ASD is diagnosed with any significant SVC-RA step-up. A significant step-up exceeds ≥5-8% of O_2 saturation on averages of multiple SVC-RA samples. Grossman says,

> *"Obviously, calculations from the formula (Flamm formula) would be little changed in many cases by ignoring inferior vena cava blood altogether, and this is done in some laboratories - especially those involved in pediatric catheterization."*

See: Baim and Grossman, Chapter on "Cardiac Catheterization in Infants and Children." & Pepine, Chapter on "The Adult Patient with Congenital Disease" Keywords: Flamm equation mixed systemic venous O_2 sat. in ASD

306. Q_p/Q_s is the ratio of:

a. **Minute pulmonary ventilation / CO**
b. **Quantity of blood in the lungs / shunt blood flow**
c. **Pulmonary blood flow / systemic blood flow**
d. **Pulmonary blood flow / shunt flow**

ANSWER c. Pulmonary blood flow / systemic blood flow. Q represents quantity of flow, or cardiac output. P is for pulmonary. S is for systemic - not shunt. Note that if your have already calculated the pulmonary blood flow (Q_p) and the systemic blood flow (Q_s) you can simply take the ration of the two. Because they mean the same thing. Then Q_p/Q_s = PBF/SBF = (AO - RA O_2 sat.) /(PV - PA O_2 sat.).
See: Braunwald, chapter on "Congenital Heart Disease." Keywords: Q_p/Q_s = PBF/SBF

307. What is the formula for Q_p/Q_s (also termed the PBF/SBF ratio)?

- a. **Q_p/Q_s = (PV - PA O_2 sat.) / (AO - RA O_2 sat.)**
- b. **Q_p/Q_s = (AO - RA O_2 sat.) /(PV - PA O_2 sat.)**
- c. **Q_p/Q_s = (PV - RA O_2 sat.) / (AO - PA O_2 sat.)**
- d. **Q_p/Q_s = (AO - PA O_2 sat.) / (PV - RA O_2 sat.)**

ANSWER b. Q_p/Q_s = (AO - RA O_2 sat.) /(PV - PA O_2 sat.).
The ratio of pulmonary to systemic blood flows (Q_p/Q_s) formula is:

$$\frac{PBF}{SBF} = \frac{Q_p}{Q_s} = \frac{(SA - SV)}{(PV - PA)} = \frac{\text{Systemic AV dif.}}{\text{Pulm. A-V dif.}} = \frac{AO - RA}{PV - PA}$$

This formula which is easily derived from the Fick formulae, is the ratio of the reciprocal A-V differences of the two systems. Note how Q_p (pulmonary) is in the left numerator. But, systemic A-V difference is in the numerator - on the right side of equation. This is because of the inverse relation between A-V difference and CO. It looks weird, Q_p looks opposite to Pulmonary A-V difference. But that is the way this formula is always set up.

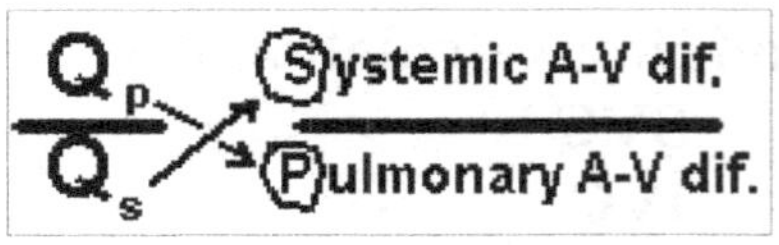

The only tricky part occurs in ASDs and PDAs. The mixing of shunt blood with non-contaminated blood, presents the question of which O_2 saturation to put into the Q_p/Q_s equation. In response, always select the samples closest to the capillary system named. E.g., AV difference across the systemic capillary bed is AO - RA (or SVC).

Ragosta says, "in most cases, the ratio Qp/Qs is used to determine the significance of the shunt. This ratio can be easily calculated by combining the equations for systemic and pulmonary flow equations and canceling all the common terms (O2 consumption, hemoglobin, and oxygen carrying capacity)...." See: Braunwald, chapter on "Congenital Heart Disease." Keywords: Q_p/Q_s = (AO-RA)/(PV-PA)

308. In a normal adult with no shunt, the Q_p/Q_s ratio is:

- a. 0
- b. 1.0
- c. 2.0
- d. 10.

ANSWER b. 1.0. Normally the pulmonary blood flow equals the systemic blood flow. The ratio of the right heart to left heart outputs is thus one. a Q_p/Q_s greater than one indicates a L-R shunt; less than one indicates a R-L shunt.
See: Braunwald, chapter on "Congenital Heart Disease." **Keywords**: Normal Q_p/Q_s = 1

309. A Q_p/Q_s ratio of 3.5 indicates:

- a. **Normal blood flow**
- b. **Increased ventilation perfusion ratio**
- c. **Right heart volume overload**
- d. **Possible cyanosis**

ANSWER c. Right heart volume overload of a L-R shunt. A Q_p/Q_s ratio > 1 indicates that pulmonary blood flow exceeds systemic flow. So blood must be entering the right side of the heart. This can volume overload and dilate the RV and flood the lungs with excess blood. The high pressures in the lungs may permanently damage the pulmonary arterioles. **See**: Braunwald, chapter on "Congenital Heart Disease." **Keywords:** Q_p/Q_s ratio > 1 is L-R shunt with possible Rt. Ht. volume overload

Shunt Calculations (not expected on RCIS exam)

310. Estimate the Q_p/Q_s for the patient shown in the box.

a. 1:4
b. 1:2
c. 2:1
d. 4:1

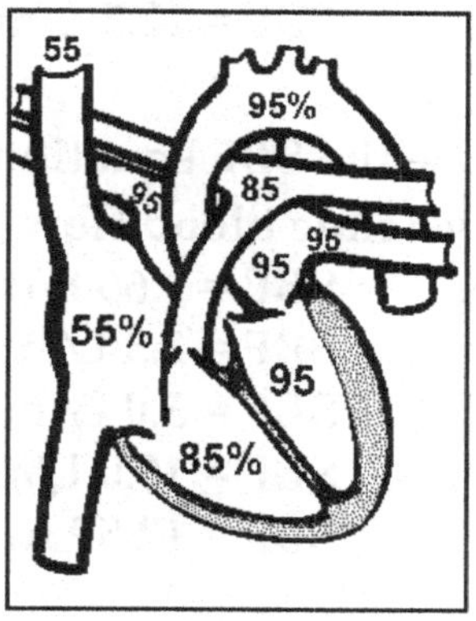

Patient #310

ANSWER d. 4:1. This is a straightforward L-R VSD. RV blood steps up from 55% to 85%. Q_p/Q_s=(95-55)/(95-85) = 40/10 = 4:1. This indicates that the PBF is 4 times the SBF, which is a large right heart volume overload. Immediate surgical correction may be indicated to prevent damage to pulmonary arterioles. Q_p/Q_s = PBF/SBF = (AO - RA O_2 sat.) /(PV - PA O_2 sat.). **See:** Kern, chapter on "Hemodynamics" **Keywords:** Calculate Q_p/Q_s

311. A child with a VSD has the cardiac outputs measured at cath as shown in the box (PBF = 3, SBF = 4, TDCO = 5). Estimate the amount and direction of the shunt.

a. 1 L/min R-L Shunt
b. 1 L/min L-R Shunt
c. 2 L/min R-L Shunt
d. 2 L/min L-R Shunt

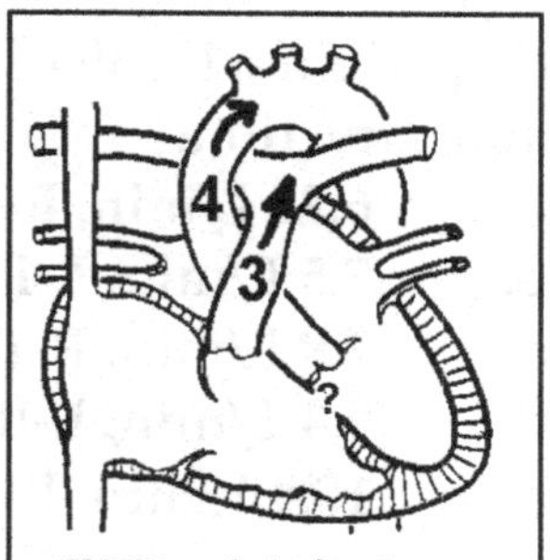

PBF = 3 L/min
SBF = 4 L/min
TDCO = 5 L/min

ANSWER a. 1 L/min R-L Shunt. Q_s=4 L/min. Q_p=3 L/min. , R-L shunt = 1 L/min. The R-L shunt adds to the blood the LV must pump and subtracts from the PA blood flow. 4 L/min comes back into the RA, 1 L/min is shunted into the LV, making aortic flow 4 L/min and pulmonary flow 3 L/minute as shown in the diagram..

Shunt formulas are: L-R shunt flow = PBF - SBF = Q_p - Q_s.

L-R shunt flow = 3 - 4 = -1 L/min. Since this shunt flow comes out negative it is the unusual direction, reversed, cyanotic, R-L shunt. TDCO is unreliable in the presence of shunts.

See: Baim and Grossman, chapter on "Shunt Detection and Measurement" **Keywords:** L-R shunt flow = PBF - SBF = Q_p - Q_s.

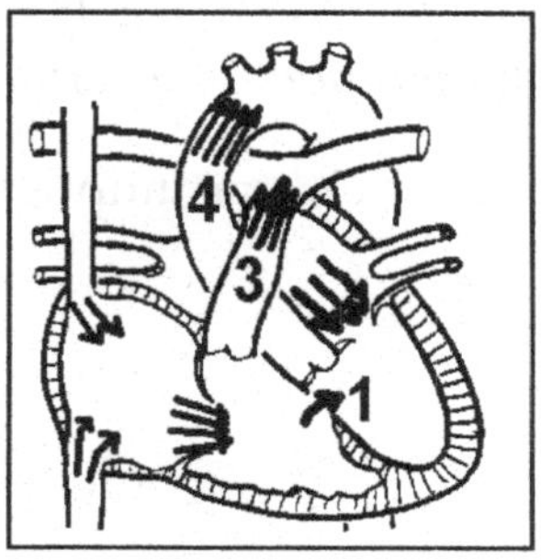

R-L VSD blood flows

USE THIS DIAGRAM FOR THE NEXT 3 QUESTIONS. These diagrams represent the O_2 saturation samples taken at heart cath. Oxygen consumption = 250 ml/min and Hgb = 14.7 gm/dL.

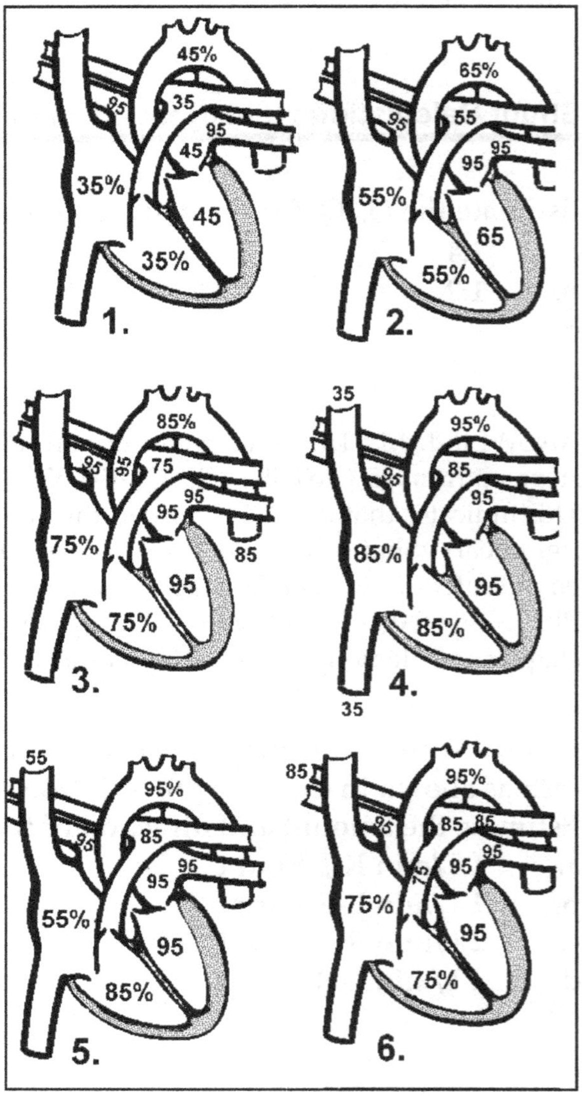

O_2 Saturations at cath, O_2 consumption = 250 ml/min, Hgb = 14.7 gm/dL

312. **Use the PBF equation to calculate the pulmonary blood flow for #1 in L/min.**

- a. PBF = 2.08 L/min
- b PBF = 3.12 L/min
- c. PBF = 6.25 L/min
- d. PBF = 12.5 L/min

313. **Use the SBF equation to calculate the systemic blood flow for #1 in L/min.**

- a. SBF = 1.66 L/min
- b. SBF = 2.5 L/min
- c. SBF = 5.0 L/min
- d. SBF = 10.0 L/min
- e. SBF = 12.5 L/min

314. **From the blood flow calculations above on patient #1, calculate the shunt flow and direction.**

- a. 6.25 L/min, R-L shunt
- b. 7.5 L/min, L-R shunt
- c. 7.9 L/min, R-L shunt
- d. 9.4 L/min, L-R shunt
- e. 10.4 L/min, R-L shunt

BE ABLE TO CORRECTLY MATCH ALL ANSWERS BELOW: ➤

ALL OTHER ANSWERS LISTED TOGETHER BELOW:

312.ANSWER a. 2.08 L/min = PBF = Q_p. Identify the pulmonary venous O_2 sat at 95% and the pulmonary arterial Sat. at 35%. Then, use the Fick principle to calculate PBF:

PBF = O_2 consumption/ (PV sat - PA sat.) 1.36 x Hgb x 10)

PBF = 250 (.95 - .35) 1.36 x 14.7 x 10) = 250/(.60 x 1.36 x 14.7 x 10) = 250 / 120 = **2.08 L/min**.

The mixing of shunt blood with non-contaminated blood, presents the question of which O_2 saturation to put into the Q_p/Q_s equation. In response, always select the samples closest to the **capillary system** named. In diagram #1 which sample best represents the Pulmonary venous O_2 sat? 45% or 95%? Well 95% is closer to the lung capillary system, so 95% is the pulmonary venous O_2 sat, before the shunt dumps in.

See: Braunwald, chapter on "Congenital Heart Disease." **Keywords:** ID direction and location of shunts, L-R, VSD

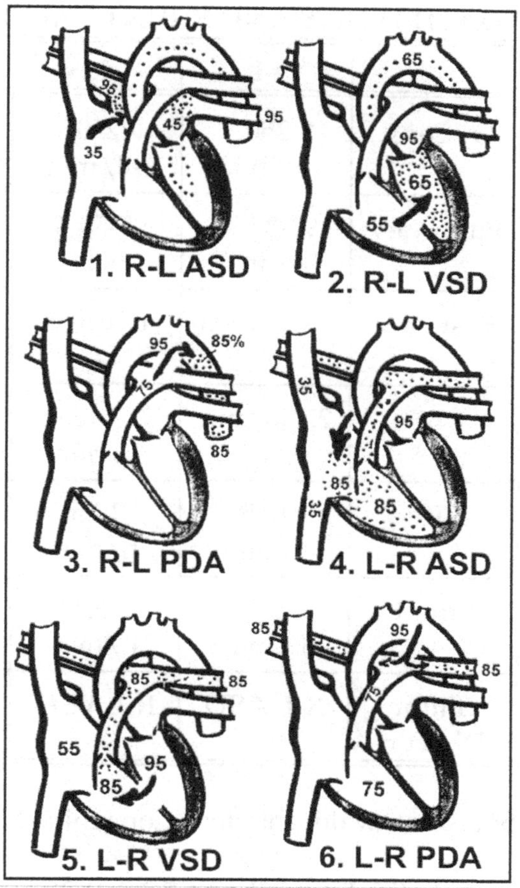

313. ANSWER e. 12.5 L/min = SBF = Q_s. Identify the systemic arterial O_2 sat at 45% and the systemic venous at 35%. Then, use the Fick principle to calculate SBF:

SBF = O_2 consumption/ (SA sat - SV sat.) (1.36 x Hgb x 10)

SBF = 250 (.45 - .35)/ (1.36 x 14.7 x 10) = 250/(.10 x 1.36 x 14.7 x 10) = 250 / 20 = **12.5**

These formulas are used, where:

SA = Systemic Arterial (usual AO)
SV = Systemic venous (usually SVC)
PV = Pulm. venous (usually PV)
PA = Pulm. arterial (usually PA)

PBF = O_2 consumption/(PV - PA) x 10
SBF = O_2 consumption/(SA - SV) x 10
∴SBF=O_2 consumption/(AO - SVC) x 10

Note the dotted blood in the diagram represents the mixed arterial and venous blood downstream from the shunt. These shunts are exaggerated and simplified for teaching purposes.

Note how the side of the heart from which the shunt originates always has constant saturation. E.g. in all R-L shunts the Right heart O_2 sat is always the same in RA, RV, & PA, with only slight variation due to streaming and incomplete mixing. Conversely, in all L-R shunts the O_2 sat. is the same in LA, LV, and AO. Also, note that Pulmonary venous saturation is 95% regardless of the direction of shunt. This is true if the lungs are oxygenating well. (Grossman says you can usually estimate PV at 98% sat. even if you can not get the catheter in to sample PV or LA)

314. ANSWER e. 10.4 L/min, R-L shunt. First Identify the type of shunt from O_2 sat data. Normally the LA should be fully saturated blood and an average between the 4 PV samples. Note the drop in saturation from a PV of 95% to an LA of 45%. This is a large drop in saturation. It must be a large R-L shunt. The step-down begins in the LA, so it must be an ASD coming into the LA from right to left. The amount of the shunt is estimated by subtracting SBF from PBF. If the result is negative, it is the least common type, a R-L shunt.

BLOOD FLOWS AND SHUNT CALCULATIONS IN THE 6 PATIENTS ABOVE:

	#1	#2	#3	#4	#5	#6
O_2 Cons.	250 ml/min	250 ml/min	250 ml/min	250 ml/min	250 ml/min	250 ml/min
Pulm. a-v	95-35 % sat	95-55 % sat	95-75 % sat	95-85 % sat	95-85 % sat	95-85 % sat
Syst. a-v	45-35% sat	65-55 % sat	85-75% sat	95-35% sat	95-55% sat	95-75% sat
PBF	2.1 L/min	3.12 L/min	6.25 L/min	12.5 L/min	12.5 L/min	12.5 L/min
SBF	12.5 L/min	12.5 L/min	12.5 L/min	2.1 L/min	3.12 L/min	6.25 L/min
Shunt	-10.4 L/min	-9.4 L/min	-6.25 L/min	10.5 L/min	9.4 L/min	6.25 L/min
Shunt Direct'n	**R-L ASD**	**R-L VSD**	**R-L PDA**	**L-R ASD**	**L-R VSD**	**L-R PDA**

See: Braunwald, chapter "Congenital Heart Disease." **Keywords:** Calculate Q_p/Q_s

USE THIS DIAGRAM FOR BOTH QUESTIONS.
This diagram shows a <u>bidirectional</u> ASD shunt and blood oxygen saturations.

315. Calculate net PBF and SBF.

	PBF	**SBF**
a.	**3.8 L/min**	**5.0 L/min**
b.	**5.0 L/min**	**3.8 L/min**
c.	**2.5 L/min**	**6 L/min**
d	**5.9 L/min**	**2.4 L/min**

316. Estimate the R-L shunt and the L-R shunt.

	R-L shunt	**L-R shunt**
a.	**0.3 L/min,**	**3.8 L/min**
b.	**3.8 L/min**	**0.3 L/min**
c.	**3.5 L/min**	**6.0 L/min**
d.	**6.0 L/min**	**3.5 L/min**

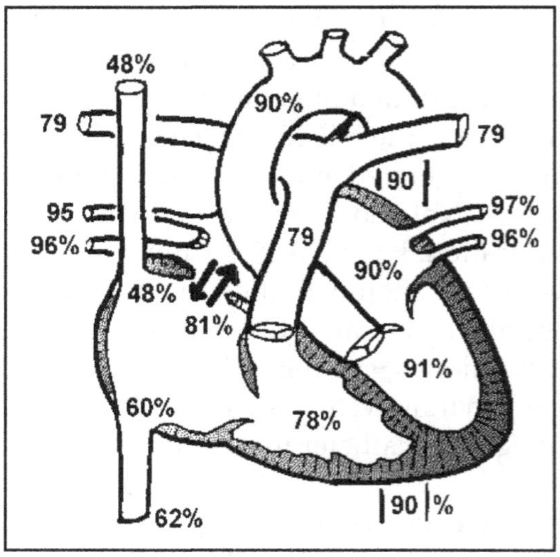

O_2 consumption = 200 , Hgb = 14.7,
SA = .98, SV = .48, PA = .79, PV = .96

315. ANSWER d. 5.9 L/min R-L and 2.4 L/min L-R. Bidirectional ASD. shunts show both step-up in Rt. Heart and step-down in Lt. Heart The RA shows a 30% step-up (Big L-R ASD). The LA shows a PV average of 96% which drops to 90% in the LA. This is a 6% step-down, indicating a small R-L shunt. Calculate PBF and SBF as usual:

Q_p = PBF = 200/[(.96 - .79) 1.36 x 14.7 x 10] = 200/[.17 x 1.36 x 14.7 x 10] = 200/34= 5.9 L/min.

Q_s = SBF = 200/[(.90 - .48) x1.36 x 14.7 x 10)] = 200/[.42 x 1.36 x 14.7 x 10] = 200/84 = 2.4 L/min

Q_p = PBF = $\frac{O_2 \text{ consumption}}{[(\textbf{PV - PA}) \times 10]}$

Q_s = SBF = $\frac{O_2 \text{ consumption}}{[(\textbf{SA - SV}) \times 10]}$

Here:

PV(pulm. venous)	= .96 x cap.
PA(pulm. art.)	= .79 x cap.
SA (syst. art.) =AO	= .90 x cap.
SV (syst. ven.) = SVC	= .48 x cap.

where cap.=O_2 Capacity = 1.36 x Hgb=20

The difference between PBF and SBF indicates a net 3.5 L/min L-R shunt, but tells us nothing about the bidirectional shunts. **To calculate bidirectional shunts a special formula for Q_{eff} must be used. See next question.** Here, calculation of Q_p/Q_s is misleading and low because it only measures **net** flow results. (E.g. It is possible to have a net shunt of 0 and a Q_p/Q_s of 1.0, if the L-R and R-L shunts are equal.) **See:** Baim, chapter on "Shunt Detection and Measurement." **Keywords:** Bi-directional ASD

316. ANSWER a. R-L shunt = 0.3 L/min, L-R = 3.8 L/min. This special Fick formula for effective blood flow (Q_{eff}) uses the AV difference from the inlet chambers PV and RA(SVC). Since the inlet chambers PV and SVC are used to calculate Q_{eff}, step-up and step-down data is not included. Thus, Q_{eff} estimates the amount of blood flow (CO) as if NO shunts were present.

Effective blood flow (Q_{eff}) is a kind of average between Q_p and Q_s. It is a theoretical flow used only for a quick bidirectional shunt approximation. Q_{eff} is then subtracted from the actual Q_p and Q_s to estimate the amount of each bidirectional shunt. This diagram shows how Q_{eff} is the same as Q_p and Q_s when no shunts are present and when good mixing occurs. Note, that the net shunt found by subtracting SBF from PBF can also be found by subtracting L-R and R-L shunts. Also note that the saturation data makes it clear that the L-R shunt predominates. There is a HUGE O2 step up in the RA.

Q_{eff} = $\frac{O_2 \text{ consumption}}{[(\textbf{PV - SV}) \times 10]}$

R-L shunt = Q_s - Q_{eff}

L-R shunt = Q_p - Q_{eff}

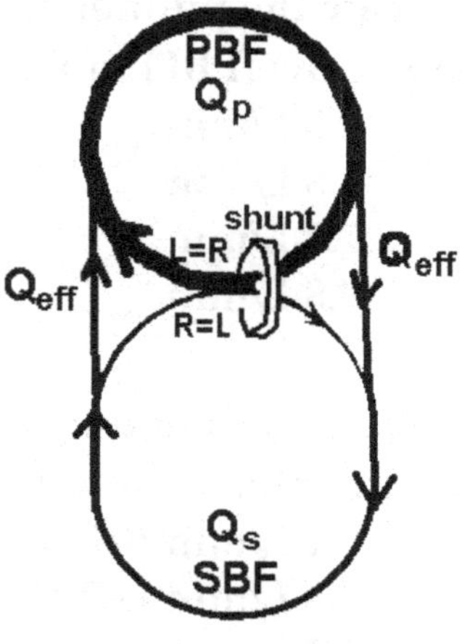

Q_{eff} = 200/[(.96-.48)x1.36 x 14.7 x 10)]= 200/96 = 2.1 L/min

R-L shunt = 2.4 - 2.1 = 0.3 L/min

L-R shunt = 5.9 - 2.1 = 3.8 L/min

Use the Fick principle to calculate PBF and SBF as above then subtract Q_{eff} from each as shown to get the actual R-L and L-R shunts. **See**: Baim, chapter on "Shunt Detection and Measurement." **Keywords:** Bidirectional shunt calculation

317. **A patient has a large** VSD **shunt on angio, yet the Qp/Qs ratio calculation is only 1.1/1. This low Qp/Qs ratio suggests a:**

a. **Small R-L shunt**
b. **Low cardiac output**
c. **Bidirectional shunt**
d. **Second shunt location**

ANSWER: c. Bidirectional shunt may be present where the L-R part of the shunt almost equals the R-L portion. Remember, it is possible to have a net shunt of 0 and a Q_p/Q_s of 1.0, if the L-R and R-L shunts are equal. Cyanosis or pulmonary volume overload may still be present because of the mixing of blue and red blood in a common ventricle. **See:** explanation on previous question, also, Baim, chapter on "Shunt Detection and Measurement." **Keywords:** Bi-directional VSD

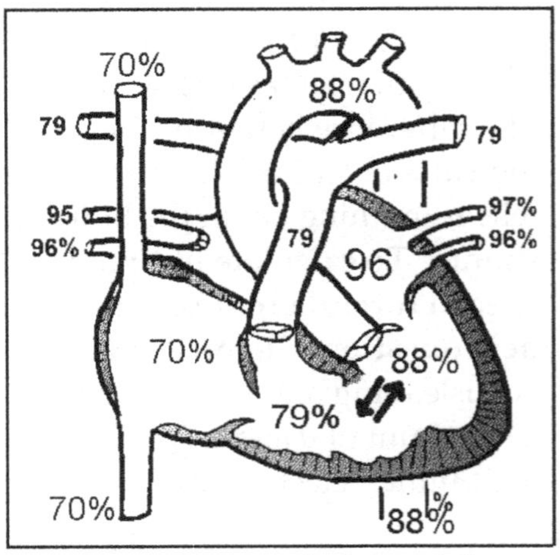

Bidirectional VSD, balanced flow

THREE QUESTIONS BELOW REFER TO THIS DIAGRAM:
In these 4 patients the O_2 consumption is 150 ml/min and Hgb = 16 gm/dL.

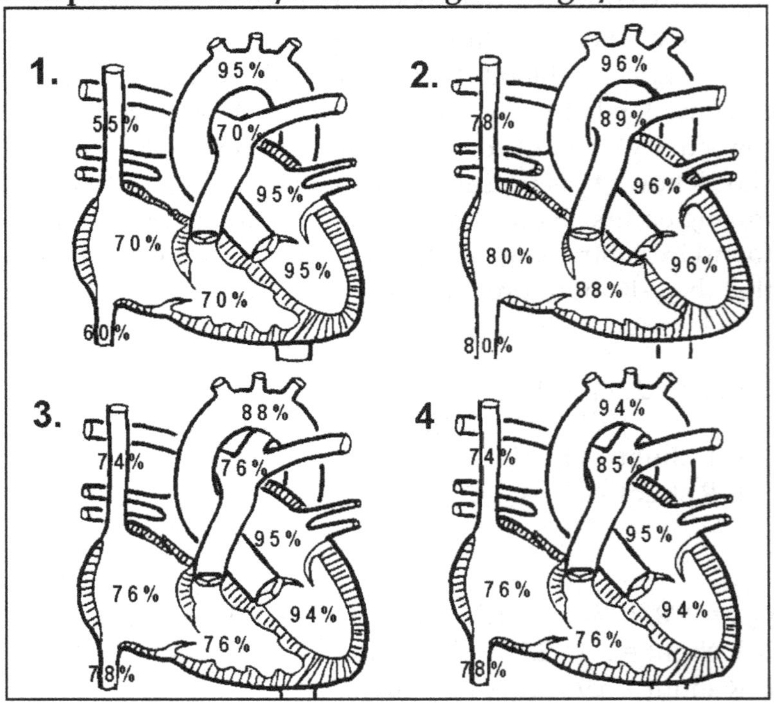

Congenital defects (shunt orifice not shown)
Oxygen consumption = 150 ml/min, Hgb = 16 gm/dL

318. **Estimate the systemic blood flow in #2.**

a. **4.0 L/min**
b. **4.3 L/min**
c. **4.9 L/min**
d. **5.3 L/min**

319. **Estimate the pulmonary blood flow (PBF) in #2.**

a. **4.3 L/min**
b. **5.8 L/min**
c. **7.2 L/min**
d. **9.8 L/min**

320. **Estimate the amount, site, and direction of shunt #2.**

a. **3.1 L/min R-L VSD**
b. **4.3 L/min L-R PDA**
c. **5.5 L/min L-R VSD**
d. **6.7 L/min R-L PDA**

THREE ANSWERS LISTED TOGETHER BELOW:
318. ANSWER b. 4.3 L/min = SBF. Use the Fick formula for systemic blood flow:

SBF = O_2 cons / [(SA - SV) x1.36 x Hgb x 10)]

SBF = 150/ [(.96 - .80) 1.36 x 16 x 10] = 150 / .16 x 1.36 x 16 x 10 =
150 / 34.8 = 4.3 L/min. **See**: Braunwald, chapter on "Congenital Heart Disease."
Keywords: SBF formula

319. ANSWER d. 9.8 L/min. Use the Fick formula for pulmonary blood flow.

PBF = O_2 cons / [(PV - PA) x1.36 x Hgb x 10)]

PBF = O_2 cons /[(LA - PA) 1.36 x 16 x10] = 150/ [(.96 - .89) 1.36 x 16 x 10] = 150 / .07 x 1.36 x 16 x 10 = 150 / 15.2 = 9.8 L/min.

This is a very large PBF. The ratio of PBF/SBF = Q_p/Q_s = 9.8/4.3 = 2.3. In a L=R VSD oxygenated blood enters the RV. The formula for PBF is: PBF = O_2 consumption / [(Pulmonary venous - pulmonary arterial O_2 cont.) x 10] Note that the samples needed are the vessels supplying and draining the lungs. PA blood is easy to get, but pulmonary venous blood may be difficult to sample unless the catheter can pass through the shunt and into the LA. A LA sample is preferred because it is the last chamber before the shunt dumps into the LV. If LA cannot be entered, the pulmonary venous blood may have to be estimated at 95-98% O_2 saturation.
See: Braunwald, chapter on "Congenital Heart Disease." **Keywords:** PBF calculation

320. ANSWER c. 5.5 L/min. Calculate the amount of the shunt: Shunt flow = PBF - SBF = 9.8 - 4.3 = 5.5 L/min. Since the saturation step-up occurs in the RV this is a L-R VSD.
See: Braunwald, chapter on "Congenital Heart Disease." **Keywords:** Shunt calculation

BLOOD FLOWS AND SHUNT CALCULATIONS IN THE 4 PATIENTS ABOVE:

Calculation	Pt. #1	Pt. #2	Pt. #3	Pt. #4
Pulm. a-v diff.	.95 - .70	.96 - .89 = .07	.95 - .76 = .19	.95 - .85 = .10
Q_p = PBF	2.76 L/min	9.86 L/min	3.63 L/min	6.90 L/min
Syst. a-v diff.	.95 - .55 = .40	.95 - .76	.88 - .76 = .12	.94 - .76 = .18
Q_s = SBF	1.73 L/min	3.63 L/min	5.75 L/min	3.83 L/min
Shunt flow	1.03 L/min	5.55 L/min	-2.12 L/min	3.07 L/min
Shunt	L-R ASD	L-R VSD	R-L PDA	L-R PDA

See: Braunwald, chapter on "Congenital Heart Disease in Infants and Children."
Keywords: Calculate R-L shunts

321. When calculating the amount of shunt in a L-to-R VSD, the best mixed systemic venous blood sample is the:

a. **Left atrium**
b. **Right atrium**
c. **Right ventricle**
d. **Pulmonary capillary wedge (LA)**

Answer: b. Right atrium. To estimate the shunt, you need an O2 sat. from the chamber just proximal to where the shunt blood enters - the RA. Many different saturations enter the RA (SVC, IVC, & CS), and it is often difficult to get a good average Sat. there. For the mixed systemic venous blood, many RA samples should be taken and averaged to get the RA O2 saturation. Grossman says, "VENTRICULAR SEPTAL DEFECT, In this case, the O2 saturation of mixed venous blood is calculated by averaging the right atrial O2 saturations because the right atrium is the chamber immediately proximal to the O2 step-up." The RA average should be close to the Flamm equation average (3x SVC + IVC)/4
See: Grossman, chapter on "Shunt Detection and Quantification" Keywords: Best mixed venous =chamber immediately proximal to shunt entry

322. During a pediatric heart cath diagnostic run on a young girl with mild cyanosis finds these O2 sats. SVC = 63%, IVC = 65%, high RA sat = 64%, mid RA = 66%, low RA = 67%, RV = 66%, PA = 66%, LA = 95%, LV = 85%. What type of shunt is this?

a. **L- R ASD**
b. **L- R VSD**
c. **R-L ASD**
d. **R-L VSD**

Answer: d. R-L VSD. An O2 saturation step-down in the LV means that dark venous blood is entering the LV through a VSD. RV pressures would have to be high (pulmonary hypertension) to overcome the high LV pressure. Since the girl is cyanotic the shunt is R-L as expected. Remember, central cyanosis occurs when significant amounts of dark right sided blood enter the systemic circuit. See: Braunwald, chapter on "Congenital Heart Disease" Keywords: R-L shunt = O2 step down

323. -Which ratio below is the "Flamm" Formula?

a. **(3 SVC + 1 IVC) / 4**
b. **(2 SVC + 3 IVC) / 5**
c. **(1 SVC + 2 IVC) / 3**
d. **(1 SVC + 1 IVC) / 2**

Answer: a. (3 SVC + 1 IVC) / 4. The formula is an average for mixed systemic venous O2 Sat. The Flamm formula weighs the SVC as 3 times more important than the IVC blood sat. This formula is only used to average RA saturation in presence of a L-R ASD. Remember, the CS blood from the heart and SVC from the brain are both low in O_2. The SVC blood from the liver is higher in O_2. Since there are three widely different O_2 sats. dumping into the RA where there is poor mixing, we need a theoretical average of mixed venous blood -

like this Flamm equation.

Braunwald says, "The mixed venous oxygen content is the average oxygen content of the blood in the chamber proximal to the shunt. When assessing a left-to-right shunt at the level of the right atrium, one must calculate mixed venous oxygen content on the basis of the contributing blood flow from the IVC, SVC, and coronary sinus. The most common method used is the FLAMM formula: MVO_2=(3 SVC O_2 cont.+ 1 IVC O_2 cont.) / 4". For simplicity sake, some physician use SVC as the mixed venous RA, instead of the Flamm average. See: Braunwald, chapter on "Congenital Heart Disease" Keywords: Flamm =(3 SVC + 1 IVC) / 4

324. The Flamm formula (1 IVC + 3 SVC) / 4 is used to estimate:

a. Systemic venous O_2 saturation in L-R ASD
b. Pulmonary venous O_2 saturation in R-L ASD
c. Systemic venous pressure in L-R ASD
d. Pulmonary venous pressure in R-L ASD

Answer: a. Systemic venous O_2 saturation in L-R ASD. This is because the RA is compromised with the red shunt blood and a true average sample of the systemic venous blood is impossible to measure. This formula is an average which weighs the SVC as 3 times more important than the IVC blood sat. That is why many pediatric cardiologists use only the SVC sat in a L-R ASD instead of the Flamm Formula. See: Braunwald, chapter on "Congenital Heart Disease" Keywords: Flamm =(3 SVC + 1 IVC) / 4

REFERENCES

Pappano & Wier, *Cardiovascular Physiology*, 10th Ed., Mosby Year Book, 2013

Braunwald, Eugene, Ed., HEART DISEASE A Textbook of Cardiovascular Medicine, 9th Ed., W. B. Saunders Co., 2012

Baim, D. S. and Grossman W., Cardiac Catheterization, Angiography, and Intervention, 7th Ed., Lea and Febiger, 2006

Darovic, Gloria O., Hemodynamic Monitoring: Invasive and Noninvasive Clinical Application, 2nd Edition, W.B. Saunders Co., 1995

Egan, Donald F., *Fundamentals of Respiratory Therapy*, 2nd Ed., Mosby-Year Book, Inc., 1973

Guyton, A. C., *Functions of the Human Body*, WB Saunders Co., 1974

Kern, M. J., Ed., The Cardiac Catheterization Handbook, 6th Ed., Mosby-Year Book, Inc., 2016

Peterson, and Nicad, *Cardiac Catheterization Methods, Diagnosis, and Therapy*, 1st edition, W.B. Saunders Co., 1997

Pepine, J. C., and Hill, J. A., et. al., *Diagnostic and Therapeutic Cardiac Catheterization*, 2nd Ed., Williams and Wilkins, 1994

Tilkian, A. G., and Daily, E, J, *Cardiovascular Procedures, Diagnostic Techniques and Therapeutic Procedures*, C. V. Mosby Company, 1986

Tortora, G. J., *Introduction to the HUMAN BODY*, Harper and Row Pub., 1988

Underhill, S. L., Ed., *CARDIAC NURSING*, 2nd Ed., J. B. Lippincott Co., 1989

West, J. B., *Pulmonary Physiology - The Essentials*, 3rd Ed., Williams and Wilkins Co., 1981

Yang, Bentivoglio, Maranhao, and Goldberg, *From Cardiac Catheterization to Hemodynamic Parameters*, 3rd edition, F.A. Davis Co., 3rd edition, 1988

OUTLINE: FICK CARDIAC OUTPUT

1. CO General
   a. Definitions
      i. TDCO (Thermodilution CO)
      ii. Fick CO = Average Pulmonary CO measured via oxygen extraction
      iii. LVMF = Quantitative angiographic CO (Left Ventricular Minute Flow)
      iv. CI = Amount of blood pumped by the heart adjusted to body size (Cardiac Index)
      v. VO_2: Oxygen consumption rate in ml/min
      vi. V dot O_2 = O_2 Consumption rate
      vii. SaO_2 = Saturation of arterial Oxygen, as measured by oximetery
      viii. CaO_2 = Content of arterial Oxygen, as calculated from O_2 sat. & Hgb
      ix. FIO_2 = Fraction of inspired Oxygen, normally 21% unless pt. is on O_2
      x. PaO_2 = Partial pressure of arterial oxygen, as in arterial blood gas PO_2
   b. Units
      i. Q = flow rate = L/min
      ii. O_2 Consumption units= ml/min
      iii. A-V difference units = vol. % or ml/decaliter
      iv. P O_2 = mmHg
      v. Hemoglobin = gm/deciliter or gm %
   c. CI = Cardiac Index = CO/BSA
   d. BSA = Body Surface Area in M^2
   e. BSA nomogram
2. BLOOD OXYGEN
   a. Normal values
      i. Hgb = 15 gm %
      ii. Arterial O_2 Content = 18-22
      iii. Venous O_2 Content
      iv. Lowest O_2 Cont. = CS
      v. Highest Rt. Ht. O_2 Cont. = IVC
      vi. Mixed venous (RA) O_2 Cont. = SVC
      vii. O_2 Capacity = 19-23
         (1) reduced in anemia
      viii. A-V difference = 4-5 vol.%
      ix. CI = 2.0 - 4.5 L/min/M2
         (1) CI, Reduced with standing
         (2) CI, Reduced with age
   b. Calculations
      i. O_2 Content in Vol %
      ii. Oc Capacity in Vol %
      iii. % O_2 Saturation
   c. Blood Sampling
      i. Air-tight syringe, bubble free, heparinized
      ii. Stored: iced and capped
      iii. For Fick CO: PA & any artery
   d. Blood O_2 Analyzers
      i. Van Slyke
      ii. Clark Electrode (P O_2)
      iii. Spectrophotometer
      iv. O_2 Saturation
   e. Oxygen Capacity & Saturation
      i. Capacity = maximum O_2 content (100% sat.)
      ii. Arterial Cap. = Venous Cap.
      iii. O_2 Saturation = Content/Capacity
      iv. O_2 Dissociation Curve
         (1) P O_2 vs. O_2 Sat.
         (2) Used if only given PO_2
3. OXYGEN CONSUMPTION
   a. Ambient air % O_2 = 21 %
   b. Ambient air P O_2
   c. PiO_2
   d. STPD
   e. Assumed O_2 Consumption
      i. Errors = 20% SD
   f. Metabolic Rate Meter
   g. Douglas Bag method
   h. If Patient on O_2
   i. R-L shunt exists if still desaturated on 100% O_2
4. FICK CO
   a. Best (Gold Standard) in low CO states
5. FICK CALCULATIONS
   a. CO = O_2 Consumption/(a-v difference)x 10
   b. Uses AO & PA blood (if no shunt)
   c. Wide a-v difference = low CO
   d. CO using estimated O_2 Consumption
   e. CI = CO/BSA
6. SHUNT CALCULATIONS
   a. Estimates using oximetry
   b. From Fick method
      i. PBF
      ii. SBF
   c. Methods
      i. Oximetry
      ii. Angiography
      iii. Dye dilution curves
      iv. Radioactive tracers
   d. Cyanotic shunts
      i. R-L shunt
      ii. Sat. Step down in Lt. Ht.
      iii. Q_p/Q_s <1
   e. Acyanotic shunts
      i. L-R shunt
      ii. Sat. Step up in Rt. Ht.
      iii. Q_p/Q_s >1
   f. Flamm equation
   g. Q_p = PBF
   h. Q_s = SBF
   i. Q_p/Q_s = PBF/SBF
   j. Q_p/Q_s = (AO-RA)/(PV-PA)
   k. Normal Q_p/Qs = 1
   l. ASD, VSD, PDA
   m. Shunt flow = PBF - SBF
   n. PBF = VO_2/(PV-PA)10
   o. SBF = VO_2/(SA-SV)10
   p. Bidirectional shunt
      i. Q_{eff}

Indicator Dilution CO

INDEX: E7

Thermodilution equipment

BOTH QUESTIONS BELOW REFER TO THIS DIAGRAM.

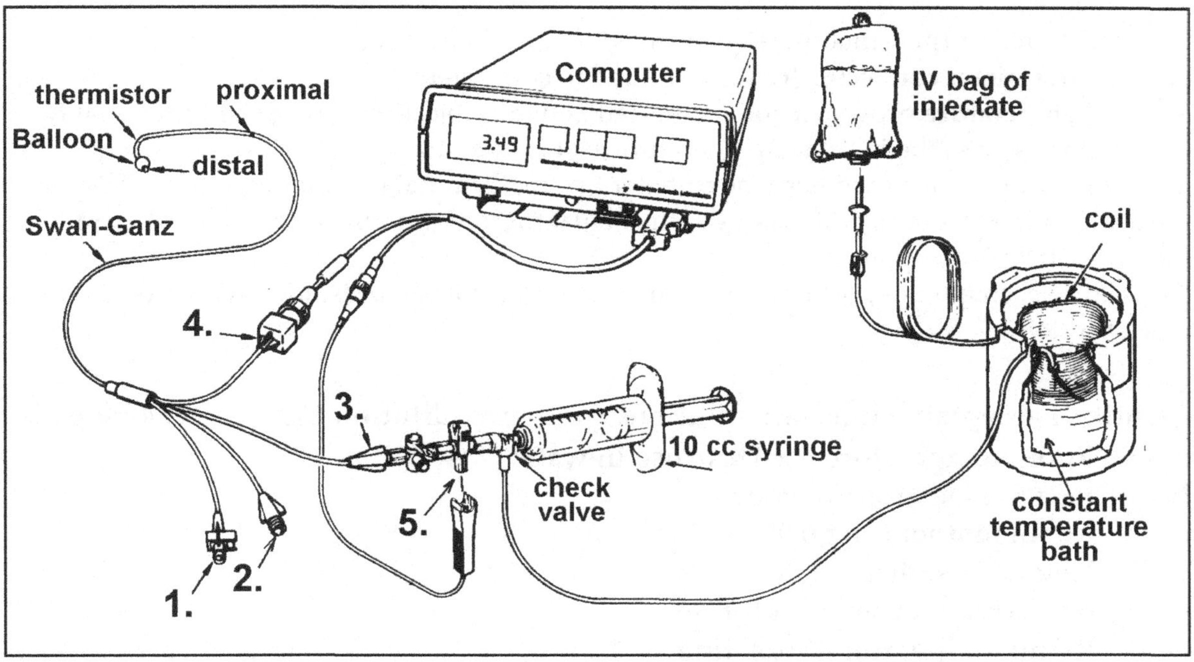

One type of thermodilution system, after, Edwards Co., Swan Ganz package insert

325. What type of TDCO system is shown in the diagram above?

a. Iced injectate, open system
b. Iced injectate, closed system
c. Room temperature injectate, open system
d. Room temperature injectate, closed system

326. Identify the Swan-Ganz catheter port labeled #1 in the diagram above.

a. PA pressure monitoring lumen (distal port)
b. Balloon lumen (stopcock)
c. Thermistor connector (red)
d. RA lumen (proximal port)
e. Temperature probe/sensor

BOTH ANSWERS LISTED TOGETHER BELOW.
325. ANSWER b. Iced injectate, closed system. The styrofoam bath contains ice at 0 to 4 degrees C. This cools the injectate prior to injection. This system is closed (not exposed to air) to reduce the risk of contamination. The open system uses several syringes, each filled and left in an ice basin until they are needed (seldom used now). **See**: Darovic, chapter on, "Monitoring Cardiac Output." **Keywords**: Identify closed-iced TDCO system

326. ANSWER b. Balloon lumen (stopcock). This tail of the catheter is for inflating/deflating the balloon. It should be deflated for TDCO determination.
BE ABLE TO CORRECTLY MATCH ALL ANSWERS:
1. **Balloon lumen (stopcock):** is for inflating/deflating the balloon
2. **PA pressure monitoring lumen (distal port):** connected to right heart manifold (not shown)
3. **RA lumen (proximal port):** connected to injection syringe
4. **Thermistor connector (red):** connected to computer
5. **Temperature probe/sensor:** connected between injection syringe and proximal RA port, senses the injectate temperature as it is injected.

The thermistor bead shown near the catheter tip senses initial body temperature. Then as the cooled blood from the RA passes it, the actual thermodilution curve is recorded and measured by the computer.
See: Darovic, chapter on, "Monitoring Cardiac Output." **Keywords**: Identify closed-iced TDCO system

327. Identify 4 acceptable injectate solutions for thermodilution CO. (Select 4 below.)
- a. **Room temperature 5% Dextrose in water**
- b. **Iced 5% Dextrose in water**
- c. **Room temperature 0.9% saline**
- d. **Iced 0.9% saline**
- e. **Iced Ringers Lactate solution**
- f. **Room temperature 5% saline**

ANSWERS: a, b, c, & d. Both iced and room temperature injectates give comparable results. However, Darovic says that only D5W and NS injectates may be used:

> *"5 percent dextrose in water or 0.9 percent saline. These are the only two acceptable injectate solutions; other types of fluids have varying specific heats and densities that affect the accuracy of the cardiac output measurement."*

See: Darovic, chapter on, "Monitoring Cardiac Output." **Keywords**: acceptable TDCO injectate solutions are D5W and NS

328. A correction factor is entered into the computer for each type of thermodilution catheter used. This factor mainly corrects for:
- a. **Blood lost to the other branch of the PA**
- b. **Variability in thermistor sensitivity**
- c. **Variations in specific heat of different injectates**
- d. **Loss of heat (indicator)**

ANSWER d. Loss of heat (indicator). This factor corrects for cold (calories) that does not find its way into the PA to be measured. For example the 20-40 cm of catheter between the sheath and the stopcock contains injectate that was not injected - and its heat (cold) lost to the atmosphere. The first injection especially, just cools the catheter down and should be discarded. Pepine says,

> *"The correction factor, CF . . . , attempts to account for this unmeasured loss of indicator, and is determined for each catheter model by the manufacturer under standardized conditions. Loss of indicator is greatest for the first injection of a series, since the catheter and the fluid it contains are closest to body temperature. Accordingly, the first cardiac output may be higher than subsequent outputs, especially when iced injectate is used. The factor supplied by the manufacturer assumes that (a) repeat injections are performed 1-2 minutes after the previous output is displayed by the computer, (b) injection rate is 10 cc within 4 seconds, (c) the first injection is disregarded, and (d) the catheter is not aspirated between injections."*

Pepine, Chapter "The Adult Patient with Congenital Disease **Keywords**: Correction factor

Thermodilution techniques

329. Which of the following may lead to inaccurate thermodilution cardiac output? (Select 3.)

a. **Tricuspid regurgitation (TR)**
b. **Cardiac shunt**
c. **Aortic stenosis**
d. **AV fistula in arm**
e. **Rapid IV infusion**

ANSWERS: a, b, & e. TDCO is considered accurate to within 5-10% unless an abnormal flow enters or leaves the right heart. Many dialysis patients have an AV fistula in their arm, shunting from brachial artery to brachial vein. This is not a cardiac shunt so does not effect the direction of intracardiac flow. AV fistulas may increase the cardiac output above normal, but does not interfere with accurate CO measurement. Darovic says,

> *"To record an accurate cardiac output and inscribe a normal curve, all of the cold injectate must enter the right ventricle and then pass the thermistor bead located near the catheter tip in the pulmonary artery. When tricuspid regurgitation or intracardiac shunt exists, recirculation and dilution of the cold injectate before the first pass through the pulmonary artery distort the curve and invalidate the accuracy of values. . . . Rapid intravenous fluid infusions during the cardiac output measurement procedure may artifactually reduce cardiac output measurements."*

See: Darovic, chapter on, "Monitoring Cardiac Output."

330. In which of the following patients would the thermodilution cardiac output method be inaccurate?

a. **Patient is febrile**
b. **Patient with a intracardiac shunt**
c. **Patient with right heart hypertrophy (CHF)**
d. **Patient with stenotic valves, tricuspid or pulmonic**

Answer: b. Patient with a intracardiac shunt. Shunts, leaky Pulmonic Valve, Large bore IV infusion or very low COs (<3 L/min) -all invalidate thermodilution CO. In a intracardiac shunt, blood is either lost or gained between the RA and PA which invalidates the idicator dilution method. See: Kern, chapter on "Hemodynamic Data" Keywords: intracardiac shunts invalidate TDCO

331. Most bolus thermodilution catheter systems use two thermistors to measure temperature difference. Where are the 2 thermistors?

a. **Catheter tip (PA) and injection manifold**
b. **Catheter tip (PA) and display computer**
c. **Catheter tip (RV) and injection manifold**
d. **Catheter tip (RV) and proximal port (RA)**

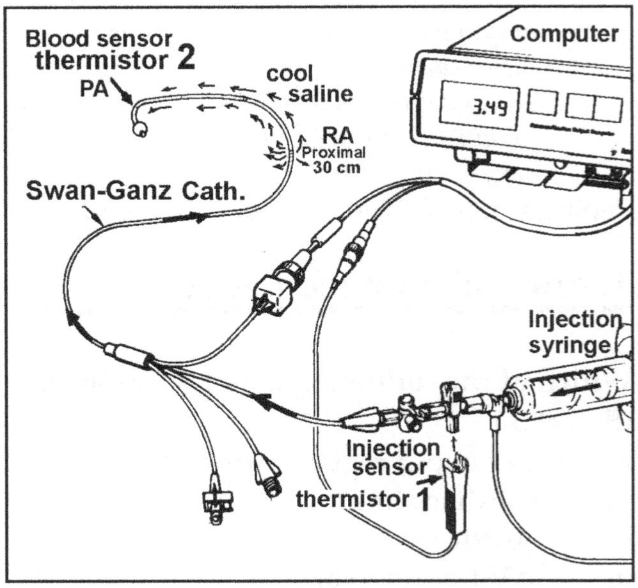

Answer: a. Catheter tip (PA) and injection manifold. One thermistor measures PA blood temperature in PA (thermistor 2). The other measures the temperature of the injectate coming from the injection syringe into the manifold and RA port (thermistor 1). This second thermistor accounts for any warming of the injectate between the cool injectate bath (usually room temperature) and the injection syringe.

By the time the 10 ccs of cool saline is mixed with the warm right heart blood the temp difference, which initially was about 13 degrees (37 - 24 degrees C) may be only a few degrees C. So, the temp change or peak shown on the thermodilution graph may only be one or two degrees cooler than normal blood. These temperatures are all measured accurately by sensors in the catheter and at the injectate syringe manifold. They are essential for accurate calculation of CO. The computer then takes these temperatures and calculates the area under the temperature difference curve and calculates CO. See: Kern, chapter on "Hemodynamic Data" Keywords: PA and injection syringe thermistors

332. A notch or irregularly shaped thermodilution curve is usually due to:

a. **R-L shunt**
b. **L-R shunt**
c. **Uneven injection**
d. **Catheter motion within the PA**

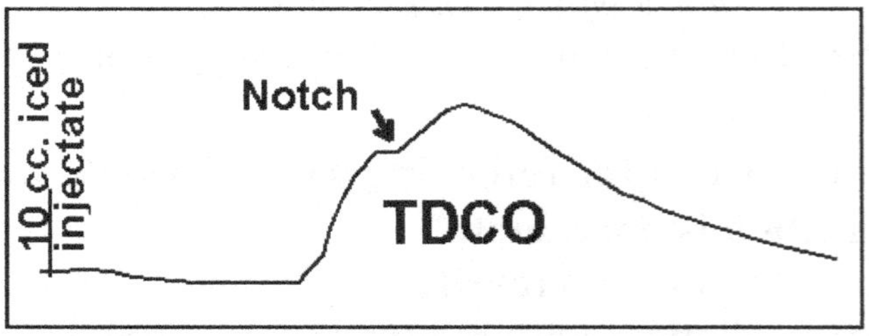

ANSWER c. Uneven injection. The injectate must be injected rapidly and smoothly. If the injector hesitates, an irregular curve may result. Such curves should be discarded and repeated. Darovic says,

> "*The cardiac output curve should be inspected for deviations from the expected normal shape; the computed/calculated readout should never be accepted without question. Faulty technique may cause an artifactual curve variation in which the peak may be notched or the upstroke may not be well defined and is slow. When this occurs, the measurement results should be discarded and the cardiac output measurement procedure repeated.*"

See: Darovic, chapter on, "Monitoring Cardiac Output."

333. Which of the following are recommended for reproducible and accurate thermodilution CO measurement? (Select 3 below.)

a. Inject rapidly and forcefully
b. Aspirate the catheter between injections
c. Throw out the first TDCO reading
d. Wait 30-40 seconds between successive injections
e. Synchronize all injections to the patients expiratory cycle

ANSWERS: a, c, & e. The end of expiration is the most stable hemodynamic phase. That is why pressures should be recorded at end expiration. However, if your patient is short of breath, has a rapid respiratory rate, or gasping respirations it may be impossible to synchronize the injections so the results are completed before the next inhalation. It is acceptable to throw out the 1st reading because the catheter is warm. Most authors recommend that you wait 90 seconds between successive injections. Few physicians are that patient. Darovic says,

> "*Random measurement of cardiac output with the respiratory cycle may produce variability in results because pulmonary artery blood temperature decreases during inspiration, particularly during mechanical ventilation, sighing, or labored breathing. End-expiration is used, when possible, for consistent measurement of cardiac output because absence of chest wall movements provides a convenient determination for injection time. It may, however, be impossible to uniformly time the injection at the same point in the respiratory cycle in a patient with rapid, labored or irregular breathing. . . . When the computer signals READY, a bolus of prepared solution is injected smoothly, rapidly (within 4 seconds), and preferably at end-expiration. The procedure is repeated three times, at least 90 seconds apart, to permit restoration of steady blood flow.*"

Pepine says,

> "*The factor supplied by the manufacturer assumes that (a) repeat injections are performed 1-2 minutes after the previous output is displayed by the computer, (b) injection rate is 10 cc within 4 seconds, © the first injection is disregarded, and (d) the catheter is not aspirated between injections. . . . Reproducibility will be improved in dyspneic or mechanically ventilated patients if injection is timed to begin at the-expiration or peak -inspiration. However, thermodilution outputs performed in this manner may not accurately reflect the average cardiac output throughout the respiratory cycle.*"

See: Darovic, chapter on, "Monitoring Cardiac Output" and Pepine, Chapter on "The Adult Patient with Congenital Disease **Keywords**: inject on expiration

334. Which statement is true about bolus thermodilution?

- a. **The patient's body temperature must be carefully measured prior to injection**
- b. **Always confirm the presence of a PA waveform before injecting**
- c. **Bolus injection must be completed within 10 seconds**
- d. **Tricuspid stenosis reduces the accuracy of bolus TDCO measurement**
- e. **The balloon must be left inflated during TDCO measurement**

ANSWER b. Always confirm the presence of a PA waveform before injecting. Darovic says: "To obtain accurate cardiac output measurement, the thermistor bead located near the tip of the pulmonary artery catheter, must be located in either the left or right mean pulmonary artery. ... Spontaneous distal migration of the catheter tip is suggested by damping of the pulmonary artery waveform. Periodic evaluation of the position of the pulmonary artery catheter tip is also done as a safety measure because current leakage from the thermistor bead can induce ventricular arrhythmias if th catheter tip is in the right ventricle when the thermistor port is connected to the cardiac output computer."
See: Darovic, chapter on "Monitoring Cardiac Output"

335. Which of the following statements about bolus thermodilution is most correct?

- a. **The PA temperature should decrease to about 15° C following injection of room temperature injectate**
- b. **The PA temperature should decrease to about 2° C following injection of iced temperature injectate.**
- c. **The accuracy of injection technique and cardiac output values should be evaluated by the appearance of curve**
- d. **The downslope of the cardiac output curve reflects the bolus injection technique.**

ANSWER c. The accuracy of injection technique and cardiac output values should be evaluated by the appearance of curve - especially the upstroke. Darovic says: "The cardiac output curve should be inspected for deviations from the expected normal shape; the computed/calculated readout should never be accepted without question. Faulty technique may cause an artifactual curve variation in which the peak may be notched or the upstroke may not be well defined and is slow. When this occurs, the measurement should be disregarded and the cardiac output measurement procedure repeated."
See: Darovic, chapter on "Monitoring Cardiac Output"

336. Which one of the following statements regarding bolus thermodilution cardiac outputs is FALSE?

a. **The cardiac output constant reflects the specific catheter used, the injectate temperature and the injectate volume.**
b. **A cardiac output curve with a slow gradual decline best insures proper injection technique.**
c. **Cardiac output determinations in the presence of tricuspid regurgitation or septal defects are commonly erroneous.**
d. **The injectate should be infused in less than 4 seconds.**

ANSWER b. A cardiac output curve with a slow gradual decline best insures proper injection technique is false. It is the upstroke that you are most concerned about smoothness, because this reflects a smooth rapid injection technique (<4 sec.). You want the downstroke to be smooth and gradual with an exponential decay. Notched curves are bad. TR, PR, MR or shunts may alter the flow over the thermistor or shunt some of the indicator into the other side of the heart. All the iced injectate must pass the thermistor once.
See: Darovic, chapter on "Monitoring Cardiac Output"

337. Which one of the following conditions is a cause of inaccurate thermodilution cardiac output measurements?

a. **Injecting 5 ml instead of 10 ml of injectate solution.**
b. **Injecting D5W instead of saline for the injectate solution.**
c. **Injecting room temperature instead of iced temperature injectate solution.**
d. **Injecting with the balloon inflated.**

ANSWER d. Injecting with the balloon inflated. If the balloon is inflated flood flow through the lungs decreases, in fact stops in the area where the balloon is wedged. D5w and Saline are appropriate injectates. In pediatric cases the thermodilution computer may be set to inject 5 ml. instead of the usual 10 ml.
See: Darovic, chapter on "Pulmonary Artery Pressure Monitoring"

338. -The continuous thermodilution CO system (CCO) uses a:

a. **Continuous slow cool saline infusion**
b. **Periodic bolus injection of iced saline**
c. **Doppler transducer at the tip of a balloon catheter**
d. **Warm bolus created by electrically heating a coil on the catheter**

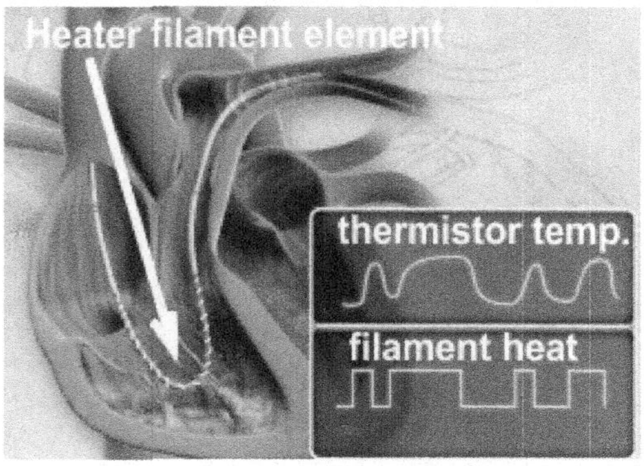

Continuous CO catheter & output

ANSWER d. Warm bolus created by electrically heating a coil (filament) on the catheter wall, instead of the usual cool bolus injection. In both cases the washout curve predicts the patients CO. Edwards Co. Says, "The thermal filament provides a unique input signal. The change in blood temperature resulting from the input signal from the thermal filament is subsequently measured downstream in the PA by the thermistor." It uses time averaging to obtain washout curves from several intermittent [heated] bolus measurements and then averaging the values to obtain the CO. These periodic heated boluses produce a continuous trend in CO. It is also available with a SvO2 fiber optic sensor.

The CCO is commonly used post-op cardiac surgery. Note in the diagram, how a series of square heater filament pulses result in a series of small washout curves sensed by the thermistor. Each curve area gives a CO, all of which are averaged for one TDCO.

See: Edwards.com

Keywords: Continuous CO, heated filament thermodilution

Thermodilution CO (TDCO) measurement

339. What 4 measurements must be made (usually by the computer) to measure thermodilution CO?

a. Injectate temperature (ice C°)
b. Patient body temperature (C°)
c. Amount of injectate (ml)
d. Catheter volume
e. Indicator appearance time
f. Area under curve

ANSWERS: a, b, c, & f. The CO computer tells you when to inject, but no measurement is taken from the time of injection to the appearance of indicator in the blood. Two ml of injectate is the standard amount for an adult. Pepine says,

> "*The variables that must be measured at the time of each measurement are the temperature of blood and injectate and the area under the temperature-time curve. In practice, analog cardiac computers are routinely used to integrate the temperature-time curve and calculate cardiac output.*"

See: Yang, chapter on "Cardiac Output." **Keywords**: things needed to calculate TDCO

340. When 10 ml of iced saline is injected to measure thermodilution CO, the cardiac output is:

a. **Directly proportional to the appearance time of iced saline at the thermistor**
b. **Inversely proportional to the appearance time of iced saline at the thermistor**
c. **Directly proportional to area under TDCO curve**
d. **Inversely proportional to area under TDCO curve**

ANSWER d. Inversely proportional to area under TDCO curve. The bigger the curve the lower the CO. Septic patients with high CO, may have very small TDCO curve areas. The formula for TDCO is:

$$CO = \frac{K\,V_i\,(T_b - T_i)}{\text{Area under curve} \times C}$$

Where: V_i = volume of injectate
T_b = temperature of body
T_i = temperature of injectate
Area = $\int T\,dt$ or(temperature time integral)
K and C = constants

Darovic says,

"The volume of cardiac output is inversely proportional to the area observed under the curve. A high cardiac output characteristically has a small area under the curve. The rapid rise of the curve is due to the rapid appearance of the cold indicator and the small area under the curve is produced by rapid blood flow through the central circulation. In patients with a low cardiac output, the upstroke of the curve may be slurred, and the area under the curve is large because wash-out of the cold indicator is prolonged."

We do not expect that actual calculation of thermodilution CO will be on the CV exams. **See**: Darovic, chapter on, "Monitoring Cardiac Output." **Keywords**: TDCO inversely proportional to area under time deflection curve

BOTH QUESTIONS BELOW REFER TO THESE TDCO MEASUREMENTS.

341. Thermodilution CO readings are shown in the box. How should the average CO be reported?

a. **2.95 L/min**
b. **3.1 L/min**
c. **3.2 L/min**
d. **3.3 L/min**
e. **Do not report, do another injection**

TDCO READINGS	
1st injection	= 3.5 L/min
2nd injection	= 3.0 L/min
3rd injection	= 2.9 L/min

342. In the patient above, a 4th TDCO injection was made as shown (2.7 L/min). How should the average CO be reported?

a. **2.9 L/min**
b. **3.1 L/min**
c. **3.2 L/min**
d. **3.3 L/min**
e. **Do not report, do another injection**

TDCO READINGS	
1st injection	= 3.5 L/min
2nd injection	= 3.0 L/min
3rd injection	= 2.9 L/min
4th injection	= 2.7 L/min

BOTH ANSWERS LISTED TOGETHER BELOW.

341. ANSWER e. Do not report, do another injection. The first injection 3.5 is 0.5 L/min away from the next closest reading. This is more than a 10% variation. (10% of 3.5 = 0.35 L/min). The first injection should be thrown out and injections repeated until three come within 10% of each other. Darovic says,

> *"Thermodilution cardiac output always should be based on the average of at least three individual measurements that are within 10 percent of each other. . . . An average of three injections determines the cardiac output. The readings should fall within a 10 percent range; if not, a technical error may have occurred and the fourth syringe should be used to perform an additional measurement. If there is wide scatter of results, all three measurements may have to be repeated with careful attention to technique."*

It may be difficult to obtain this degree of reproducibility if the patient is unstable. **See**: Darovic, chapter on, "Monitoring Cardiac Output." **Keywords**: TDCO variability should not exceed 10%.

342. ANSWER a. 2.9 L/min. The first injection should be thrown out because it is not within 10% of the others. The last 3 injections average to 2.87 L/min. Average TDCO = (3.0 + 2.9 + 2.7)/3 = 2.86 rounded to 2.9 L/min.
See: Darovic, chapter on, "Monitoring Cardiac Output." **Keywords**: Average TDCOs that are within 10% of each other.

343. From the data in the diagram calculate the cardiac index (CI).

- **a. 2.30 L/min/M²**
- **b. 4.26 L/min/M²**
- **c. 7.88 L/min/M²**
- **d. Do not report, do another injection**

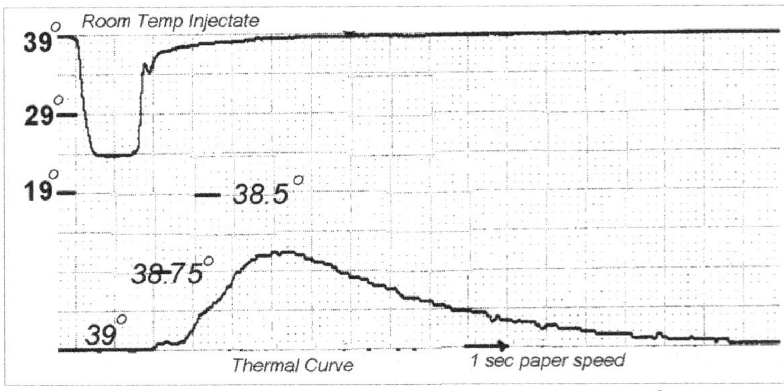

Thermo. CO = 4.26 L/min, BSA = 1.85 M^2

ANSWER a. 2.30 L/min/M^2.
CI is simply CO/BSA = 4.26/1.85 = 2.30 L/min/M^2.
This is the printout from Braun's Dualtherm ® Thermodilution catheter. Note that the injectate temperature is sensed at the proximal RA catheter port, as opposed to externally in the injectate reservoir or injection syringe. Thus no injectate (heat) is lost by remaining in the dead space of the catheter. This is reported to increase the accuracy and reproducibility of the cardiac outputs. **See:** Williams, Steven, and Deckelbaum, Effect of Injectate Temperature and Thermistor Position on Reproducibility of Thermodilution Cardiac Output Determination, Chest, Sept. 1994; 106; 3, 895-898 **Keywords:** Calculate CI from TDCO

Green Dye - NOT TESTED ON RCIS

344. These are GREEN DYE CURVES. Indocyanine green dye was injected in the RA and sampled from the AO. Identify the type of shunt detected by the curve labeled #3.

- **a. Normal**
- **b. L-R shunt**
- **c. R-L shunt**

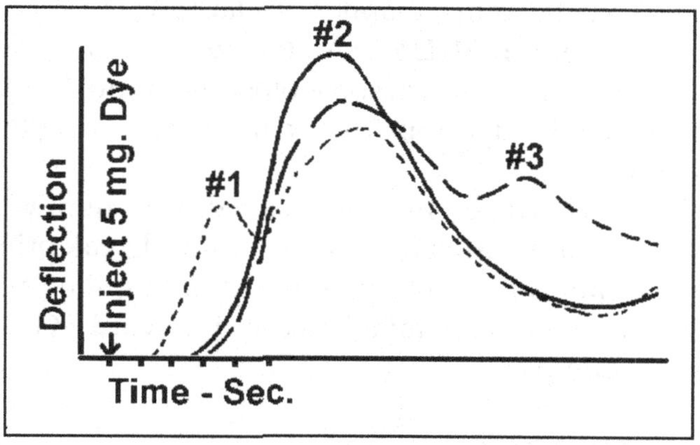

Green Dye curves (IVC→AO)

ANSWER b. L-R shunt causes this late bump. Although some labs still use green dye curves, they have been largely replaced by thermodilution CO because they are so much easier to perform. But, shunt identification by green dye is still a classic test question. Conway says:

> *Dye-dilution has been the basis of accurate determination of cardiac output for many years. It has a repeatability of 5% and has replaced the Fick method as a 'standard'. It requires venous catheterization (with injection near the right atrium) and arterial catheterization with a catheter of sufficient size to allow for the withdrawal of blood at 15-20 ml/min."*

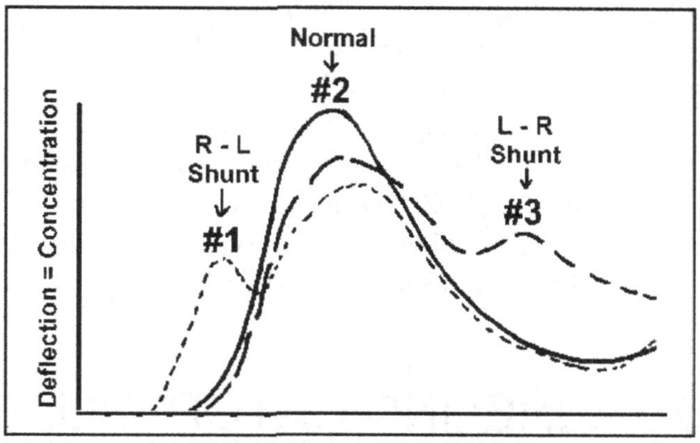

Green Dye curves (IVC→AO)

GREEN DYE CURVES SHOWN ARE:

#1. R-L SHUNT: The dye divides in the right heart as shunted blood appears early in the left heart - making a distinctive early appearance in the aorta (early bump). Small R-L shunts show the small "early bump" shown. While large L-R shunts show large "early bumps." The size of the early bump is proportional to the amount of shunt.

At present this sensitive method of R-L shunt detection is the only major application for green dye curves. Note in the diagram that the dye divides (#1 & 2) at the VSD shunt. As it passes into the aorta, you see two concentrations of dye (#1 & 2 in AO). The amount of the R-L shunt seen at #2 accounts for the curves early hump.

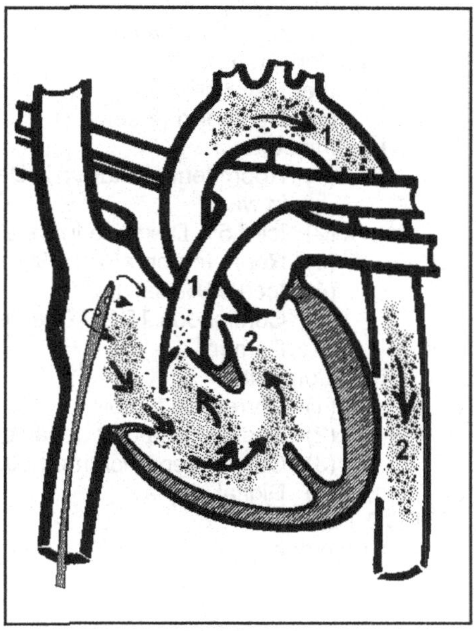

R-L VSD - Shunted Dye (#2) appears early in LV and AO

#2. NORMAL: The curve rises rapidly to a peak and decays exponentially. As the dye returns through the right and left heart on it's second pass it creates the low recirculation curve seen. These were the first indicator dilution curves, before thermodilution. Cardiac output was calculated in a manner similar to TD CO.

#3. L-R SHUNT: All the dye circulates through the right heart but as it passes through the left heart, some blood is shunted back into the right heart again. This recirculating dye appears as a hump following the primary curve, on the recirculation curve.

This diagram shows a **small** R-L shunt with distinct secondary bump. Instead of a "bump" large L-R shunts show reduced peak primary curve concentration and prolonged the disappearance of dye at the sampling site (AO). **See**: Pepine, Chapter on "The Adult Patient with Congenital Disease" **Keywords:** Green dye curves - R-L shunt detection = early bump

REFERENCES

Pepine, J. C., and Hill, J. A., et. al., *Diagnostic and Therapeutic Cardiac Catheterization,* 2nd Ed., Williams and Wilkins, 1994

Yang, Bentivoglio, Maranhao, and Goldberg, *From Cardiac Catheterization to Hemodynamic Parameters,* 3rd edition, F.A. Davis Co., 3rd edition, 1988

Baim, D. S. and Grossman W., *Cardiac Catheterization, Angiography, and Intervention,* 6th Ed., Lea and Febiger, 2006

Darovic, G.O., *Hemodynamic Monitoring: Invasive and Noninvasive Clinical Applications,* 2nd Ed., W.B. Saunders Co., 1995

Conway, J., Clinical assessment of cardiac output, in *Cardiac Output Measurement",* Edited by Robetson and Birkenhager, W. B. Saunders Co., 1991

OUTLINE: INDICATOR DILUTION CO

1. TDCO EQUIPMENT
   a. Open/closed system
   b. Ice/Room temp. injectate
   c. TDCO Swan Ganz catheter
      i. Ports/lumen
      ii. thermistor sensor
         (1) Duotherm (2 sensor)
      iii. Injectate
         (1) Room temperature 5% Dextrose in water
         (2) Iced 5% Dextrose in water
         (3) Room temperature 0.9% saline
         (4) Iced 0.9% saline
         (5) Continuous TDCO - heated filament
      iv. Computer
         (1) Correction factor
         (2) Analog computer decay constant
         (3) Curve integration methods
         (4) Digital display
2. TDCO TECHNIQUES
   a. Curve shape
      i. Unsteady injection
   b. Reproducibility
      i. Throw out 1st reading
      ii. Inject during expiration
      iii. Duplicates acceptable ± 10%
3. TDCO MEASUREMENTS
   a. Measurements needed
      i. Injectate temperature (ice C°)
      ii. Patient body temperature (C°)
      iii. Amount of injectate (ml)
      iv. Area under curve
   b. ↑ Curve area = ↓ CO
   c. ↓ Curve area = ↑ CO
4. GREEN DYE CURVES
   a. Early hump = R-L shunt
   b. Late hump = L-R shunt
   c. Same theory as TDCO
   d. "Standard" indicator dilution CO

QUANTITATIVE LV ANGIOGRAPHY

INDEX: E8

General LV Volumes

345. Match the hemodynamic abbreviation labeled #1 (SV) with its definition below.

a. Amount of blood ejected out the LV with each systole
b. Total amount of blood pumped by the LV per minute
c. Maximum volume of blood in the ventricle when filled
d. Percentage of blood ejected out the ventricle with each beat
e. Net forward amount of blood pumped by LV per minute
f. Minimum volume of blood in the ventricular chamber
g. Amount of blood regurgitating (reverse flow)
h. Ratio of regurgitation to total LV flow

Hemodynamic Abbreviations

*1. SV
2. RV
3. EF
4. CO
5. EDV
6. ESV
7. LVMF
8. RF

ANSWER a. Amount of blood ejected out the LV with each systole = SV. There are actually two types of SV, forward SV from Fick CO and total SV measured from quantitative angiography.

BE ABLE TO MATCH ALL BELOW:
Hemodynamic Abbreviations

*1. **SV** = Amount of blood ejected out the aortic valve with each systole (Stroke Volume in ml)
2. **RV** = Regurgitant Volume = Amount of blood regurgitating (reverse flow)
3. **EF** = Percentage of blood ejected out the ventricle with each beat (Ejection Fraction in %)
4. **CO** = (Cardiac Output in L/min) Net amount of blood pumped by the LV per minute. It is NET or forward flow, because CO only measures average forward flow and does not include the increase in flow necessary to compensate for valvular regurgitation.
5. **EDV** =Maximum volume of blood in the ventricle when filled (End Diastolic Volume in ml)
6. **ESV** = Minimum volume or residual blood left in the ventricle after contraction

(End Systolic Volume in ml)

7. **LVMF** = (Left ventricular minute flow in L/min) Total amount of blood pumped by the LV per minute. It is TOTAL because some of this blood may leak back during valvular regurgitation. Sometimes called the "Angio CO" or "Total CO. "
8. **RF:** Regurgitant Fraction = Ratio of regurgitation to total LV flow

See: Baim chapter on "Ventricular Volumes,..." **Keywords:** CO definitions

346. Identify the correct formulas for stroke volume. (Select 3 below.)

a. **SV = CO/HR**

b. **SV = EF x EDV**

c. **SV = CO x HR**

d. **SV = 1 - ESV/EDV**

e. **SV = EDV - ESV**

ANSWERS: a, b, & e.

FORMULAS LISTED ARE:

1. **SV = CO/HR**: **YES.** This SV is estimated from the minute CO. If Fick CO is used, this SV is an average SV. Since Cardiac output = Stroke Volume x Heart **rate the formula can be rearranged to give SV=CO/HR.**
2. **SV = EF x EDV: YES. This is a rearrangement of the EF formula: EF = SV/EDV.**
3. **SV = CO x HR: NO. This is a ms-statement of #1. It is SV = CO / HR**
4. **SV = 1 - ESV/EDV: NO. This is a mis-statement of the formula for ejection fraction. The true formula for EF is: EF = 1 - ESV/EDV = (EDV - ESV)/EDV = SV / ED**

5 **SV =EDV - ESV: YES.** This is measured directly from one LV angio beat. This chapter is about measuring these angiographic volumes. Since this SV is measured from one beat it may not take into account phasic variations in heart rate and breathing. To accurately estimate minute CO or LVMF from this one beat, one must select a representative average SV since any error will be multiplied by the heart rate.

See: Sheehan, "Cardiac Angiography" in Marcus, *Cardiac Imaging, A companion to Braunwald's Heart Disease.*" Baim chapter on "Ventricular Volumes,..."**Keywords**: stroke volume

347. The amount of blood pumped from the left ventricle during a single systole can be calculated by:

a. **EDV - SV**

b. **ESV - SV**

c. **EDV - ESV**

d. **ESV - EDV**

ANSWER c. EDV - ESV = SV. Stroke index is the amount of blood the heart pumps with each beat. SV is the difference between the full ventricle (EDV) and the almost empty ventricle (ESV).

SV = EDV - ESV

E.g.: 150 ml - 80 ml = 70 ml

See: Kern, chapter on "Hemodynamics" **Keywords:**: Define stroke volume

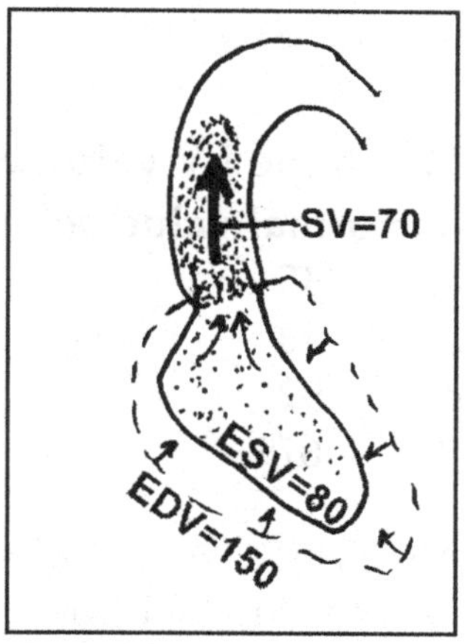

SV = EDV - ESV

348. Identify all the correct formulas for ejection fraction (EF). (Check 3 below.)

a. EF = 1 - (ESV/EDV)
b. EF = (CO x HR) / EDV
c. EF = (EDV - ESV)/ EDV
d. EF = SV/EDV
e. EF = EDV/SV

ANSWERS: a, c, & d.
a. YES: EF = 1 - (ESV/EDV)
b. NO: EF = (CO x HR) / EDV (This formula could be corrected by dividing by the HR instead of multiplying times it. E.g., EF = (CO / HR) / EDV = SV/EDV.)
c. YES: EF = (EDV - ESV) / EDV
d. YES: EF = SV / EDV
e. NO: this formula is inverted and would result in a.
Note that since SV = EDV - ESV, it can be substituted into the EF equation:
EF = SV/EDV = (EDV - ESV)/EDV = 1 - (ESV/EDV)
See: Baim chapter on "Ventricular Volumes,..." **Keywords:** EF formulas

349. The formula to calculate CO using quantitative LV angiography (LVMF) is:

a. LVMF = (LVEDP) x SVR
b. LVMF = SV / EDV
c. LVMF = SV x HR
d. LVMF = (EDV - ESV) x SV

ANSWER c. LVMF = SV x HR. Left ventricular minute flow (LVMF) is the angiographic stroke volume times heart rate. Since SV is the amount pumped per beat, and HR is the number of beats/min, the product is amount pumped/min. SV is usually measured in ml/beat, HR in beats/min.

LVMF = SV ml/beat x HR b/min = ml/min

To change LVMF (ml/min) into L/min, divide by 1000 ml/L.
In the previous example LVMF = SV x HR = (70 ml/beat) x (60 beats/min) / (1000 ml/L) = 4.2 L/min.

See: Braunwald, Chapter on "Evaluation of LV Function" **Keywords:** LV Performance LVMF = SV x HR

350. Match the LV volume #1 (EDVI) in the box with its normal value below.

a. 45
b. 70
c. 92
d. 67%

Normal LV Volume Data for		
***1.**	**EDV Index**	**(ml/m²)**
2.	Stroke Index	(ml/m²)
3.	Mass	(gm/m²)
4.	Ejection Fraction (%)	

ANSWER b. 70 ml/m^2 = EDV index.
Braunwald's table 14-1 indicates normal values as follows:

1. End Diastolic Vol. Index = 70 ± 20 ml/m^2
2. Stroke Volume Index = 45 ± 13 ml/m^2
3. LV Mass Index = 92 ± 16 ml/m^2
4. Ejection Fraction = 0.67 ± 0.08

Note normal ESV can be found by subtracting normal SV from normal EDV. Actual normal volumes for your patient can be found by multiplying these indexed values times the patients BSA. E.g., with a BSA of 1.7 m^2, normal stroke volume values would be: 45 x 1.7 = 76 ml. Note that EF is not indexed to body size since it is the ratio of two volumes. **See**: Braunwald, Chapter on "Evaluation of LV Function." **Keywords:** Normal EDV = 70 ml/m^2 ± *20*

Normals for BSA of 1.7 m²	
EDV	119 (ml)
ESV	43 (ml)
SV	76 (ml)
Mass	150 (gm)
EF	67 (%)

351. The cutoff between normal and abnormal resting ejection fraction (EF) is approximately:

a. 10-20%
b. 30-35%
c. 50-55%
d. 70-75%

ANSWER c. 50-55%. The normal EF is around 66%. Sheehan uses 55% as the cutoff point. But the cutoff for abnormal is usually considered to be an EF less than <50%. Peterson suggests 45 to 50% as the cutoff. He says,

> *"Ejection fraction (EF) is the most commonly used measure of left ventricular ejection performance because of its prognostic value; it is expressed in percentages.... In normal subjects an excessive rise in afterload may reduce the EF to a value of 50% or slightly less. A more severely reduced EF (≤ 45%) can be considered as an indicator of depressed myocardial function, regardless of the cardiac disorder and loading conditions present."*

From the above table normal EF = .67 ± .08 SD. Two standard deviations below normal would include 95% of all normals. So 0.67 - .16 = 0.51% cutoff point. **See:** Peterson, chapter on "Left and Right Contrast Ventriculography" also, Sheehan, "Cardiac Angiography" in Marcus, *Cardiac Imaging, A companion to Braunwald's Heart Disease."* **Keywords:** Normal EF = >50%

352. When measured simultaneously all cardiac outputs should be equal (Fick CO = TDCO = LVMF) <u>EXCEPT</u> in cases of:

a. Low CO
b High CO
c. Valvular stenosis
d. Valvular regurgitation

ANSWER d. Valvular regurgitation. In normal conditions, if all methods of CO and SV were done accurately and at the same time, they should be equal. Braunwald says,

> *"In the absence of valvular regurgitation or intracardiac shunt, the angiographic SV should correlate closely with an independent measurement of SV (cardiac output/heart rate) using the Fick or thermodilution cardiac method. In the presence of valvular regurgitation or shunt, the total SV determined by angiocardiography is greater than the effective forward SV determined by the Fick or indicator dilution method. The difference between the two represents the regurgitant (or shunt) flow per cardiac cycle."*

See: Braunwald, chapter on "Coronary Arteriography" **Keywords:** LVMF = Fick = TDCO unless regurgitation present

353. In the LV pressure - volume curve drawn in the box, what cardiac event occurs at #7 in the diagram?

a. Systolic ejection
b. AO valve opens
c. Diastolic filling
d. Mitral valve closure
e. Isometric contraction
f. AO valve closes
g. Isometric relaxation
h. Mitral valve opens

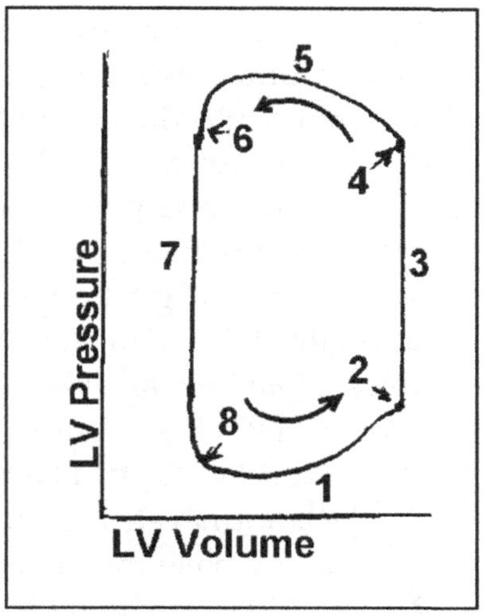

LV P-V Loop

ANSWER g. Isometric relaxation is the beginning of diastole. The heart relaxes after the AO valve closes. So the LV is relaxing without changing its volume - against closed valves. This rapid down slope of the LV pressure curve is termed "isotonic" or "isometric", because the volume is constant. LV pressure is still too high to allow the mitral valve to open. At point #8 the mitral valve opens and allows diastolic filling. Be able to match all answers.

The Pressure - Volume loop is an X-Y plot of the LV pressure on the Y-axis against LV volume on the X-axis. The loop progresses counterclockwise representing all phases of LV hemodynamics. This graph may look foreign to you, but study it. Note how it resembles systole of an LV pressure (drawn on the right). The aortic valve opens in the upper right corner. If you reverse the systolic ejection phase of a pressure curve, it begins to resemble the top of the PV curve. Each corner is associated with a valvular event (marked with a •). Systolic ejection occurs in a Rt-Lt direction across the top of the box.

BE ABLE TO MATCH ALL BELOW:

1. Diastolic filling
2. Mitral valve closure
3. Isometric contraction
4. AO valve opens
5. Systolic ejection
6. AO valve closes
7. Isometric relaxation
8. Mitral valve opens

See: Berne & Levy, chapter on "Cardiac Pump **Keywords:**: Wiggers, PV Loop

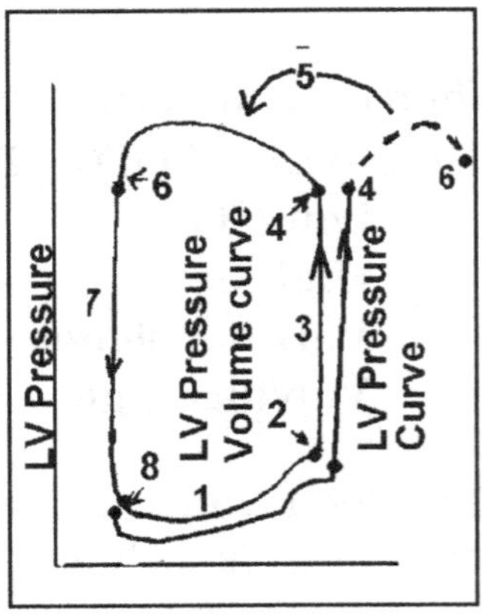

LV PV loop & pressure

354. Match the pressure-volume curve #1 with its pathology.

a. **MS**
b. **MR**
c. **AS**
d. **AR**

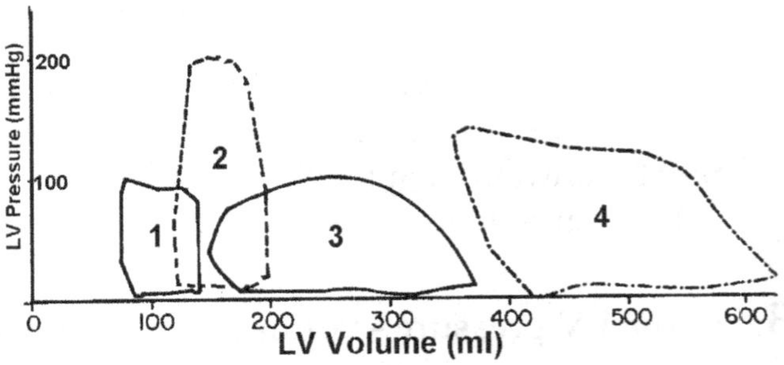

Pressure Volume curves from various pathologies (after Sheehan, fig. 9-36)

ANSWER a. MS. When LV pressure is plotted against LV volume throughout the heart cycle, a pressure volume curve results. It moves counter-clockwise, up and to the left in systole, and down and to the right in diastole. The area inscribed within the loop represents the amount of LV stroke work (P x V). Valvular stenosis patients have small LV volumes because blood has difficulty entering the LV through the tight mitral valve. Patients with regurgitation tend to have sloping or rounded isovolumetric periods as the blood regurgitates. They also tend to have large stroke volumes with dilated end-diastolic volumes. Note how as disease progresses the curves move to larger volumes (LV dilation) and larger EDVs (LV failure).

MATCH ANSWERS BELOW:

1. **MS:** normal stroke volume, and stroke work (area within curve). In MS the LA and RV have the increased work load. Average EDV = 83 ml/m^2, SV = 43 ml/m^2.
2. **AS**: Generate high LV pressures to overcome the tight aortic valve. Compensatory LV hypertrophy develops. Average EDV 84 ml/m^2, SV = 44 ml/m^2
3. **MR:** Average EDV = 160 ml/m^2, SV = 87 ml/m^2
4. **AR:** These are the largest LVs with the largest stroke volumes. Average EDV = 193 ml/m^2, SV = 92 ml/m^2.

See: Sheehan, "Cardiac Angiography" in Marcus, *Cardiac Imaging, A companion to Braunwald's Heart Disease*" **Keywords:** Quantitative LV Pressure volume curves in MS

355. The Kennedy/Dodge area length method of quantitative LV volume measurement simplifies the shape of the LV chamber to that of a/an:

a. **Sphere**
b. **Truncated cone**
c. **Cylinder**
d. **Ellipse of rotation**

ANSWER d. Ellipse of rotation. When an ellipse (2 dimensional shape) is rotated, it inscribes a football (3 dimensional) shape, termed an ellipsoid or ellipse of rotation. Peterson says,

> "*Geometric methods for estimation of left ventricular volume assume that the left ventricular shape is that of an ellipsoid. Although the shape of the left ventricular cavity is complicated by the presence of the papillary muscles, its relatively convex, or football-shaped, geometry permits the use of simplified mathematic models.... For both single-plane and biplane left ventricular volume estimation, these formulas have been shown to be valid even when the shape of the ventricle deviates from the assumed uniform ellipsoid.*"

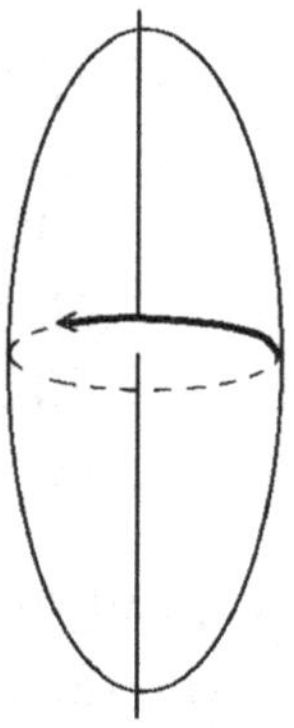

Ellipse

See: Peterson, chapter on "Left and Right Contrast Ventriculography."
Keywords: LV= ellipsoid

356. -Calculate regurgitant fraction when LVMF = 10.4 L/min and Fick C.O. = 4.1 L/min

a. **0.15**
b. **0.25**
c. **0.39**
d. **0.61**

Answer: d. 0.61 RF is the regurgitant flow divided by the Total CO. Or it is the difference between the Total and forward CO divided by the Total CO usually RF = (LVMF-FICK CO)/ LVMF. Here RF = (10.4 - 4.1) / 10.4 = 6.3/10.4 = .61 = 61% Remember Total CO, is the largest CO which is the LVMF. The largest number goes in the denominator. See: Grossman chapter on "Volumes, EF..." Keywords: RF = (LVMF-FICK CO)/ LVMF

357. Calculate the LV ejection fraction from EDV= 175 cc, ESV=145 cc, HR = 67, LV EDP=12 mmHg

a. **17%**
b. **21%**
c. **29%.**
d. **71%**

Answer: a. 17% = (175 - 145) / 175 = .17 or 17% The difference between EDV and ESV is the SV of 30 cc. EF is the ratio of SV / EDV = 30 / 175 = .17 This is a very low EF, suggesting the patient is in heart failure. Normal is > 50 %. See: Grossman chapter on "Volumes, EF..." Keywords: EF = SV / EDV

LV ANGIOGRAPHY MEASUREMENTS

358. For single plane quantitative angiography (area-length method of Dodge) the LV must be filmed in the _____ angiographic view:

a. **30 degree RAO**
b. **60 degree RAO**
c. **30 degree LAO**
d. **60 degree LAO**

ANSWER a. In the 30 degree RAO the hearts long axis is perpendicular to the X-ray beam. This is the standard view for the long axis which must be measured for LV volumes and ejection fractions.
See: Baim chapter on "Ventricular Volumes,..."
Keywords: Long axis = 30 degree RAO

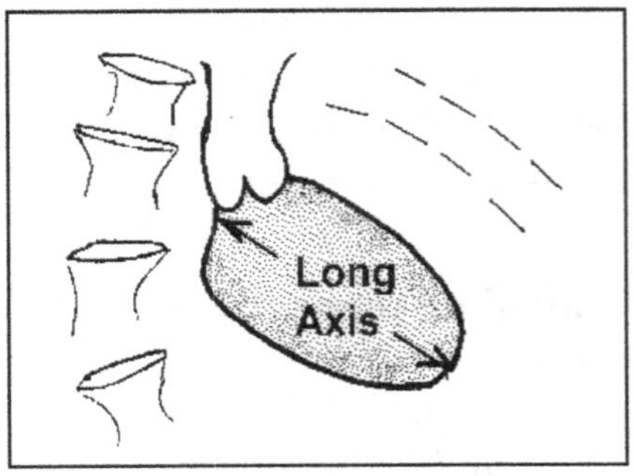

LV long axis = 30° RAO

359. For accurate LV volume calculations what must be added to the catheterization procedure?

a. **One additional LV gram to get biplane images**
b. **Quality control X-ray film with sensitometry**
c. **Calibrate the system with LV casts of known volume**
d. **Film a calibration grid, ball or a banded catheter**

ANSWER d. Film a calibration grid, ball or a banded catheter. All cath labs should routinely quantitate their LV angiography. It requires no additional case time, only the calibration of the system with a calibration grid, ball, or catheter. Sheehan says,

> *"When the end-diastolic and end-systolic contours have been delineated, it is possible to calculate rapidly the end-diastolic, end-systolic, and stroke volumes; cardiac output; ejection fraction; and wall motion. the only adjustment to the cardiac catheterization routine needed is either filming of a grid at the end of the procedure or performance of biplane ventriculography with a banded catheter to correct for magnification.... Because of its accuracy, volume determination by contrast ventriculography is the gold standard by which other imaging modalities are judged."*

See: Sheehan, "Cardiac Angiography" in Marcus, *Cardiac Imaging, A companion to Braunwald's Heart Disease."* Baim chapter on "Ventricular Volumes,..." **Keywords:** Quantitative LV angiography only requires addition of calibration grids

360. **This LV gram shows prominent trabeculations and papillary muscles. Which outline is correctly drawn for end-systolic volume?**

a. #1 lower rib margin

b. #2 drawn around epicardial outline

c. #3 drawn at base of trabeculi and papillary muscles

d. #4 drawn inside trabeculi and papillary muscles

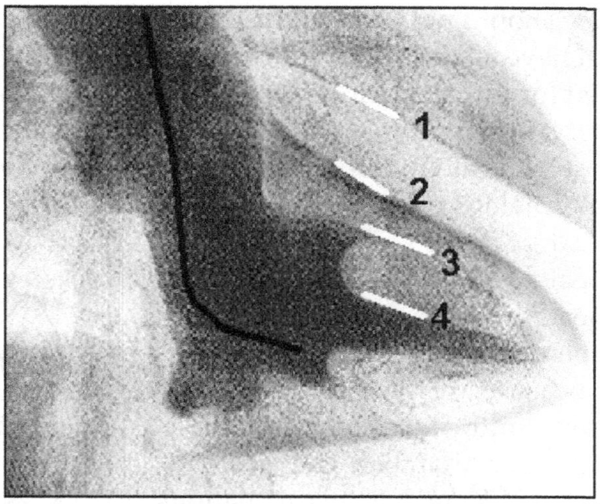

30° RAO LVgram ESV

ANSWER c. #3 drawn at base of trabeculi and papillary muscles, to include any whiff of contrast. #2 is the epicardial outline, not the LV chamber. #4 is wrong, because the outline should include the papillary muscles. Baim says,

> "*In the first step in calculating left ventricular chamber volume, the left ventricular outline or silhouette is traced. The ventricular silhouette should be traced at* ***the outermost margin of visible radiographic contrast*** *so as to include trabeculations and papillary muscles within the perimeter. The aortic valve border is defined as a line connecting the inferior aspects of the sinuses of Valsalva.*"

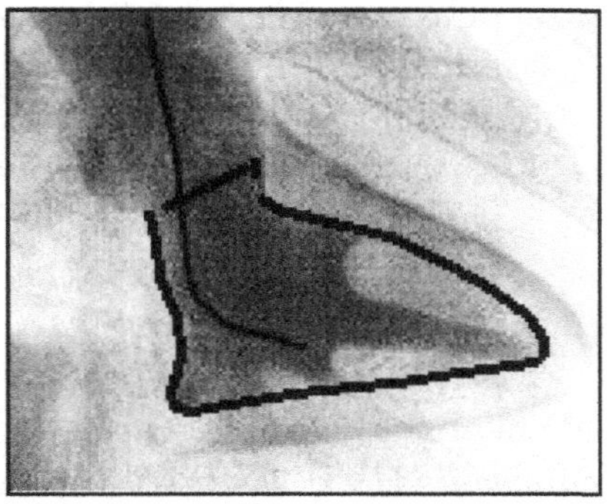

LV perimeter & Pap. muscles

See: Baim chapter on "Ventricular Volumes,..." **Keywords:** draw ESV to include papillary muscles and contrast perimeter

THIS DIAGRAM SHOWS 6 CINE FRAMES TRACED AT 6 POINTS ON THE ECG.

361. **Which frames would you choose to analyze for EDV and ESV?**

a. #1 and #2

b. #3 and #4

c. #4 and #5

d. #5 and #6

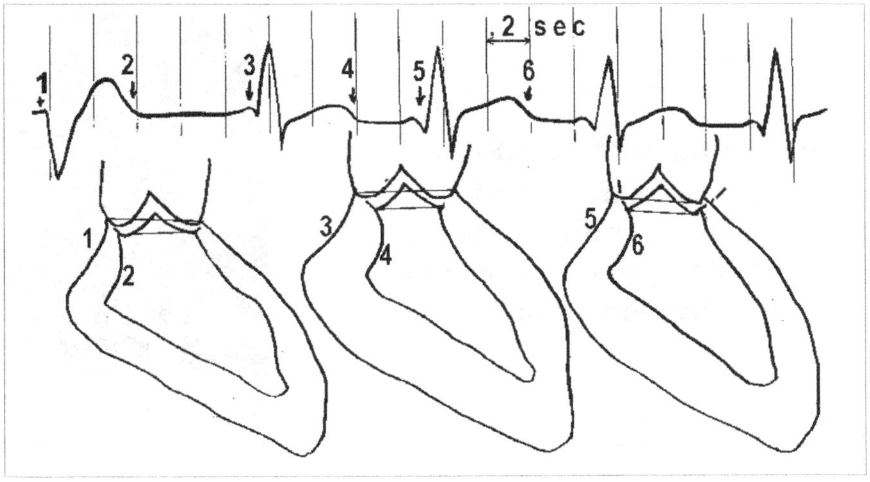

ANSWER d. #5 and #6. The PVC at #1 occurs early. Ventricular filling ends prematurely thus reducing preload and systolic ejection. PVCs don't conduct or contract normally. They should not be used for EF calculation. Beat #3 follows a compensatory pause and will have an artificially elevated EDV and EF due to increased preload. It should not be used for EF calculation. The first normal beat after the PVC is #5 and #6. Use the RR interval preceding #5, because it is most associated with EDV #5, and ESV #6 which is most associated with EDV #5. Note the wide variation in EF in conjunction with these abnormal RR intervals:

Beat #1 and 2	est. EF = 70%
Beat #3 and 4	est. EF = 90%
Beat #5 and 6	est. EF = 80%

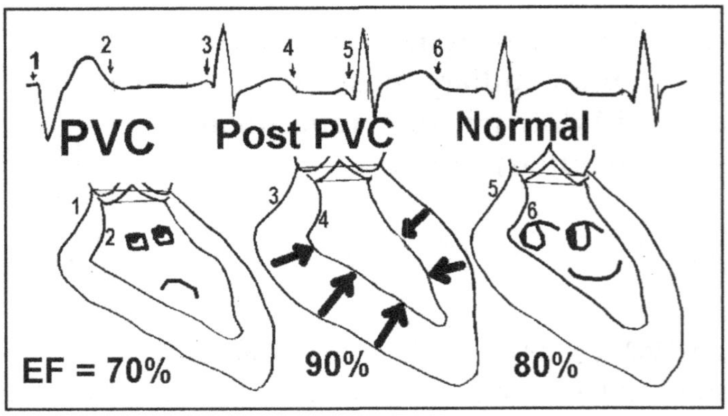

If there is no ectopy, the best beats to measure are the earliest beats before contrast washes out of the ventricular chamber. The most accurate EF and LVMF calculations average several normal beats. See Sheehan,

> "*Care must be taken to avoid ectopy, which is undesirable for several reasons. First, contrast is wasted. Second, the normal beat following it is usually not analyzed because function is potentiated and therefore nonrepresentative. Finally, this potentiated beat empties the ventricle of much of its remaining contrast, so the ensuing normal sinus beats are poorly opacified.... Because of the cardiodepressive effect of the contrast agent, analysis should be performed on the earliest possible beat following contrast injection.*"

See: Sheehan, "Cardiac Angiography" in Marcus, *Cardiac Imaging, A companion to Braunwald's Heart Disease.*" Baim chapter on "Ventricular Volumes,..." **Keywords:** Do not analyze PVCs or Post PVC beats

BOTH QUESTIONS BELOW REFER TO THIS DIAGRAM.

362. Calculate the ejection fraction of this LV.

- **a.** 68%
- **b.** 79%
- **c.** 86%
- **d.** 92%

363. What is wrong with the EF calculation?

- **a.** Measured after a PVC
- **b.** No grid or calibration
- **c.** EDV length measured too long
- **d.** ESV traced too small

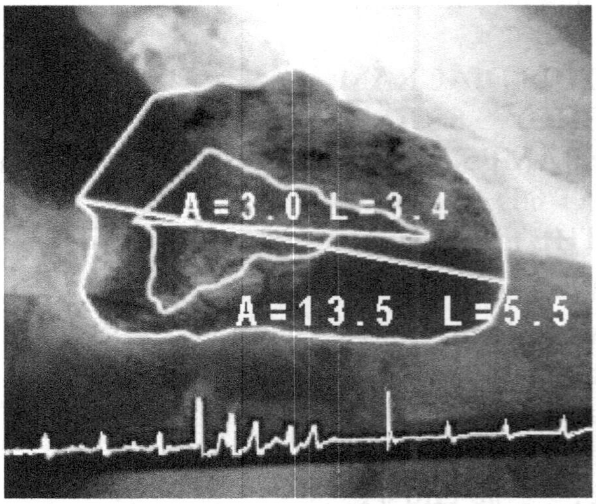

Patient #362 30° RAO, LV-EDV and ESV

BOTH ANSWERS LISTED TOGETHER:

362. ANSWER d. 92%. Use the short formula for ejection fraction without correction factors (explained in section on "Formulas" below). Note that the two areas are superimposed on the diagram. The larger area is end diastole and the smaller is end systole. A is the planimetered area of each. L is the long axis of each.

$EF = 1 - (Aes / Aed)^2 \; (Led / Les)$

$EF = 1 - \left(\frac{3.0}{13.5}\right)^2 \left(\frac{5.5}{3.4}\right) = 1 - (.22)^2 (1.6) = 1 - (.049)(1.6) = 1 - 0.08 = .92 = 92\%$

See: Peterson, chapter on "Left and Right Contrast Ventriculography." **Keywords:** Calculate EF

363. ANSWER a. Measured after a PVC. Note the run of PVCs on the ECG. The ECG marker indicates that the EDV was drawn on the first R wave after the run of V tach. The compensatory pause artificially increases the EDV and ejection fraction. Here the pigtail catheter can be seen almost touching the inferior wall. An angled pigtail can avoid this problem. Baim says,

> "*Attention to catheter position and injection rate minimizes the occurrence of ventricular ectopy during contrast studies; this is important because analysis of extrasystoles and posextrasystolic beats cannot be used for proper assessment of basal ventricular function.*"

See: Baim chapter on "Ventricular Volumes,..." **Keywords:** Do not analyze PVCs or Post PVC beats for EF

CORRECTION FACTORS

364. Pincushion distortion on LV angiography is:

a. Grid distortion near center of film

b Magnification at edges and corners of film

c. Uneven film density due to heel effect

d. Quantum mottle due to low film density

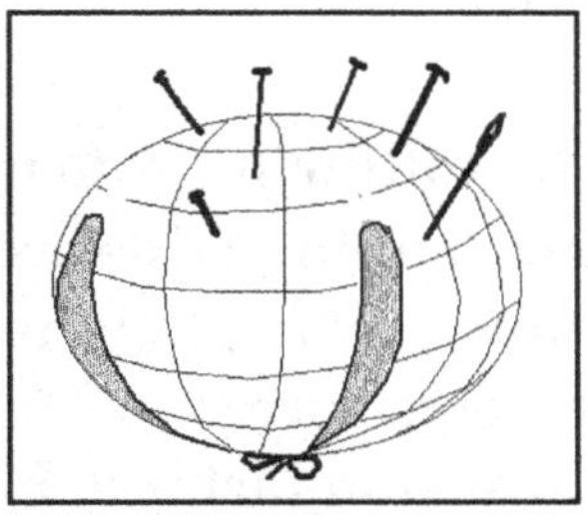

Pincushion

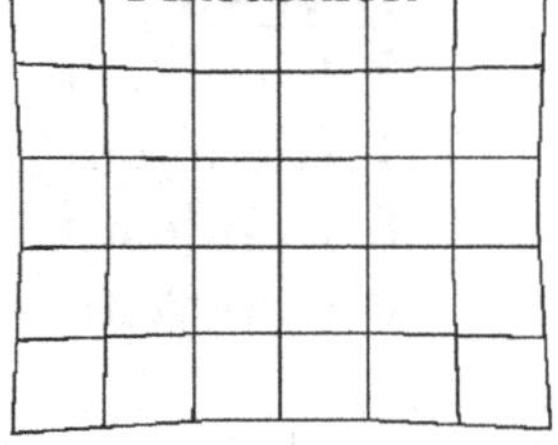

ANSWER b. Magnification at edges and corners of film. Note in the filmed grid that the squares near the corners are distorted and magnified more than those at the center. This is pincushion distortion. It is inherent in all image intensifier systems. Consider a piece of cloth, where corners are drawn around to the back, and sewn together. It would form a pincushion as shown. Peterson says,

> "*The size and region of the calibration grid used should be chosen to overlap with the ventricular silhouette... This is important because the peripheral region of the image intensifier has pincushion distortion, and... may contribute 6% to 30% of the calculated volume.*"

See: Peterson, chapter on "Left and Right Contrast Ventriculography." **Keywords:** Pincushion distortion

365. A metal calibration ball is 5.0 cm in diameter. When filmed in the patients axilla, it is magnified to 6.0 cm on the cine screen as shown. What is the cubic correction factor (CF^3)?

a. $CF^3 = 0.496\ cm^3/cm^3$
b. $CF^3 = 0.578\ cm^3/cm^3$
c. $CF^3 = 0.694\ cm^3/cm^3$
d. $CF^3 = 0.833\ cm^3/cm^3$
e. $CF^3 = 1.20\ cm^3/cm^3$

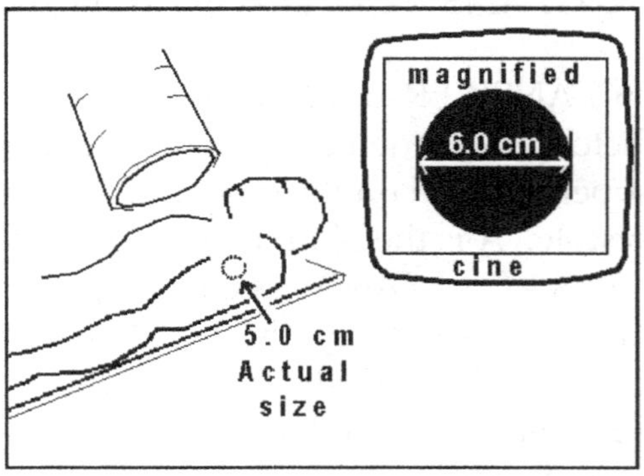

Cine of 5 cm calibration ball

ANSWER b. $CF^3 = 0.578\ cm^3/cm^3$ is the cubic correction factor. First calculate the linear correction factor as the true length over the cine length. CF = 5.0/6.0 = 0.833 cm/cm. Using this factor linear cine measurements can be multiplied by the CF of 0.83 to get the true length. However, a cubic correction factor is needed to convert the final calculated volumes into true cm^3. Simply cube the linear factor to get the cubic correction factor. $CF^3 = 0.833 \times 0.833 \times 0.833 = 0.578\ cm^3/cm^3$. Correction factors are set up so the true measurement is in the numerator and the measured value is in the denominator: CF = true length / measured length. Kern says,

> "*To obtain absolute volumes, correction must be made for distortion caused by divergence of the x-ray beams and the magnification of the image during projection of the film. Correction factors are obtained from a grid of square centimeters filmed at the level of the patient's heart during the procedure in both the RAO and LAO projections. Utilizing the planimetered area of the projected grids, a linear correction factor (CF) for each plane is calculated....*"

See: Kern Appendix VI on "Ventricular Volume and Mass." **Keywords:** cubic correction factor

366. The following data uses a calibration grid made from overlapping wires exactly 1 cm apart. The 30 boxes shown were planimetered to be 60 square cm. What is the area correction factor (CF^2) and the cubic correction factor (CF^3) for LV volume calculation?

	Area CF^2	Volume CF^3
a.	$2.0\ cm^2/cm^2$,	$2.83\ cm^3/cm^3$
b.	$1.41\ cm^2/cm^2$,	$2.83\ cm^3/cm^3$
c.	$0.5\ cm^2/cm^2$,	$0.71\ cm^3/cm^3$
d.	$0.5\ cm^2/cm^2$,	$0.35\ cm^3/cm^3$

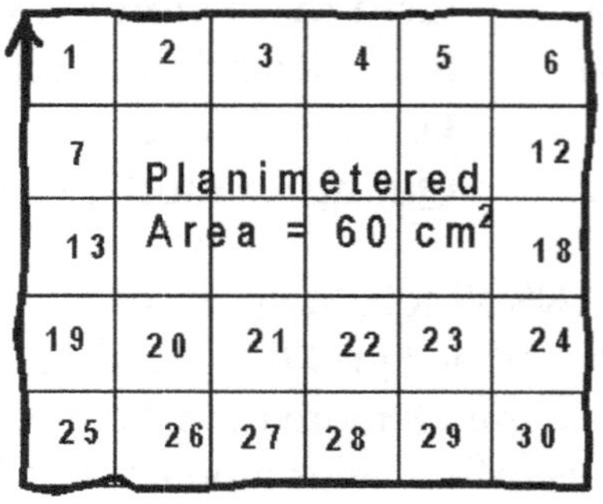

30 cm calibration grid

ANSWER d. $0.5\ cm^2/cm^2$, $0.35\ cm^3$ The area correction factor is $CF^2 = 30/60 = 0.5\ cm^2/cm^2$. However, a cubic correction factor is needed to convert the measurements into volume or cm^3. First convert the area CF^2 into a linear CF by taking its square root. $CF = \sqrt{CF^2} = \sqrt{0.5} = 0.707$ cm/cm . Then, simply cube the linear factor to get the cubic correction factor. $CF^3 = (0.707)^3 = 0.35\ cm^3/cm^3$. Correction factors are always set up so the true measurement is in the numerator and the measured value is in the denominator.
Baim says,

"If the projected (planimetered) area is A_p, and the actual area (number of squares) is A_{true}, then the linear correction factor CF is $CF = \sqrt{(A_{true}/A_p)}$.... In the single-plane formula, the cube of the linear correction fraction adjusts the volume for magnification."

He adds that calibration discs and catheters may be used instead of a grid and do not significantly alter the calculated correction factor. Note that most authors do not recommend planimetering a square grid for CF. They planimeter the actual squares on which the LV lies. This compensates for distortion at the edges of the film. **See:** Baim chapter on "Ventricular Volumes,..." **Keywords:** cubic correction factor

367. The elliptical LV volume model tends to overestimate the true left ventricular volume. The mathematical model must be adjusted by comparing its result to the volume of real postmortem LV chamber casts. These adjustments are termed:

a. Magnification corrections

b. Pincushion distortion

c. Regression equations

d. In vitro adjustments

ANSWER c. Regression equations. Regression equations are corrections made to mathematical models to adjust the final calculations to fit experimental data. These empiric adjustments are sometimes called "fudge factors." LV casts were made within human ventricles obtained at autopsy. The true LV volume was measured by how much water each cast displaced. Then the casts were filmed and planimetered as if they were live LV angiograms. Usually, the volumes calculated from cine exceed the true cast volumes. This is because the papillary muscles and trabeculations were planimetered and included within the calculated cine volume. The true volume is usually about 80% of the measured cine volume. This implies that about 20% of the LV is filled with papillary muscle and trabeculation.

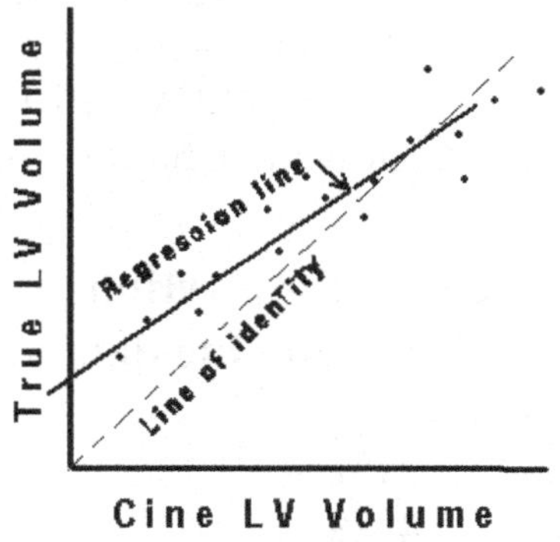

When the true LV volume is plotted graphically against the measured cine volume, even after magnification correction and pincushion distortion is accounted for, it is not a 45° line of identity. The equation of the "line of best fit" that results from this graph is termed the "regression equation." Various authors have derived different regression equations for these various techniques. When the corrected mathematical model equation is corrected for regression the final equation below results. Most computers are programmed to use the Kennedy et. al. regression equations for RAO single-plane angiography. Vol. = 0.81 x (cine volume) + 2 cc.

This brings the final equation to:

$$\text{LV Vol.} = \frac{0.682\ A^2\ CF^3}{L} + 2\text{ cc.}$$

This is the equation I will use for all volume calculations in this chapter.

See: Peterson, chapter on "Left and Right Contrast Ventriculography." **Keywords:** Regression equation

SAMPLE LV ANGIOGRAPHY PROBLEMS

368. Calculate the ejection fraction using data in the box?

a. 47%
b. 53%
c. 56%
d. 70%

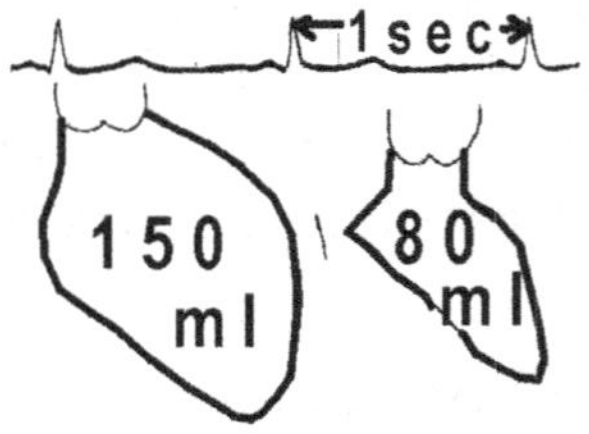

Patient #368
LV Volumes
EDV = 150 ml
ESV = 80 ml
HR = 60 / min

ANSWER a. 47%. Ejection fraction is the ratio of stroke volume to end diastolic volume. It is the ratio of the amount pumped by the LV to its total filled volume. Because the denominator EDV is dependent on body size, it need not be adjusted to BSA. Normal EF is 67 %. When it falls below 50%the heart is probably in failure. EF is the most important measure of LV function, and a vital number to know before heart surgery is performed. It may be measured by angiographic, ultrasonic, or nuclear methods.

The ejection fraction calculation is made as follows:

SV = EDV - ESV = 150-80 = 70 ml

EF = SV/EDV = 70/150 = .466 = 47% (below normal)

EF = SV/EDV

See: Braunwald, Chapter on "Evaluation of LV Function" **Keywords**: calculate EF

369. Calculate the ejection fraction using the data in the box.

a. 31%
b. 44%
c. 55%
d. 69%

Patient #369	Area	Length
End Diastole=	50 cm^2	14 cm
End Systole =	35 cm^2	10 cm

ANSWER a. 31%. No grids, correction factors or regression equations are needed if you use the ratio of elliptical formulas below:

$$EF = 1 - \frac{(Aes)^2\ (Led)}{(Aed)^2\ (Les)} = 1 - \frac{35^2 \times 14}{50^2 \times 10} = 1 - \frac{17150}{25000} = 1 - .69 = 31\%$$

This EF is below normal and indicates probable heart failure. Be sure to subtract the large fraction from one.

$$EF = \mathbf{1} - \frac{(Aes)^2\ (Led)}{(Aed)^2\ (Les)}$$

See: Peterson, chapter on Left and Right Contrast Ventriculography." **Keywords:** EF calculation no correction factors

BOTH QUESTIONS BELOW REFER TO THE DATA IN THIS BOX.

370. Calculate the angiographic cardiac output (LVMF) of this patient.

- a. **4.8 L/min**
- b. **6.0 L/min**
- c. **7.5 L/min**
- d. **8.0 L/min**

Patient #370 Data on patient with MS & MR

RR interval = 0.75 sec.

Thermodilution CO = 4.8 L/min

Quantitative LV angiography Data:

EDV = 100 cc.

ESV = 25 cc.

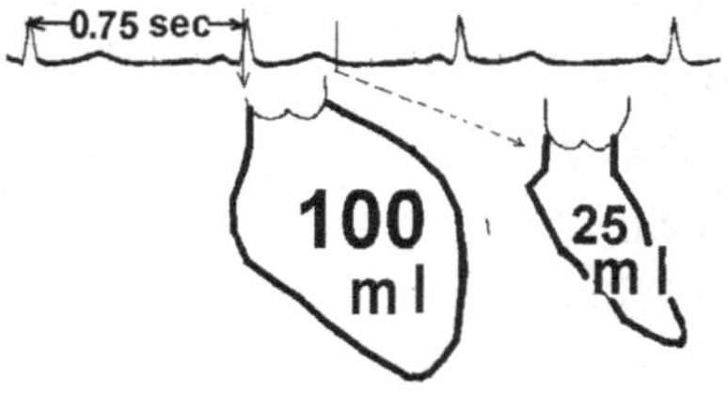

371. What is this patient's angiographic ejection fraction (EF)?

- a. 25%
- b. 45%
- c. 60%
- d. 75%

372. This man's BSA is 1.7 m². Evaluate his LV ejection.

- a. **Normal EF with small LV volumes**
- b. **Normal EF with large LV volumes**
- c. **Low EF with small LV volumes**
- d. **Low EF with large LV volumes**

ANSWERS FOR ABOVE QUESTIONS ARE LISTED TOGETHER BELOW:

370. ANSWER b. 6.0 L/min. The formulas needed are:

HR = 60/RR interval = 60/0.75 = 80 b/min

SV = EDV - ESV = 100-25 = 75 ml.

LVMF = angio. CO = SV x HR

LVMF = 75 ml x 80 bpm = 6000 ml/min = 6.0 L/min

Note that LVMF is how much blood the LV pumps. This is not necessarily the forward CO since some blood may leak backward or otherwise be lost to shunts. In this example the LVMF = 6 while the TDCO = 4.8. This discrepancy implies 1.2 L/min of regurgitation.
See: Kern, chapter on "Hemodynamics" **Keywords:** calc. LVMF

371. ANSWER d. 75%. Stroke volume is EDV-ESV. This (angio. SV) is the difference between the largest (EDV) and the smallest (ESV) LV volume. Ejection fraction is the ratio of stroke volume to end diastolic volume. There is certain to be a question calculating EF because it is the most important measure of LV function. Become familiar with the terms involved and these calculations:

SV = EDV - ESV = 100-25 = 75 ml

EF = SV/EDV = 75/100 = .75 = 75%

See: Kern chapter on "Hemodynamics." **Keywords:** calculate EF

372. ANSWER. a. Normal EF, with small LV volumes.

Normal values are approximately 120 ml and 40 ml, for an EF of 66%. His heart

contracts well, but contracts down to an excessively small volume. Low ESV.
See: Kern chapter on "Hemodynamics." **Keywords:** normal LV values EF

BOTH QUESTIONS BELOW REFER TO THE DATA IN THIS BOX.

373. Use the single-plane LV volume equation Vol. = (0.682 A^2/L) (CF^3)+ 2 ml to calculate the EDV and ESV using the data in the box.

	EDV	ESV
a.	71 cc,	and 39 cc
b.	71 cc,	and 57 cc
c.	124 cc,	and 86 cc
d.	155 cc,	and 95 cc

374. Using the data in the box calculate LVMF.

- a. **2.4 L/min**
- b. **4.8 L/min**
- c. **5.9 L/min**
- d. **6.4 L/min**
- e. **7.5 L/min**

Patient #373	End Diastole	End Systole
Planimetered area =	50 cm^2	35 cm^2
Measure long axis =	14 cm	10 cm
Cubic correction factor (CF^3) = 1.0 cm^3/ cm^3		
RR interval	= 0.94 sec	

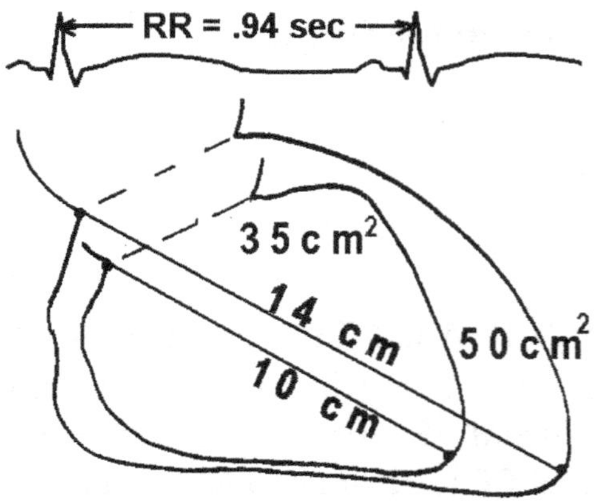

Cine projected on screen and magnified

BOTH ANSWERS LISTED TOGETHER BELOW:

373. ANSWER c. 124 cc and 86 cc. Substitute areas and lengths into the Kennedy Dodge formula:

LV-E DV = (0.682 A^2/L) (CF^3)+ 2 = (0.682 x 50^2 / 14)(1) + 2 = 122 + 2 = 124 cc.

LV-ESV = (0.682 A^2/L) (CF^3)+ 2 = (0.682 x 35^2 / 10) + 2 =84 + 2 = 86 cc.

See: Baim chapter on "Ventricular Volumes,..." **Keywords:** calculate EDV using Kennedy single plane formula

374. ANSWER a. 2.4 L/min.

. First calculate the heart rate:

HR = 60/RR interval = 60/0.94 = 64 b/min.

Next calculate SV. Then calculate LVMF by multiplying SV x HR:

SV = EDV - ESV = 124 - 86 = 38 ml

LVMF = 38 ml x 64 b/min = 2432 ml/min = 2.4 L/min **See:** Baim chapter on "Ventricular Volumes,..." **Keywords:** calculate EDV using Kennedy single plane formula

USE THESE TWO CINE FRAMES FOR THE NEXT 4 QUESTIONS.

375. **Use the Kennedy/Dodge area-length single-plane formula to calculate this end systolic volume (ESV). (Draw and measure long axis. Note 5 cm ball measures 2.9 cm.)**

a. 31 cc
b. 42 cc
c. 56 cc
d. 68 cc

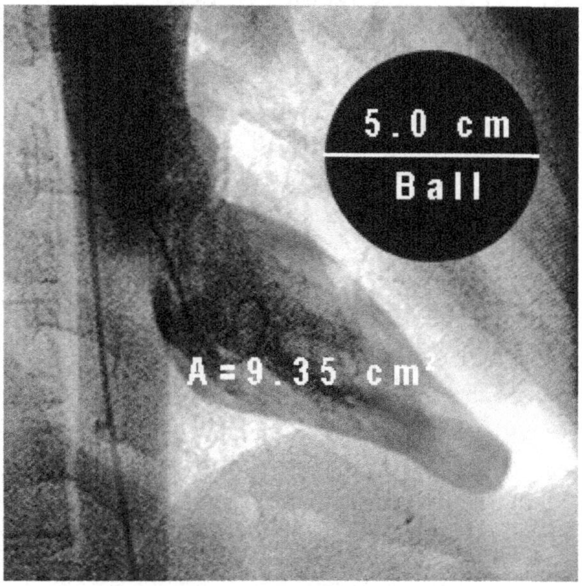

LV - ESV planimetered from this print

376. **Calculate the stroke volume (SV).**

a. 45 cc
b. 56 cc
c. 69 cc
d. 77 cc

377. **From the ECG calculate the heart rate.**

a. 60 beats/min
b. 70 beats/min
c. 80 beats/min
d. 90 beats/min

378. **Calculate the LVMF.**

a. 3.6 L/min
b. 4.2 L/min
c. 5.5 L/min
d. 6.2 L/min

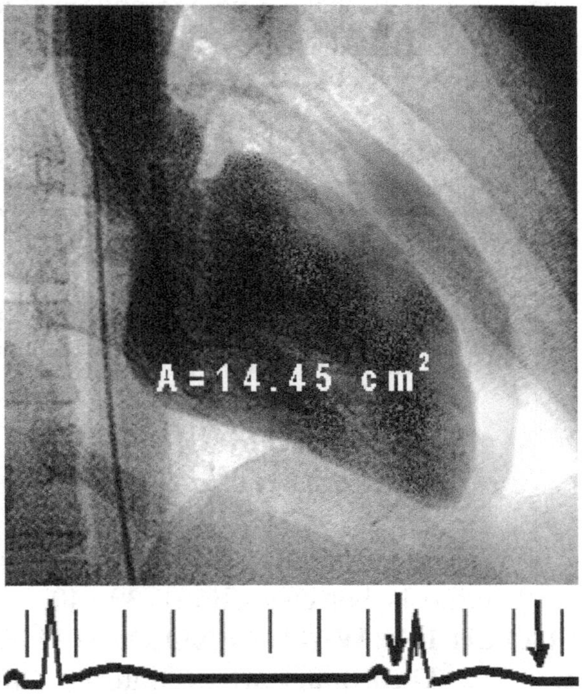

LV-EDV time lines 0.1 sec

379. **Calculate the EF.**

a. 39%
b. 48 %
c. 55%
d. 66%

ALL FOUR ANSWERS BELOW:
375. ANSWER c. 56 cc = ESV.
Calculate linear CF = 5 cm/2.9 cm = 1.72
Calculate cubic $CF^3 = 1.72^3 = 5.1$
Measure systolic length L_s = 5.6 cm
Measure diastolic length L_d = 5.8 cm
Then since $V = .682\ (A^2 / L)\ CF^3 + 2$ cc
ESV = .682 (9.35^2/5.6) 5.10 +2 = 56 cc
EDV = .682 (14.45^2/5.8) 5.10 +2 = 125 cc

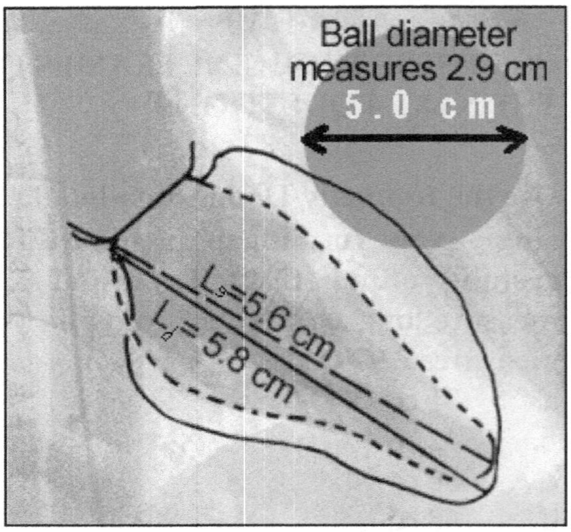

EDV, ESV (dotted), & calibration ball

376. ANSWER c. 69 cc = SV = EDV - ESV
SV= 125 - 56 = 69 cc

377 ANSWER c. 80 beats/min = HR.
Measure RR interval = 0.75 sec
HR = 60 / rr int = 60/0.75 = 80 b/min

378. ANSWER c. 5.5 L/min = LVMF.
LVMF = SV x HR = 69 x 80 = 5.52 L/min
See: Sheehan, "Cardiac Angiography" in Marcus, Cardiac Imaging, A companion to Braunwald's Heart Disease. and Baim, chapter on "Stenotic Valve Calculations." **Keywords**: Calculate ESV, EDV, HR, and LVMF

379. ANSWER c. 55% EF = SV/EDV = 69 cc/ 125 cc = .55 or 55%

LV Wall Motion

380. What coronary artery obstruction would cause the LV wall motion abnormality seen at #2 (LAO)?.
- **a. Right coronary artery**
- **b. LAD coronary artery**
- **c. Circumflex coronary artery**

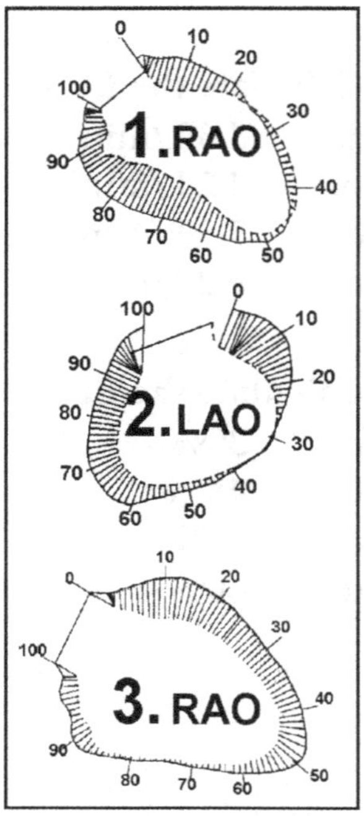

Superimposed LV-EDV and ESV

ANSWER c. Circumflex coronary artery. Note postero-lateral wall akinesis between chords 30 - 40.

MATCH THE WALL ABNORMALITIES:
1. **LAD coronary artery:** anterior wall dyskinesis (Note that the bulge occurs between lines 25-45 in the RAO view)
2. **Circumflex coronary artery**: postero-lateral wall akinesis
3. **Right coronary artery:** Inferior wall akinesis

In the 100 chord method of Sheehan, 100 chords are constructed perpendicular to, and evenly distributed along, a "centerline" drawn midway between the EDV and ESV contours. Sheehan says,

"The territories of the left anterior descending artery (LAD), right coronary artery (RCA), and the circumflex artery (CFX) were defined as the sequence of contiguous chords having significantly depressed wall motion in patients with isolated stenosis of the respective artery. The LAD and RCA territories are well visualized in the 30-degree RAO projection and the CFX in the 60-degree LAO projection."

See: Sheehan, "Cardiac Angiography" in Marcus, Cardiac Imaging, A companion to Braunwald's Heart Disease." Baim chapter on "Ventricular Volumes,..." **Keywords:** Circumflex MI Wall motion

381. This 30° RAO LV wall motion diagram uses the "100 chord centerline method" of Sheehan, Kennedy, and Dodge. What LV wall motion abnormality is graphed in the box?

a. RCA chronic ischemia pattern

b. RCA acute MI with compensatory anterior hyperkinesis

c. LAD chronic ischemia pattern

d LAD acute MI with compensatory hyperkinesis

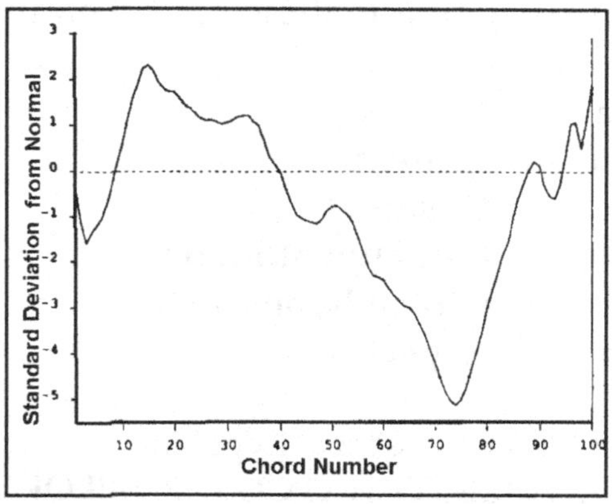

30° RAO, LV wall chord length graph

ANSWER b. RCA acute MI with compensatory anterior hyperkinesis. Chords 50-80 correspond to the LV inferior. These chords are severely depressed - more than 2 standard deviations below normal. This indicates inferior wall hypokinesis due to myocardial infarction. However, the first 30 chords here (anterior wall) show hyperkinesis as a compensation for the inferior MI induced akinesis. Sheehan says,

"Motion in the wall opposite the site of acute infarction is frequently increased.... The influence of compensatory hyperkinesis during acute myocardial infarction often results in a normal (>55 percent) ejection fraction."

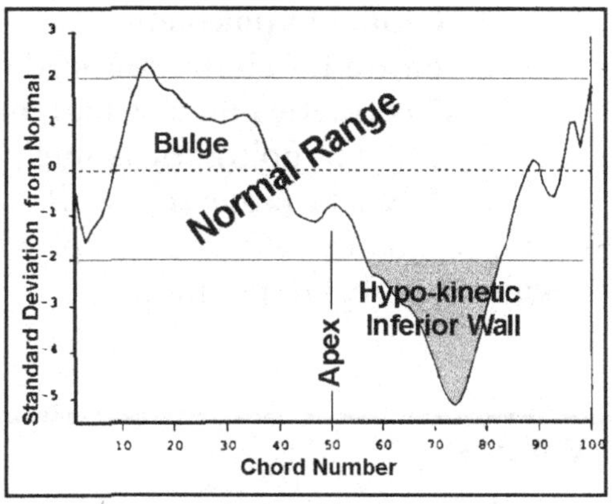

30° RAO, LV wall chord length graph

This LV diagram is a composite of EDV and ESV frames from which the chord length graph was derived. The outer solid line is the end diastolic volume. Note the inferior hypokinesis (even slightly dyskinetic) and the compensatory anterior wall hyperkinesis. The initial chord diagram shows chord shortening plotted in "standard deviations" from normal. Normal is the dotted "0" standard deviation line on the graph. Hyperkinetic motion is graphed above normal, and hypokinetic motion is graphed as below normal motion.

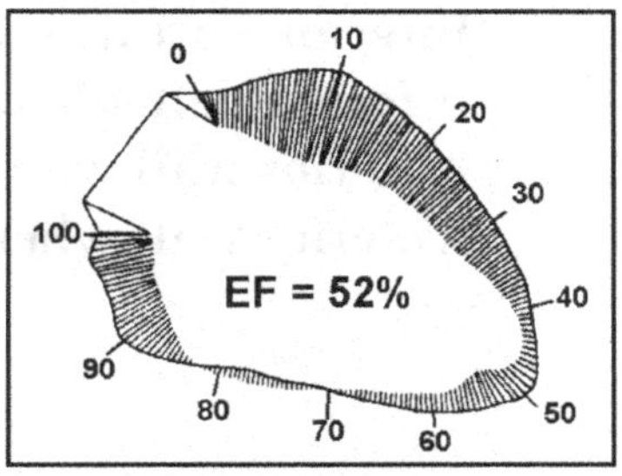

30° RAO, EDV-ESV 100 chord centerline method of Sheehan

Most of us are used to seeing angiograms. But, when chord shortening is related to a normal population, like this, it is much more objective and accurate.
See: Sheehan, "Cardiac Angiography" in Marcus, _Cardiac Imaging, A companion to Braunwald's Heart Disease._ **Keywords:** inferior MI wall motion

382. These diagrams show the various patterns of LV regional wall motion in systole. The outer line is the EDV outline. The inner line is the ESV. What type of LV wall motion is shown at # 3 on the diagram?

- a. **Normal**
- b. **Akinetic**
- c. **Dyskinetic**
- d. **Local hypokinetic**
- e. **Global hypokinetic**
- f. **Asynchronous**

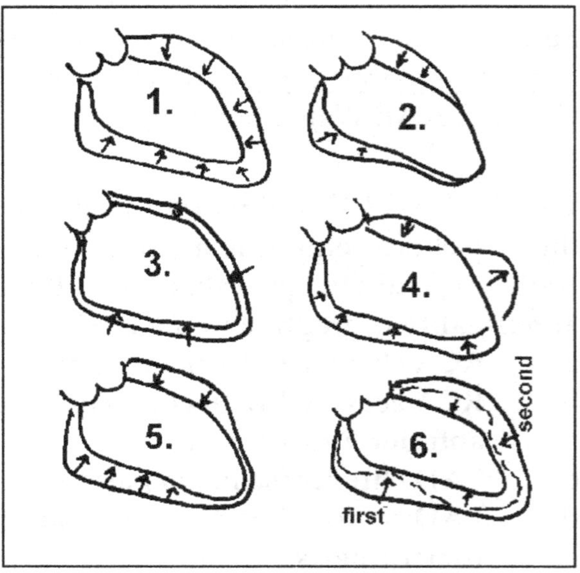

Abnormal LV Angio wall motion, Superimposed LV EDV and ESV

ANSWER e. Global hypokinetic.
BE ABLE TO MATCH ALL BELOW:

1. **Normal**
2. **Akinetic (no motion)**
3. **Global hypokinetic (entire LV shows reduced motion)**
4. **Dyskinetic (aneurysmal bulging motion)**
5. **Local hypokinetic (some portion of the LV shows reduced motion)**
6. **Asynchronous (LV walls beat at different rates and times)**

See: Kern, chapter on "Angiography" **Keywords:** LV wall motion abnormalities, akinesis, dyskinesis, global hypokinesis...

LV Mass

383. Where should heart thickness be measured for the most accurate LV mass measurement?

- a. **Inferior wall where epicardium is best visible**
- b **Inferior wall where endocardium is best visible**
- c. **Anterior wall where endocardium is best visible**
- d. **Anterior wall where epicardium is best visible**

ANSWER d. Anterior wall where epicardium is best visible. Sheehan says,

"The thickness of the myocardium is measured along the anterior wall, in the neighborhood of the hemiaxis between the middle and distal third of the long axis, where the epicardium is visible."

The best heart thickness is made during end diastole where papillary muscles and trabeculi are less prominent. The endocardium easier to see.

See: Sheehan, "Cardiac Angiography" in Marcus, <u>*Cardiac Imaging, A companion to Braunwald's Heart Disease.*</u> **Keywords:** measure anterior LV wall **in diastole**

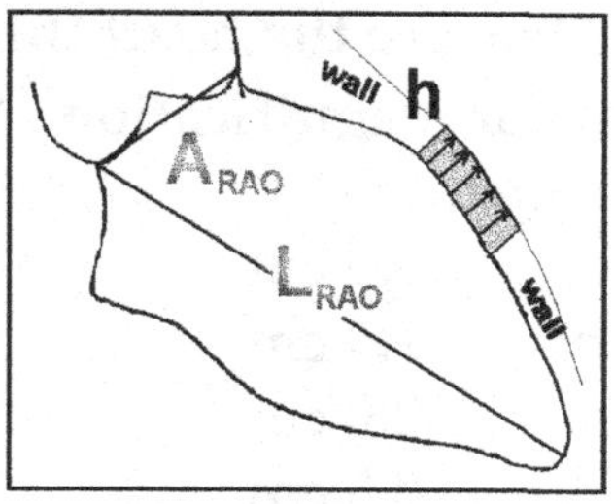

Measuring LV wall

384. Which of the following pathologies would be expected to have the LOWEST Mass/EDV volume ratio?

a. **AS, Compensated pressure overload (concentric hypertrophy)**
b. **Decompensated hypertensive dilated heart**
c. **Compensated volume overload (chronic AI) with hypertrophy (concentric)**
d. **Decompensated volume overload (acute ruptured chordae)**

ANSWER d. Decompensated volume overload (acute ruptured chordae).
This will be the most dilated heart. Being acute it has had no opportunity to hypertrophy.
LV mass related to EDV, like this, helps one evaluate hypertrophy in dilated hearts.
See: Braunwald, Chapter on "Evaluation of LV Function." **Keywords**: acutely ruptured chordae tendineae occurs in low mass/vol ratio

385. What is the specific gravity of myocardial tissue? To convert LV wall thickness to muscle mass, the muscle volume must be multiplied by this factor.

a. **.89 gm/cc**
b **1.00 gm/cc**
c. **1.05 gm/cc**
d. **1.19 gm/cc**

ANSWER c. 1.05 gm/cc is the specific gravity of myocardium. Once the LV muscle volume is calculated then it must be multiplied by 1.05 gm/cc. **See:** Baim chapter on "Ventricular Volumes,..." **Keywords:** Specific gravity of myocardium = 1.05 gm/cc

BOTH QUESTIONS BELOW REFER TO THIS DIAGRAM

386. Measure the heart thickness and correct it for magnification. Linear CF = 1.72 cm/cm.

a. 0.9 cm
b. 1.5 cm
c. 2.0 cm
d. 2.5 cm

387. What is a normal heart (LV wall) thickness?

a. 0.4 cm
b. 0.8 cm
c. 1.1 cm
d. 1.5 cm

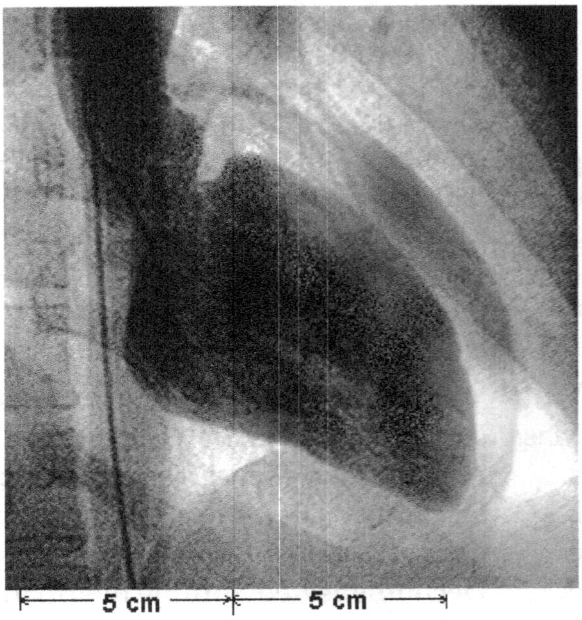

EDV filmed in 30° RAO with calibration

386. ANSWER b. 1.5 cm. Measure The average heart thickness (h) on the anterior wall between epicardium and endocardium at 0.9 cm. When this is multiplied times the linear correction factor 1.72 cm/cm it gives 1.5 cm. **See:** Sheehan, "Cardiac Angiography" in Marcus, *Cardiac Imaging, A companion to Braunwald's Heart Disease.* **Keywords**: measure LV wall thickness

387. ANSWER 1.1 cm. Sheehan says the mean normal LV wall thickness is 10.9 mm ± 2 mm Our patient's heart is 15 mm indicating significant LV hypertrophy. This is explained by this patient's chronic aortic stenosis.
See: Sheehan, "Cardiac Angiography" in Marcus, *Cardiac Imaging, A companion to Braunwald's Heart Disease.* **Keywords**: Normal LV wall thickness = 1.1 cm

---

REGURGITANT VOLUME AND FRACTION

388. Match the LV output #3 (Regurgitant Volume) in the box with its formula below.

a. **Regurgitant vol./Total SV**
b. **Total SV/EDV**
c. **Fick CO/HR**
d. **Total SV - Forward SV**
e. **Cine EDV - Cine ESV**

LV volumes and fractions

1.	Total Stroke volume SV	(ml)
2.	Forward Stroke volume	(ml)
***3.**	**Regurgitant volume**	**(ml)**
4.	Ejection Fraction	(%)
5.	Regurgitant Fraction	(%)

ANSWER d. Total SV - Forward SV.

BE ABLE TO MATCH ALL RESPONSES BELOW:

1.	Total Stroke volume SV	(ml)	= Cine EDV - Cine ESV
2.	Forward Stroke volume	(ml)	= Fick CO/HR
*3.	Regurgitant volume	(ml)	= Total SV - Forward SV
4.	Ejection Fraction	(%)	= Total SV/EDV
5.	Regurgitant Fraction	(%)	= Regurgitant vol./Total SV

Sheehan says,

> "*Since the angiographic stroke volume is volume output from the left ventricle, but the Fick or dilution stroke volume is the forward output, the difference between them is the regurgitant flow per beat. The severity of regurgitation may be expressed as a percentage of the angiographic stroke volume.*"

Where a patients has left sided regurgitation, the LVMF should be the largest CO, because it includes forward and reverse blood flow. Whenever you see "total" it refers to the largest CO which is usually the LVMF. Whenever you see "forward" if refers to the smaller, Fick CO, or occasionally the thermodilution CO. Note that EF is a ratio based on heart volume, while RF is a ratio based on flows.

See: Sheehan, "Cardiac Angiography" in Marcus, *Cardiac Imaging, A companion to Braunwald's Heart Disease.* and Baim, chapter on "Stenotic Valve Calculations." **Keywords**: Regurgitant volume

BOTH QUESTIONS BELOW REFER TO THE DATA IN THIS BOX:

389. A patient with MS and MR has the hemodynamic data shown in the box. Calculate regurgitant flow.

a. **1.0 L/min**
b. **1.2 L/min**
c. **1.6 L/min**
d. **1.8 L/min**

390. What is this patient's regurgitant fraction?

a. 15%
b. 20%
c. 48%
d. 80%

Patient # 389 has MS and MR
LVMF = 6.0 L/min
TDCO = 4.8 L/min
HR = 100 /min

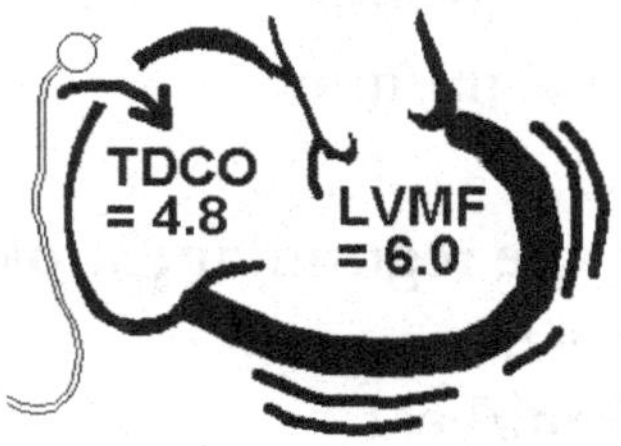

TDCO = Thermodilution CO

390. ANSWER b. 1.2 L/min. First calculate the regurgitant volume by subtracting the measured forward CO from the total CO:

> Regurgitant flow = Total Angio CO - Forward CO
> = LVMF - (Fick or thermo CO)

Regurgitation/min = LVMF - TD CO.
Regurgitation/min = 6.0 - 4.8 L/min = **1.2 L/min**

See: Kern, chapter on "Hemodynamics." **Keywords:** calc. Reg. flow = LVMF - TDCO or Fick

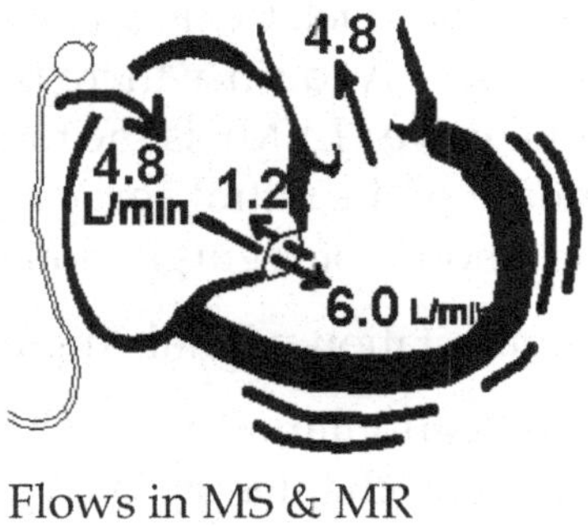

Flows in MS & MR

390. ANSWER b. 20% Then regurgitant fraction is that regurgitant flow divided by the LVMF.

RF = (Regurgitation/min) / (LVMF)

RF = 1.2 / 6.0 = .20 = 20%

RF can also be calculated on a per beat basis using stroke volume and regurgitant volume/beat. See next problem.

In this example assuming the heart rate was 100/min during both CO measurements, 60 ml is pumped by the LV with each beat but only 48 ml. goes forward out the AO. The difference 12 ml. leaks back during each beat. To clarify the total, forward, and regurgitation numbers draw two pictures of the heart with arrows as shown. On the first diagram label each arrow with the CO data (LVMF = largest CO, Fick = Forward CO, and regurgitation = LVMF-Fick = backwards arrow). Then on the second diagram label the arrows with the appropriate stroke volume. It is easy here, because the heart rate is 100/min, you just move the decimal point.

See: Kern, chapter on "Hemodynamics." **Keywords:** calc. Reg. Fraction = RV/TSV

BOTH QUESTIONS BELOW REFER TO THE DATA IN THIS BOX:

391. The patient has severe AS, AI and TI. Several types of resting cardiac outputs were done during heart catheterization as shown in the box. From the data in the box estimate the aortic regurgitation flow/min.

a. **1,000 ml/min**
b. **2,500 ml/min**
c. **3,000 ml/min**
d. **3,900 ml/min**

Patient # 391
CARDIAC OUTPUTS
HR = 80 beats/min
LVMF = 10.4 L/min
FICK = 6.5 L/min.
TDCO =7.4 L/min

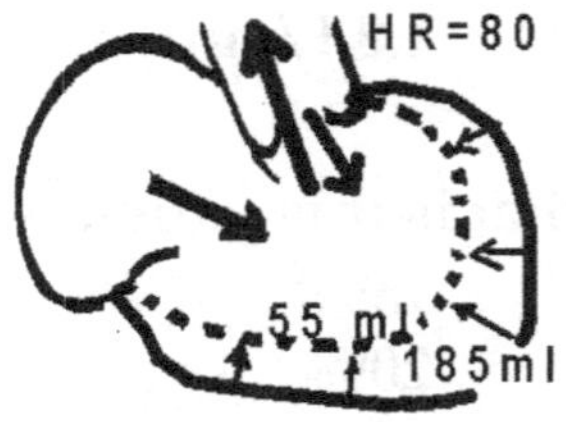

392. Estimate the regurgitant stroke volume through the aortic valve.

a. **49 ml/beat**
b. **55 ml/beat**
c. **92 ml/beat**
d. **130 ml/beat**

BOTH ANSWERS LISTED TOGETHER BELOW:

391. ANSWER d. 3,900 ml/min. In tricuspid regurgitation the thermodilution CO is unreliable. Fick CO is the best (gold standard) average forward flow entering the LA from the lungs. And since there is no shunt Fick CO is also the average forward flow across the aortic valve. LVMF is the total flow out of the LV. In this case LVMF is increased by the amount of the mitral aortic regurgitation. Regurgitant flow = Total LVMF - Forward CO. The amount of regurgitation is estimated by subtracting angio and Fick CO's.

Regurgitation = Total Angio CO - Forward CO = LVMF - Fick CO

Here Regurgitation = LVMF - Fick CO = 10.4 - 6.5 = 3.9 L/min

See: Baim, chapter on "Stenotic Valve Calculations." **Keywords**: Regurg vol. in AI

392. ANSWER a. 49 ml/beat. Using a per minute basis, the Reg. Vol. is simply the regurgitant flow divided by heart rate. RV = 3900/80 = 48.75 ml. Forward Stroke Volume = FSV = Fick CO / HR= 6500/80 = 81.25 ml/beat.

FORWARD FLOWS	TOTAL FLOWS
Forward CO = Fick CO:	Total CO = LVMF:
FSV = Fick CO/ HR	TSV = EDV - ESV

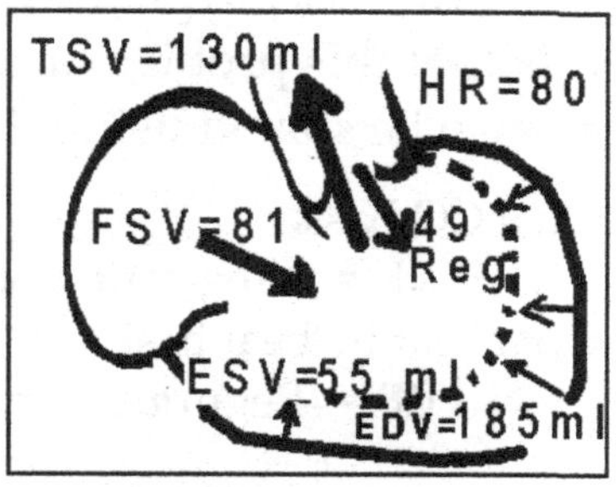

Length of arrows indicate magnitude of flow

Forward LA SV is the average forward SV across the competent mitral valve. Total Stroke Volume = TSV = EDV - ESV = 185 - 55 = 130 ml. This is the total amount the LV pumps per beat. Here TSV is increased by the amount of the regurgitation through the aortic valve into the LV during diastole. The difference between total stroke volume and forward SV is the regurgitant stroke volume. RSV = TSV - FSV = 130 - 81.25 = 48.75 ml. This is the regurgitation per beat. To clarify these numbers it is helpful to write them next to their arrow in the diagram as shown. **See:** Baim, chapter on "Stenotic Valve Calculations." **Keywords**: Regurg vol. in AI

BOTH QUESTIONS BELOW REFER TO THE DATA IN THIS BOX:

393. From the angiographic volumes and cardiac output data shown in the box, estimate the regurgitant volume (RV).

a. **15 ml**
b. **20 ml**
c. **25 ml**
d. **30 ml**

Patient # 393 has MR
Fick CO = 6.0 L/min
HR = 100 /min
EDV = 200 ml
ESV = 125 ml

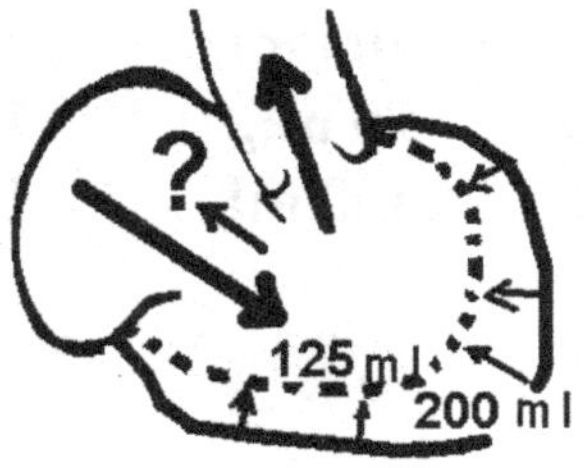

394. Estimate the regurgitant fraction (RF).

a. **20 %**
b. **30%**
c. **40%**
d. **50%**

BOTH ANSWERS LISTED TOGETHER BELOW:

393. ANSWER a. 15 ml. To calculate the forward stroke volume divide the HR into the Fick CO.

Fd. SV= Fick CO/HR = 6,000/100 = 60 ml

Then calculate the total stroke volume from angiographic data:

Total SV = EDV - ESV = 200 - 125 = 75 ml

Calculate regurgitant volume by subtracting forward SV from total SV.

RV = Total CO - Forward CO = LVMF - Fick = 75 - 60 = 15 ml/beat. To clarify these numbers it is helpful to write them next to their arrow in the diagram as shown.

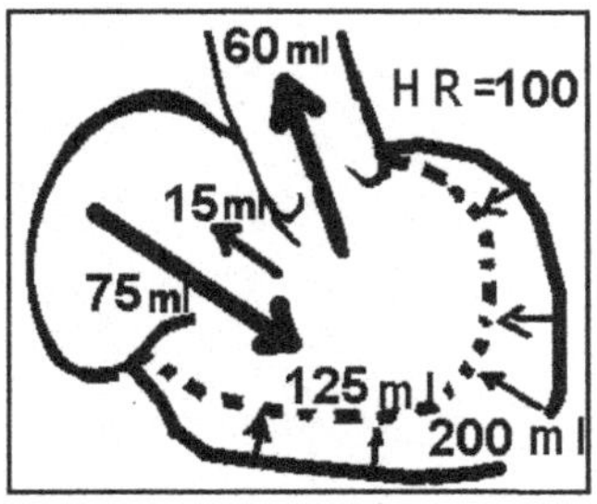

See: Baim chapter on "Ventricular Volumes,..." **Keywords:** Calculate regurgitant volume

394. ANSWER a. 20 %. Regurgitant fraction is the regurgitant volume (RV) divided by the total stroke volume (LVMF).

RF = Regurgitant volume / Total angio. stroke volume = 15/75 = .20 = 20%. Note that this problem asks only for the per beat stroke or regurgitant volumes. It can also be solved using the CO data, as in the previous problem.

On a CO basis:

RF = (Regurgitation/min) / (LVMF) = (LVMF-Fick)/LVMF

On a beat by beat basis:

RF = (Regurgitation/beat) / (Total SV) = $(SV_{angio} - SV_{foward})/SV_{angio}$

Note the regurgitant fraction (RF) is related to the total flow (LVMF) or its stroke volume, while ejection fraction (EF) is related to the volume of the heart (EDV). And although they are both fractions, they are calculated on a different basis.
See: Baim chapter on "Ventricular Volumes,..." **Keywords:** Calculate regurgitant fraction

BOTH QUESTIONS BELOW REFER TO THE DATA IN THE BOX BELOW:

395. From the data in the box on a patient with MS and MR calculate the total stroke volume and the forward stroke volume. (Here forward SV is the SV out the competent AO valve.)

	Tot. SV	Fd. SV out AO valve
a.	70 ml,	30 ml
b.	100 ml,	70 ml
c.	70 ml,	100 ml
d.	100 ml,	130 ml

<u>Patient # 395</u>
<u>with MS and MR</u>
HR = 100 /min
EDV = 200 ml
ESV = 100 ml
Fick CO = 7.0 L/min

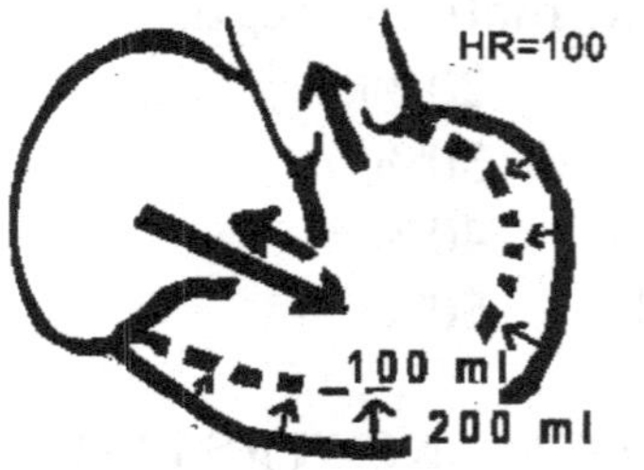

396. From the data in the box on the same patient with MS and MR calculate the regurgitant volume and regurgitant fraction through the mitral valve.

<u>Reg. Vol.</u> <u>Reg. Fraction</u>

a. **30 ml, 30%**
b. **30 ml, 43%**
c. **70 ml, 35 %**
d. **70 ml, 70 %**

BOTH ANSWERS FOLLOW:

395. ANSWER b. 100 ml, 70 ml. Total LV angio SV = TSV = EDV-ESV= 200 - 100 = 100 ml. Fick and Thermo are considered to be the forward COs (7 L/min). Forward SV is simply the Fick CO/HR = 7000/100 = 70 ml.

TOTAL FLOWS	FORWARD FLOWS
Total CO = LVMF	Forward CO = Fick CO
Tot.SV = EDV-ESV	Fd. SV = Fick CO/ HR

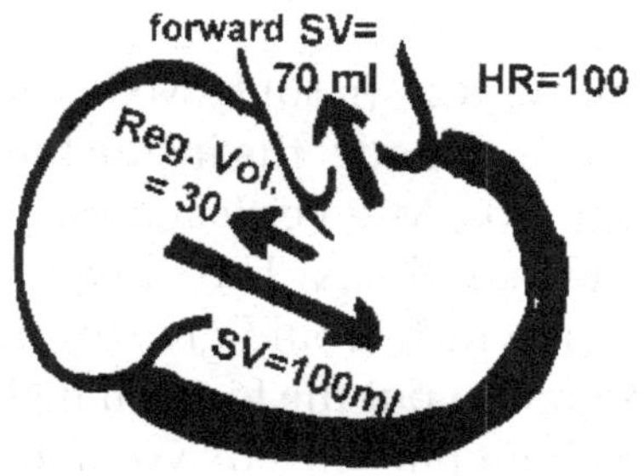

LVMF and forward C.O.

In the diagram note that the mitral valve diastolic inflow is large. This is the LV-angio stroke volume. It is the sum of what leaks back and what is pumped out the aorta each beat. Regurgitation is simply the difference between these "total" and "forward" numbers. **See:** Baim, chapter on "Stenotic Valve Calculations" **Keywords**: Forward SV in MI

396. ANSWER a. 30 ml, 30%. You know the total and forward stroke volumes from the previous question. The difference between them is the regurgitant volume: RV =100-70 = 30 ml. These volumes/beat are labeled in the second diagram.

The regurgitant fraction is this difference (RV) divided by the total SV. RF = 30/100 = 30%. So, 30% of the blood pumped by the heart is leaking backwards. Here we calculated everything in stoke volumes/beat. You would get the same answers if you used CO's/minute: RF = (LVMF-Fick)/LVMF = (10-7)/10 = 30%. Just keep your units straight.

Also, don't get regurgitant fraction (RF) confused with ejection fraction (EF). Here the EF = 100/200 = 50%. **See:** Baim, chapter on "Stenotic Valve Calculations."

Advanced LV Volume Formulas - (May be beyond scope of RCIS & CIT exams)

397. The formula for calculating the volume of an ellipsoid using the axes labeled in the diagram is:

a. (π/6) LxMxN
b. (π) LxMxN
c. (π/6) $(LxM)^2$ / L
d. (π) $(LxM)^2$ / L

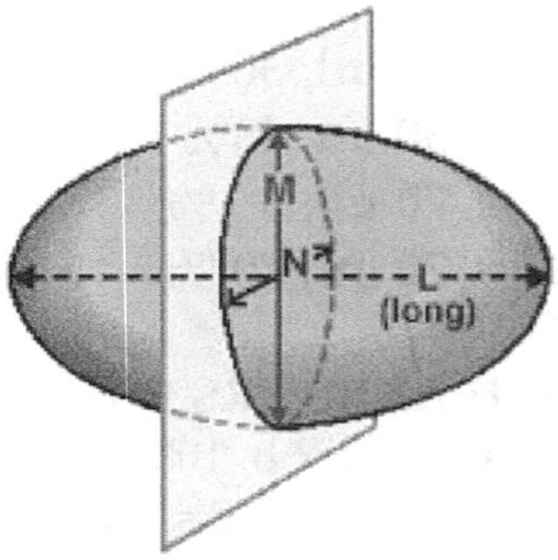

Ellipsoid model
(after Baim p. 316)

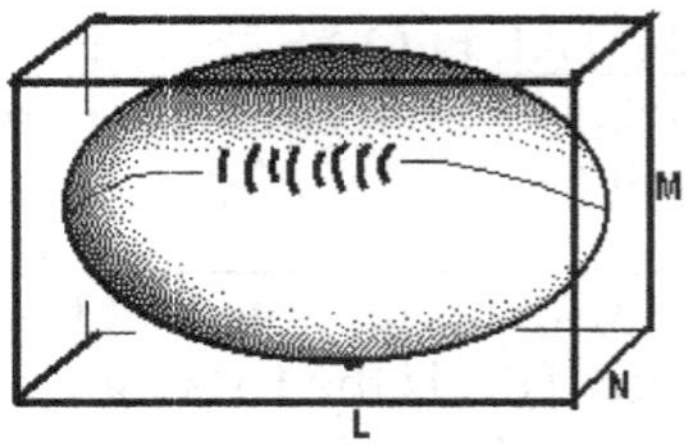

Football in a box

ANSWER a. (π/6) LxMxN. This ellipsoid of revolution or "football" model fits inside the LV to estimate its volume. L = Long axis, M = vertical minor axis, N = horizontal minor axis. Note that M = N. The three axes are multiplied times each other, which would give the area of a rectangular box just big enough to put the football inside. But the football will only fill about half the box volume (3.14/6). This is the basic mathematical model for LV volume calculations. It provides accurate results when correction factors are applied. **See:** Baim chapter on "Ventricular Volumes,..." **Keywords:** Ellipsoid of revolution

398. For the area length method of single plane LV angiography, the long axis of the ellipse is measured. Why is the short axis M (diameter) not measured?

a. Because the two short axis are equal
b. Because they cancel out of the equation
c. It is assumed to be half of the long axis
d. It is calculated from the ellipse area formula

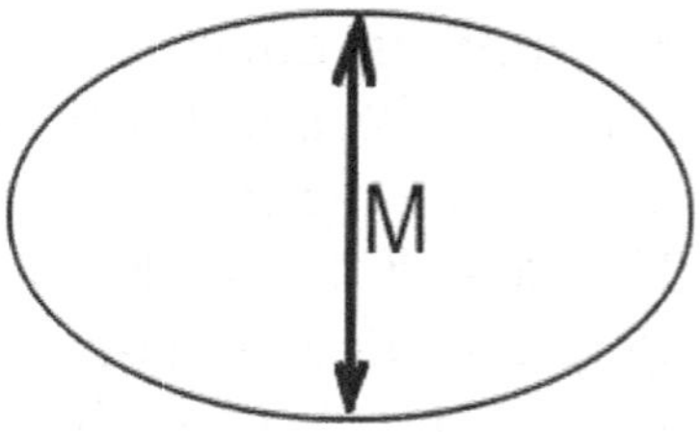

Short axis M

ANSWER d. It is calculated from the ellipse area formula.
The ellipse area formula is rearranged to solve for the short axis M = 4 A/π L. And since the two short axes L and M are assumed equal, their product is M^2 in the formula below.

$$\text{LV Vol.} = \frac{\pi L M^2}{6} = \frac{\pi L}{6}\left(\frac{4A}{\pi L}\right)^2 = \frac{8A^2}{3\pi L} = 0.849\ \frac{A^2}{L}$$

Note, in the middle equation how one L in the numerator cancels out leaving only one L in the denominator. The final theoretical equation is 0.849 (A^2/ L) for the volume of an ellipse. This same equation is used for EDV and ESV after correction factors are applied. Note also, that area squared yields units of cm^4, that is then divided by length yielding cm^3 or ml. **See:** Baim chapter on "Ventricular Volumes,..."

399. When simultaneous biplane ventriculography is used in orthogonal RAO and LAO positions, LV volume can be calculated using Dodge's area-length method. This biplane LV volume formula is:

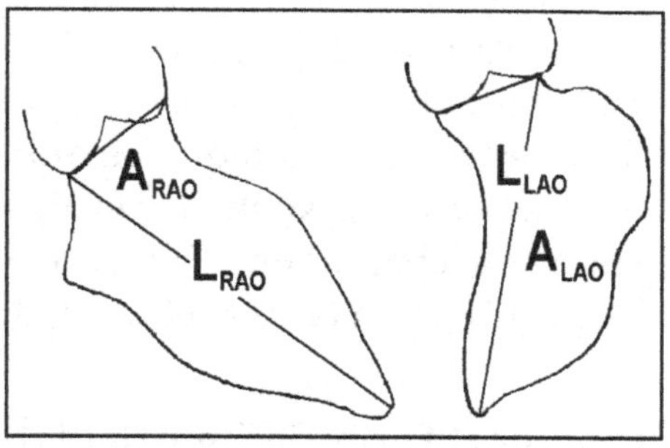

a. $\frac{8}{3\pi} \frac{(A_{RAO} A_{LAO})}{(L_{min})}$

b. $\frac{\pi}{6} \frac{(A_{RAO} A_{LAO})}{(L_{min})}$

c. $\frac{8}{3\pi} \frac{(A_{RAO} A_{LAO})^2}{(L_{max})}$

d. $\frac{\pi}{6} \frac{(A_{RAO} A_{LAO})^2}{(L_{max})}$

ANSWER a. $(8/3\pi)(A_{RAO} A_{LAO} / L_{min})$. As in the single plane formula the areas in the numerator are squared, yielding units of cm^4. This is then divided by the **minimum** long axis (usually the LAO long axis), measured in cm. L_{max} which was in the original formula, cancels out of the equation. This yields the needed volume units cm^3 or ml. As with the single plane method, grids must be filmed in both planes, then magnification and regression corrections are applied. This method is reportedly more accurate than the simpler single plane method.

Biplane LV Vol. = $\frac{8}{3\pi} \frac{(A_{RAO} A_{LAO})}{L_{min}}$

See: Baim chapter on "Ventricular Volumes,..." **Keywords:** Biplane LV volume formula

400. The Simpson rule method of approximating LV volumes assumes that the heart is composed of a series of:

a. **Pixels (digital dots)**
b. **Ellipses (footballs)**
c. **Discs (coins)**
d. **Triangles**

ANSWER c. Discs (coins). This method adds up the volume of a series of discs. Its rather like slicing a potato and calculating the volume of each slice, then adding all the volumes together to get the volume of the potato. In the biplane method, the coins or discs may be oval in shape. Yang says,

> **"Modified Simpson's Rule Method of Chapman and Associates.** *Based on the assumption that the cross-section outline of the left ventricle is approximately circular or elliptic, this method requires successive measurements of corresponding horizontal axes at 1-mm intervals from the biplane cine images. The left ventricle is thus divided into slices, all 1 mm in thickness (on the film, and not corrected for image distortion.) The volume of each slice is calculated by the following equation: V = h(A x B)/4 where V = volume of each segment in ml, h = thickness of each*

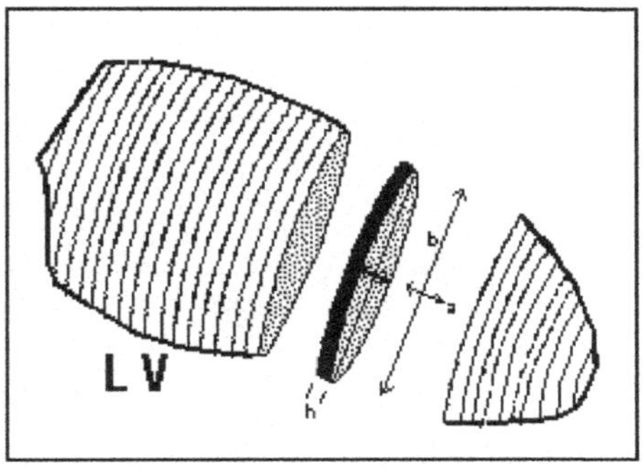

Simpson's method of LV Volume

segment (0.1 cm), A = axis in one view, in cm, and B = axis in the other view, at the same level in cm.... The total left ventricular volume is given by summing up the volume of all segments.... The formidable amount of measurements and calculations required for this method necessitates the use of a digitizer interfaced with a computer."

This method is reported to be more accurate than the area-length method, but is seldom used because the Kennedy/Dodge area-length method has gained general acceptance. **See**: Yang, chapter on "Cardiac Chamber Volume and Left Ventricular Mass." **Keywords**: Simpson's LV volume method = dicing a potato

401. The Short formula for calculating LV ejection fraction from single-plane RAO view, without using calibration grids is: (Note Aes = Area of end systolic LV angiogram and Aed = area of end systolic LV angiogram)

a. **$EF = 1 - (Aes/Aed)^2\ (Les/Led)$**
b. **$EF = 1 - (Aes/Aed)^2\ (Led/Les)$**
c. **$EF = 1 - (Aes/Aed)\ (Led/Les)^2$**
d. **$EF = 1 - (Aes/Aed)\ (Led/Les)^2$**

ANSWER b. $EF = 1 - (Aes / Aed)^2\ (Led / Les)$. Peterson says,

> *"When single-plane analysis is used alone for calculation of ejection fraction, it is unnecessary to know or correct for magnification, because it cancels from both the numerator and the denominator."*

The simplified method for measuring ejection fraction is planimeter the systolic and diastolic areas and measure the LV lengths in cm. Then the formula becomes:
This formula is easily derived from the basic ellipse formulas for end systole and end diastole where $EF = 1 - ESV/EDV$.

$$EF = 1 - \left(\frac{\cancel{.684\ CF^3}\ Aes^2 / Les}{\cancel{.684\ CF^3}\ Aed^2 / Led} \right) \text{ thus:}$$

$$EF = 1 - \frac{(Aes)^2\ (Led)}{(Aed)^2\ (Les)} = 1 - \left(\frac{Aes}{Aed} \right)^2 \frac{Led}{Les}$$

Note how the correction factors cancel out, leaving the smaller systolic area to be squared in the numerator, but the larger diastolic length in the numerator. That is the beauty of this method, there is no correction needed. It's all in ratios. **See**: Peterson, chapter on "Left and Right Contrast Ventriculography." **Keywords:** EF equation no corrections

REFERENCES

Baim, D. S. and Grossman W., Cardiac Catheterization, Angiography, and Intervention, 7th Ed., Lea and Febiger, 2006

Braunwald, Eugene, Ed., HEART DISEASE A Textbook of Cardiovascular Medicine, 9th Ed., W. B. Saunders Co., 2012

Kern, M. J., Ed., The Cardiac Catheterization Handbook, 6th Ed., Mosby-Year Book, Inc., 2016

Peterson, and Nicod, *Cardiac Catheterization Methods, Diagnosis, and Therapy,* 1st edition, W.B. Saunders Co., 1997

Pepine, J. C., and Hill, J. A., et. al., *Diagnostic and Therapeutic Cardiac Catheterization,* 2nd Ed., Williams and Wilkins, 1994

Sheehan, "Cardiac Angiography" in Marcus, *Cardiac Imaging, A companion to Braunwald's Heart Disease.,* W.B Saunders, 1991

Tilkian, A. G., and Daily, E, J, *Cardiovascular Procedures, Diagnostic Techniques and Therapeutic Procedures,* C. V. Mosby Company, 1986

Yang, Bentivoglio, Maranhao, and Goldberg, *From Cardiac Catheterization to Hemodynamic Parameters,* 3rd edition, F.A. Davis Co., 3rd edition, 1988

OUTLINE: QUANTITATIVE LV ANGIOGRAPHY

1. GENERAL QUANTITATIVE LV ANGIO.
   a. Abbreviations & Definitions
      i. SV = Amount of blood ejected out the aortic valve with each systole (Stroke Volume in ml)
      ii. RV = Regurgitant Volume = Amount of blood regurgitating (reverse flow)
      iii. EF = Percentage of blood ejected out the ventricle with each beat (Ejection Fraction in %)
      iv. CO = (Cardiac Output in L/min) Net amount of blood pumped by the LV per minute
      v. EDV =Maximum volume of blood in the ventricle when filled (End Diastolic Volume in ml)
      vi. ESV = Minimum volume or residual blood left in the ventricle after contraction (End Systolic Volume in ml)
      vii. LVMF = (Left ventricular minute flow in L/min) Total amount of blood pumped by the LV per minute. It is TOTAL because some of this
      viii. RF = Regurgitant Fraction = Ratio of regurgitation to total LV flow
   b. Stroke Volume formulas
      i. SV = CO/HR
      ii. SV = EF x EDV
      iii. SV = EDV - ESV
   c. CO = LVMF = SBF = PBF unless regurg. or shunt present
   d. LVMF = SV x HR.
   e. Normals
      i. EDVI = 70 ± 20 ml/m^2
      ii. SVI = 45 ± 13 ml/m^2
      iii. LV Mass Index = 92 ± 16 ml/m^2
      iv. EF = 0.67 ± 0.08
      v. Normal EF > 50%
      vi. Normally Fick CO = LVMF = TDCO(unless shunt or regurg.)
   f. LV Volumes
      i. Pressure Volume curves
      ii. PV curves in disease: MS, AS...
      iii. Ellipse of rotation
      iv. Area Length method of Kennedy & Dodge
2. LV ANGIOGRAPHY MEASUREMENTS
   a. Single-plane Area-length method of Dodge
   b. Long axis = 30 degree RAO
   c. Tracing LV outline
      i. Include papillary muscles & trabeculi
   d. Do LV angio prior to coronary arteriography
   e. Avoid PVCs & Post-PVC beats
   f. EF formula - no correction factors
3. LV ANGIOGRAPHY CORRECTION FACTORS
   a. Use of grids
      i. square wire grid
      ii. Metal sphere
      iii. Catheter bands or diameter
   b. LV angio Distortion
      i. Pincushion distortion
      ii. Magnification
   c. Linear correction factor = CF
   d. Square correction factor = CF^2
   e. Cubic correction factor = CF^3

f. Use of Grid to calculate CF^2
g. Calculation of CF^3
h. Regression equation

4. SAMPLE LV ANGIOGRAPHY PROBLEMS
   a. EF = SV/EDV
   b. SV = EDV - ESV
   c. Area length formula
   d. $EF = = \mathbf{1} - \frac{(Aes)^2 \ (Led)}{(Aed)^2 \ (Les)}$
   e. LVMF = SV x HR
   f. HR = 1/ rr interval
5. LV MASS
   a. Wall thickness (ant. wall)
   b. Mass calculation
   c. Specific gravity myocardium =1.05
   d. Mass/Volume ratio
6. LV WALL MOTION
   a. Associated coronary obstruction
      i. inferior = RCA
      ii. Anterior = LAD
      iii. Lateral = Cx
   b. Chord-length graph interpretation
   c. Wall motion abnormalities
      i. Normal
      ii. Akinetic (no motion)
      iii. Global hypokinetic (entire LV shows reduced motion)
      iv. Dyskinetic (aneurysmal bulging motion)
      v. Local hypokinetic (some portion of the LV shows reduced motion)
      vi. Asynchronous (LV walls beat at different rates and times)
7. REGURGITANT VOLUME AND FRACTION
   a. Definitions
   b. Total Stroke volume SV (ml) = Cine EDV - Cine ESV
   c. Forward Stroke volume (ml) = Fick CO/HR
   d. Regurgitant volume (ml) = Total SV - Forward SV
   e. Ejection Fraction (%) = Total SV/EDV
   f. Regurgitant Fraction (%) = Regurgitant vol./Total SV
   g. Regurgitant Flow = LVMF - Forward CO
   h. Forward Flow = Fick CO or TDCO
   i. Forward SV = Fick SV
   j. Forward CO = Fick
   k. Total CO = LVMF
   l. Total SV = LVMF SV
   m. Total EF
8. ADVANCED LV ANGIOGRAPHY FORMULAS
   a. Long Axis
   b. Short Axis
   c. Single plane formula
   d. Biplane formula
   e. Simpson's rule formula, sliced potato
   f. Short formula for EF, derived

Resistance Calculations

INDEX: E9

Resistance - General

402. What is the normal value for the vascular resistance #1 (Absolute SVR in dyne sec cm^{-5}) in the box?

a. 0.84
b. 14
c. 67.
d. 1130

NORMAL VASCULAR RESISTANCE
*1. Absolute SVR in dyne sec cm^{-5}
2. Hybrid SVR in HRUs
3. Absolute PVR in dyne sec cm^{-5}
4. Hybrid PVR in HRUs

ANSWER d. 1130 dyne sec cm^{-5} (dsc^{-5}).
Normal PVR is low, around 1.0 HRUs, while the normal SVR is 10-20 times greater. The absolute metric units of resistance are the HRU units multiplied times x 80.
MATCHED NORMAL VASCULAR RESISTANCES ARE:
*1. Absolute SVR = 1130 dsc^{-5}
2. Hybrid SVR = 14 HRUs
3. Absolute PVR = 67.0 dsc^{-5}
4. Hybrid PVR = 0.84 HRUs

Understand the units of resistance. Wood units = Hybrid Resistance Units (HRU)= mmHg/L/min. Absolute CGS units are dsc^{-5} which is 80 x the Wood unit.
See: Kern, chapter on "Hemodynamics." **Keywords:** Ratio SVR/PVR = 12:1

403. When you calculate systemic resistance, you have the option to report it in different units. When you report a vascular resistance in the units below, which one will have a resistance value 80 times higher than the others?

a. Wood units
b. Hybrid resistance units (HRUs)
c. mmHg/L/min
d. dyne sec cm^{-5}

ANSWER d. Dyne sec cm^{-5}. The hybrid resistance units developed by Wood, are in mmHg/L/min. They are the easiest to calculate. Just divide the pressure gradient in mmHg by the CO in L/min. The absolute units for resistance are calculated by

Hybrid units = HRUs = Wood Units = mmHg/L/min
Absolute units = metric units = dyne sec cm^{-5} (DSC^{-5})

multiplying the HRUs times 80. Thus 80 HRUs = 1 dsc^{-5}. This 80 factor is a constant that comes from converting mmHg into metric units.
See: Baim, chapter on "Clinical Measurement of Vascular Resistance **Keywords**: Absolute resistance units dsc^{-5} use x80

404. In the adult, what is the normal ratio of Systemic Vascular Resistance to Pulmonary Vascular Resistance? (SVR/PVR ratio)
a. 1:7
b. 2:1
c. 6:1
d. 12:1

ANSWER d. 12:1. Since the ratio of pressures gradients across each capillary bed is the same as the ratio of resistances (assuming the right sided CO equals the left sided CO) it follows that the ratio of resistances is the same as the ratio of pressures (using Kern's normals below):

SVR/PVR = (AO mean pressure - RA mean) /(PA mean pressure - LA or PAW).
(85-2.8) / (15-7.9) = 12:1

Note some authors quote this ratio as 10:1, perhaps because it is easy to remember.
See: Kern, chapter on "Hemodynamics." **Keywords:** Ratio SVR/PVR = 12:1

405. As infants grow, the normal PA pressure tends to _____ and the systemic BP tends to ______.
a. Increase, Increase
b. Increase, Decrease
c. Decrease, Decrease
d. Decrease, Increase

ANSWER d. Decrease, Increase. PA pressure tends to decrease from 90/55 at birth to 25/10 mmHg during teen years; while the systemic BP rises from 85/50 at birth to 120/70 mm Hg during teenage.

Remember that at birth the RV = LV pressure and the two ventricular walls are the same thickness. During the first few years of life the PA pressure continues to drop and the RV continues to thin. With the first breath the

CARDIOVASCULAR PRESSURES IN CHILDREN

Age	PVR	PA(mmHg)	AO(mmHg)
Preemie	8-10	±90/55	±85/50
Neonate	1-3	±50/25	±96/60
Teenage	0.5-1	±25/10	±120/70

Pulmonary Pressures Drop and Systemic Rise with age

pulmonary resistance drops and the ostium secundum closes. And, within 3 days the PDA closes. This separates the right and left heart so that thereafter each side develops to meet its individual needs. The AO must drive into the high resistant systemic circuit and thus builds a stronger left heart and pressure. Braunwald says, "

> "*CHANGES AT BIRTH.... Inflation of the lungs at the first inspiration produces a marked reduction in pulmonary vascular resistance owing partly to the sudden suspension in air of fetal pulmonary vessels previously supported by fluid media. The reduced extravascular pressure assists new vessels to open and already patent vessels to enlarge. The rapid decrease in pulmonary vascular resistance is related more importantly to vasodilatation owing to the increase in oxygen tension to which pulmonary vessels are exposed rather than to physical expansion of alveoli with gas. . . . Systemic vascular resistance rises when clamping of the umbilical cord removes the low-resistance placental circulation. Increased pulmonary blood flow increases the return of blood to the left atrium and raises left atrial pressure, which in turn closes the foramen ovale.*"

See: Daily, Chapter on "Hemodynamic Monitoring of Children." **Keywords:** as infants grow PA decreases AO increases

406. How does increasing SVR effect the heart?

a. Increased myocardial O_2 consumption & increased stroke volume
b. Increased myocardial O_2 consumption & decreased stroke volume
c. Decreased myocardial O_2 consumption & increased stroke volume
d. Decreased myocardial O_2 consumption & decreased stroke volume

ANSWER b. Increased myocardial O_2 consumption & decreased stroke volume. Increasing SVR is associated with increased afterload. Darovic says: "As afterload increases, stroke volume falls and myocardial oxygen consumption rises proportionate to the increased load placed on the heart. As afterload decreases, stroke volume rises and myocardial oxygen consumption falls proportionate to the decreased load placed on the heart."
See: Darovic, chapter on "Pulmonary Artery Pressure Monitoring."

407. According to Poiseuille's law, changes in vascular resistance are most sensitive to changes in the:

a. Length of capillary bed
b. Average arteriolar radius
c. Blood viscosity
d. Number of recruited capillaries

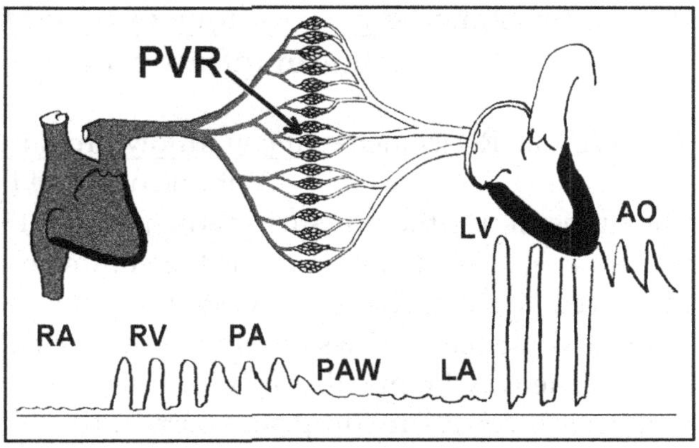

Pulmonary circulation and related pressures (after Rushmer Fig. 1-17)

ANSWER b. Average arteriolar radius. Vasodilation opens up the arterioles, causing a reduction in vascular resistance. This results in increase flow through the system and reduced driving pressures across it. The rearranged Poiseuille's law is:

$R = 8(\text{Viscosity})(\text{Length})/(\pi)(\text{radius})^4$

Note that the radius is to the 4th power. This is the most important factor in the equation. Small changes in radius dramatically affect the resistance.

To use Poiseuille's law we would have to calculate the length and radius of every vessel in the circulation - an impossible task. It is much easier to utilize Ohms law for fluids and calculate the ratio of pressure change to flow, $R = \Delta P/Q$.

Darovic says,

> "*The resistance to flow through the systemic and pulmonary circulations is the result of friction between flowing blood and the vascular walls. The diameter of the blood vessels is the principal factor determining resistance to blood flow. The resistance to blood flow disproportionately increases by a reduction in the cross-sectional area of the vascular bed. For example, if vasoconstriction decreases the cross-sectional area of the arterial circulation by one half, resistance to flow increases by 16 times.*"

Damage to arterial endothelium (e.g. atherosclerosis) may retard the normal endothelial vaso-active properties mediated through Nitric Oxide, endothelin, etc.)

See: Darovic, chapter on "Pulmonary Artery Pressure Monitoring." **Keywords:** Resistance, Poiseuille

---

Formulas

408. The general formula to calculate vascular resistance is:

a. **Resistance = $\dfrac{\text{(mean inflow pressure - mean outflow pressure)}}{\text{volume of blood flow per minute}}$**

b. **Resistance = $\dfrac{\text{(mean outflow pressure - mean inflow pressure)}}{\text{volume of blood flow per minute}}$**

c. **Resistance = $\dfrac{\text{volume of blood flow per minute}}{\text{(mean outflow pressure - mean inflow pressure)}}$**

d. **Resistance = $\dfrac{\text{volume of blood flow per minute}}{\text{(mean inflow pressure - mean outflow pressure)}}$**

ANSWER a. Resistance = $\dfrac{\text{(mean inflow pressure - mean outflow pressure)}}{\text{Volume of blood flow per minute}}$

The numerator is the pressure gradient across the circulation being measured (systemic or pulmonary). The denominator is the volume blood flow through the circulation being measured [systemic blood flow(SBF) or pulmonary blood flow (PBF)]. But, unless there is a shunt, these blood flows are simply the cardiac output (CO).

The way I remember this formula is to remember Ohms law. $R = V/I$, where voltage is the pressure drop, and current (I) is the blood flow.

See: Darovic, chapter on "Pulmonary Artery Pressure Monitoring." **Keywords**: Vascular resistance = pressure gradient/flow

409. The formula to calculate SVR (systemic vascular resistance) is:

a. **$SVR = CO / (\overline{AO} - \overline{PV})$**
b. **$SVR = SBF / (\overline{AO} - \overline{RA})$**
c. **$SVR = (\overline{AO} - \overline{PV})/CO$**
d. **$SVR = (\overline{AO} - \overline{RA})/SBF$**

ANSWER d. $SVR = (\overline{AO} - \overline{RA}) / SBF$ = (mean AO - mean RA pressure) / Systemic blood flow. Using the Ohms law analogy Resistance = voltage drop / current flow, or Poiseuille resistance = pressure drop / flow. The pressure drop across the systemic circulation is the difference between systemic arterial and systemic venous pressure, or AO - RA mean pressures. The flow must be the actual cardiac output across the systemic capillary bed. In the case of a shunt this is the systemic blood flow (SBF).

$$SVR = (\overline{AO} - \overline{RA})/SBF$$
$$PVR = (\overline{PA} - \overline{LA})/PBF$$

Since normally CO = SBF = PBF (unless shunt is present) CO is usually used in the denominator. Note that a line over a number indicates mean or average. **See**: Baim, chapter on "Clinical Measurement of Vascular Resistance." **Keywords**: SVR formula

410. The hemodynamic effect of increasing a patient's systemic vascular resistance (SVR) is to: (Assume constant CO and negligible CVP.)

a. **Increased BP**
b. **Decreased BP**
c. **Increased HR**
d. **Decreased HR**

ANSWER a. Increased BP. The formula BP = CO X SVR demonstrates the direct proportionality between CO and SVR. In the SVR formula (AO-RA) is the difference between the mean aortic and right atrial pressures. This is the driving pressure across the peripheral capillary bed. For simplicity we often leave out mean RA pressure because it is usually negligible. Then the equation becomes simply:

$$SVR \cong \overline{AO}/CO \qquad \text{where } \overline{AO} = \text{mean Aortic BP.}$$

If CO doubles so does BP. If resistance doubles so does BP. That is why administration of vasoconstrictors raises the BP.

The resistance is normally closely regulated by the baroreceptor reflex, through vasoactivity. Reflexes also regulate the CO by altering the HR and SV. For example, the SVR lowers in exercise to allow increased blood flow with only slight elevation of the BP.

Note: SVR (Systemic Vascular Resistance) is sometimes also termed PVR. "**Peripheral**" Vascular **R**esistance - often confused with **"Pulmonary" V**ascular **R**esistance." **See:** Berne & Levy, chapter on "Hemodynamics." **Keywords:** SVR, Resistance, BP

411. **The formula to calculate SVRI (systemic vascular resistance index) is:**

a. **$SVR = CO / (\overline{AO} - \overline{PV})\ BSA$**
b. **$SVR = SBF / (\overline{AO} - \overline{RA})\ BSA$**
c. **$SVR = (\overline{AO} - \overline{PV})/CI$**
d. **$SVR = (\overline{AO} - \overline{RA})(BSA)/ SBF$**

ANSWER d. $SVR = (\overline{AO} - \overline{RA})\ (BSA)/ SBF$ = (mean AO - mean RA pressure) (BSA)/ Systemic blood flow. This can be written more simply as $SVR = (\overline{AO} - \overline{RA}) / CI$. Here the SBF or CO must be divided by the BSA not the numerator. Baim says,

> "*The normalized resistance, however, is NOT obtained by dividing resistance . . . by body surface area. Rather, normalized resistance is calculated by substituting blood flow index for blood flow in the resistance formula.*"

Note that when resistance is "indexed" it is MULTIPLIED times BSA, not divided by it. This is because CI has BSA in the denominator. And since CI is already in the denominator or the SVR equation, it must be inverted and multiplied times the pressure gradient.
See: Baim, chapter on "Clinical Measurement of Vascular Resistance **Keywords**: SVRI multiplied by BSA - not divided

---

Calculations

BOTH QUESTIONS BELOW REFER TO THESE HEMODYNAMIC MEASUREMENTS

412. **Calculate the PVR (pulmonary vascular resistance) from the data in the box.**

a. **0.22 HRUs**
b. **0.5 HRUs**
c. **2 HRUs**
d. **4 HRUs**

CATH. HEMODYNAMIC MEASUREMENTS	
Systemic Mean Pressure	= 95 mm Hg
Pulmonary Artery Mean Pressure	= 28 mm Hg
PA Wedge Mean Pressure	= 8 mm Hg
Right Atrial Mean Pressure	= 5 mm Hg
Cardiac Output	= 5 L/min

413. **Calculate the SVR (systemic vascular resistance) from the data in the box above.**

a. **2 HRUs**
b. **4 HRUs**
c. **9 HRUs**
d. **18 HRUs**

BOTH ANSWERS LISTED TOGETHER BELOW.

$$SVR = (\overline{AO} - \overline{RA})/CO$$
$$PVR = (\overline{PA} - \overline{LA})/CO$$

412. ANSWER d. 4 HRUs. Assuming there is no shunt and $Q_p = Q_s$, you can substitute CO for SBF and PBF to get the formula in the box. Most labs use PAWP instead of LA in the formula. $PVR = (\overline{PA} - \overline{LA})/CO$ = (28 - 8 mmHg) / 5.0 L/min = 20/5 = 4 mmHg/L/min = 4 HRUs. **See**: Baim, chapter on "Clinical Measurement of Vascular Resistance." **Keywords**: calculate PVR

412- 413- 414- 415-

413. ANSWER d. 18 HRUs. SVR = $(\overline{AO} - \overline{RA})/CO$ = (95 - 5 mmHg) / 5.0 L/min = 90/5 = 18 mmHg/L/min = 18 HRUs. **See**: Baim, chapter on "Clinical Measurement of Vascular Resistance." **Keywords**: calculate SVR

414. Calculate the flow (CO) through a vascular bed when an average pressure of 100 mmHg is applied across 33 HRUs?

- a. **⅓ L/min**
- b. **1 L/min**
- c. **3 L/min**
- d. **33 L/min**

ANSWER c. 3 L/min. Rearrange the resistance formula where R = pressure gradient/flow, to flow or CO = pressure gradient/R = 100 mmHg/33 mmHg/L/min = 3. L/min. Fluid flow problems are analogous to simple electric circuits, where current flow equals fluid flow. In fact I use Ohm's law to remember the resistance equation. **See**: Baim, chapter on "Clinical Measurement of Vascular Resistance **Keywords**: Ohms law for fluids

> **Ohm's Law:** I = V/R, or
> Flow = (Δ pressure)/ Resistance

Hemodynamic findings from a heart cath on a child are shown in the box.

415. Calculate the pulmonary vascular resistance (PVR).

- a. **2.0 Hybrid Resistance Units**
- b. **4.2 Hybrid Resistance Units**
- c. **8.0 Hybrid Resistance Units**
- d. **10.0 Hybrid Resistance Units**

HEMODYNAMICS ON CHILD		
CO	=	2.2 L/min.
RA	=	6/8/(4) mmHg
RV	=	36/4/6 mmHg
PA	=	35/15/(28) mmHg
PA wedge	=	7/10/(6)mmHg

ANSWER d. 10 Hybrid Resistance Units.

$$PVR = \frac{\text{(PA mean pressure - Wedge Mean)}}{\text{PBF or CO}}$$

Mean PA pressure is 28 mmHg. Mean LA is mean PA wedge of 6 mmHg.

PVR = (28-6)/2.2 = 22/2.2 = 10 mmHg/L/min, HRUs, or Wood units.

This is an elevated PVR. Normal PVR is less than 1.0 HRU.

This child may be UNABLE to benefit from corrective surgery unless the PVR can be reduced. However, if PVR drops significantly with O_2 or vasodilators - then corrective surgery may be considered and her prognosis improved. One goal of the pediatric cardiologist is to prevent this fixed pulmonary vascular resistance and hypertension. **See:** Braunwald, chapter on "Congenital Heart Disease." **Keywords:** Calculate PVR

BOTH QUESTIONS BELOW REFER TO THESE HEMODYNAMIC MEASUREMENTS

416. **From the data in the box, calculate the shunt flow and direction.**

a. 1.7 L/min R-L shunt
b. 3.4 L/min R-L shunt
c. 1.7 L/min L-R shunt
d. 3.4 L/min L-R shunt

HEMODYNAMICS ON CHILD

BSA	=	0.6	M^2
SBF (Q_s)	=	5.3	L/min
PBF (Q_p)	=	7.0	L/min
AO	=	120/70,90	mmHg
PAW	=	5,6,5	mmHg
PA	=	21/10,12	mmHg
RA wedge	=	4,3,3	mmHg

417. **From the data in the box above, calculate #2, PVR (pulmonary vascular resistance) in HRU units.**

a. 1.0
b. 16.4
c. 80.
d. 1313

VASCULAR RESISTANCE UNITS

1. SVR in hybrid units
*2. PVR in hybrid units
3. SVR in absolute metric units
4. PVR in absolute metric units

BOTH ANSWERS LISTED TOGETHER BELOW.

416. ANSWER c. 1.7 L/min L-R shunt. You can easily estimate a shunt by subtracting the systemic and pulmonary blood flows.
Shunt = 7.0 - 5.3 L/min = 1.7 L/min. It must be entering into the right side of the heart since the pulmonary blood flow is the largest. So, it is a left-to-right shunt. This points out that you can not just plug in a CO into the resistance formula. It must be the specific flow through the system you are measuring. **See**: Baim, chapter on "Clinical Measurement of Vascular Resistance **Keywords**: calculate shunt flow

417. ANSWER a. 1.0 mmHg/L/min, or HRUs.

Hybrid SVR	=	$(\overline{AO} - \overline{RA})$/SBF
Hybrid PVR	=	$(\overline{PA} - \overline{LA})$/PBF
Absolute SVR	= 80 x	$(\overline{AO} - \overline{RA})$/SBF
Absolute PVR	= 80 x	$(\overline{PA} - \overline{LA})$/PBF

BE ABLE TO MATCH ALL ANSWERS BELOW:

1. SVR = 16.4 hybrid units (mmHg /L/min)
2. PVR = 1.0 hybrid units (mmHg/L/min)
3. SVR = 1313 absolute metric units (dyne sec cm^{-5})
4. PVR = 80. absolute metric units (dyne sec cm^{-5})

See: Baim, chapter on "Clinical Measurement of Vascular Resistance **Keywords**: calculate PVR

418. From the data in the box calculate the hybrid PVR and SVR.

HEMODYNAMICS on a child			
BSA	=	0.6	M^2
CO	=	3.7	L/min
AO	=	120/62/84	mmHg
PAW	=	35,30,27	mmHg
PA	=	82,32,51	mmHg
RA	=	5,8,4	mmHg

a. PVR = 3.24 HRUs, SVR = 11.3 HRUs
b. PVR = 11.3 HRUs, SVR = 3.24 HRUs
c. PVR = 6.48 HRUs, SVR = 22.7 HRUs
d. PVR = 22.7 HRUs, SVR = 6.48 HRUs

ANSWER c. PVR = 6.48 HRUs, SVR = 22.7 HRUs. Note that since there is no shunt the SBF = PBF = CO . Then the resistance formulas are:

PVR = $(\overline{PA} - \overline{LA})/CO = (51-27)/3.7 = 24/3.7 = 6.48$

SVR = $(\overline{AO} - \overline{RA})/CO = (84-4)/3.7 = 80/3.7 = 22.7$

Note the elevated wedge pressures. This child may have mitral stenosis, cor-tri-atriatum, or other LV inlet obstruction. PVR is commonly elevated in mitral stenosis patients due to a "2nd stenosis" in the pulmonary arterioles. This develops to protect the lungs from excessive PA pressure. **See**: Baim, chapter on "Clinical Measurement of Vascular Resistance **Keywords**: calculate PVR

419. From the data in the box above where BSA = 0.6 M^2 and CO = 3.7 L/min, calculate #3 SVRI (systemic vascular resistance index) in absolute dsc^{-5} units.

VASCULAR RESISTANCE INDEX
1. SVRI in hybrid units
2. PVRI in hybrid units
*3. SVRI in absolute metric units
4. PVRI in absolute metric units

a. 3.9 dsc^{-5}
b. 13.6 dsc^{-5}
c. 311 dsc^{-5}
d. 1090 dsc^{-5}

ANSWER d. 1090 dsc^{-5} systemic vascular resistance index (SVRI). In absolute metric units (dyne sec M^2 cm^{-5}). Note that vascular resistance index is pressure drop per cardiac index or mmHg/CI. The hybrid HRU units are mmHg/L/min/M^2 or mmHg /[(L/min)/ BSA]. When this is simplified it becomes (mmHg x min x M^2/ Liter). **Note that when resistance is "*indexed*" it is *multiplied* times BSA, not divided by it as CI is.**

BE ABLE TO MATCH ALL ANSWERS BELOW:

1. SVRI in Wood or hybrid units (mmHg/L/min/M^2) = 22.7 x 0.6 = 13.6
2. PVRI in Wood or hybrid units (mmHg/L/min/M^2) = 6.48 x 0.6 = 3.9

* 3. SVRI in absolute metric units (dyne sec cm^{-5} M^2) = ((84-4)/3.7) x .6 x 80 = 1090

4. PVRI in absolute metric units (dyne sec cm^{-5} M^2) = 3.9 x 0.6 x 80 = 311

See: Baim, chapter on "Clinical Measurement of Vascular Resistance" **Keywords**: SVRI

420. **A child has the hemodynamic findings shown in the box. Calculate the pulmonary vascular resistance (PVR).**

HEMODYNAMIC FINDINGS	
PBF = 2.2 L/min., SBF = 3.6 L/min	
PA press. =	35 / 15 , 28 mmHg
RV press. =	36 / 0 , 5 mmHg
PA wedge =	7, 10, 6 mmHg

a. **1 Hybrid Resistance Unit**
b. **4.2 Hybrid Resistance Units**
c. **8.0 Hybrid Resistance Units**
d. **10.0 Hybrid Resistance Units**

ANSWER d. 10.0 wood or Hybrid Resistance Units. Formula for Pulmonary Vascular Resistance is:

PVR = (PA mean pressure - Wedge Mean) / CO

PVR = (28-6)/2.2 = 22/2.2 = 10 mmHg/L/min, HRUs, or Wood units
This is an elevated PVR (0.6-1 is normal). she will be UNABLE to tolerate and benefit from corrective surgery unless the PVR can be reduced. If it drops to 1 HRU with vasodilators or O2 administration then corrective surgery may be considered and her prognosis improved.
See: Braunwald, chapter on "Congenital Heart Disease." **Keywords:** Calculate PVR

421. **Determine the systemic vascular resistance in ARU (not hybrid units). CO = 5.20 L/min, AO mean = 118, PA mean =33, PA wedge mean = 9, RA mean = 4, HR = 75 beats/min, Hgb = 14.0, AO sat = 99%, PA sat = 79%.**

a. **16 dcs^{-5}**
b. **21 dcs^{-5}**
c. **1308 dcs^{-5}**
d. **1754 dcs^{-5}**

Answer: d. 1754 dyne cm sec^{-5}. This absolute resistance scale is a factor of 80 times greater than the hybrid unit scale (mmHg/L/min). Calculate the SVR in ARU then multiply by 80 to get dyne cm sec^{-5}. You need to memorize the resistance formula as $\Delta P/CO$. SVR = 80 (mean AO - mean RA) / CO = (118 - 4) / 5.20 = 80 x 114 / 5.2 = 1754 dcs^{-5} (dyne cm/sec^{5}). This weird unit (dcs^{-5}) is commonly used in cath reports.
See: Kern, chapter on "Hemodynamic Data" Keywords: calculate SVR

422. **What pressures are used to calculate systemic vascular resistance (SVR)?**

a. **AO mean - PA mean**
b. **AO mean - RA mean**
c. **AO systolic - Wedge mean**
d. **AO systolic - LV systolic**

Answer b. AO - RA mean pressures are subtracted to give the average systemic driving pressure. Aortic blood passes through the systemic resistance bed into the RA. This pressure gradient is then divided by the cardiac output to yield SVR. It is a variation of

Ohms law R = (V)/(I). It makes sense. If the CO drops, this suggests the Resistance is high. If the pressure gradient across the peripheral capillary bed raises, this suggests the resistance is high.
See: Grossman chapter on "Resistance" Keywords: SVR = (AO mean - RA mean)/CO

423. Estimate the aortic blood pressure if a patient's CO is 5 L/min and his peripheral resistance (SVR) is 20 hybrid or Wood units.

a. **200/133 (120) mmHg**
b. **160/100 (120) mmHg**
c. **120/90 (100) mmHg**
d. **100/70 (80) mmHg**

ANSWER c. 120/90 (100) mmHg. The formula is: mean BP = CO x SVR. Substituting CO and SVR into this equation:

$\overline{BP} \cong CO \times SVR$

mean BP = 5.0 x 20 = 100 mmHg

So a mean BP of 100 mmHg is correct. The systolic and diastolic can only be estimated. But usually systolic BP is twice the distance above the mean as diastole is below the mean. This is estimated by the formula: Mean BP = [systole + (2 x diastole)] / 3 (This is a handy formula to know but less accurate than measuring the mean pressure with a catheter and transducer)

I just picked a likely diastolic BP of 90 and substituted it and the known mean of 100 into this formula to derive an estimated systolic BP of 120 mmHg. (140/80 with mean 100 mmHg would also be a correct answer)
See: Braunwald, chapter on "Systemic Hypertension." **Keywords:** Calculate mean BP = CO x SVR

Applications

424. Increases in the systemic vascular resistance (SVR) chiefly cause:

a. **Increased LV preload**
b. **Decreased LV preload**
c. **Increased LV afterload**
d. **Decreased LV afterload**

ANSWER c. Increased LV afterload. Afterload is the resistance to pumping blood out the aorta during systole. This resistance is measured chiefly by the systemic vascular resistance (SVR) in a steady state. Since the CO is not likely to change dramatically, increasing SVR usually increases the BP. Resistance numbers are especially useful when discussing vaso-active drugs.
See: Todd, Vol. I, chapter on "Contractility and Frank Starling Law" and Braunwald, chapter on "Assessment of Cardiac Function." **Keywords:** Afterload, SVR

425. **A cyanotic cardiac shunt implies a:**
- a. **Low systemic vascular resistance (SVR)**
- b. **High systemic vascular resistance (SVR)**
- c. **Low pulmonary vascular resistance (PVR)**
- d. **High pulmonary vascular resistance (PVR)**

ANSWER d. High (PVR) pulmonary vascular resistance. Shunts go from high pressure to low pressure areas. For a shunt to be cyanotic, it must shunt from the right side of the heart to the left side (diluting the red blood). Cyanotic lesions must have high pressures on the right side of the heart. The right sided pressures usually build up over the years to overcome high resistance in the pulmonary arterioles and capillaries.

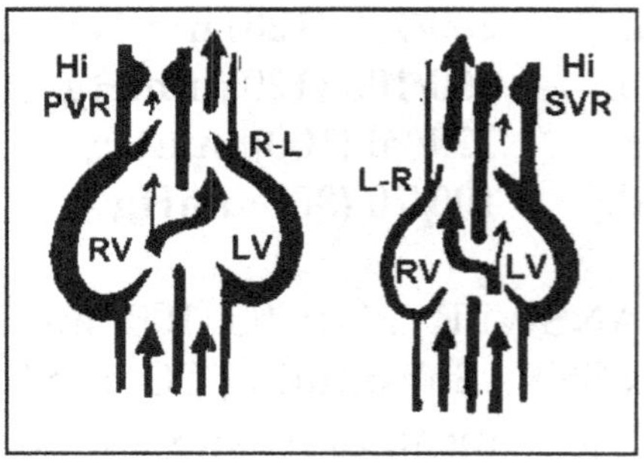

High Pulm. resistance

Shunts are like a river. If the river bifurcates and one leg of the river is dammed, shunt flow will be diverted to the other leg. That is why most shunts redirect blood from the left to the low pressure right side of the heart. When the pulmonary resistance exceeds the systemic resistance the cardiac shunts will redirect blood into the left side of the heart. **See:** Todd, Vol. I, chapter on "Congenital Heart Disease" Braunwald, chapter on "Congenital Heart Disease."
Keywords: Cyanotic shunt = high PVR

426. **In pulmonary hypertension it is essential to distinguish between reversible and irreversible pulmonary vascular resistance. The most accurate diagnostic test for evaluating vascular resistance is:**
- a. **Clinical evaluation**
- b. **Doppler echocardiography**
- c. **Two dimensional echocardiography**
- d. **Cardiac catheterization**

ANSWER d. Cardiac catheterization. Resistance can only be measured from the right heart cath hemodynamic data. There is general agreement that all newborns with cyanotic heart disease and/or CHF should be cathed. Braunwald says,

> *"Clinical and electrocardiographic observations do not distinguish between reversible and irreversible elevations in pulmonary vascular resistance. Echocardiography and Doppler interrogation of the heart may enable one to diagnose the presence of pulmonary hypertension but do not provide an accurate estimate of pressure or a reliable calculation of pulmonary vascular resistance. Thus,* ***hemodynamic measurements at cardiac catheterization are the mainstay in assessing the pulmonary vascular bed, especially its reactivity.*** *The premium on accuracy is high because the presence, degree, and reactivity of pulmonary vascular obstruction determine the feasibility and long-term outcome of operation."*

See: Braunwald, chapter on "Congenital Heart Disease" and "Pulmonary Hypertension."
Keywords: Cath to assess reactivity of high PVR

427. At peak exercise a normal individual's mean blood pressure does not significantly elevate, even though CO may increase up to seven times. This regulation of BP in exercise is due to ___________ vascular resistance.

a. Increased systemic
b. Decreased systemic
c. Increased pulmonary
d. Decreased pulmonary

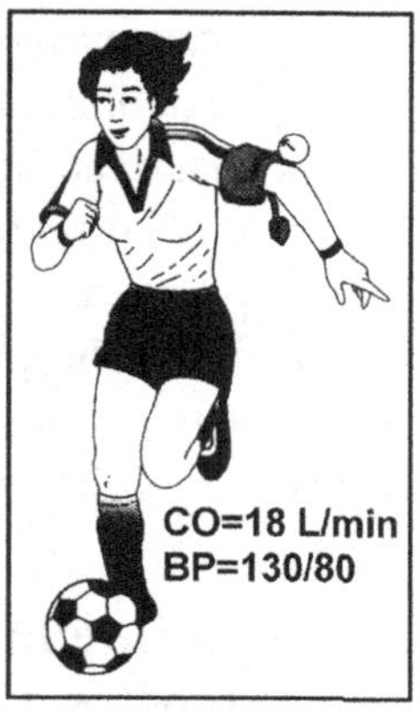

In exercise high CO and reduced SVR equalize BP

ANSWER b. Decrease systemic vascular resistance (↓SVR). Because BP = CO X SVR, to keep a constant BP while the CO increases 4-6 times, the SVR must decrease 4-6 times. This peripheral vasodilation allows blood to pass the capillary bed more easily and not significantly elevate the BP. The same auto-regulation occurs in the pulmonary system on exercise. Braunwald says,

> "*In normal individuals, when pulmonary blood flow is doubled, the pulmonary vascular resistance is halved, resulting in no change in pulmonary artery pressure. Pulmonary artery pressure does not rise until pulmonary blood flow increases by four to sixfold.*"

Note that the pulmonary resistance (PVR) primarily affects PA pressure, whereas systemic resistance (SVR) affects the systemic BP. Note that in CAD the coronary circulation cannot dilate to adequately increase flow to ischemic areas during exercise. Because of this diseased hearts may have to switch to anaerobic metabolism during exercise. **See**: Berne & Levy section on exercise. **Keywords:** Resistance, exercise, BP

428. How does hypoxemia effect the two vascular systems? In the systemic circulation decreased PO_2 causes ________, and in the pulmonary system it causes ________.

a. Vasodilation, Vasodilation
b. Vasodilation, Vasoconstriction
c. Vasoconstriction, Vasodilation
d. Vasoconstriction, Vasoconstriction

ANSWER b. Vasodilation, Vasoconstriction. The **systemic vasodilator** effect is opposite to the potent **pulmonary vasoconstrictor** effect. Remember that in the lungs, nonventilated areas become ischemic and need to be shut down or cyanosis may result. Thus, blood flow is diverted away from atelectatic (collapsed) alveoli. Whereas, in the tissues, ischemic areas need more perfusion and thus vasodilate.
See: Darovic, chapter on"Intro. to CV and Pulm. Anatomy and Physiology."
Keywords: Hypoventilation

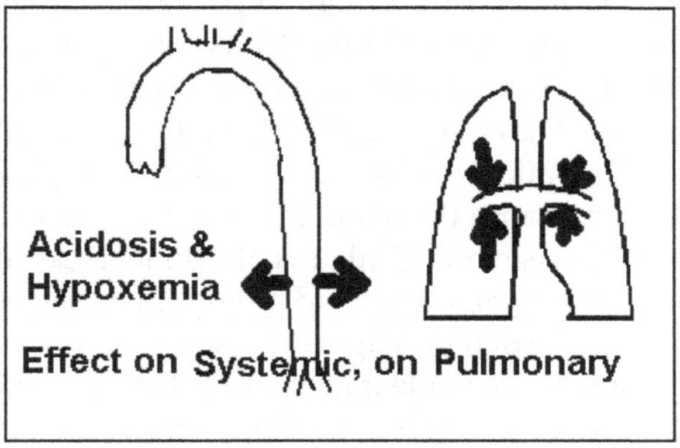

Effect of ischemia & acidemia

429. Which of the following IV medications would be most likely to reduce systemic vascular resistance (SVR)?

- **a. Dopamine (high dose)**
- **b. Norepinephrine**
- **c. Nitrates (Nitroprusside)**
- **d. Phenylephrine**

ANSWER c. Nitrates (Nitroprusside). All the nitrate drugs are vasodilators. Darovic, says,

> *"Nitroprusside is an extremely potent direct-acting dilator of both veins and arteries of the systemic coronary, pulmonary, and renal circulations. . . . Decreased afterload (mediated by arteriolar dilation) results in a reduction in systemic and pulmonary vascular resistance and an increase in stroke volume. . . . Reflex tachycardia may result from decreased blood pressure."*

Dopamine, Norepinephrine, and Phenylephrine are vasoconstrictors or pressors.
See: Darovic, chapter on "Pharmacologic Influences on Hemodynamic Parameters."
Keywords: Nitroprusside reduces SVR

430. All the following drugs reduce PVR and pulmonary pressures EXCEPT:

- **a. 100% oxygen administration**
- **b. Adenosine and epoprostenol**
- **c. Nitric oxide (NO)**
- **d. Angiotensin and epinephrine**

ANSWER d. Angiotensin and epinephrine are both pulmonary vasoconstrictors used to evaluate pulmonary reactivity. Other agents listed are vasodilators. Baim says,

> *"Pulmonary vascular resistance may be decreased by oxygen, adenosine, isoproterenol, alpha-antagonists such as phentolamine or tolazoline, inhaled nitric oxide, prostacyclin infusions, and high doses of calcium channel blockers. These vasodilators may be used to test for fixed, irreversible pulmonary hypertension. A practical approach use in may labs to test for responsiveness and determine therapeutic dosage uses IV epoprostenol..."*

Nitric oxide (NO) is an endothelially generated vasodilator. The role of endothelial factors in regulating flow is very important. A Texas Heart Institute publication says, "Nitric oxide has also been used clinically as a diagnostic tool in patients with PHT [Pulmonary HyperTension] and congenital heart disease. The main role for this application has been in the cardiac catheterization laboratory to evaluate the reactivity of the pulmonary vascular bed in patients with PHT. A relatively high incidence of serious side effects has been reported with the use of nonselective vasodilators for evaluating pulmonary vascular resistance, making inhaled NO an ideal screening agent. Inhaled NO has been particularly useful in evaluating candidates for cardiac or cardiopulmonary transplantation."

"Another diagnostic use of NO is in the evaluation of the postoperative cyanotic infant. Nitric oxide may be useful in determining if cyanosis is related to anatomic obstruction to pulmonary blood flow or related to pulmonary vasoconstriction. Adatia and coworkers studied 15 patients aged 1 to 52 days with PHT or excessive cyanosis compatible with elevated pulmonary vascular resistance after cardiac surgery. ...The infants who did not respond to the NO trial were subsequently found to have anatomic obstruction to pulmonary blood flow."

See: Kovalchin, et al, "Nitric Oxide for the Evaluation and Treatment of Pulmonary Hypertension in Congenital Heart Disease", Texas Heart Institute Journal 1997 at: http://www.ncbi.nlm.nih.gov/pmc/articles/PMC325473/pdf/thij00027-0078.pdf
See: Baim, chapter on "Clinical Measurement of Vascular Resistance" and Braunwald, chapter on " Normal pulmonary Circulation," **Keywords**: pulmonary vasodilators

Pathology

431. A man with a chronic cyanotic shunt and pulmonary hypertension (PA = 65/30/42) is evaluated for corrective surgery. While breathing 100% O2 small amounts of nitric oxide his PA pressures falls to 30/15/22 mmHg. This indicates a ________ pulmonary resistance, and that surgery ______ considered

a. Reversible, WILL NOT BE
b. Reversible, MAY BE
c. Irreversible, WILL NOT BE
d. Irreversible, MAY BE

ANSWER b. Reversible, SURGERY MAY BE CONSIDERED. This is the main reason we test for pulmonary vascular resistance reactivity. Since PVR = (PA-LA)/CO the resistance appears to have dropped in half. Accurate calculations for PVR should be made. But, since it is unlikely the CO or LA pressures changed dramatically, the PVR is proportional to PA mean pressure (PVR $\propto$ mean PA). This patients drop in PVR is a good indication that he will be able to adapt to corrective surgery. Baim says,

> *"When pulmonary hypertension has been present for many years, permanent obliterative changes in the pulmonary vasculature occur, and reactive vasoconstriction is less significant. Oxygen inhalation may also be of value in assessing pulmonary vascular reactivity. Patients with high pulmonary vascular resistance (i.e. greater than or equal to 600 dynes-sec-cm^{-5}) in association with a central shunt (e.g. a ventricular septal defect) should be given 100% oxygen by face mask before concluding that the changes are fixed."*

A new test for pulmonary hypertension done in the cath lab measures PVR while breathing small amounts of nitric oxide. Again if the PVR drops significantly, the PVR may be reversible. **See:** Baim, chapter on "Clinical Measurement of Vascular Resistance."
Keywords: O2 reversibility of high PVR, surgery may now be considered

432. High PVR leading to severe pulmonary hypertension and reversal of a L-R shunt into a R-L (cyanotic) shunt is termed:

a. Kawasaki syndrome
b. Total anomalous venous return
c. Eisenmenger complex
d. Tetralogy of Fallot

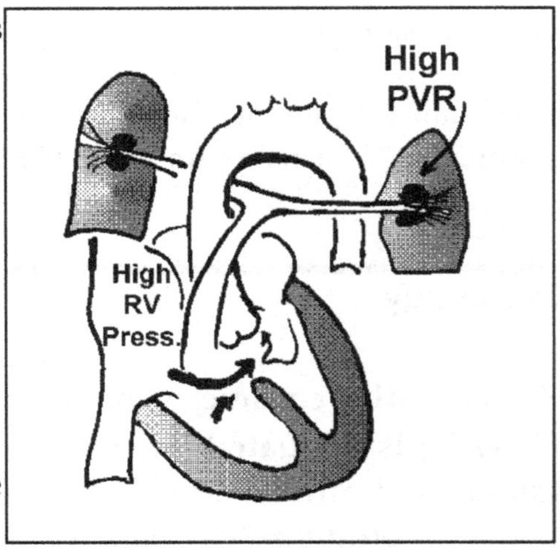

Eisenmenger Complex

ANSWER c. Eisenmenger complex. "Eisenmenger" has come to represent the end stage of a shunt in which the pulmonary arterioles have reacted to the high pulmonary pressure with fixed hypertrophy. When this resistance increases to the point where RV pressure exceeds LV pressure, the shunt will reverse and switch to a R-L shunt. Then cyanosis becomes evident. When this high PVR becomes fixed and irreversible it is too late for corrective surgery. The irreversible PVR will not readjust, and pulmonary hypertension remains despite corrected anatomy. For this reason "Eisenmenger" often refers to the end stage of a congenital shunt which has become irreversible. It is a most important condition to prevent.
Braunwald says,

> *"Surgery must not be offered to patients with severe, fixed pulmonary vascular obstruction, even when the cardiac defect is anatomically correctable. Such patients either do not survive operation or, if they do, are not benefitted and more often than not are harmed."*

The NO inhalation test screens these patients to see if a patient's pulmonary hypertension is relieved with this local vasodilator. If so surgery may proceed.
See: Braunwald, chapter on "Congenital Heart Disease" and "Pulmonary Hypertension."
Keywords: Eisenmenger complex

433. In acyanotic shunt patients, surgical repair should be limited to patients in whom the net shunt is __________and/or the ratio of PVR to SVR is __________.

- **a. Left-to-right, greater than 0.2**
- **b. Left-to-right, less than 0.5**
- **c. Right-to-left, greater than 0.2**
- **d. Right-to-left, less than 0.5**

ANSWER b. Left-to-right, less than 0.5. Longstanding L-R shunt patients may develop Eisenminger's syndrome with elevated fixed pulmonary resistance. Such patients do not do well with total repair surgery. One of the goals in pediatric cardiology is carefully monitor these children to prevent L- R shunts from getting to this point.
Baim says,

> *"surgical repair should be limited to patients in whom the net shunt is left-to-right and the pulmonary vascular resistance is less than systemic vascular resistance, preferably with a resistance ratio less than 0.50."*

Of course R-L shunts may be surgically repaired, because the lungs are not flooded with damaging high pressure blood flow.
See: Baim, chapter on "Clinical Measurement of Vascular Resistance." **Keywords**: pulmonary

434. **Clinical factors that increase SVR include all the following EXCEPT:**

a. **Anemia**
b. **Hypothermia**
c. **Hypovolemia**
d. **Low CO syndrome**

ANSWER a. Anemia causes compensatory increase in HR and CO due to the lower oxygen delivery of arterial blood. This requires the systemic arterioles to open up and DECREASE the SVR. Darovic says: "Clinical factors that decrease SVR and left ventricular afterload include vasodilator therapy, hyperdynamic sheptic shock, cirrhosis, compensated aortic regurgitation, anemia, and anaphylactic shock. Clinical factors that increase SVR and left ventricular afterload include hypovolemia, hypothermia, low cardiac output syndrome, and excessive catecholamine release and/or adminstration."
See: Darovic, chapter on "Pulmonary Artery Pressure Monitoring"

435. **Clinical factors that increase PVR include all the following EXCEPT:**

a. **Pulmonary embolism**
b. **Pulmonary edema**
c. **Oxygen administration**
d. **CO_2 administration**

ANSWER c. Oxygen administration vasodilates the pulmonary capillaries (remember is it opposite in the systemic tissue beds). And oxygen administration may used in the cath lab to measure how much it dilates the pulmonary beds and reduces PVR. Remember that In the lungs, nonventilated areas become ischemic and need to be shut down or cyanosis may result. Thus, blood flow is diverted away from atelectatic (collapsed) alveoli. Oxygen has the happy effect of dilating these capillaries. Darovic says: "Factors that may increase PVR and in turn, right ventricular afterload include massive pulmonary embolism, cardiogenic and noncardiogenic pulmonary edema, sepsis, , acidemia, hypoxemia, idiopathic primary pulmonary hypertension, and some congenital or valvular heart diseases. Factors that may decrease pulmonary vascular resistance and right ventricular afterload include use of vasodilator drugs, as well as correction of hypoxemia or acidemia."
See: Darovic, chapter on "Pulmonary Artery Pressure Monitoring"

REFERENCES:

Baim, D. S. and Grossman W., *Cardiac Catheterization, Angiography,* and Intervention, 7th Ed., Lea and Febiger, 2006

Pappano & Wier.,(previously Berne & Levy) *Cardiovascular Physiology,* 10th Ed., Mosby Year Book, 2013

Kern, M. J., Ed., *The Cardiac Catheterization Handbook,* 6th Ed., Mosby-Year Book, Inc., 2016

Braunwald, Eugene, Ed., *HEART DISEASE A Textbook of Cardiovascular Medicine,* 9th Ed., W. B. Saunders Co., 2012

Daily, E. K., and Schroeder, J. S., *Techniques in Bedside Hemodynamic Monitoring,* 4th Ed., C. V. Mosby Company, 1989

Darovic, G.O., *Hemodynamic Monitoring: Invasive and Noninvasive Clinical Application,* WB Saunders, 1995

Pepine, J. C., and Hill, J. A., et. al., *Diagnostic and Therapeutic Cardiac Catheterization,* 2nd Ed., Williams and Wilkins, 1994

Underhill, S. L., Ed., *CARDIAC NURSING,* 2nd Ed., J. B. Lippincott Co., 1989

OUTLINE: RESISTANCE CALCULATIONS

1. General Resistance
   a. Units
      i. Hybrid = Wood = mmHg/L/min
      ii. Absolute = dsc^{-5}
      iii. Normal values
         (1) Absolute SVR = 1130 dsc^{-5}
      iv. Hybrid SVR = 14 HRUs
      v. Absolute PVR = 67.0 dsc^{-5}
      vi. Hybrid PVR = 0.84 HRUs
      vii. SVR/PVR =12:1
   b. Changes with growth
      i. ↓ PVR, ↓ PA pressure
      ii. ↑ SVR, ↑ AO pressure
   c. Poiseuille's Law
      i. Arteriolar resistance
      ii. Vascular Resistance
      iii. R = 8(Viscosity)x (Length)/(π)(radius)^4
   d. Resistance = (outflow pr. - inflow pr.)/ Blood flow per minute
   e. SVR = $(\overline{AO} - \overline{RA})$ / SBF
   f. PVR = $(\overline{PA} - \overline{PAW})$ / PBF
   g. ↑ SVR = ↑ BP
   h. ↑ PVR = ↑ PA pressure
   i. Resistance Index
      i. Multiplies by BSA
2. FORMULAS
   a. PVR = $(\overline{PA} - \overline{LA})$/CO
   b. SVR = $(\overline{AO} - \overline{RA})$/CO
   c. PVRI = $(\overline{PA} - \overline{LA})$/CI
   d. SVRI = $(\overline{AO} - \overline{RA})$/CI
3. CALCULATIONS
   a. PVR in HRUs
   b. PVR in dsc^{-5}
   c. SVR in HRUs
   d. SVR in dsc^{-5}
   e. Above indexed
   f. Ohms Law: R = (P1 - P2)/CO
   g. Shunt flow and direction (using O2 Sat.)
4. APPLICATIONS
   a. SVR = afterload
   b. ↑ PVR increased likelihood of R-L shunt
   c. Pulmonary hypertension
   d. Exercise = ↓ SVR and ↓ PVR
   e. Hypoxemia = ↑ SVR, ↓ SVR
   f. Vasodilators
      i. Nitrates
   g. Vasoconstrictors
      i. Dopamine, Norepinephrine, and Phenylephrine
5. PATHOLOGY
   a. Oxygen challenge
   b. Eisenminger's Syndrome
   c. Fixed high pulmonary resistance
   d. Tolerate closure of L-R shunt
      i. If PVR/SVR < 0.5

VALVE AREA

INDEX E10:

General Valve Area

436. What left heart valve pressure abnormality is labeled #3 .

a. MS
b. MR
c. AS
d. AR

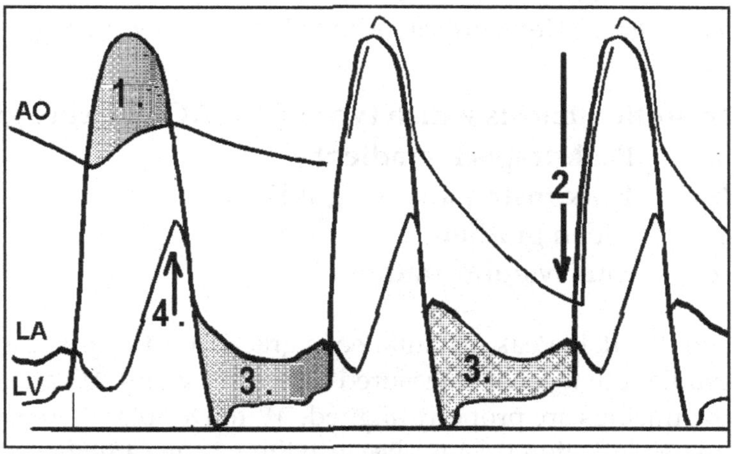

Simultaneous LV, AO, LA x 200

ANSWER a. MS. The shaded areas are the areas of gradient. The mitral valve gradient is seen in diastole between the simultaneous LA and LV pressures. Compare this to the normal Wiggers diagram, and note the diastolic LA and LV pressures should be the same.

MATCHING ANSWERS ARE:

1. AS (Aortic Stenosis) LV-AO gradient in systole
2. AR (Aortic Regurgitation) wide AO pulse pressure, low AO diastole
3. MS (Mitral stenosis) LA-LV gradient in diastole
4. MR (Mitral regurgitation) LA or PAW elevated "v" wave at end systole

See: Baim and Grossman, chapter on "Assessment of Stenotic Valves." **Keywords:** AS, MS gradient

437. Baim and Grossman say that the "gold standard" for assessing the severity of valvular stenosis is:

a. **Gorlin valve area**
b. **Hakki valve area**
c. **M-Mode echocardiography**
d. **Two dimensional transthoracic echocardiography**

ANSWER a. Gorlin valve area. Baim and Grossman say ,

"the Gorlin formula remains the "gold standard" for assessing the severity of stenotic

cardiac valves."

The invasive Gorlin formula remains the standard to judge all other techniques. Certainly echocardiography techniques give better qualitative assessment of valvular stenosis by imaging the pliability, degree of calcification, and the shape of the valve orifice. And Doppler can accurately evaluate the gradient. Braunwald says,

> *"It is possible to make a semiquantitative assessment of AS with 2-D echocardiography by judging the mobility of the leaflets, especially in the short-axis view. Although transthoracic 2-D echocardiography is rarely used to quantitate AS, there is renewed interest in using transesophageal echocardiography to measure the cross-sectional area of the aortic valve and thus quantitating it... The best ultrasonic technique for quantifying AS utilizes continuous-wave Doppler. Using the modified Bernoulli equation, it is possible to measure the pressure gradient across the aortic valve."*

Noninvasive and invasive mitral valve area can also be easily estimated using the "half time" technique described later in this chapter.

See: Pressure ½ time question in this chapter, and Baim, chapter on "Calculation of Stenotic Valve Area" **Keywords**: Gorlin valve area is "gold standard"

438. In aortic stenosis which type of LV-AO pressure gradient is the largest?

a. **Peak-to-peak gradient**

b. **Peak instantaneous gradient**

c. **Mean gradient**

d. **End systolic gradient**

ANSWER b. Peak instantaneous gradient is the greatest gradient that can be measured between LV and AO after the tracings are properly aligned. With Doppler there is no need to align tracings because there is no catheter delay. Instantaneous gradient is very important because it is the gradient Doppler provides.

The mean gradient is usually the smallest of the gradients measured in AS. It is measured by integrating the gradient area. Gradient = mean LV (in systole) - minus mean AO (in systole). It is the area of the shaded box (SEP x mean gradient). This box is the same area as the ∫(LV-AO) systolic gradient.

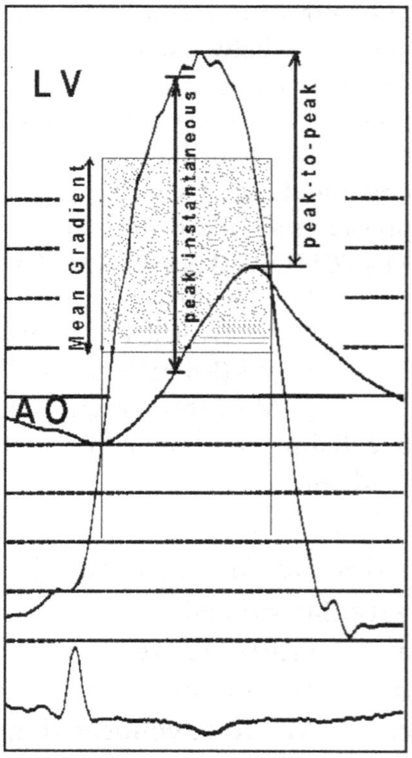

Braunwald says,

> *"In the cardiac catheterization laboratory it is customary to measure the aortic valve gradient as the difference between the peak left ventricular pressure and the peak aortic pressures (the "peak-to-peak gradient) This gradient actually does not exist at any instant in time because the peak aortic pressure occurs later than the peak left ventricular pressure. The peak instantaneous pressure gradient measured by the Doppler technique is invariably larger. If one measures the more accurate mean gradients both in the cardiac catheterization lab and with the Doppler examination, then the measurements are quite similar."*

See: Kern, chapter on "Hemodynamics." **Keywords**: peak instantaneous gradient

439. In aortic stenosis how accurate is the mean simultaneous LV-FA gradient when recording FA from the sheath sidearm? When FA is shifted and aligned with LV upstroke the gradient is _________; when FA is not shifted or aligned with LV upstroke the gradient is _____.

- a. **Accurate, overestimated**
- b. **Accurate, underestimated**
- c. **Overestimated, underestimated**
- d. **Underestimated, overestimated**

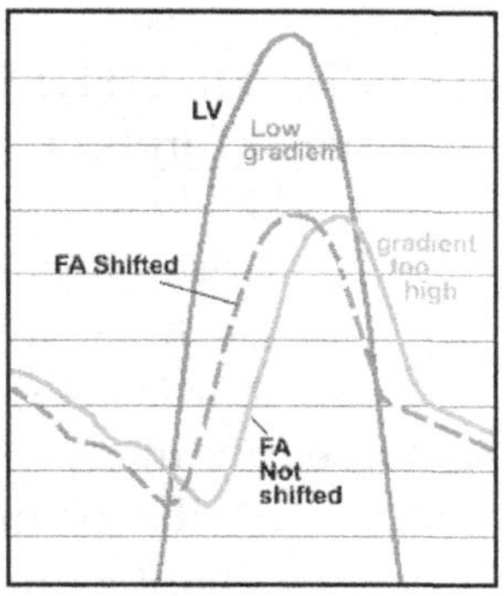

ANSWER d. Underestimated, overestimated . Remember the femoral and radial artery systole is increased above true AO pressure due to wave reflection. If the FA is shifted left, as shown, the gradient is artificially reduced and the calculated valve area increased. It FA must be used Kern recommends not shifting it. But, it is more accurate to get an aortic arch pressure with another catheter or use a pressure wire in the LV.

Peterson says, "*The least desirable approach is to estimate the aortic valve pressure gradient by using a simultaneous registration of the left ventricular and femoral or brachial artery pressure pulses. These latter pressures are altered by the impedance characteristics of the arterial vascular tree.... In 26 patients, Folland and colleagues studied the aortic valve left ventricular-ascending aortic gradient and compared it with the left ventricular-femoral artery pressure gradient, with and without realignment.* ***Without realignment there was a systematic overestimation, and with realignment an underestimation of the left ventricular-ascending aortic gradient****.... In cases where the valve orifice area is marginally severe (e.g., 0.7 to 1.0 cm^2), the errors inherent in the left ventricular-femoral artery measurements can become crucial. Thus, we prefer ..., simultaneous measurements of left ventricular and ascending aortic pressures, to estimate the valve orifice size.*"

The other problem is the clearance between the sheath sidearm and the LV catheter. Pepine recommends that the sheath be **at least one French size larger than the catheter**, to reduce the intrinsic sheath gradient.

See: Kern, chapter on "Hemodynamics" and Pepine, chapter on "Valve Function."

Valve Area Equation

440. Match #1 in the box (Hakki or "quick" aortic valve area) to its formula below.

- a. **Flow / 44.5 √ Mean gradient**
- b. **Flow / 38 √ Mean gradient**
- c. **CO / √ (Peak - peak gradient)**
- d. **Mean gradient / (CO / SEP)**

Hemodynamic Formulas

*1. Hakki formula for aortic valve area
2. Gorlin formula for mitral valve area
3. Gorlin formula for aortic valve area
4. Aortic valve resistance

ANSWER c. CO / √ (Peak - peak Gradient.)
Hakki developed a simplified formula for the calculation of stenotic cardiac valve areas. The simplified Hakki formula is:

Valve area = cardiac output in L/min / √(peak - peak pressure gradient in mmHg

This simplified formula provides quick in-lab determination of aortic valve area. Simply take the square root of the LV-AO peak-to-peak pressure difference, and divide that into the cardiac output. Grossman suggests that this simplified valve area may overestimate the valve area in bradycardic MS patients and tachycardic AS patients. A correction factor is available - see Baim.

MATCH THE OTHER HEMODYNAMIC FORMULAS:

Name of formula	Hemodynamic Formula
1. Hakki formula for aortic valve area	**= CO / √ (Peak - peak gradient)**
2. Gorlin formula for mitral valve area	**= Flow / 38 √ Mean gradient**
3. Gorlin formula for aortic valve area	**= Flow / 44.5 √ Mean gradient**
4. Aortic valve resistance	**= Mean gradient / (CO / SEP)**

All these formulas are useful to assess valvular stenosis and should be memorized. Some authors describe the mitral emperic constant as 37.7 or 0.85 x 44.5.

See: Baim, chapter on "Calculation of Stenotic Valve Orifice Area" and Kern, chapter on "Hemodynamics." **Keywords**: Hakki formula, Gorlin formula, Valve resistance

441. Estimate the aortic valve area using the Hakki formula from the simultaneous AO-LV pressure tracings recorded on X200 below. CO = 5.0 L/min.

a. **0.25 cm^2**

b. **0.50 cm^2**

c. **1.0 cm^2**

d. **2.5 cm^2**

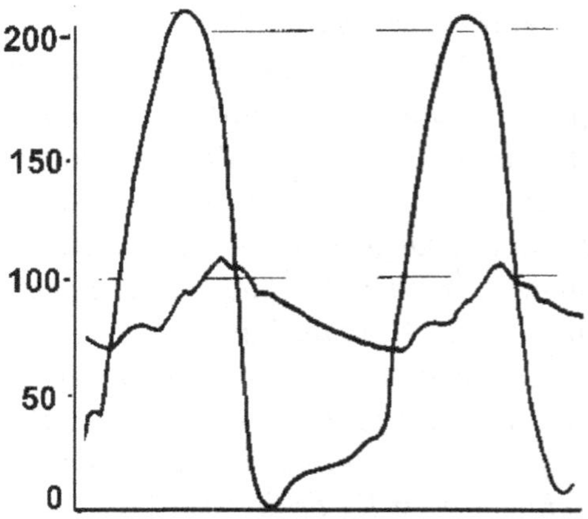

Simultaneous LV& AO X200

ANSWER b. 0.5 cm^2. This Hakki or "quick and easy" valve area formula estimates the valve area in cm^2. First the peak - peak gradient of AS is measured between the systolic LV and AO pressures.

AS peak - peak gradient = $LV_{systole} - AO_{systole}$

Peak AO is 110 mmHg. Peak LV is 210 mmHg. This makes the difference between these two peaks 210 - 110 = 100 mmHg.

The Hakki formula is also called the "quick and easy" formula.

Hakki valve area formula = $\dfrac{\textbf{CO (in L/min)}}{\sqrt{\textbf{(peak - peak gradient in mmHg)}}}$

Since the square root of 100 = 10, the formula becomes VA = 5.0 / 10 = 0.50 cm^2. It appears to be less accurate than the Gorlin formula in brady or tachycardia situations. But it can be done quickly in the lab. Note, some authors suggest using the square root of the mean gradient, instead of the peak-to peak-gradient.

See: Kern, chapter on "Hemodynamics." **Keywords**: measure peak to peak gradient

442. What is the empiric constant (K) in the denominator of the Gorlin valve area formula used for #1 (Aortic Stenosis)?

a. 32
b. 34.5
c. 38
d. 44.5

Type of stenosis
***1. Aortic Stenosis**
2. Mitral Stenosis
3. Pulmonic Stenosis

ANSWER d. 44.5. This constant comes from the derivation of the formula which assumes a constant gravity driven pressure. Note that the constants are all 44.5 except in the mitral valve area calculation where it is 38. **BE ABLE TO MATCH ALL ANSWERS BELOW.**

Type of stenosis	Empiric constant
1. Aortic Stenosis	44.5
2. Mitral Stenosis	38 (0.85 of 44.5)
3. Pulmonic Stenosis	44.5

This empiric constant corrects for viscous properties of blood and complexities of the geometry of the orifice and converts the pressure units to mmHg. Kern states that the empiric constant for tricuspid stenosis is not validated. Most authors call "C" the constant and multiply it by 44.5. The aortic "C" is 1.0 x 44.5 = 44.5. The mitral "C" is 0.85 x 44.5 = 37.7.
See: Kern, chapter on "Hemodynamics." **Keywords**: empiric constant

443. From the data in the box calculate the numerator or "Flow" for use in the Gorlin aortic valve area formula.

a. 125 ml/sec
b. 145 ml/sec
c. 179 ml/sec
d. 215 ml/sec

Patient # 443
CO = 5.0 L/min
SEP = 0.40 sec/beat
HR = 70 / min
Mean Gradient=65

ANSWER c. 179 ml/sec. The "Flow" that is for the numerator of the Gorlin valve area is calculated by this formula:

AO Flow = CO / (HR x SEP)
or

$$\text{Flow(ml/sec)} = \frac{\text{CO (ml/min)}}{\text{HR (b/min) x SEP (seconds)}}$$

Flow = CO / (SEP x HR) = (5000 ml/min) / (0.40 sec/bt. x 70 bts./min) = 179 ml/systolic sec. The CO is converted to ml/sec by multiplying by 1000 ml/L. The product of SEP x HR must then be divided into that CO. The resulting "flow" is how many ml/sec would flow through the valve if it were open continuously. Exams usually give you the flow number.

After calculating Flow you can substitute it into the numerator of the Gorlin valve area formula. Note how the units cancel into flow in ml/sec beat. Some authors call this the flow in ml/systolic second for aortic flow or ml/diastolic second for mitral flow. An acronym for the Flow formula: "Flow is CO over HR x SEP"is: "Flo is Cried-Out / HeR SEParation," or "Flow = CO over HR x SEP."
See: Kern, chapter on "Hemodynamics." **Keywords**: aortic valve "Flow" calculation

444. The difference between the valve "flow" in the mitral and aortic Gorlin valve area formulas is that mitral valve "flow" uses:

a. **48 instead of 32**
b. **32 instead of 44.5**
c. **SEP instead of DFP**
d. **DFP instead of SEP**

ANSWER d. DFP instead of SEP. Mitral valve area uses the diastolic filling period (DFP) because mitral forward flow only occurs in diastole. The systolic ejection period is used in the aortic valve area "flow" formula. The two valve area formulas are the same except for two things:

- switch SEP and DFP (used in the "flow" formula)
- switch empiric constants 48 and 38 (used in denominator of Gorlin formula)

See: Kern, chapter on "Hemodynamics."

445. According to Gorlin's formula the patient's calculated valve area:

a. **Increases as the peak to peak pressure gradient increases**
b. **Increases as the mean pressure gradient increases**
c. **Decreases as the peak to peak pressure gradient increases**
d. **Decreases as the mean pressure gradient increases**

Answer: d. Decreases as the mean pressure gradient increases. Gorlins Formula uses the square root of the mean pressure gradient in the denominator. This means when the gradient increases, the calculated valve area decreases (inverse relationship). E.g., Higher gradient means smaller valve. It is the Hakki formula that uses peak-to-peak pressures.

Gorlin's mitral VA formula is: MVA = [CO / (DFP x HR)] / 38 √ Mean gradient, where the 3 term numerator in brackets [] is sometimes called "FLOW." For aortic valve area replace 38 with 44.5. See: Grossman chapter on "Valve area"

446. You have a Swan-Ganz catheter in the PA, a pigtail catheter in the LV, and a short femoral artery sheath to measure arterial pressure. With the tracing shown, how would you most accurately measure the pressure gradient for accurate calculation of aortic valve area?

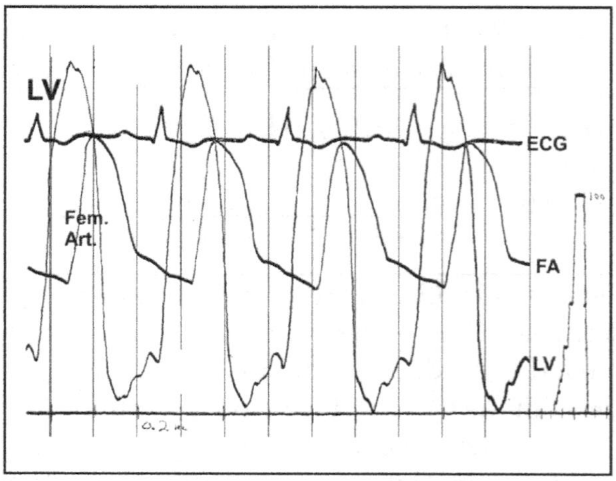

Simultaneous LV & Fem. Art. Via sheath

a. **Measure peak to peak LV-FA gradient on exercise.**
b. **Administer dobutamine to increase CO, then rerun simultaneous LV-FA pressures.**
c. **Don't accept this pressure recording. Record simultaneous pressures again, using a second catheter in the ascending AO instead of FA.**
d. **Shift the aortic tracing left to compensate for FA pressure delay.**

ANSWER c. Don't accept. Record from a second catheter in the ascending AO instead of FA. This tracing shows excessive phase delay in the femoral artery tracing. FA sheaths pressure will give inaccurate readings. These errors are caused by: tight sheath and peripheral amplification of the FA systolic pressure due to wave reflections in descending AO.

Kern says, "The delay in pressure transmission and pressure wave reflection from the proximal aorta to the femoral artery artificially increases the mean gradient. Femoral pressure overshoot (amplification) reduces the true gradient. If femoral arterial pressure is used, phase shifting of the femoral arterial pressure to the left ventricle upstroke may be important. In patients with low gradients (i.e., <35 mm Hg), more accurate valve areas were obtained with unadjusted LV-Ao pressure tracings. Optimally a second catheter can be positioned directly above the aortic valve to reduce transmission delay and femoral pressure overshoot (amplification)." See: Kern, chapter on Hemodynamic Data,

Valve Area Measurement

447. In the simultaneous LV, AO and PAW pressures shown, which area should be measured to get the mean gradient in aortic valve area?

- **a.** 1
- **b.** 2
- **c.** 3
- **d.** 4

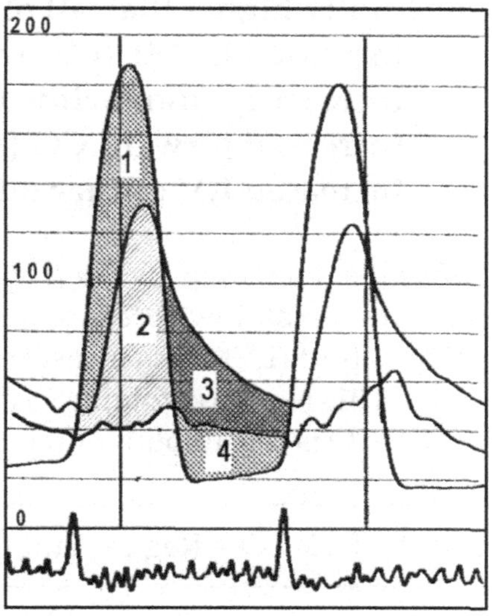

Simultaneous LV, AO, PAW Pressures X200

ANSWER a. 1. The aortic stenotic systolic gradient is between LV (on top), AO pressures (on bottom), and LV-AO pressure crossover points on either side. Unless you use a computer to integrate this gradient, you must use a planimeter to measure the gradient area and gradient "mean" for the Gorlin formula. Note that this AO tracing appears slightly delayed. The LV and AO upstroke needs to be realigned by shifting the AO slightly to the left. Area 4 above is planimetered for the mitral valve area.

See: Baim and Grossman, chapter on "Assessment of Stenotic Valves." **Keywords**: Area to planimeter for aortic valve area

448. From this ECG recorded with 0.1 second time lines, determine the heart rate.

- **a.** **50 bpm**
- **b.** **66 bpm**
- **c.** **72 bpm**
- **d.** **83 bpm**

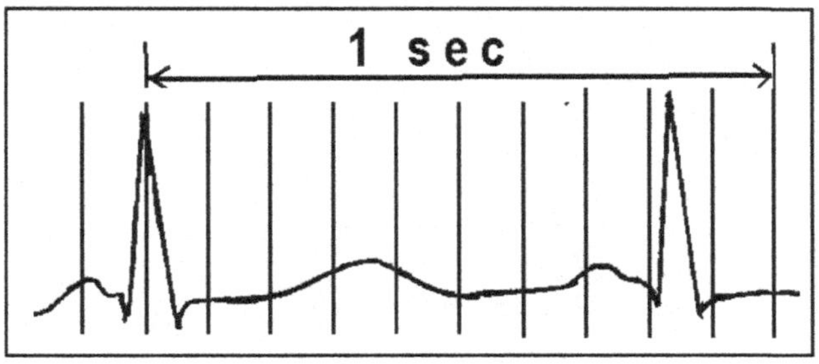

ECG recorded at time lines 0.1 sec

ANSWER c. 72 bpm

RR interval is 0.83 sec. If the paper speed is 100 mm/sec or the time lines are 0.1 as shown, it is EASY to calculate the rr interval and heart rate. Just use the time lines to count up the rr time interval, as shown.

HR = 60/ r-r interval

Know the heart rate formula:

Here the rr interval is 8.3 time lines.

HR (Bts/min) = 60 (sec/min) / r-r interval in (sec)

HR = 60 sec/min / 0.83 sec = 72. Note the unit cancellation resulting in beats/min.

You may include a paper speed factor in the numerator to convert the r-r interval measurement from mm. to seconds.

HR (bts./min) = 60 (sec/min) x paper speed (mm/sec) / r-r interval (mm)

See: Baim and Grossman, chapter on "Assessing Valvular Stenosis." **Keywords:** calc. HR

449. In patients with mitral or aortic regurgitation, which type of cardiac output is significantly higher than all others?

a. **Increased LVMF (LV Angio CO)**

b. **Increased radionuclide CO (Technetium)**

c. **Increased forward CO (Fick CO)**

d. **Increased RV cardiac output (Thermodilution CO)**

ANSWER a. Increased LVMF (LV Angio CO). Left Ventricular Minute Flow (LVMF) is termed the "total flow" because it includes the amount of regurgitation. Quantitative LV cardiac output (LVMF) is measured by calculating and LV volumes at end diastole and end systole. This is stroke volume (SV). Then LVMF = SV x HR. The difference between LVMF and Fick CO is the amount of regurgitation.

LVMF - Fick CO = Regurgitant flow

See: Baim and Grossman, chapter on "Evaluation of Ventricular Volumes, EF, ..."

Aortic Valve Area Calculation

USE THIS SIMULTANEOUS PRESSURE FOR THE NEXT FOUR QUESTIONS:

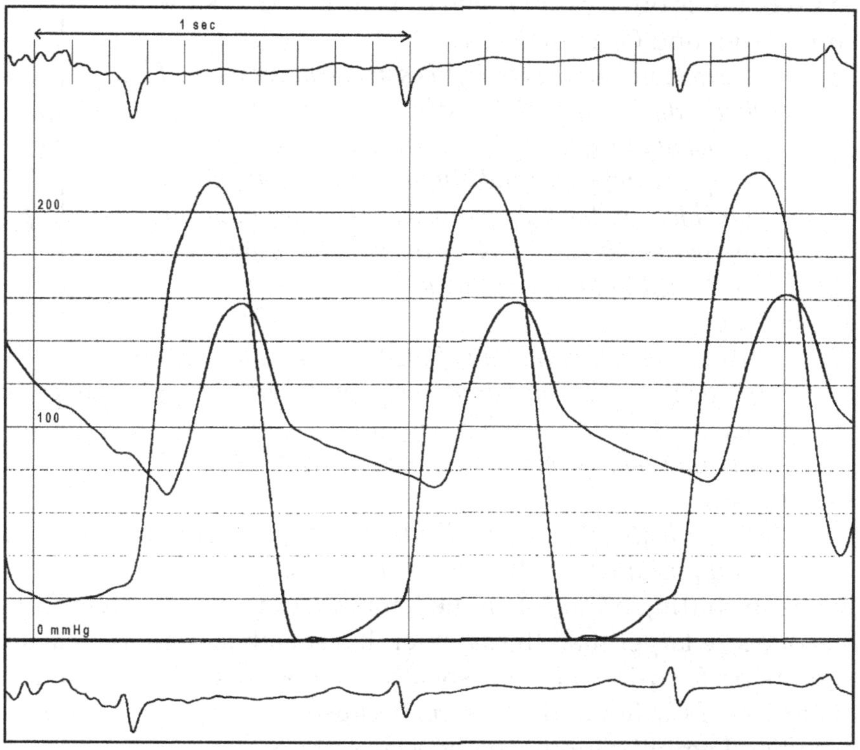

450 Simultaneous LV & AO pressures, x 200 scale, 100 mm/sec speed, CO=6.06

450. Determine the heart rate in this patient # 450 above.

a. 75 beats/min
b. 82 beats/min
c. 89 beats/min
d. 97 beats/min

451. Before the aortic stenosis gradient above is measured, how should the AO tracing above be shifted?

a. Not moved unless it is a radial artery tracing
b. Moved left so dicrotic notch intersects LV downslope
c. Moved left so diastole intersects LV up slope
d. Moved left to align ECG "r" wave with beginning systole

BOTH ANSWERS TOGETHER BELOW:

450. ANSWER HR b. 82 beats/min. Measure the rr interval with the time lines provided. Use the standard formula: HR = 60/ r-r interval.
So: HR= 60/.73 sec=82 bpm
If you prefer to measure the rr interval with a cm ruler the rr interval must be divided by paper sped to convert to seconds. Use the HR formula:

HR (bts./min) = 60 (sec/min) x paper speed (mm/sec) / r-r interval (mm)

See: Baim, chapter on "Calculation of Stenotic Valve Orifice Area" and Pepine, chapter on "Valve Function." **Keywords:** Measure HR

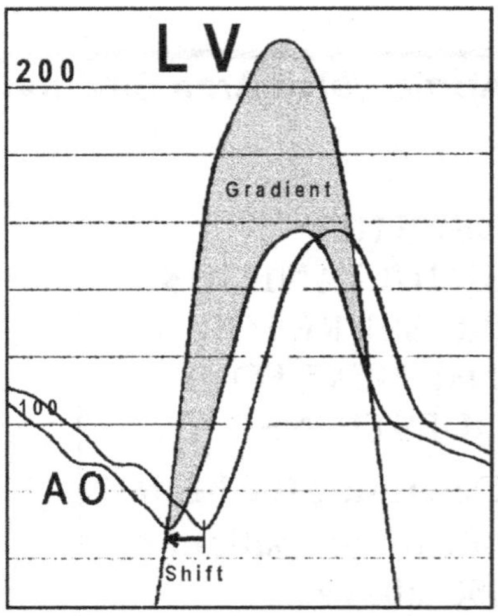

451. ANSWER c. Moved left so diastole intersects LV up slope. The AO dip preceding systole should be aligned with the LV upstroke as shown. This corresponds with the opening of the aortic valve. The dicrotic notch could be used, but is often poorly seen or is rounded as shown here. Baim and Grossman say,

> "*the femoral artery tracing is somewhat delayed... Fig... shows the LV and RFA tracings realigned to correct for the delay in transmission time. This is accomplished using tracing paper and aligning the arterial upstroke to coincide with the LV upstroke.... The most accurate approach however, involves the use of a second catheter positioned in the ascending aorta,...*"

Pepine says,

> "*Accurate determination of the transvalvular pressure gradient requires simultaneous, high-fidelity, properly damped pressure recordings from the chambers upstream and downstream from the valve in question. Pullback gradients are not accurate enough and should not be used.*"

Kern says,

> *"In patients with low gradients (i.e., <35 mm Hg), more accurate valve areas were obtained with unshifted LV-Ao pressure tracings."*

Errors in shifting occur when the femoral artery sheath pressure is used for the AO, even if it is one size larger than the catheter. If a sheath is used to measure arterial pressure many authors prefer using a LONG sheath that goes over the arch to reduce the pressure lag and distortion of the femoral pressure, because peripheral amplification usually occurs in FA tracings which reducers the apparent gradient. **See:** Baim, chapter on "Calculation of Stenotic Valve Orifice Area" and Pepine, chapter on "Valve Function" & Kern chapter on Hemodynamic Data. **Keywords**: LV - AO alignment mismatch in AS

USE THIS DIAGRAM FOR THE NEXT THREE QUESTIONS - Same patient as above.

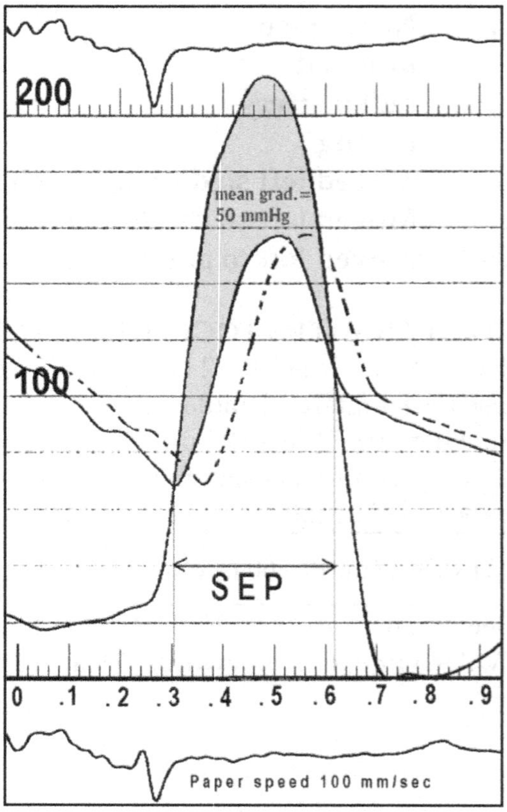

LV - AO x 200 scale, speed 100 mm/s

452. From these simultaneous pressure tracings, estimate the SEP between pressure crossover points.

a. **0.28 sec**
b. **0.31 sec**
c. **0.36 sec**
d. **0.41 sec**

453. **Calculate the FLOW for use in the Gorlin Valve area formula (CO = 6.06 L/min).**

a. **7.4 L/min**
b. **740 ml/sec**
c. **2.38 L/min**
d. **238 ml/sec**

THREE ANSWERS FOLLOW:

451. ANSWER b. 0.31 sec. SEP. From the pressure crossover points, draw vertical lines down to the time lines. Read 0.313 sec for the systolic ejection period (SEP). This is the time the valve is open, and when systolic flow and the gradient occurs.
See: Kern, chapter on "Hemodynamics."

452. ANSWER Flow d. 238 ml/sec. = 6060/(238 x 82)

FLOW = (CO ml/min) / (SEPsec x HRb/min)

See: Baim and Grossman, chapter on "Assessing Valvular Stenosis." **Keywords:** calculate FLOW

453. **Calculate the Gorlin aortic valve area for the above patient whose data is summarized in this box.**

a. **0.76 cm^2**
b. **0.85 cm^2**
c. **0.98 cm^2**
d. **1.14 cm^2**

Patient # 453	**Cath Data**
Fick CO	= 6.06 L/min
SEP = .31 sec	
Heart Rate	= 82 bt/min
Mean gradient	= 50 mmHg

ANSWER a. 0.76 cm^2.

Flow = CO/(SEP x HR) = 6060/ (.31 x 82) = 238 ml/sec
VA = Flow/(44.5 x $\sqrt{}$m.grad) = 238/(44.5 x $\sqrt{50}$) = 238/(44.5 x 7.07) = 0.76 cm^2

For a Gorlin valve area calculation you need the following data:

-SEP (or dfp) =time between pressure crossover points
-Mean gradient = gradient area via digital integration in mmHg. This area is usually averaged over several beats, 10 beats if in AF.
-CO in L/min. This is converted to ml/min by multiplying by 1000.

$$\text{Gorlin Area} = \frac{(\text{CO in ml/min})/[(\text{SEP in seconds}) \times (\text{HR in b/min})]}{(\text{Emperic Constant})\sqrt{(\text{mean gradient in mmHg})}}$$

See: Baim and Grossman, chapter on "Assessing Valvular Stenosis." **Keywords:** calculate Gorlin VA

USE THIS DIAGRAM FOR THE NEXT THREE QUESTIONS

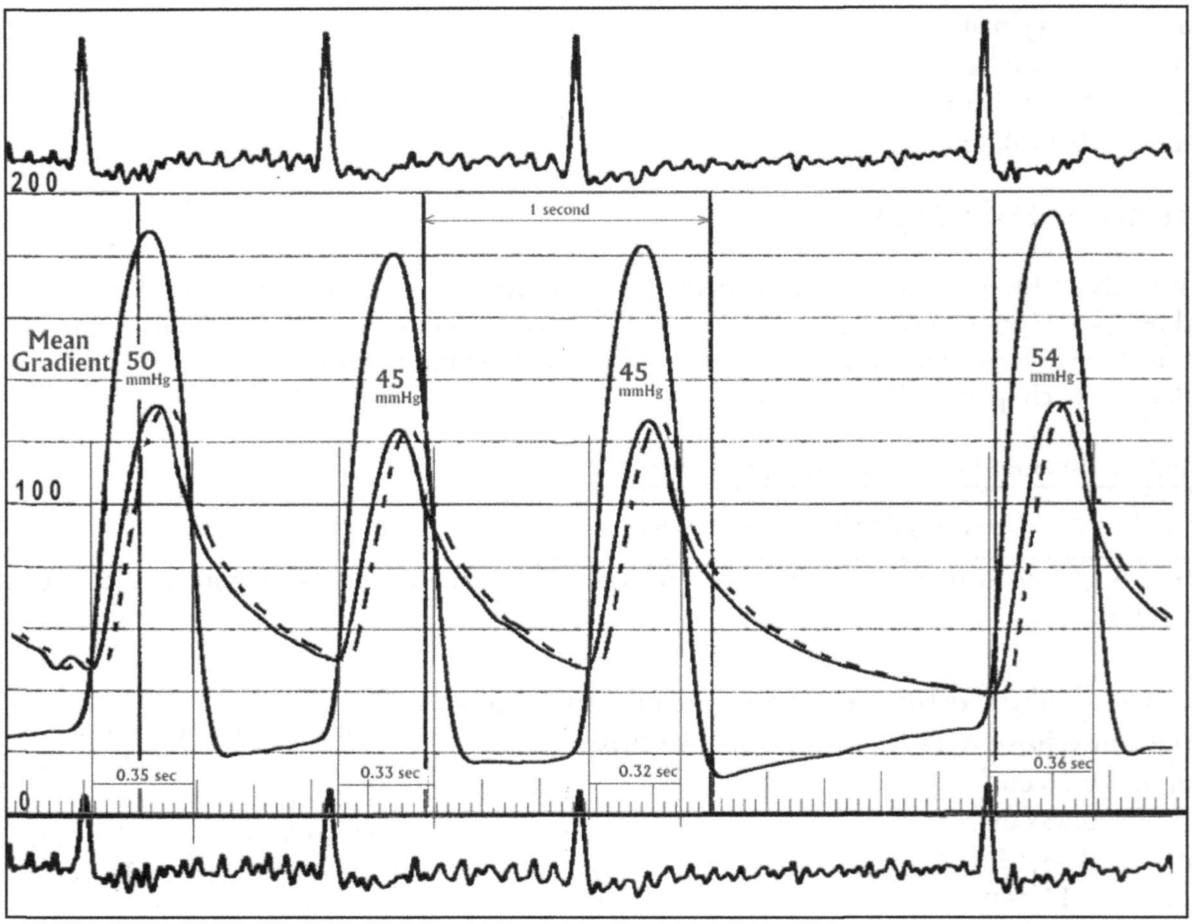

454. **On this patient estimate the mean gradient of the last 3 beats. Mean Gradient is:**
- a. 27 mmHg
- b. 34 mmHg
- c. 40 mmHg
- d. 48 mmHg

455. **On this patient estimate the SEP, on the last 3 beats?**
- a. 29.0 sec.
- b. 31.3 sec.
- c. 33.6 sec.
- d. 36.6 sec.

456. **On this patient estimate the average heart rate?**

a. **60.3 beats/min**
b. **65.5 beats/min**
c. **70.0 beats/min**
d. **75.5 beats/min**

Patient # 456 Cath Data
TDCO = 3.45 L/min
Fick CO (assumed) = 5.53 L/min
Mean gradient = 48 mmHg

457. **On the above patient calculate the FLOW for Gorlin Aortic valve area.**

a. **155 ml/sec**
b. **161 ml/sec**
c. **170 ml/sec**
d. **181 ml/sec**

458. **On the above patient calculate the Gorlin Aortic valve area.**

a. **0.42 cm^2**
b. **0.55 cm^2**
c. **0.71 cm^2**
d. **0.99 cm^2**

ALL ANSWERS TOGETHER BELOW:

456. ANSWER d. Mean gradient = 48 mmHg. as marked in the area of gradient.
Average area of last 3 beats = (45 + 45 + 54) / 3 = 48.0 mmHg
I used the last 3 beats because we do not have a full RR interval for the first beat.
Remember, the EDV, SEP, and gradient are determined by the preceding rr interval.
See: Kern, chapter on "Hemodynamics." **Keywords**: calculate mean gradient

457. ANSWER c. SEP = 33.6 sec. As marked between pressure crossover points.
Avg. SEP = (33 + 32 + 36)/3 = 33.6 sec
Note that this patient is in atrial fibrillation. Since the RR interval varies with each beat, measuring just one or even five beats will not yield a representative valve area. Kern says, in sinus rhythm it is OK to "*Planimeter 5 aortic-LV gradients and average (if atrial fibrillation, planimeter 10 beats)*" **See:** Kern, chapter on "Hemodynamics." **Keywords**: average 10 beats in atrial fib.

458. ANSWER a. HR = 60.3 beats/min. RR intervals are .85, .88 & 1.44 sec. Each RR interval is divided into 60 sec/min yields heart rates of 71, 68 & 42 b/min. The average of these 3 HR = 60.3 beats/min. (71 + 68 + 42)/3 = 60.3 beats/min

459. ANSWER c. FLOW = 170 ml/sec
FLOW is CO/ (SEP X HR)
here FLOW = 3450 / (33.6 x 60.3) = 170 ml/sec

460. ANSWER b. AVA = 0.55 cm^2. This is below the 0.7 cm^2 cutoff that requires valve replacement. Gorlin VA = FLOW/(44.5 x √48) =170/ (44.5 x 6.93) = 0.55 cm^2
Watch your unit cancellation. It is also helpful to develop a form to be sure you measure and calculate valve area the same & correct way each time. See Baim and Grossman's form. **See:** Kern, chapter on "Hemodynamics." **Keywords**: aortic Gorlin calculation

461. After the LV-gram, the pigtail catheter is pulled back from the LV to the aorta while recording pressures. This phasic pullback may be used to measure LV-AO:

a. Mean pressure gradient for the quick Hakki valve area formula
b. Mean pressure gradient for the Gorlin valve area formula
c. Peak-to-peak pressure gradient for the quick Hakki valve area formula
d. Peak-to-peak pressure gradient for the Gorlin valve area formula

Answer: c. Peak-to-peak pressure gradient for the quick Hakki valve area formula. For the Gorlin formula you need simultaneous LV-AO pressures, recorded with 2 catheters, 2 transducers and superimposed tracings, recorded at fast speed. For the quick Hakki formula you only need the peak-to-peak gradient measured on pullback. In the above example where Gorlins AVA = 0.55 cm^2, the Hakki formula gives 3.45 /√59 = 0.45 cm^2

Kern says, "The mean pressure gradient is measured by planimetry of the superimposed aortic and LV pressure tracings. [needed for Gorlin formula] Peak-to-peak pressure gradients are easily seen and are often used as an estimate of the severity of stenosis. The peak-to-peak gradient is not equivalent to mean gradient....Simplified formulas provide quick in-laboratory determination of aortic valve area. Aortic valve area can be estimated closely as CO divided by the square root of the LV-aortic peak-to-peak pressure difference."
Quick valve area (Hakki formula) = (CO L/min) / √ (LV-aortic peak-to-peak gradient)"

Kern says that this quick method *differs from the Gorlin* aortic valve area by approximately 18% in low-flow states (CO<2.5 L/min) or tachycardia (>100 beats/min). However, the Gorlin formula is not perfect either, it *overestimates* the severity of valve stenosis in low-flow states, and should be modified with empirically derived constants. Some authors list the Hakki formula using the mean pressure gradient instead of the peak-to-peak gradient. See: Kern, chapter on "Hemodynamic Data" Keywords: Can use peak-to-peak pullback gradient for the Hakki aortic valve area formula

---

Mitral Valve Area Calculation

462. In mitral stenosis with atrial fibrillation an accurate pressure gradient must be recorded for Gorlin valve area calculation. For this, the most accurate pressure recordings would be provided by:

a. Pullback of PAW catheter to PA
b. Pullback of a transseptal LV catheter into LA
c. Simultaneous LV and LA (via pigtail and transseptal catheters)
d. Simultaneous LV and PAW (via pigtail and Swan-Ganz catheter)

ANSWER c. Simultaneous LV and LA via pigtail and transseptal catheters. Kern says, *"Using direct LA pressure with transseptal measurements is the most accurate method.*

Transseptal catheterization should be performed to confirm large pressure gradients, especially for suspected prosthetic mitral stenosis. However, if the wedge pressure/LV pressure tracings show no significant gradients, transseptal catheterization is unnecessary."

See: Kern, chapter on "Hemodynamics."

463. How should the simultaneous pressure recordings be run for hand calculation of mitral valve area?

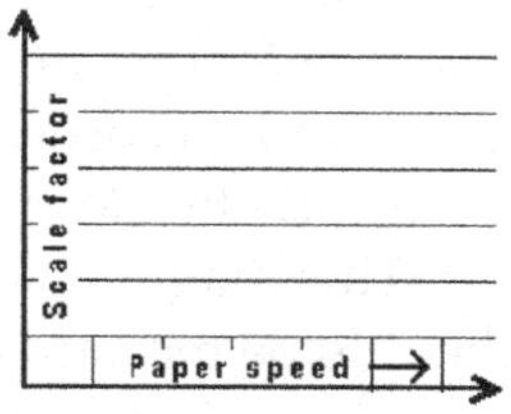

a. x 25 or x 50 scale on speed 25 mm/sec
b. x 25 or x 50 scale on speed 100 mm/sec
c. x 100 or x 200 scale on speed 25 mm/sec
d. x 100 or x 200 scale on speed 100 mm/sec

ANSWER b. x 25 or x 50 scale on speed 100 mm/sec. In MS the diastolic gradient must be planimetered in order to estimate the mean gradient. This gradient may be only 5-10 mmHg. So it must be magnified by recording on high sensitivity and paper speeds. A calibration of x 25 or x 40 full scale gain will amplify the diastolic portion of the tracing. This will "peg" the LV channel so it goes off the top of the paper. Rapid paper speeds of 50 or 100 mm/sec will spread the recording out horizontally. Gradients amplified like this are easier to see and make planimetery more accurate. Also, record these pressures with appropriate reference time and pressure grid lines. Pepine says,

"Recordings should be made at a paper speed of 100 mm/sec and at a gain which produces a recorded image of the gradient which is large enough to measure accurately. Average gradients should be determined by planimetric methods."

NOT ON EXAM. For hand calculation, instead of copying both recordings through tracing paper, I prefer to make 2 Xerox copies of the valve areas to be measured. Then place them both on a window or light table so that both tracings show through. For accuracy you must superimpose the two pressure grids and carefully slide the tracings horizontally until the time delay is corrected. Then redraw the PAW over the LV tracing. This prevents errors in retracing the LV and keeps the scale and time line information on one page. Then you can planimeter the gradient seen. **See:** Baim, chapter on "Calculation of Stenotic Valve Orifice Area" and Pepine, chapter on "Valve Function."

464. The mean gradient of mitral stenosis is the average pressure difference between what 2 pressures?

a. LA end diastolic and LV end diastolic
b. Mean PAW and mean LV
c. Average systolic LA and average systolic LV
d. Average diastolic LA and average diastolic LV

ANSWER d. Average diastolic LA (or PAW) - average diastolic LV. This is the area of gradient during the diastolic filling period shown shaded. It can be measured with planimeter - a device that measures square cm area by drawing around an area, but all hemodynamic recorders do this automatically by electronic integration.

This diagram shows the actual gradient to be measured on the right. Once this area is measured, it is divided by the diastolic filling period (dfp) measured between pressure crossover points.

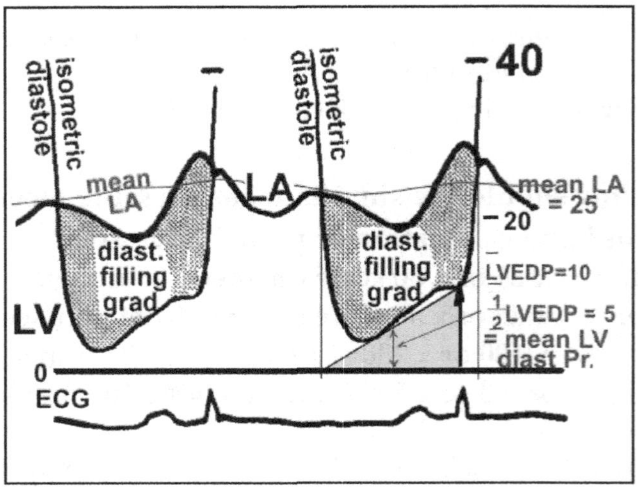

Cui estimate of mean LA-LV gradient in MS.

ESTIMATE MEAN MS GRADIENT:

Kern notes a quick estimation of the MS gradient by subtracting ½ the LVEDP from the mean LA or wedge pressure as shown. We normally record the mean wedge or LA and the LVEDP. So, just take ½ of the LVEDP from the average mean pressure for the MS gradient. This is the Cui method. The diagram shows how a triangle follows the diastolic LV pressure. The measured LVEDP was 10 mmHg, so ½ of 10 is 5 mmHg. Subtract this from mean LA to get the mean mitral gradient of 5 mmHg to be used in the simplified Hakki equation.

Kern says: "Cui et al simplified estimation of the mitral valve gradient and thus simplified the calculation of MVA from hemodynamic tracings. Because the mean mitral valve gradient is the pressure difference between the mean left atrium pressure (MLAP) and mean left ventricular pressure (MLVP) during diastole (i.e., MLVG = MLAP - MLVP), the computation of the mean mitral valve gradient depends on simply knowing the MLVP. The MLAP is easily obtained from the electronically meaned LA signal on the hemodynamic recorder. The area under the LV pressure during diastole is roughly a triangle with the three corners formed from the intersections of the DFP starting and ending points (mitral valve closure and opening) marking the vertical lines intersecting with the LV pressure line (rising diagonally across diastole). This triangular area can be estimated from the rectangular area LVEDP × DFP divided by 2. Thus, the MLVPdiast. is equal to the LVEDP/2. From this key calculation, the mitral valve gradient is therefore simplified as MVG = MLAP - LVEDP/2."

This quick estimation method works well in MS if the LV diastole is triangular. **See**: Kern, chapter on Hemodynamic Data

465. A patient with MS is sent to cath because of inconclusive echocardiography results. While measuring LV-PAW gradients, it is important to:

a. Confirm that the balloon is in the anterior lung zone (zone 1)

b. Confirm good wedge waveforms and wedge blood sample > 95% O2 sat.

c. Confirm that the LV waveform is not critically damped or ventricularized

d. Use the same transducer for separate LV & wedge measurements

ANSWER b. Confirm good wedge waveforms and wedge blood sample > 95% O2 sat. Ragosta says, "Importantly, if the PCWP is used, the operator must pay meticulous attention to detail and confirm the wedge pressure using oximetry sampling to demonstrate an arterial saturation >95%. Patients with evidence of significant gradient using the PCWP who have discrepant noninvasive studies, poor-quality wedge pressure waveforms, pulmonary hypertension, or prior prosthetic valve surgery should be considered for transseptal catheterization to confirm the gradient with a left atrial pressure measurement before making a major decision related to the mitral valve stenosis." Wedge should be in posterior lung zone and critically damped. Two transducers should be used for simultaneous pressures. See Ragosta, chapter on "Mitral Valve Disorders" Keywords: MS requires good wedge

USE THIS DIAGRAM FOR THE NEXT SIX QUESTIONS.

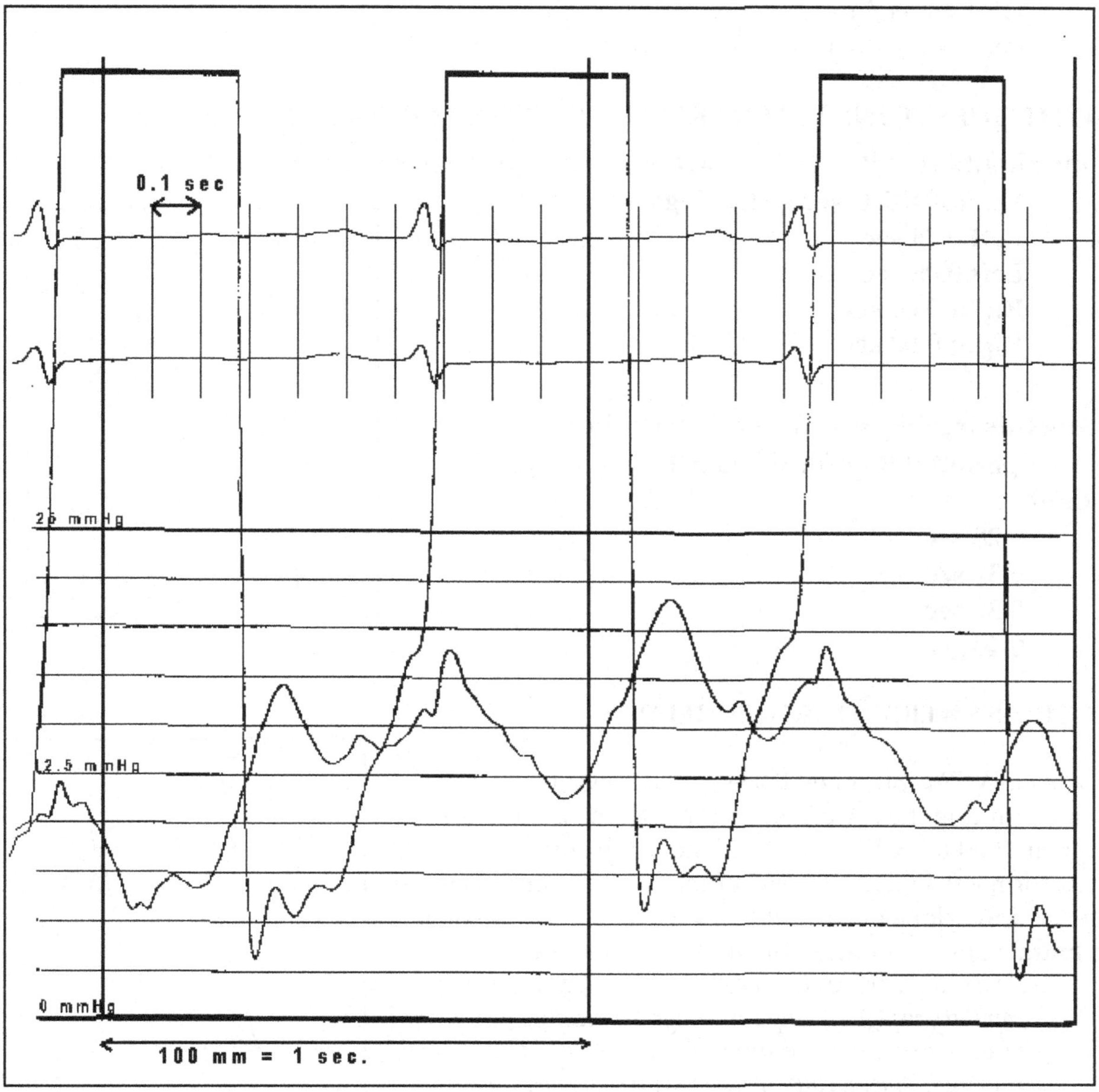

Patient # 466 - 472: LV and PAW x 25 at speed 100 mm/sec, CO = 3.75 L/min

466. **Estimate the heart rate of the above patient.**

- a. **64 beats/min**
- b. **78 beats/min**
- c. **86 beats/min**
- d. **128 beats/min**

ANSWER b. 78 beats/min. RR interval is 0.78 sec. If the paper speed is 100 mm/sec and the time lines are 0.1 as shown, it is EASY to calculate the rr interval and heart rate. Just use the time lines to count up the rr time intervals, as shown, then divide each into 60 sec/min.

Know the heart rate formula: HR = 60/ r-r interval

RR interval = 0.78 sec/beat
HR (Bts/min) = 60 (sec/min) / r-r interval in (sec/bt)
HR = 60 sec/min / 0.78 sec = 78 beats/min.
See: Baim and Grossman, chapter on "Assessing Valvular Stenosis."

BOTH QUESTIONS BELOW REFER TO THE SAME PATIENT ABOVE.

467. **How should this PA wedge tracing be shifted to measure mitral valve area?**

- a. **Do not shift wedge tracings**
- b. **Left 0.04 sec**
- c. **Left 0.08 sec**
- d. **Right 0.04 sec**
- e. **Right 0.08 sec**

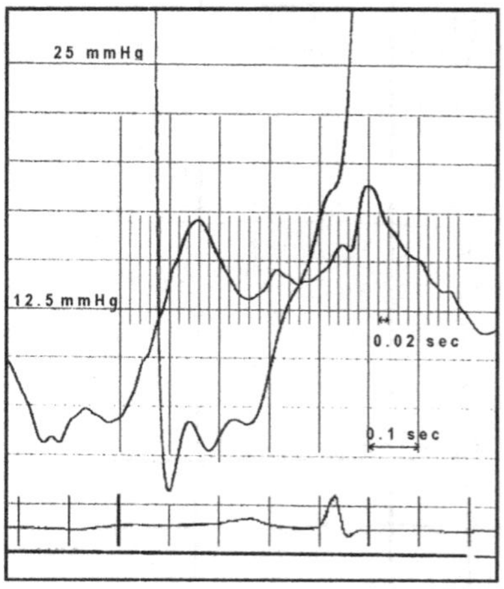

468. **From this tracing, estimate the diastolic filling period (DFP) for the Gorlin valve area formula.**

- a. **0.28 sec**
- b. **0.32 sec**
- c. **0.36 sec**
- d. **0.40 sec**

BOTH ANSWERS TOGETHER BELOW:

467. ANSWER c. Shift Left 0.08 sec. There is often a delay in transmitting the LA pressure through the pulmonary capillary bed to PCW. Trace and move the entire waveform left so that the peak of the "v" wave intersects the LV downslope or peak of the R wave. This is the time of mitral valve opening. Baim and Grossman say,

"the a and v waves in an optimally damped pulmonary capillary wedge tracing are delayed typically by 50 to 70 msec compared with a simultaneous left atrial pressure tracing. Thus, ideally the wedge pressure should be realigned with the left ventricular pressure (using tracing paper) by shifting it leftward by 50 to 70 msec."

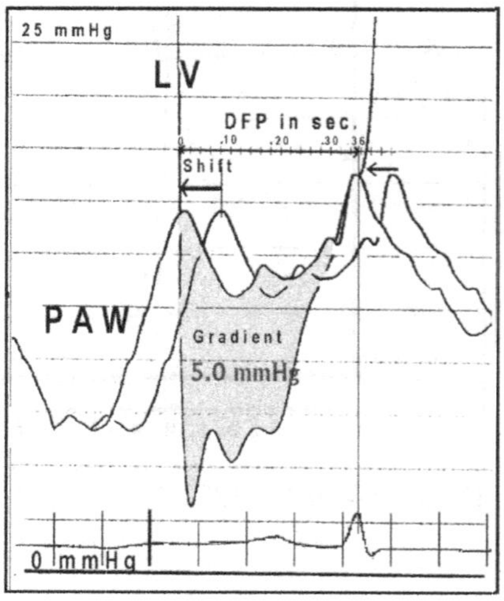

This PAW tracing shown was taken with a Swan-Ganz catheter which has especially bad damping and delay characteristics. The long formula using a planimeter to estimate the mean gradient is: Mean Gradient = (Gradient area in cm^2 x Scale factor in mmHg/cm) / (filling period in cm / paper speed in cm/sec.) Note that the units cancel out to give the average gradient in mmHg. Instead of tracing paper I prefer to make 2 Xerox copies of the valve areas to me measured. Then place them both on a window or light table so that both tracings show through. For accuracy you must superimpose the two pressure grids and carefully slide the tracings horizontally until the time delay is corrected. Then redraw the PAW over the top tracing. This prevents errors in retracing the LV and keeps the scale and time line information on one page.
See: Baim, chapter on "Calculation of Stenotic Valve Orifice Area."

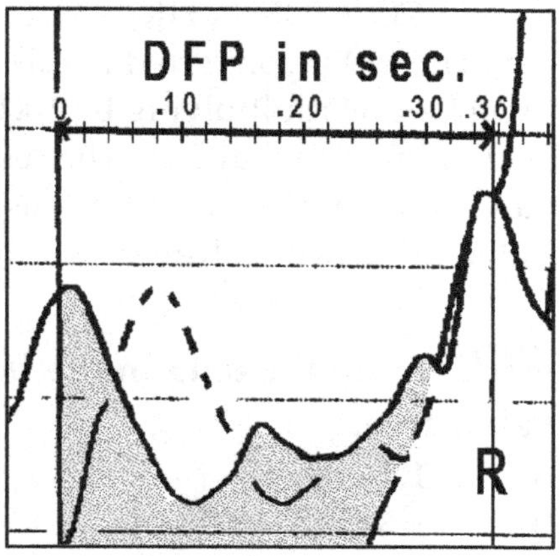

468. ANSWER c. DFP=0.36 sec. Baim and Grossman say,

> "*The diastolic filling period begins at mitral valve opening and continues until end diastole.... using the average measured length between initial PCW - LV crossover in early diastole and end diastole (peak of the R wave by ECG).*"

In this example the end diastolic pressure crossover point appears somewhat delayed as pressures equalize during the atrial kick. This makes it difficult to know where to place the end of diastole. But, the end of diastole is traditionally marked by the peak of the R wave. It is essential to draw accurate vertical lines from these pressure crossover points to accurately measure horizontally between them for the DFP. Although only one beat is measured here, in sinus rhythm 5 beats should be measured to get an average DFP, 10 beats if patient in atrial fibrillation.

Pepine says, "*Since transvalvular flow enters the equation linearly and the pressure gradient enters the equation as a square root function, the valve area calculation is more strongly influenced by the cardiac output and the **flow time measurements**. Thus it is particularly important that these measurements be precise.*"

The DFP may be measured in seconds as shown here, or in millimeters and then converted to seconds by dividing by the paper speed.
See: Baim, chapter on "Calculation of Stenotic Valve Orifice Area" and Pepine, chapter on "Valve Function." **Keywords:** Measure DFP in MS

469. Using the data in the box calculate the FLOW for the numerator of the Gorlin valve area equation.

a. **117. ml/diastolic sec**
b. **128. ml/diastolic sec**
c. **134. ml/diastolic sec**
d. **142. ml/diastolic sec**

Patient # 469	Cath Data
Fick CO	= 3.75 L/min
DFP	= .36 sec/beat
Mean Gradient	= 5 mmHg
HR	= 79 beats/min

ANSWER c. 134. ml/diastolic sec. The formula for the numerator of the Gorlin formula is also termed "Flow."

Flow = CO / (DFP x HR)

Flow = CO / (DFP x HR) = (3750 ml/min) / (0.36 sec/bt. x 78 bts./min) = 134 ml/systolic sec. The CO is converted to ml/sec by multiplying times 1000 ml/L. The CO is converted to ml/sec by multiplying by 1000 ml/L. The product of Sep x HR (termed SEP) must then be divided into that CO. The resulting "flow" is how many ml/sec would flow through the valve if it were open continuously. **See:** Baim and Grossman, chapter on "Assessing Valvular Stenosis." **Keywords:** aortic valve "Flow" calculation

470. From the data in the box on the patient above, calculate the Gorlin mitral valve area.

a. **1.1 cm^2**
b. **1.6 cm^2**
c. **2.5 cm^2**
d. **3.1 cm^2**

#470	Cath Data
Flow	= 134. ml/diast. sec.
Mean gradient	= 5 mmHg
HR	= 78 b/min

ANSWER b. 1.6 cm^2. Once the "Flow" and mean gradient are found simply substitute them into the Gorlin mitral valve area (MVA) formula: (Note the square root of 5 = 2.24)

$$MVA = \frac{Flow}{38 \sqrt{\text{Mean gradient}}}$$

MVA = 134/ 38 $\sqrt{5}$ = 134/85.1 = 1.57 cm^2 This not critical MS, as it is above the 1-1.5 cm^2 cut point. Delay surgery. Many computers will not calculate a valve area if the gradient is less than 5 mmHg, because this gradient is insignificant and because the valve area calculation becomes inaccurate with low gradients.

The diagram below shows how mitral stenosis may look from the LV. Note that normally there are several orifices through which blood may enter the LV. These are termed secondary orifices in the spaces between the chordae tendinea. **See:** Kern, chapter on "Hemodynamics." **Keywords**: calculate Mitral valve area

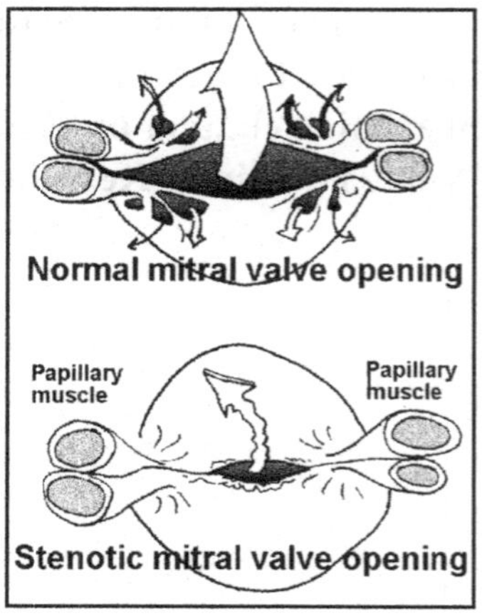

471. **Compared to the Gorlin formula for mitral valve area, the short Hakki formula is most inaccurate when:**

- a. **HR > 100 /min**
- b. **Atrial fibrillation is present**
- c. **Aortic regurgitation is also present**
- d. **Mean gradient is less than 5 mmHg**

ANSWER a. HR > 100 / min. Ragosta says, "When compared to the traditional Gorlin formula, the simplified formula may lead to significant disparity, especially if tachycardia is present (heart rate >100 beats/ min)(or bradycardia). Therefore, the simplified formula should be used with great caution." See: Ragosta, chapter on "Mitral Valve Disorders"
Keywords: Hakki most inaccurate in tachycardia

USE THIS DIAGRAM FOR THE NEXT FIVE QUESTIONS

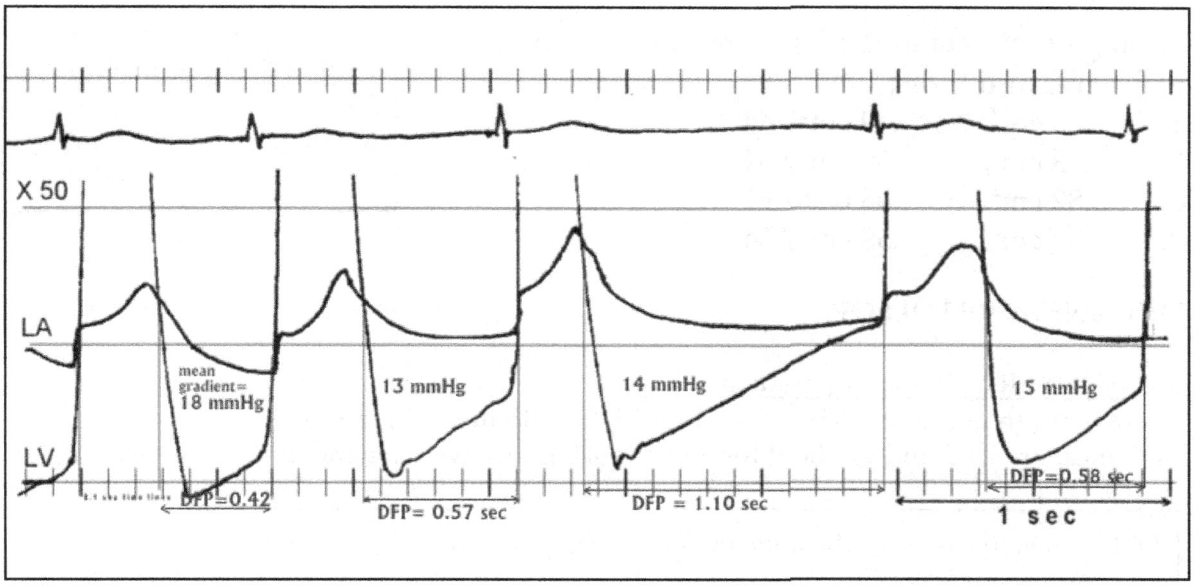

Patient # 472 - 476: Mitral Stenosis: Simultaneous LA & LV X 50, with 0.1 sec time lines

472. **From the 4 MS gradient areas shown, estimate the mean gradient?**

- a. **8 mmHg**
- b. **11 mmHg**
- c. **15 mmHg**
- d. **20 mmHg**

473. **In the patient above measure the average of 4 diastolic filling periods (DFP)?**

- a. **DFP = 0.67 sec**
- b. **DFP = 0.74 sec**
- c. **DFP = 0.82 sec**
- d. **DFP = 0.90 sec**

474. **In the patient above measure the average heart rate (HR)?**
a. **40 beats/min**
b. **48 beats/min**
c. **55 beats/min**
d. **61 beats/min**

475. **From the patient data in the box, compute mitral valve FLOW for use in the numerator of the Gorlin valve area formula.**
a. **108 ml/diastolic sec**
b. **117 ml/diastolic sec**
c. **125 ml/diastolic sec**
d. **134 ml/diastolic sec**

Patient # 475	Cath Data
Fick CO	= 5.5 L/min
HR	= 61 b/min
DFP	= .67 sec
Mean gradient	= 15 mmHg

476. **From patient data in the box compute the mitral valve area and index.**
a. **.68 cm^2, .40 cm^2/M^2**
b. **.75 cm^2, .38 cm^2/M^2**
c. **.82 cm^2, .48 cm^2/M^2**
d. **.92 cm^2, .53 cm^2/M^2**

Patient # 476	Cath Data
Flow	= 135 ml/sec
Mean gradient	= 15 mmHg
BSA	= 1.70 M^2

FIVE ANSWERS FOLLOW:

472. ANSWER c. 15 mmHg gradient.
Average mean gradient = (18 + 13 + 14 + 15)/4 = **15 mmHg gradient**
Here measure DFP and gradient for all 4 beats because we have the full RR intervals and

> DFP(sec) is the average diastolic time between pressure crossover points

associated gradient for all four beats. Although we only have 4 beats, a total of 10 beats should be recorded and measured in patients with atrial fibrillation. **See:** Kern, chapter on "Hemodynamics."

473. ANSWER a. DFP = 0.67 sec. The average dfp of 4 beats was measured above.
Measured DFP average = (0.42 + 0.57 + 1.10 + .58)/4 = 0.67 sec.
See: Kern, chapter on "Hemodynamics." **Keywords**: calculate mean DFP

474. ANSWER d. HR = 61 beats/min. When the heart rate varies like this, you need to measure the average over several beats. In atrial fibrillation Kern recommends the average of 10 beats. Measure the length of each RR interval in seconds (note ten small 0.1 sec divisions) The HR formula becomes:

> HR (bts./min) = [60 sec/min]/ r-r interval (sec)

Average RR interval is (.70 + .91 + 1.38 + .94)/4 =0.98 sec
HR = (60 sec/min) / (0.98 sec) = 61 beats/min

See: Baim and Grossman, chapter on "Assessing Valvular Stenosis."

475. ANSWER d. FLOW= 135 ml/diastolic sec. The numerator of the Gorlin formula is also termed "Flow." Its formula is:

Flow = CO / (DFP x HR)

Flow = CO / (DFP x HR) = (5500 ml/min) / (0.67 sec/bt. x 61 bts./min) = 135 ml/diastolic sec. The CO is converted to ml/sec by multiplying by 1000 ml/L. The average DFP is multiplied times the heart rate and then is divided into the CO. The resulting "flow" is how many ml/sec would flow through the valve if it were open continuously.
See: Kern, chapter on "Hemodynamics." **Keywords**: mitral valve "Flow" calculation

476. ANSWER d. 0.92 cm^2, 0.53 cm^2 / M^2. Once the "Flow" and mean gradient are found simply substitute them into the Gorlin formula: (Note the square root of √15 = 3.87) MVA = 135/ 38 √15 = 135 / (38 x 3.87) =0.92 cm^2 which is slightly below the critical MVA of 1.0 cm^2. Surgery is indicated. MVA index = MVA / BSA = 0.92 cm^2 / 1.7 M^2 = 0.48 cm^2/ M^2. **See:** Kern, chapter on "Hemodynamics."

Gorlin Mitral Valve Area

$$MVA = \frac{Flow}{38 \sqrt{\text{Mean gradient}}}$$

MVAI = MVA/BSA

USE THESE SIMULTANEOUS PRESSURES FOR THE NEXT QUESTION.

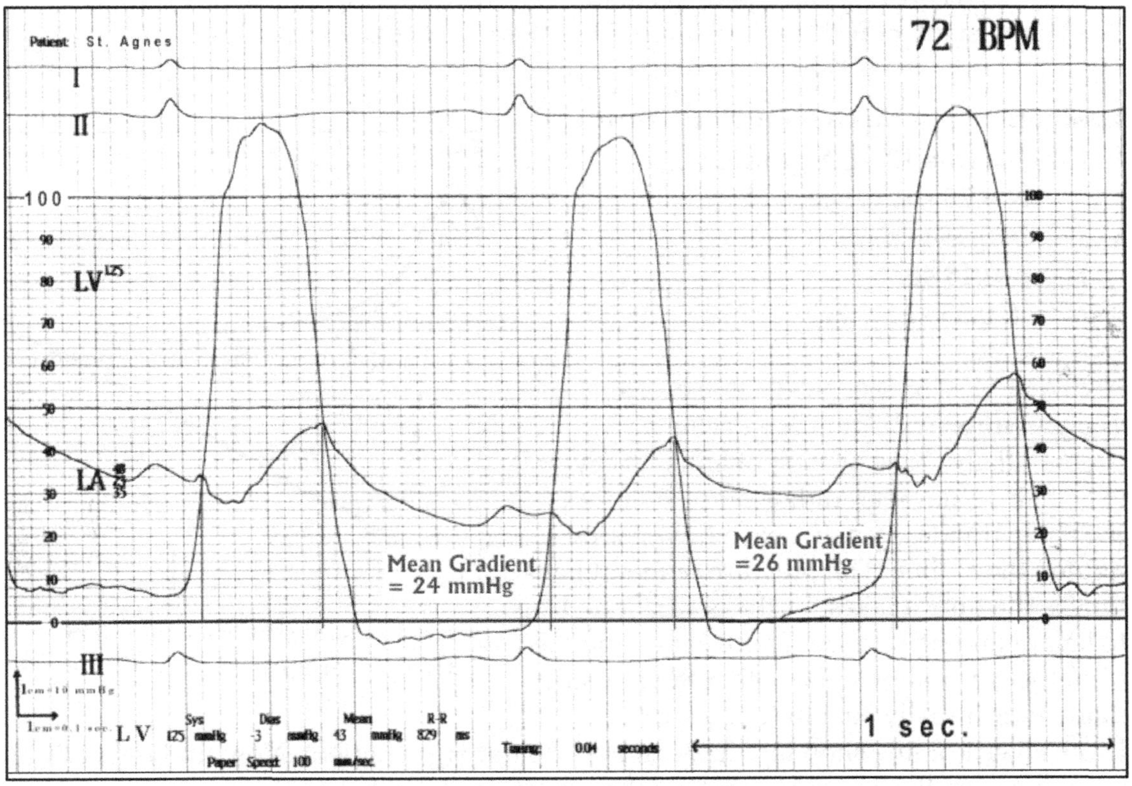

477. The MS patient above had a left heart and transseptal cath done. From the data calculated and this Fick CO data, calculate the Gorlin mitral valve area?

a. 0.27 cm^2
b. 0.38 cm^2
c. 0.48 cm^2
d. 0.59 cm^2

Patient # 477	Cath Data
O2 Cons. (ml O2/min)	207
Arterial O2 Content (vol%)	20.1
Venous O2 Content (vol%)	9.5

ANSWER a. 0.27 cm^2.

Fick CO = 207 / [10 x (20.1-9.5)] = 207 / 106 = 1.95 L/min
Average dfp time = .53 sec
Average mean gradient = (24 + 26)/ 3 = 25. mmHg
Average HR = 60 / 0.82 sec = 73 bpm (HR printed from recorder is close.)
Flow= CO/(DFP x HR) =1950/(0.53 x 73) = 50.4 ml/diastolic sec
Gorlin VA = Flow/(38 x $\sqrt{25}$.) = 50.4 / (38 x 5.0) = 0.27 cm^2

This is a critically narrowed mitral valve (< 1.0 cm^2) and needs surgery.
(for your info. Hakki VA = 1.95 / $\sqrt{27.4}$ = 0.38 cm^2)
The patient's LV should not go below zero like this. He may have taken a deep breath during this recording. Have patients hold their breath during critical recordings.
See: Kern, chapter on "Hemodynamics." Keywords: calculate mean gradient

478. Evaluate the hemodynamic pressure ½ time of this LV-LA gradient.

a. 0.25 sec
b. 0.35 sec
c. 0.45 sec
d. 0.55 sec

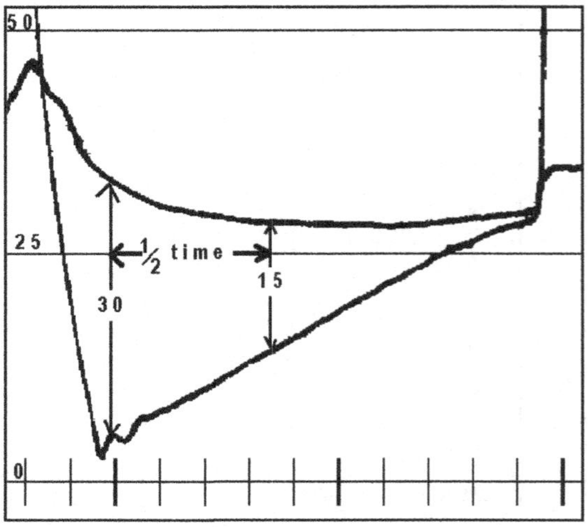

LV & LA x 50, 0.1 sec time lines,
Calculate pressure ½ time

ANSWER b. 0.35 sec. **NOT ON EXAM.**
The pressure gradient in MS declines exponentially. Like any exponential decay (e.g., half value layer, radioisotope half time) the value divides in half - each time period - termed the ½ time. The pressure gradient half-time is the time it takes for the gradient to drop to half of an initial value. This can be estimated from the curve shown. Note that the pressure gradient is initially 30 mm (or 30 mmHg).
Draw a vertical line showing the 30 mm (or 30 mmHg) gradient. Now find the vertical point between the 2 pressures where the gradient is ½ of that or 15 mm or (15 mmHg). Draw a vertical line showing the 15 mm (or 15 mmHg) gradient. Now measure the time between the 2 vertical lines you have drawn. That is termed the pressure half time. If the rate is fast and/or "a" waves are present to distort the "y" descent the gradient can be plotted out on semilogarithmic paper where the decline will appear as a straight line. When you have extrapolated the line to where it does falls to ½ of an initial value, measure

this ½ time.

In mild MS the pressure ½ time is about 0.1 sec.
In moderate MS ½ time is about 0.2 sec.
In severe MS it is greater than 0.3 sec.
(ours at .35 sec is severe)

Note that no CO measurement is required. The Doppler technique of measuring mitral valve area utilizes this same simple half time principle. Simply divide the pressure half time (from Doppler mitral flow) into 220 to get the valve area. Eg. Doppler MVA = 220/ (pressure ½ time in msec) = 220 / 350 = .63 cm^2. In the diagram, note the sloping mitral Doppler in MS. When using Doppler, the half time is measured when its value falls to $1/\sqrt{2}$ or 70% of its initial value. This method is much easier than the Gorlin equation and not reliant upon inaccurate CO measurements.

See: Yang, chapters on "Assessment of ventricular Inflow and Outflow Obstruction." and "Noninvasive Data Relevant to Cardiac Catheterization" **Keywords**: Pressure ½ time

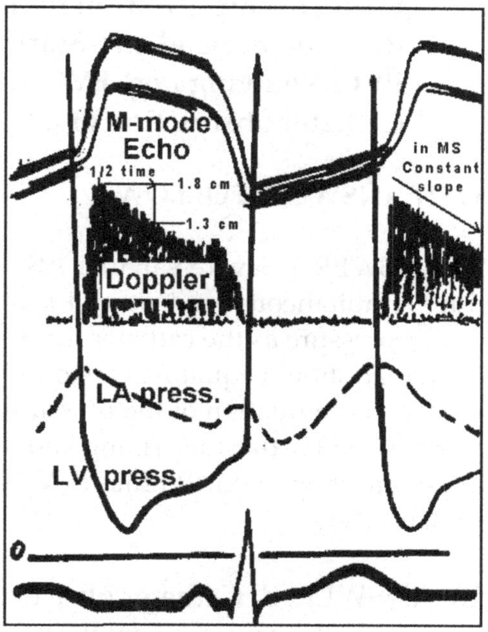

Simultaneous MS hemodynamics: mitral echo, Doppler & pressures

Other

BOTH QUESTIONS BELOW REFER TO THE PRESSURE TRACING BELOW.

479. **This pressure pullback tracing shows: (Note higher AO systolic after pullback.)**

- a. **Severe valvular AS**
- b. **HOCM/IHSS**
- c. **Peripheral pressure amplification**
- d. **False gradient due to unequal sensitivities**

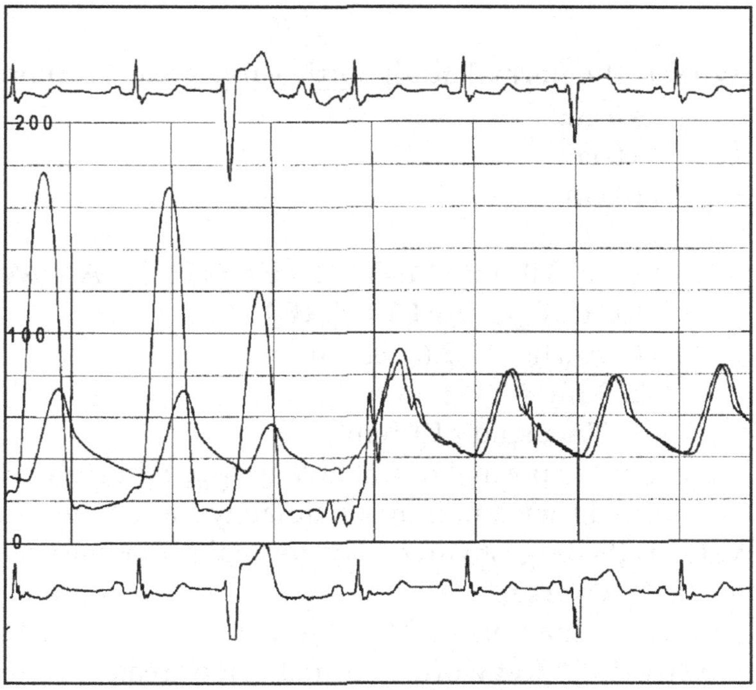

LV pullback and AO x 200, Carabello's sign

480. This recording of simultaneous LV-FA pressures with pullback shows Carabello's sign. The initial AO pressure is falsely low due to:

- a. **Pressure amplification in the periphery**
- b. **Reduced preload and Starling effect**
- c. **PVCs showing post PVC accentuation**
- d. **Catheter obstruction of a tight aortic valve**

BOTH ANSWERS FOLLOW:

479. ANSWER a. Severe valvular AS. The classic valvular aortic stenosis tracing is seen with a simultaneous gradient of 100 mmHg. The pullback then shows a 90 mmHg drop in systolic pressure as the catheter tip crosses the AO valve. In a normal LV-AO pullback, the LV systolic should equal AO systolic. This patient had a PVC during pullback, with normal post PVC accentuation of the pressure. The compensatory pause following the PVC allows for increased LV diastolic filling and increased Starling effect post PVC. **See:** Baim and Grossman, chapter on "Profiles in Valvular Heart Disease." **Keywords:** AS pullback gradient, PVC

480. ANSWER. d. Catheter obstruction of a tight aortic valve. Here is one case of when a simultaneous gradient is misleading and inaccurate. Note the jump in aortic pressure immediately after pullback. This is Carabello's sign. It is a rise in peak arterial pressure during LV catheter withdrawal, associated with **critical** aortic stenosis. It is caused by the retrograde catheter partial obstructing a very narrowed aortic orifice. This increased obstruction is relieved when the catheter is withdrawn. In these cases the gradient is increased by the catheter crossing the valve. A solution would be to record LV via transseptal catheter, and AO via retrograde catheter. **See:** example in Todd, Vol. 3 chapter C3 and Baim and Grossman, chapter on "Profiles in Valvular Heart Disease." **Keywords:** Carabello's sign in severe AS

481. What is the normal adult <u>aortic valve area</u> (#1 in box)?

- a. **3.0 cm^2**
- b. **5.0 cm^2**
- c. **10 cm^2**

<u>VALVE</u>
***1. Aortic**
2. Mitral
3. Tricuspid

ANSWER a. 3.0 cm^2. **MATCH THE OTHER ANSWERS:**

NORMAL	VALVE AREA
1. Aortic	2.6 - 3.5 cm^2
2. Mitral	4 - 6 cm^2
3. Tricuspid	10 +cm^2

Note that the normal mitral area is approximately twice the normal aortic area, and the normal tricuspid is approximately three times the aortic area. The tricuspid valve is the largest valve. The normal pulmonary valve area is very close to the aortic valve area.

See: Yang, chapters on "Assessment of ventricular Inflow and Outflow Obstruction." **Keywords**: normal valve areas

482. Surgery is generally warranted for #1 (AS) when the valve area is less than ______ (critical valve area).

a. **<0.7 - .8 cm^2**
b. **<1.0 - 1.5 cm^2**
c. **<1.5 - 2.0 cm^2**

VALVE
***1. Aortic**
2. Tricuspid
3. Mitral

ANSWER a. <0.7 - .8 cm2. This is the critical number range where symptoms usually begin, and valve surgery or valvuloplasty should proceed. **MATCH THE OTHER ANSWERS:**

VALVE	CRITICAL AREA	
1. Aortic	0.7-.8 cm^2	(or 0.5 - 0.8 cm^2/M^2)
2. Mitral	1 - 1.5 cm^2	(or 1.0 cm^2/M^2)
3. Tricuspid	1.5 - 2.0 cm^2	

Baim and Grossman say,

> ***"An aortic valve area of 0.7 cm² is generally considered severe enough to account for the symptoms of angina, syncope, or heart failure."***

Note that the critical aortic valve area is about ½ of the mitral critical orifice size and average critical areas increase by approximately 0.5 cm^2 (.75 → 1.25 → 1.75 cm^2). Braunwald recommends indexing critical valve areas to BSA. Valve replacement may proceed prior to these critical numbers, depending of the patients's symptoms. Better diagnostic and surgical techniques have made cardiologists and surgeons more confident about doing early surgery for valvular stenosis. **See:** Baim and Grossman, chapter on "Stenotic Valve Calculations" and Braunwald, chapter on "Valvular Heart Disease."
Keywords: Critical AS <0.7 or .8 cm^2

483. This patient has the combined valvular stenosis and insufficiency labeled #1 (MS and MR). When calculating the Gorlin valve area, which CO would you use in the numerator of the FLOW formula ?

a. **FICK CO**
b. **LVMF**
c. **TDCO**
d. **LVMF - Fick CO**
e. **Unable to estimate flow**

Combined Stenosis & Regurg.
***1. MS and MR with high CO**
2. MS and AR with high CO
3. AS and AR with low CO
4. AS and MR with low CO
5. MS, AR, and MR with high CO

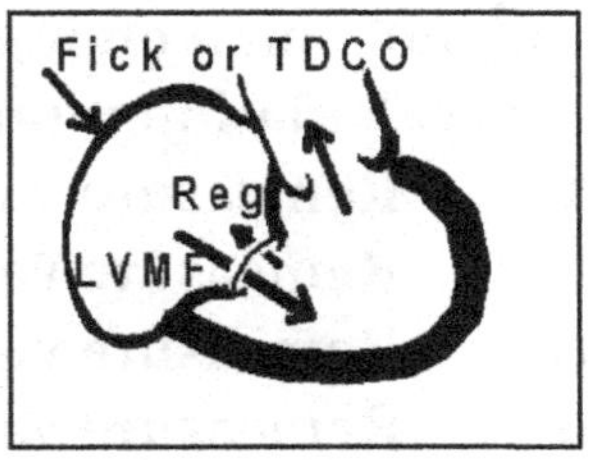

Flows in MS & MR

ANSWER b. LVMF. The total diastolic flow across this regurgitant mitral valve in ventricular diastole is large. Since this valve is also regurgitant, much of that total flow leaks back into the LV during diastole. Here the Total flow (LVMF) is increased by the amount of the regurgitation (Reg.). It clarifies the flows to draw a diagram like this. Label the arrows, total (LVMF), forward (Fick or TDCO), and regurgitation (LVMF - Fick or TDCO). The actual flows can be inserted, either in L/min or as stroke volumes. I like to draw a circle around the stenotic valve to show it is tight, as shown. Then it is clear that the flow needed to calculate the valve area is the large

LVMF through the mitral valve, because it is this large total flow passing through the tight orifice that causes the MS gradient. It turns out that when the stenosis and regurgitation are in the same valve, as here, the flow used in the Gorlin formula is the Total or LVMF flow. When the stenosis and regurgitation are in different valves the flow used in the Gorlin formula is the forward or Fick or thermodilution CO. Fick and thermodilution are the two "net" or "forward" CO methods. The TDCO is relatively more accurate in high COs or when the Fick accuracy is reduced with an *estimated* O_2 consumption. The Fick CO given is most accurate at low COs, or when there is right sided regurgitation fouling up the TDCO. Braunwald says:

> *"The Fick method of determining cardiac output is the most accurate for assessing cardiac output, especially in low-output states. As noted previously, both the dye-dilution technique and the thermodilution technique may provide inaccurate cardiac output data when cardiac output is reduced or when concomitant aortic, mitral, or tricuspid regurgitation is present. In patients with mixed valvular disease (stenosis and regurgitation) of the same valve, the use of forward flow as determined by the Fick method or thermodilution technique will overestimate the severity of the valvular stenosis. This is because the Gorlin formula depends on total forward flow across the stenotic valve, not net forward flow. If valvular regurgitation is present, the angiographic cardiac output is the most appropriate measure of flow. If both aortic and mitral regurgitation are present, flow across a single valve cannot be determined and neither aortic valve area nor mitral valve area can be assessed accurately."*

MATCH OTHER VALVE DISEASES WITH THE BEST METHOD OF CO BELOW.

Combined Stenosis & Regurg.	Use in Gorlin Flow Formula:
1. MS and MR with high CO	use LVMF
2. MS and AR with high CO	use TDCO
3. AS and AR with low CO	use LVMF
4. AS and MR with low CO	use Fick CO
5. MS, AR, and MR with high CO	Unable to calculate

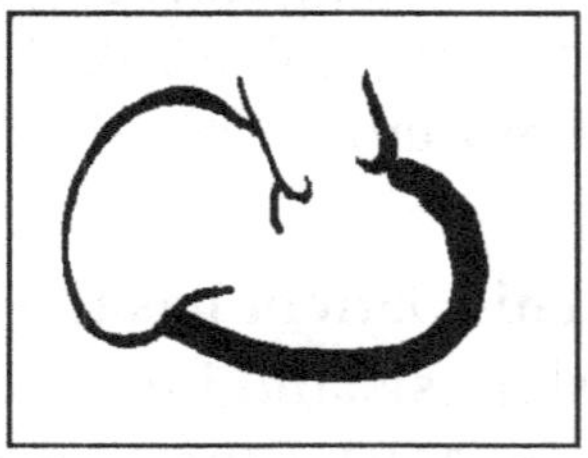
Draw flow arrows

Amount of Regurgitation = LVMF - (Fick or TDCO).

This method of calculating regurgitant volume is rather crude because it mixes two methods of measuring stroke volume. It also assumes the HR remains constant between the various methods of measuring SV. If in doubt about which CO to use and a valve calculation, calculate 2 valve areas, one for each CO method. **See**: Braunwald, chapter on "Cardiac Catheterization." **Keywords:** What Flow in combined stenosis regurgitation patients?

484. At cath, a patient with a CO =4.0 L/min has a calculated aortic valve area of 0.8 cm^2, not small enough to recommend TAVR. How can you make a repeat valve area calculation more accurate and decisive?

a. **Remeasure valve area with rapid atrial pacing**
b. **Remeasure valve area with dobutamine administration**
c. **Remeasure valve area with of adenosine administration**
d. **Remeasure valve area with inhalation of nitric oxide**

ANSWERS: b. Remeasure valve area with dobutamine administration to increase the CO and gradient. A small gradient makes the Gorlin valve area calculation inaccurate. Inaccurate valve area measurement may cause a patient to be denied surgery when he or she needs it, or prematurely push him/her into surgery.

Stenotic valves are usually rigid and cannot dilate. So, the valve area will not normally change significantly with increased cardiac output. But, increasing the cardiac output with dobutamine will increase the gradient and make the calculation of the fixed valve area more accurate and definitive.

Grossman says, "We recommend cautious hemodynamic manipulation with dobutamine or nitroprusside for patients with a cardiac output of <4.5 L/min who have a transvalvular gradient <40 mmHg and a valve resistance of <275 dyn.sec.cm-5. If patients respond substantially increasing the measured gradient, they probably have truly severe aortic stenosis and may benefit from aortic valve replacement. However, if cardiac output increases substantially but gradient increases only slightly or actually declines, the aortic stenosis is" **See**: Braunwald, chapter on "Valvular Heart Disease."
↑↑ gradient

485. What is wrong with this valve area calculation?

- **a. Should have used TDCO**
- **b. Should have used LVMF**
- **c. Should use Hakki formula**
- **d. Too great a difference between peak and mean gradients**

Patient # 485	**Cath Data on Patient with AS and AR**	
Heart Rate	(beats/min)	56
O2 consumption	(assumed ml/min)	140
A-V O2 difference	(vol %)	2.0
Fick Cardiac Output	(L/min)	7.00
Fick Stroke Volume	(ml)	125
Thermodilution Cardiac Output	(L/min)	4.50
Thermodilution Stroke Volume	(ml)	80
Angiographic Cardiac Output	(LVMF in L/min)	7.90
Angiographic Stroke Volume	(ml)	141
Aortic Valve Calculations	**units**	
Cardiac Output used for valve area	(L/min)	7.00
Mean Gradient	(mmHg)	52
Systolic peak-peak gradient	(mmHg)	103
Peak Inst. Gradient	(mmHg)	107
Flow	(ml/sec)	318
Valve Area	(cm^2)	.0.99

ANSWER b. Should have used LVMF. Here all three CO's are significantly different. Which to use? The Fick uses an assumed O2 consumption and gives a high CO. Fick is relatively inaccurate with high CO's since the A-V difference is very narrow (2.0 vol%). The TDCO is the most accurate net forward flow into the LV. But flow out the aortic valve is more complicated. Since the aortic valve is both stenotic and regurgitant the total flow through it in systole causing the systolic gradient is the LVMF.

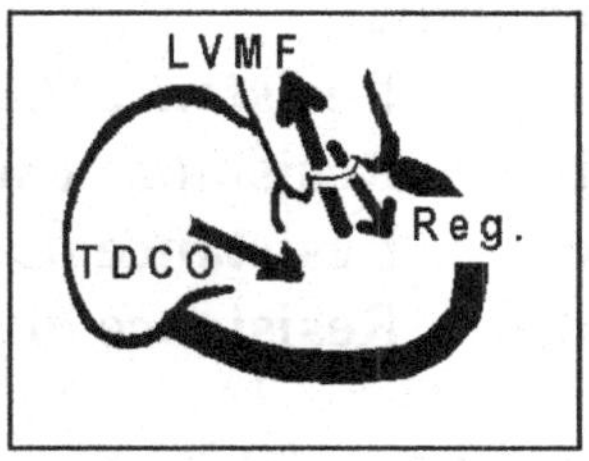

Flows in AS & AR

Kern says,

> "*Angiographic cardiac output determination provides the best estimate of cardiac output through a stenotic valve when any degree of regurgitation is present.*" *[in that valve.]*

Individuals responsible for hemodynamic calculations must be able to assess the accuracy of data, and troubleshoot questionable values. If in doubt about which CO to use for the valve area, calculate two valve areas, one for each CO. **See**: Braunwald, chapter on "Cardiac Catheterization." **Keywords:** What Flow in combined stenosis regurgitation patients?

486. What is the most accurate TOTAL cardiac output when the patient has both stenosis and regurgitation in an aortic valve (E.g., systolic aortic flow in combined AS and AI)?

- a. **Fick**
- b. **Angiographic**
- c. **Thermodilution**
- d. **Green dye**

Answer: b. Angiographic. There are two measures of flow through a leaky valve: Total and forward CO. Total flow uses the LV angio CO which is the largest of the 3 CO's. It is also termed LVMF . The Total flow passes antegrade, and some leaks back retrograde. LVMF measures how much the LV is pumping. Some of that pumped blood may go to a shunt or regurgitate. Remember, Total flow is the largest flow.

Forward flow is the smallest CO or average flow - either Fick or thermodilution CO. Fick and Thermodilution CO measure the average blood flow though the lungs. The difference between Total and forward CO is the valvular regurgitation.

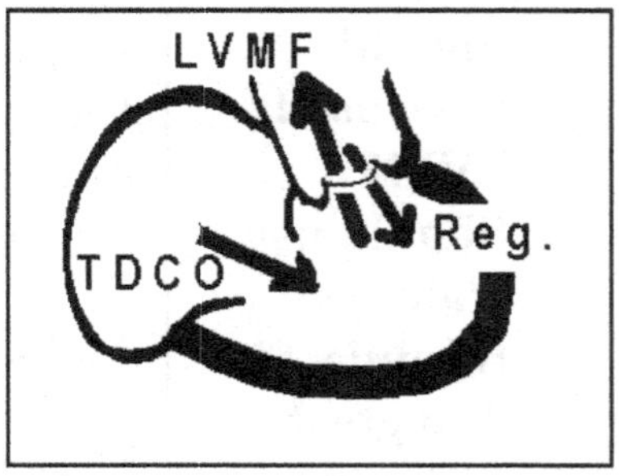

This "total" or "forward" designation becomes important when you calculate the valve area of a valve that is both stenotic and leaky, because you want the flow through the valve that causes the gradient. In the case of combined AS & AI, the systolic flow is the largest or total flow - the angiographic CO. Here, the "total CO" should be used to calculate valve area. Note, that if a valve does not leak the flow through it is always the average or forward flow (Fick or Thermodilution CO). It helps to diagram the various flows as arrows as shown. Note how the LVMF arrow is longest. See: Kern, chapter on "Hemodynamic Data" Keywords: TOTAL Cardiac Output = largest = LVMF

487. How does the calculation of valve resistance differ from the Gorlin valve area formula?

- a. **Resistance uses systemic vascular resistance**
- b. **Resistance uses ejection fraction instead of CO**
- c. **Resistance uses adjusted heart rate instead of SEP**
- d. **Resistance does not take the square root of the gradient**

ANSWERS **d. Valve resistance does not take the square root of the gradient.**

Valve Resistance = [mean gradient / (CO / SEP)] x 1.33 dynes.sec.cm^{-5}

Note that it is reciprocal to valve area, as resistance increases the valve area decreases. Resistance uses the gradient, not square of the gradient. Kern says,

"Valve resistance, a measure of valve obstruction has recently been shown to have clinical utility.... Resistance represents a complimentary index. It is not a replacement for valve area."

There is a gray area when the CO is low and the critical Gorlin valve area is between 0.7 and 1.1 cm^2. Should the patient have surgery or not? An elevated valve resistance (>250 dynes.sec.cm^{-5}) can help make that decision....Kern also says,

"Valve resistance provides an alternative method to assess valve obstruction. It is calculated using the same variables used for valve area measurement. In contrast to valve area, the mean pressure gradient is considered to be a linear variable rather than taken as square root term.... Thus, the contribution of pressure gradient to the magnitude of valve resistance is greater."

See: Kern, Chapter on "Hemodynamic Data." **Keywords**: Valve resistance, mean gradient

488. To evaluate the degree of "2nd stenosis" in severe MS calculate:

a. **RV preload**
b. **LV preload**
c. **Pulmonary arteriolar resistance**
d. **Systemic vascular resistance**

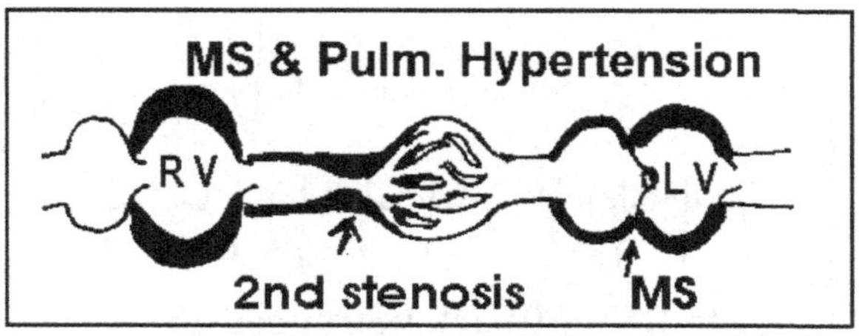

Reactive Pulm. Hypertension (after Baim)

ANSWER c. Pulmonary arteriolar resistance. This 2nd stenosis in MS is termed "Reactive Pulmonary Hypertension" and is assessed by calculating PAR. As the pulmonary arterioles hypertrophy the PAR increases. The RV pressure increases and the RV hypertrophies.

In the diagram note the mitral stenosis on the right. Then note the 2nd stenosis associated with the high pulmonary capillary resistance. Finally note the resulting RV hypertrophy. See: Braunwald, chapter on "Pulmonary Hypertension." **Keywords:** MS, Reactive pulmonary hypertension, 2nd stenosis

489. A patient with AS was cathed eight years ago. With the data shown, and the Hakki formula you can predict that his valve area has:

Patient # 489	Cath Data 2003	Cath Data 2011
Gradient	16 mmHg	36 mmHg
HR	75	80
Fick CO	4.0	6.0

a. **Decreased**
b. **Stayed the same**
c. **Increased**
d. **Inadequate information**

ANSWER b. Stayed the same. Hakki valve area is the relationship between CO and $\sqrt{}$gradient. Here the gradient went up, but the CO also went up. Using the Hakki quick formula $VA_{2003} = 4 / \sqrt{16} = 1.0\ cm^2$ and $VA_{2011} = 6 / \sqrt{36} = 1.0\ cm^2$. A Gorlin valve area calculation would be more accurate, but mean gradient and SEP will be needed. **See:** Kern,

Chapter on "Hemodynamic Data." **Keywords**: Valve area changes

490. In symptomatic pulmonary valve stenosis when is valvuloplasty recommended?

- a. **Peak systolic gradient > 10-20 mmHg**
- b. **Peak systolic gradient > 30-50 mmHg**
- c. **Pulmonary valve area > 1 cm^2**
- d. **Pulmonary valve area > 0.5 cm^2**

ANSWER b. Peak systolic gradient > 30-50 mmHg. In symptomatic patients, Ragosta recommends pulmonary valvuloplasty when the peak gradient exceeds 30 mmHg. Baim recommends it when the gradient exceeds 50-100 mmHg. Pulmonary valvuloplasty is highly successful. **See**: Baim and Ragosta **Keywords:** pulmonary valvuloplasty

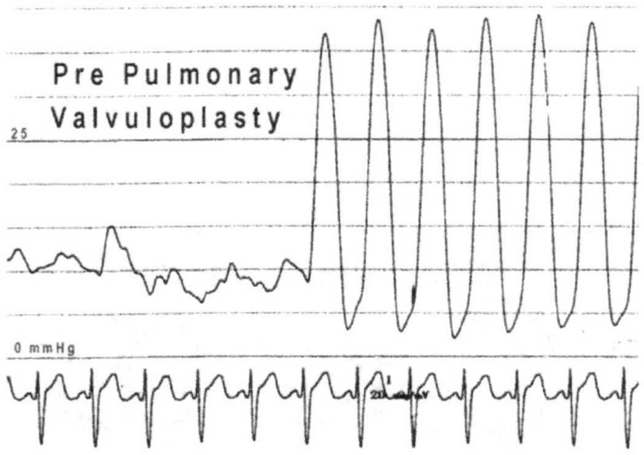

PA to RV pullback x 50 speed 25

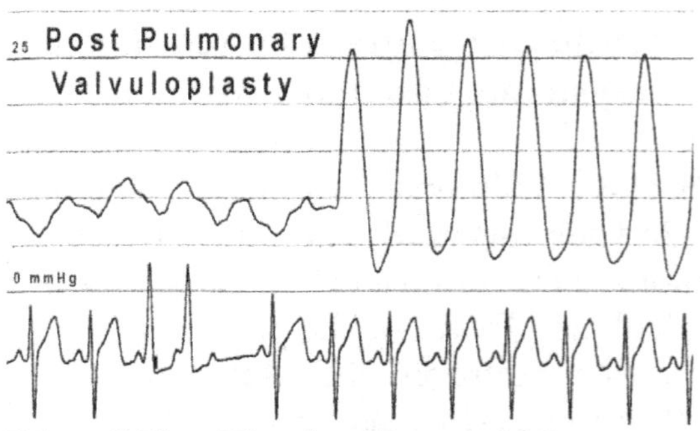

PA to RV pullback x 50 speed 25

USE THIS PA - RV PULLBACK PRESSURES FOR THE NEXT QUESTION.

491. The child above had a pulmonary valvuloplasty done during cardiac cath. Using the Hakki formula and the data given calculate any improvement in valve area. The pulmonary valve area went from an initial area of ___ cm^2 to ___ cm^2 post valvuloplasty.

Patient # 491	**Pre**	**Post**
TDCO	2.6	3.5
HR	116	114

- a. **0.23 cm^2 - 0.10 cm^2 (No improvement)**
- b. **0.10 cm^2 - 0.23 cm^2 (Significant improvement)**
- c. **0.9 cm^2 - 0.5 cm^2 (No improvement)**
- d. **0.5 cm^2 - 0.9 cm^2 (Significant improvement)**

ANSWER d. 0.5 cm^2 - 0.9 cm^2 (Significant improvement)
Estimate the peak to peak gradients of each pullback tracing. Pre and post gradients are 25 and 15 mmHg respectively. Note that although the PA pressure didn't change much post valvuloplasty, the systolic RV pressure drops from 38 to 28 mmHg indicating a reduced work load on the RV. The peak to peak gradient is almost cut in half. To estimate valve area substitute CO and gradient data into the formula below:

Hakki valve area formula =	$\dfrac{\textbf{CO (in L/min)}}{\sqrt{\textbf{(Peak - peak gradient)}}}$

Pre-valvuloplasty, Hakki VA = $2.6 / \sqrt{25} = 2.6 / 5 = \mathbf{0.52\ cm^2}$
Post-valvuloplasty Hakki VA = $3.5 / \sqrt{15} = 3.5 / 3.9 = \mathbf{0.90\ cm^2}$
This is almost a doubling of the valve area. The improved CO also indicates significant improvement. Pepine says,

> "*The hemodynamics of pulmonic stenosis are characterized by the pulmonic valve pressure gradient and the right ventricular response to the pressure load. The pulmonary artery pressure is invariably normal or low. Therefore, the right ventricular pressure is an accurate reflection of the severity of the obstruction.*"

See: Pepine, chapter on "Valve Function" and Pepine, Chapter on "The Adult Patient with Congenital Disease" **Keywords:** calculate Hakki valve area, Pulmonary valvuloplasty

492. "Valve-in-valve" TAVR is transcatheter insertion of an expandable valve into:

a. **An existing failed bioprosthetic valve**
b. **An existing failed mechanical valve**
c. **A patient's stenotic aortic valve**
d. **A patient's regurgitant aortic valve.**

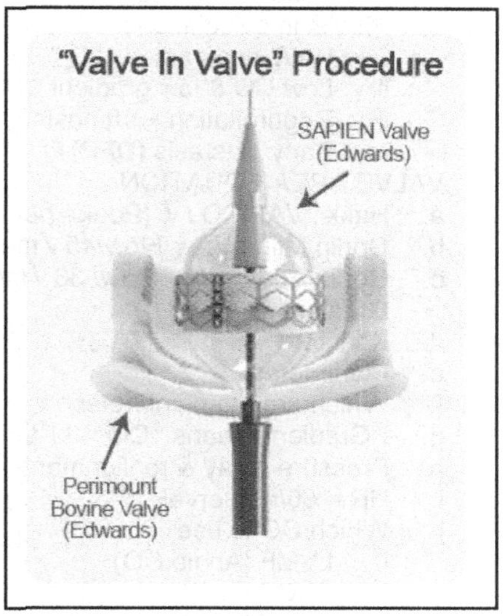

ANSWER **a. An existing failed bioprosthetic valve**. This diagram shows a Sapien TAVR within a tissue valve. Braunwald says, "Patients with a degenerated bioprosthetic heart valve might also benefit from TAVI as they would not be required to undergo cardiopulmonary bypass and cardioplegia during redo surgery. To date, however, there is limited data supporting valve-in-valve TAVI for degenerated surgical bioprostheses." It is placement of TAVR into a previously placed and surgically inserted mechanical valve. TAVR cannot be placed in a mechanical valve because metal valves are not round. See Braunwald chapter on Aortic Valvuloplasty and TAVR

REFERENCES

Baim, D. S. and Grossman W., *Cardiac Catheterization, Angiography, and Intervention*, 6th Ed., Lea and Febiger, 2006
Braunwald, et. al. Ed., *Heart Disease, a Textbook of CV Medicine*, 8th Ed., Saunders, 2008
Darovic, G.O., *Hemodynamic Monitoring: Invasive and Noninvasive Clinical Applications*, 2nd Ed., W.B. Saunders Co., 1995
Kern, M. J., Ed., *The Cardiac Catheterization Handbook*, 3rd Ed., Mosby-Year Book, 2003
Pepine, J. C., and Hill, J. A., et. al., *Diagnostic and Therapeutic Cardiac Catheterization*, 2nd Ed., Williams and Wilkins, 1994
Ragosta, Michael, Textbook of Clinical Hemodynamics, Saunders, 1st Edition, 2008
Yang, Bentivoglio, Maranhao, and Goldberg, *From Cardiac Catheterization to Hemodynamic*

Parameters, 3rd edition, F.A. Davis Co., 3rd edition, 1988

OUTLINE: VALVE AREA

1. GENERAL VALVE AREA
   a. Identify valve gradients & regurgitation
   b. Types of gradients
      i. Peak to peak
      ii. Instantaneous
      iii. Mean
      iv. End diastolic
   c. Recording gradients
      i. Use of sheath & FA
      ii. Two lumen pigtail
      iii. Pullbacks
   d. Gorlin VA = Gold Standard
      i. Echo gradient
      ii. Echo valve area
   e. Pitfalls in calculation
      i. PAW accuracy
      ii. Low CO & low gradient
      iii. Regurgitation + stenosis
      iv. Early diastasis (DFP)
2. VALVE AREA EQUATION
   a. Hakki: VA =CO / √ (Peak - peak Gradient
   b. Gorlin Mitral VA = Flow/45 √mean Gradient
   c. Gorlin Aortic VA = Flow/ 38 √mean Gradient
   d. K factor
   e. Planimeters
   f. Which area to planimeter
   g. √Gradient means ↑CO = ↑↑ Gradient
   h. Pressure delay & realignment
   i. HR = 60/rr interval
   j. Which CO to use
      i. LVMF (Angio CO)
      ii. TDCO
      iii. Fick CO
3. AORTIC VALVE AREA CALCULATION (Gorlin)
   a. LV-Ascending AO most accurate
   b. Recording speed = 100
   c. Scale factor
   d. HR
   e. Recordings
      i. Shifting AO
      ii. Use of FA
      iii. Simultaneous recordings
      iv. Pullbacks
      v. Pseudo pullbacks
   f. Flow
      i. sep measurement
      ii. SEP calculation in sec/min
   g. Planimeter LV-AO gradient
   h. Calculate mean gradient
   i. Calculate aortic valve area
4. MITRAL VALVE AREA CALCULATION (Gorlin)
   a. Recording
      i. Simultaneous LA-LV most accurate
      ii. Use of PAW
      iii. Speed 100
      iv. Expanded scale X 50
      v. Scale factor
      vi. HR
      vii. realignment of PAW
      viii. dfp measurement
      ix. DFP calculation
      x. Flow
      xi. Mitral Valve area calculation
   b. Pressure half time
      i. Echo measurement
      ii. Echo Doppler
      iii. Pressure ½ time measurement
5. OTHER
   a. Normal orifice size
   b. Critical valve area
      i. Aortic VA = 0.7-.8 cm^2 (or 0.5 - 0.8 cm^2/M^2)
      ii. Mitral VA 1 - 1.5 cm^2 (or 1.0 cm^2/M^2)
      iii. Tricuspid VA 1.5 - 2.0 cm^2
   c. Carabello's sign
      i. Catheter obstructs flow
   d. Stenosis + Regurgitation
      i. Which CO to use for flow
         (1) LVMF if same valve
   e. Marginal gradients
   f. Increasing CO
      i. Exercise
      ii. Pacing
      iii. Isuprel
   g. Valve Resistance
      i. No √ of gradient
   h. Second stenosis in MS
      i. Arteriolar
   i. Valvuloplasty
      i. Pulmonic
      ii. Mitral
      iii. Aortic
   j. Commisurotomy
   k. Valve repair
   l. Valve replacement
      i. Types of Tissue Valves
         (1) Homo-graft
         (2) Auto-graft
         (3) Hetero-graft
         (4) Xeno-graft
      ii. types of mechanical valves
         (1) Ball in cage
         (2) Disk in cage
         (3) Bi-leaflet (St. Jude)

Coronary Hemodynamics, IVUS & ICE

INDEX: E11

CORONARY PHYSIOLOGY & FLOWS

493. Left coronary blood flow occurs primarily during the ________ phase of the cardiac cycle because ________.

a. Systolic, coronary driving pressure is greatest
b. Systolic, systolic ejection opens the aortic valve
c. Diastolic, semilunar valves cover the coronary ostia in systole
d. Diastolic, diastole releases compressed endocardial capillaries

ANSWER d. Diastolic, in diastole the ventricle relaxes and releases the compressed endocardial capillaries. Most flow occurs in diastole due to the compression of LV capillaries in systole. This is why the IABP is so effective at augmenting diastolic coronary flow. Although the left coronary capillaries obstruct flow during systole, the low pressure RV capillaries are less occluded because of the lower RV pressure. A common misconception is that the open aortic leaflets occlude the coronary ostia and inhibit flow. They do not.
See: Berne and Levy, chapter on "Coronary Artery Physiology." Keywords: Coronary Flow in Diastole, capillary compression

494. Which coronary artery normally has the steadiest flow even throughout systole?

a. LAD
b. Circumflex
c. RCA
d. LCA

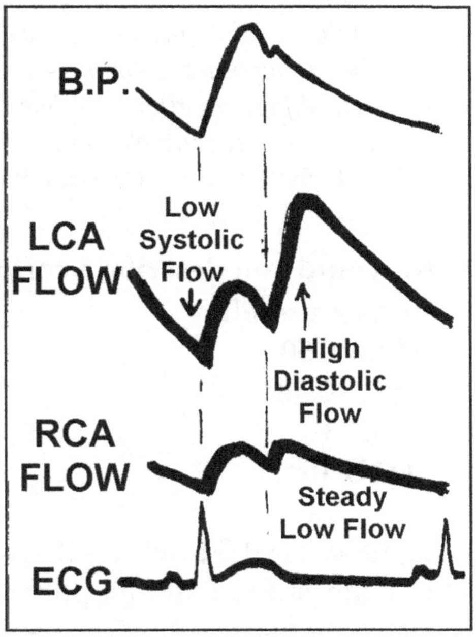

Rt. & Lt. Cor. Flows

ANSWER c. RCA. In both right and left coronary arteries the limit on coronary flow is the coronary resistance. The LV compresses the sub-endocardial capillaries in systole - the RV not so much. Since the right coronary supplies the lower pressure chambers (RV) it has less dramatic resistance change.

This compression makes it hard to force blood through LV capillaries in systole. As a result, the left coronary has almost no flow during systole. This is because of extreme LV capillary compression during

the systolic phase.
See: Berne and Levy, chapter on "Coronary Circulation." Keywords: Cor. Flow, Diastole, RCA flow

495. These are diagrams of intracoronary Doppler flow patterns from 3 major coronary arteries. Doppler pattern #1 is most likely from the:

a. Right coronary artery
b. Main left coronary artery
c. Posterior descending artery
e. Left anterior or circumflex artery

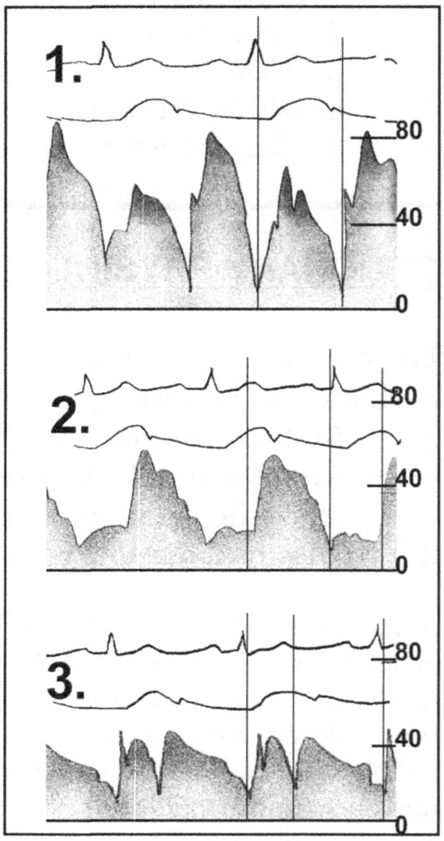

ANSWER b. Main left coronary artery. The flow patterns in the left coronary artery are similar - larger in diastole. But the main coronary often has the largest diameter and highest flow rate.
CORRECTLY MATCHED ANSWERS ARE:

1. Main left coronary artery:
2. Left anterior or circumflex artery: flow velocity down the LAD and CX arteries is virtually identical in normal anatomy.
3. Right coronary artery: Reduced flow rate with equal systolic and diastolic components. Topal says,

> *"In contrast with the flow characteristics of most arterial districts, arterial coronary blood flow has a distinctive and unique phasic pattern. Blood flow is higher in diastole and lower in systole. Large differences, however, are present between the flow pattern in the left and in the right coronary artery. . . . the systolic reduction of arterial coronary flow is due to the contraction of the heart. Squeezing of the capillary network due to the increase in tissue pressure during myocardial compression related to the high systolic intraventricular pressure. . . .The different patterns of flow during the cardiac cycle in the right and left coronary arteries is in part attributable to the greater systolic compressive force of the left ventricle . . . ."*

See: Topol, chapter on Intracoronary Doppler. Keywords: coronary flow mainly diastolic

496. How would you describe a coronary angiogram that shows wide-open fast flow through a vessel?

a. FFR >0.50
b. FFR <0.50
c. TIMI 3
d. TIMI 10

Answer: c. TIMI 3 flow. TIMI stands for "Thrombolysis in Myocardial Infarction." This is the study that first published the TIMI flow measure. It visually evaluates coronary flow from 0 to 3 as seen on angio. TIMI 0 is no flow, TIMI 3 is complete reperfusion and wide-open flow.

Kern says, "The Thrombolysis in Myocardial Infarction (TIMI) study group developed a grading scale for coronary blood flow based on visual assessment of the rate of contrast opacification of the infarct artery. The TIMI flow grade has become the standard for semiquantitative evaluation of myocardial perfusion before and after coronary reperfusion therapies. Determination of TIMI flow grade after coronary reperfusion yields important prognostic information in patients with acute myocardial infarction.... Patient's with TIMI flow grade 3 show improved regional and global left ventricular function, lower enzyme peaks, and reduced morbidity and mortality rates compared with patients with TIMI flow grades 0, 1, or 2." See: Kern, et al, Determination of Angiographic (TIMI Grade) Blood Flow by Intracoronary Doppler Flow Velocity During Acute Myocardial Infarction, Circulation, 1996

497. When measuring FFR what intracoronary drug is the standard of care and acts in the shortest time to induce a maximum coronary hyperemic response?

- a. **Adenosine**
- b. **Papaverine**
- c. **Dipyridamole**
- d. **Nitroglycerin (Tridel)**

ANSWER a. Adenosine has a 10 second half life. Baim says,

> "*Intracoronary adenosine has an extremely high safety profile in low doses and has become the pharmacologic stimulus of choice in the catheterization laboratory.*"

Topol says,

> "*In view of the extremely high safety profile of low dose intracoronary adenosine, this agent and route is the pharmacologic stimulus of choice . . . . has been reported to increase coronary blood flow velocity to four to six times the resting value in patients with normal coronary arteries.*"

See: Baim chapter on "Evaluation of Myocardial Blood Flow and Metabolism" and Topol, chapter on "Intracoronary Doppler."

498. Which invasive test uses a Doppler wire to measure the ability of the coronary vascular bed to increase coronary blood flow from resting to maximum vasodilation?

- a. **Hyperemic Doppler Flow Increase**
- b. **Coronary Flow Velocity Reserve (CFVR)**
- c. **Coronary Pressure Hyperemic Response (CPHR)**
- d. **Coronary Stress Resistance Ratio (CSRR)**
- e. **Fractional Flow Reserve (FFR)**

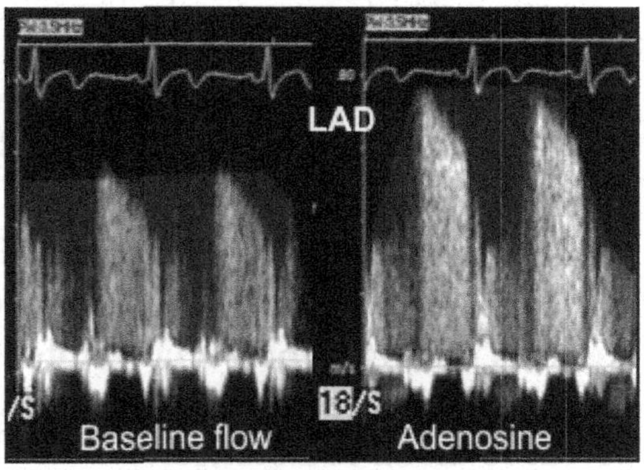

LAD Doppler Velocity after Acuson.com

ANSWER b. Coronary Flow Velocity Reserve - (CFVR). Doppler measures velocity, not flow rate. This miniature Doppler transducer is mounted on the tip of a guide wire. When

CFR is measured below a stenosis it evaluates how severely that lesion limits coronary flow. CFR is similar to FFR, but it is the ratio of maximal coronary flow to resting coronary flow, where maximal flow is measured after IC adenosine administration. In the Doppler shown, note how LAD diastolic flow predominates. A normal coronary segment can more than double its diastolic velocity with Adenosine. This CFR shown is 3.7/2.6 = 1.4 suggesting a treatable stenosis.

CFR has recently fallen out of favor, because it has motion and positioning issues. Also, it is not specific to lesion flow, because it evaluates both microvascular and epicardial stenosis together. Exams focus only on FFR, not CFR. See: Braunwald, chapter on "Coronary Blood Flow and Myocardial Ischemia"

Pressure Wire

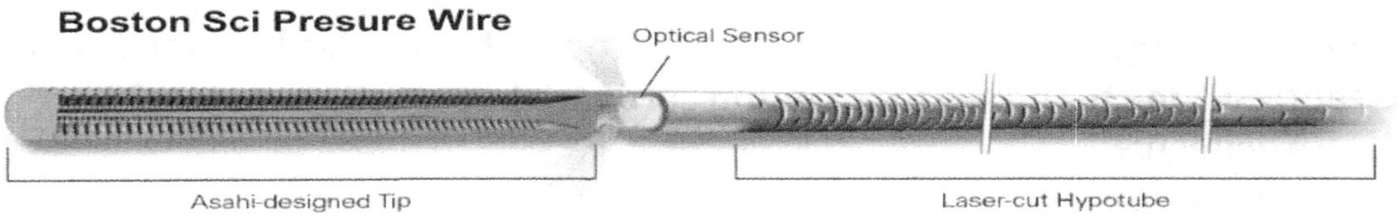

499. Which invasive test uses a pressure wire to measure the ability of the coronary vascular bed to maintain coronary perfusion pressures distal to a stenosis during maximum vasodilation?

a. Pressure Gradient Ratio (PGR)
b. Hyperemic Pressure Ratio (HPR)
c. Fractional Flow Reserve (FFR)
d. Coronary Flow Reserve (CFR)

ANSWER c. Fractional Flow Reserve (FFR) is the name for the ratio of pressures during hyperemia. Normally the coronary pressures should be the same as you move the wire down an artery. But, when you cross a lesion, a gradient will occur. This is accentuated by adenosine, which increases the flow and the gradient. The ratio of distal to proximal pressures is the FFR. Don't confuse this with coronary flow reserve (CFR) which measures hyperemic flow using the Doppler flo-wire.
See: Braunwald, chapter on "Coronary Blood Flow and Myocardial Ischemia"

500. What is the formula for Fractional Flow Reserve (FFR) as measured by a pressure guidewire placed distally to a stenosis during hyperemia? (Note Pa= Aortic pressure mean as measured by guiding catheter. Pd = Mean pressure distal to a stenosis)

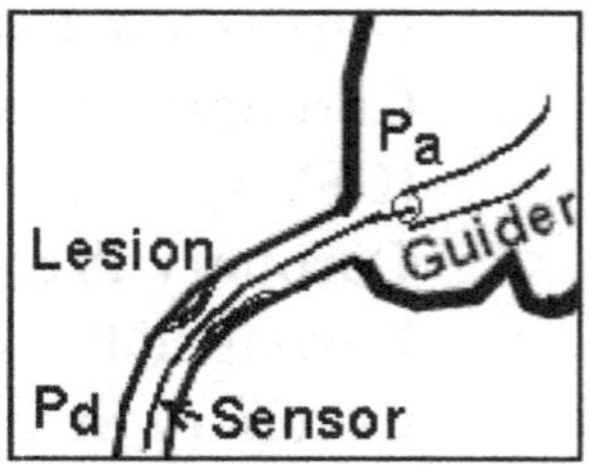

Pressure Wire

a. Pa-Pd
b. (Pd-Pa)/Pd
c. (Pa-Pd)/Pa
d. Pd/Pa

ANSWER d. Pd/Pa = Pressure distal to stenosis / Aortic pressure measured during hyperemia. A normal FFR is 1.0. Abnormal is below 0.80. If there is a stenosis, the distal pressure will be reduced due to a gradient. This index Pd/Pa represents the maximal blood flow through an artery in the presence of a stenosis, compared to the theoretical normal maximal flow in the same artery. Just as in AS the most accurate gradients are measured at high flow(we exercise the patients), so FFR gradients should be measured at high flow (Adenosine).
See: RADI Co., Coronary Pressure Measurement CD

501. When measuring FFR by pressure wire, what does the pressure waveform look like (at fast paper speeds) distal to a severe culprit coronary lesion?
- **a. Spike and dome pattern**
- **b. Ventricularization pattern**
- **c. Smoothed out and damped**
- **d. Pulsus tardus with slow upstroke**

ANSWER b. Ventricularization pattern with flattened low diastole and reduced systole. When a hemodynamically significant stenosis is stressed (hyperemia) it is mainly the diastolic pressure that drops, reflecting a ventricularized pattern. This is just like a damped main-stem left ostial lesion that shows a ventricularization pattern.

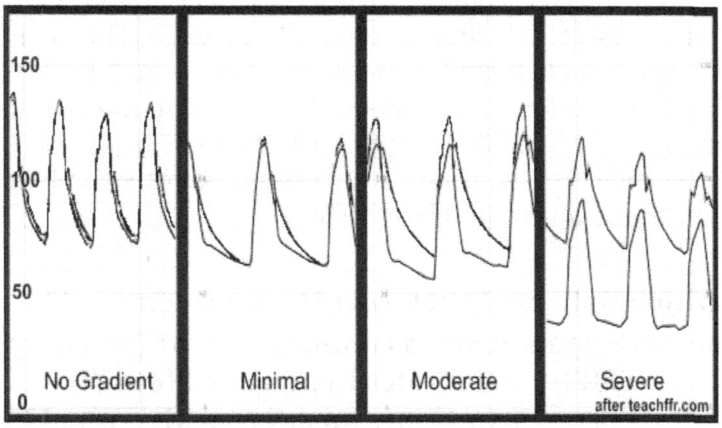

Pressure Wire

502. These simultaneous pressures were taken during adenosine induced hyperemia. Measure and calculate the Fractional Flow Reserve (FFR).
- **a. 0.68**
- **b. 0.75**
- **c. 1.50**
- **d. 48**

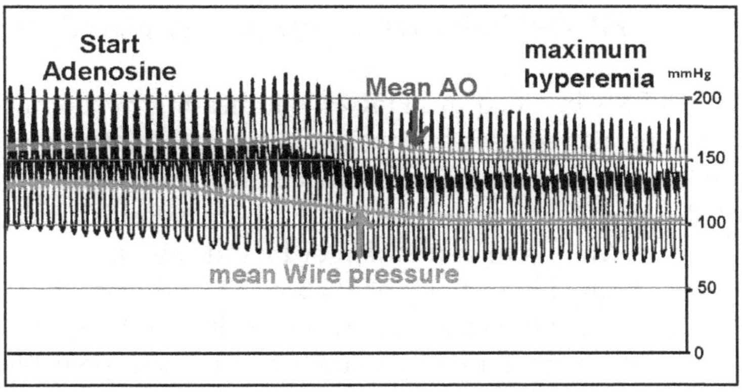

ANSWER a. 0.68 is the FFR. At its lowest point during hyperemia, the Pd wire pressure is 102 and the Pa AO pressure is 150. So the ratio of the two is simply 102/150 = 0.68. Since it is below the cutoff of 0.80, this lesion would be considered ischemic and should be revascularized. After angioplasty the ratio should rise above 0.90. With a stent it should rise even further. See: RADI Co., Coronary Pressure Measurement CD or Grossman,

Chapter on "Myocardial Blood Flow and Metabolism" Keywords: calculate FFR

503. Measure and calculate the Fractional Flow Reserve (FFR).

a. 0.38
b. 0.61
c. 0.78
d. 0.85

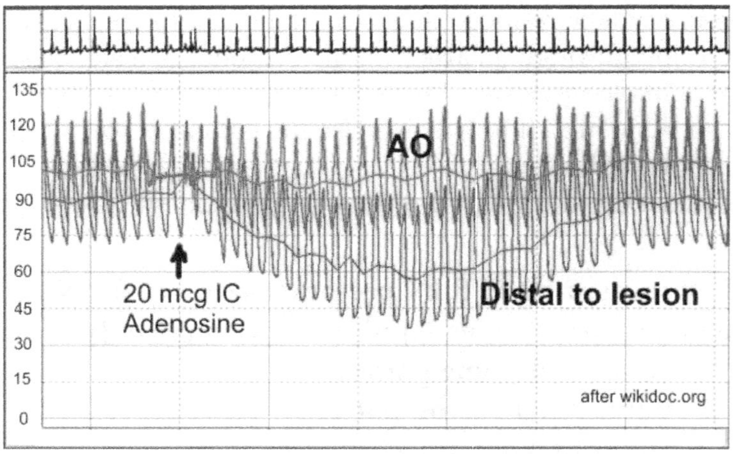

ANSWER b. 0.61 is the ratio of the mean lesion pressure to aortic mean pressures during maximum hyperemia. The lower pressure bottoms out at 60 mmHg mean with adenosine. The AO mean at the tip of the guider catheter is steady at 98 mmHg. The ratio of the 2 pressures is the FFR = 60/98= 0.61. Which is below the 0.80 cut-off for normal. This suggests that the lesion crossed is physiologically significant and should be treated.

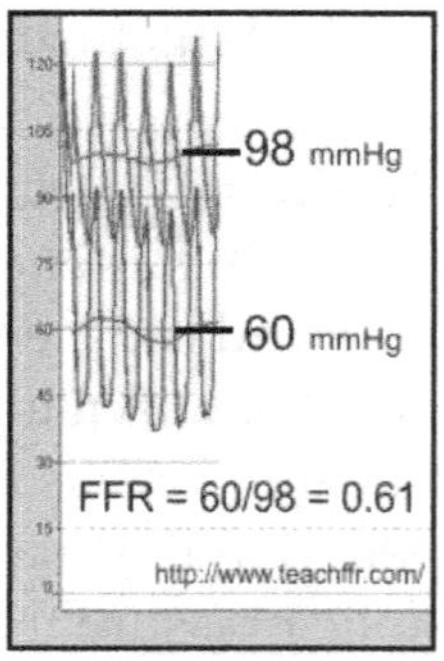

FFR measure

504. Which statements below are true concerning FFR measurements across a coronary lesion? (Select 3.)

a. **FFR > 1.0 indicates hyperemic blood flow**
b. **FFR = 1.0 indicates an artery with normal blood flow**
c. **FFR> .80 indicates that narrowing is unlikely to cause ischemia**
d. **FFR< .80 indicates that narrowing is responsible for ischemia**
e. **FFR >.80 indicates an adequately placed stent with good long term results**
f. **FFR <.80 indicates an adequately placed stent with good long term results**

ANSWERS: b, c, & d. An FFR > 1.0 indicating hyperemic blood flow is NOT correct. They are all measured with adenosine which vasodilates the arterioles and causes hyperemic blood flow to exercise levels. Since FFR is the ratio of aortic to coronary lesion pressure, **no readings should ever exceed 1.0.** St. Jude website says about the significance of FFR:

- An FFR measurement of 1.0 indicates an artery with normal blood flow
- An FFR measurement above .80 indicates that ischemia is very unlikely.
- An FFR measurement below .80 is 100% specific in identifying that the blood flow blockage caused by that narrowing is responsible for a patient's ischemia." It is these lesions that need intervention.

FFR >.90 indicates an adequately placed stent with good results

See: www.sjm.com Keywords: FFR significance: 1.0 normal, 0.8, <0.80 ischemia

Kern says, "the patients with the lowest residual FFR after stenting still have residual plaque elsewhere in the artery and, thus, are prone to more complications and major adverse events after stenting." Kern also suggests that an FFR of >0.90 is considered a successful result with low MACE rate. See: Kern, SCAI Interventional Cardiology Board Review Book

505. The 2009 FAME study showed that when coronary intervention is guided by FFR, and not angiography alone:

- **a. Procedure cost may be increased**
- **b. More and better stents are placed in patients**
- **c. Lesion morphology can guide stent placement**
- **d. There is a lower incidence of major adverse cardiac events**

ANSWER d. There is a lower incidence of major adverse cardiac events (MACE). Beside fewer complications, other benefits over angiography guided intervention include: procedure costs are reduced, fewer unnecessary stents were placed, and less dye is used on a patient.

FAME showed that, "The result was that one-third fewer stents were used in the FFR group and the difference in outcomes at one year were significant: the FFR group showed a 28% lower incidence of major adverse cardiac events (repeat procedure to open the artery, heart attack or death) -- 18.3% vs. 13.2%. The implication in these results is that placing stents in lesions that are not responsible for ischemia is not only <u>not necessary, but may cause worse outcomes</u>...

Another benefit seen in the FFR group was procedural cost. Since fewer stents were used per patient, the average cost of the procedure was $700 lower (this includes the specialized guide wire used to measure FFR). Fewer stents also meant approximately 10% less contrast dye."

However, FFR does not tell you anything about the lesion morphology/anatomy, only it's hemodynamic significance. It is IVUS that evaluates lesion morphology (lipid pools, calcium, length, etc...) and helps tailor stent placement (stent size, apposition, etc.). See: http://www.ptca.org/news/2009/0115_FFR.html Keywords: FAME study on FFR

506. Coronary lesions rated by angiography as 50% - 70% diameter stenosis are often of questionable hemodynamic significance. In which instance below is FFR <u>not</u> usually helpful in guiding PCI.

- **a. Serial stenoses**
- **b. Bifurcation lesions**
- **c. Left main lesions**
- **d. Multivessel CAD lesions**
- **e. Where no stress testing was done**
- **f. STEMI or unstable ACS lesions**

ANSWER: f. FFR is NOT helpful in STEMI or unstable ACS lesions.

SCAI guidelines say, "Fractional flow reserve (FFR). Definitely Beneficial in SIHD [Subacute Ischemic Heart Disease], when noninvasive stress imaging is contraindicated, discordant, nondiagnostic, or unavailable, FFR should be used to assess the functional significance of intermediate coronary stenoses (50–70%) and more severe stenoses (<90%). In patients with multivessel coronary disease, PCI guided by FFR measurement improves outcomes and saves resources when compared to PCI guided by angiography alone for evaluating intermediate LMCA lesions. FFR can be used to evaluate the significance of serial stenoses to guide the strategy for determining which lesion(s) should be revascularized and which should be managed medically. Observational studies have reported favorable outcomes using FFR in specific anatomic subsets, including diffuse disease, bifurcations, stent-jailed side branches...." See: Lotfi, et al., SCAI Consensus Statement on FFR , 2014

USE THIS FFR TRACING FOR THE NEXT 2 QUESTIONS

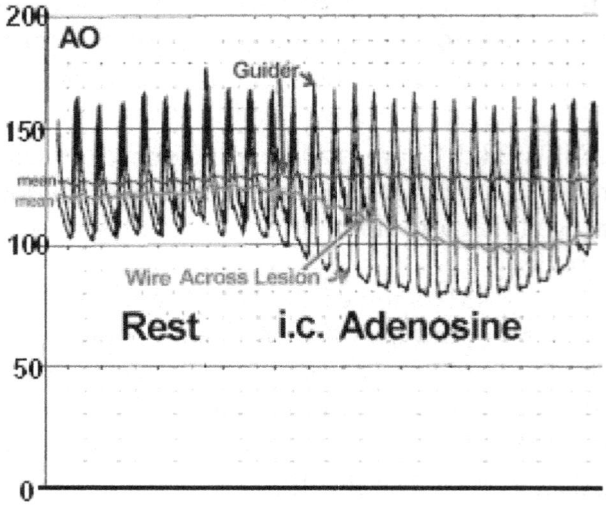

507. **This shows a pressure gradient across a coronary stenotic lesion with intracoronary adenosine administration. Estimate the maximum pressure gradient due to the lesion.**
a. 10 mmHg
b. 32 mmHg
c. 50 mmHg
d. 75 mmHg

508. **These pressure tracings were taken through a coronary guider catheter and a pressure wire. It shows the pressure gradient across a coronary stenotic lesion with intracoronary adenosine administration. Estimate the Fractional Flow Reserve (FFR) due to the lesion.**
a. 0.29
b. 0.35
c. 0.61
d. 0.75

BOTH ANSWERS LISTED BELOW:

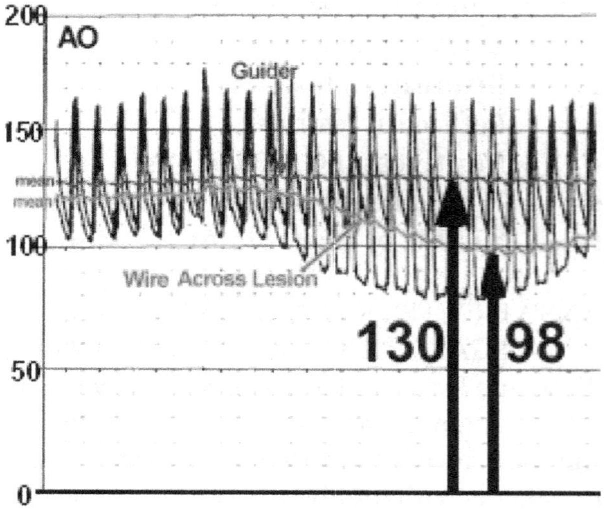

507. ANSWER b. 32 mmHg gradient. This simultaneous pressure tracing was taken during adenosine administration. Mean pressure gradient is 32 mmHg. This is measured between the blue mean AO from the guider catheter, and the red mean AO from the pressure wire across the lesion. 130 - 98 = 32 mmHg gradient. This technique evaluates the effect of a stenosis on the physiologic pressure downstream to a lesion under stress. See: Company Literature

508. ANSWER d. 0.75 is the Fractional Flow

Reserve (FFR). This is calculated by dividing the aortic mean (130 mmHg) by the mean pressure distal to the lesion (98 mmHg). FFR = 98/130 = 0.75 This technique evaluates the effect of a stenosis on the pressure distal to a stenotic lesion under stress. This lesion, falls below the 0.80 cut point, and should be stented. If the FFR falls below 0.80 it should be treated - above 0.80 not. This simple measurement is one of the best functional tests of the significance of a coronary lesion. See: Company Literature

509. This FFR on a right coronary artery lesion means that on exercise:

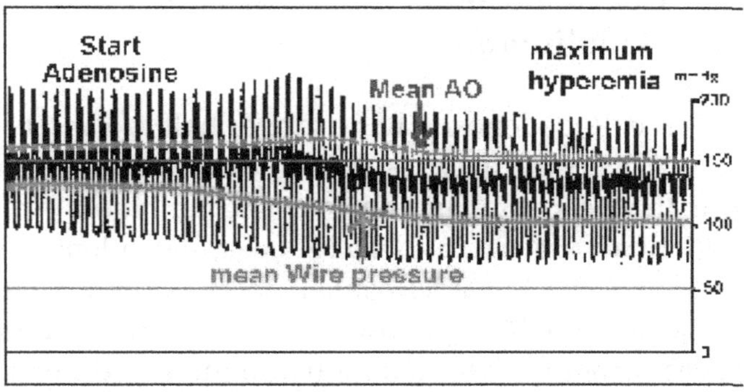

- a. **Only 66% of the needed blood flow will reach the RV**
- b. **Only 34% of the needed blood flow will reach the RV**
- c. **The RV myocardium is in the gray area (75% - 80%) and may not be ischemic**
- d. **The RV myocardium will not be ischemic**

ANSWER: a. Only 66% of the needed blood flow will reach the RV on exercise. Here Pd=102 mmHg and Pa = 150 mmHg, so FFR = 100/150 = 0.66 which is ischemic. This lesion is critical and should be treated. The ratio of these mean pressures has been shown to be the same as the ratio of blood flows down the artery on exercise compared to that at rest. There is no longer a gray area between 0.75 and 0.80. ACC standards now recommend that lesions with FFR <0.80 should get revascularized.

Kern says, "FFR is an in-lab artery specific measurement of the ischemic potential equal to what we would get if we did a stress test on this one artery." See: Kern, video in chapter on Interventional Cardiology Procedures and Kern, FFR Basics video

510. Prior to PCI you measure Fractional Flow Reserve (FFR) with a pressure wire. Lesions becomes SIGNIFICANT and should be treated when the:

- a. **FFR > 0.80**
- b. **FFR < 0.80**
- c. **FFR > 1.0**
- d. **FFR < 1.0**

ANSWER b. FFR < 0.80. When this simple ratio falls below 0.80 therapy on that lesion is recommended.

SCIA guidelines 2014 say, "FFR was first validated using a cutoff value of 0.75. With further experience with the technique, investigators appreciated that by extending the cutoff value to 0.80, the sensitivity of FFR could be improved without greatly compromising the specificity. For this reason, a cutoff value of 0.80 was used in FAME 1 and FAME 2 and shown to be clinically valid. This is now the recommended ischemic reference standard for the invasive assessment of myocardial ischemia. "
See: SCAI, Expert Consensus Statement on the Use of Fractional Flow Reserve, Intravascular Ultrasound, and Optical Coherence Tomography, in Catheterization and

Cardiovascular Interventions, 2014

511. Which new IC hyperemic agent with a half life of 2-3 minutes may replace adenosine administration during the FFR procedure because it has fewer side effects?

- a. **Papaverine**
- b. **Dobutamine**
- c. **Regadenoson**
- d. **Gadolinium**

Answer: c. Regadenoson has a longer half life and fewer side effects than adenosine.

Adenosine may result in undesirable effects including nausea, flushing, shortness of breath, chest pain, and atrioventricular block.

Bhatt & Kern say, "To reduce the incidence of side effects without affecting hyperemia, selective adenosine A2A receptor agonist agents such as regadenoson have been developed. Regadenoson is a low-affinity A2A adenosine receptor agonist that induces coronary vasodilatation and increased myocardial blood flow in a manner reportedly equivalent to adenosine. By selectively targeting the A2A receptor in coronary arteries, it has fewer adverse effects compared with adenosine. Regadenoson has a longer half-life of 2-3 minutes in the initial phase, 30 minutes in the intermediate phase, and 2 hours in the terminal phase and may prove to be easier to use than short-acting adenosine. With a single infusion bolus of regadenoson, coronary hyperemia may be achieved and maintained equivalent to that achieved with a constant infusion of adenosine. Because of these properties, regadenoson may be a promising coronary vasodilator for the measurement of FFR." See, Bhatt, chapter on "Techniques of Intracoronary Pressure Sensor Wire Measurement"

512. Your PCI patient is a severe diabetic. The LAD on angio appears diffusely diseased and narrowed all along its length. Your physician says he wants to pullback the pressure wire through the LAD. He will probably order:

- a. **40 -80 mcg adenosine IC boluses at different wire locations**
- b. **One 100-200 mcg adenosine IC bolus and pullback the wire slowly**
- c. **IV adenosine 50 mcg/Kg/min and pullback the wire slowly**
- d. **IV adenosine 140 mcg/Kg/min and pullback the wire slowly**

ANSWER d. IV adenosine 140 mcg/ Kg/ min and pullback the wire slowly.
Ragosta says, "A modification in the technique for FFR assessment is required in the setting of diffuse coronary disease. Because there is no specific, focal lesion, the pressure transducer is positioned in the distal artery and slowly pulled back during hyperemia. This technique requires sustained hyperemia that mandates the use of an intravenous infusion of adenosine at 140 mcg/ Kg/ min. The duration of hyperemia induced by IC adenosine is too brief and will likely dissipate during the course of the pullback. Typically, the lowest FFR value is at the most distal site, and a slow, progressive rise in FFR occurs as the pressure wire is withdrawn toward the guide catheter. Occasionally, the operator may note an abrupt step-up in the hyperemic pressure gradient, suggesting a more focal area of disease treatable with stenting." See: Ragosta, chapter on Coronary Hemodynamics.

513. A coronary pressure wire is placed across a suspicious lesion indicating a 10% resting pressure gradient (0.90 mean pressure ratio Pd/Pa). The physician will:
- a. **Dilate the lesion, it is a critical lesion**
- b. **Leave it alone, it is not a critical lesion**
- c. **Administer adenosine to measure FFR**
- d. **Administer nitroglycerin to see if gradient is reduced**

ANSWER: c. Administer adenosine to measure FFR. FFR is the ratio of mean distal to mean proximal pressures across the lesion during hyperemia. As it stands the lesion is not critical - only a 10% pressure reduction. IC adenosine must be administered to correctly evaluate the Fractional Flow Reserve (FFR). The gradient and flow will increase with the hyperemic state induced by IC adenosine. An FFR of 0.75-0.80 was thought to be marginal. Lower FFRs should be treated with an intervention. Kern says: "A persistently low FFR (<0.75) [now 0.80] especially if the angiographic result is suboptimal, is an indication for further inflations (either prolonged inflations or upsizing of the balloon) or stenting. An FFR >.90 is considered a successful (PCI) result.... "
See: Kern chapter on "Interventional Techniques" Keywords: FFR < 0.80 is a critical lesion

514. When is a 2-3 minute IV infusion of adenosine required to evaluate the physiologic significance of long, diffuse or sequential coronary lesions?
- a. **iFR pullback**
- b. **FFR pullback**
- c. **IVUS pullback**
- d. **OCT pullback**

Answer: b. FFR pullback, because a steady hyperemic state is required during lengthy pullbacks across diffuse long or serial lesions. Standard IV dose is 140 micrograms/ kg/ min over 3 minutes. Some patients may not tolerate a long adenosine infusion like this and may develop shortness of breath. Patients on theophyllines or smokers also may not respond appropriately.

Sandhu says, [compared to bolus adenosine administration for FFR] "IV adenosine achieves a more complete and stable vasodilatation and is more convenient for the assessment of tandem lesions, diffuse coronary artery disease and ostial lesions where a pull back of the pressure wire is needed." See: Sandhu, et al, Fractional Flow Reserve: Intracoronary Versus Intravenous Adenosine Induced Maximal Coronary Hyperemia, Indian Heart Jn, 2013

515. Your physician wishes to do an FFR on a 100 kg. patient. He asks you to set up the IV pump for adenosine administration of 140 ug/Kg/min from an IV bag with 200 mg/100 ml. Set the IV pump to:
- a. **42 ml/hr**
- b. **420 ml/hr**
- c. **70 ml/hr**
- d. **700 ml/hr**

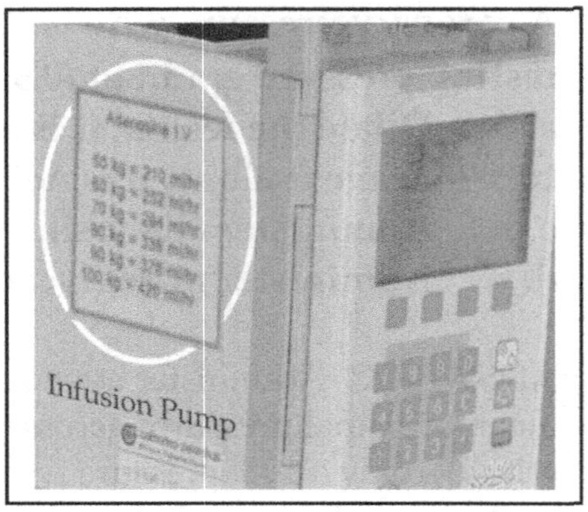

ANSWER: b. 420 ml/hr

- First convert the 140 ug/Kg/min to the units we need, milligrams and hours using unit conversion. (140 ug/Kg/min)(1 mg/1000 ug)(60 min /hr) = 8.40 mg/Kg/hr
- Then calculate the dose rate for our 100 Kg patient. (8.40 mg/Kg/hr) x 100 Kg = 840 mg/hr
- Then use the concentration in our bag to calculate infusion rate in ml/hr. (840 mg/hr)(100 ml/200 mg) = 420 ml/hr.
- You need to know: 1 mg=1000ug, 60 min=1 hr, patient weight of 100 Kg, and IV bag concentration 200mg in 100 ml. Note that the unnecessary units cancel leading to the needed infusion rate in ml/hr for our infusion pump. This image shows one labs IV bag and infusion pump with infusion rates for different sizes of patients. See: video, Dr. Nico Pijls, Radcliff Cardiology, Landmark Evidence, Ease of Use, Cost-effectiveness: The Importance of FFR in Daily Practice

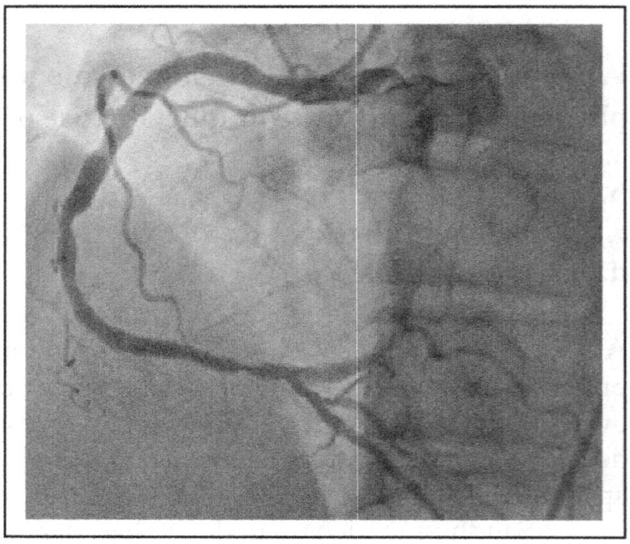

516. This patient has 2 questionable eccentric RCA coronary lesions as shown. How can you most accurately evaluate these serial lesions for potential intervention?

a. Perform an FFR on each lesion, stent any with FFR <0.80

b. If total FFR of all lesions is <0.80 stent the distal lesion 1st then proximal lesion

c. Perform a pressure wire pullback through all the lesions during hyperemia, stent the lesion with the greatest pressure gradient 1st

d. Perform a pressure wire pullback through all the lesions, stent the lesion with lowest FFR 1st

Answer: c. Perform a pressure wire pullback through all the lesions during hyperemia, stent the lesion with the greatest pressure gradient 1st. Doing single FFR on serial lesions is not accurate because multiple lesions in series add up. Do a single pullback through all the lesions and treat the lesion with the biggest pressure gradient first. Then repeat for the other lesions. See next question. See: Kern, chapter on Special Techniques

517. Your patient has 3 questionable tandem lesions in his RCA. You do a continuous pressure wire pullback across all 3 lesions with a combined FFR of 0.66 as shown. When there are significant serial coronary lesions in the same vessel like this, which lesion should you stent first? First stent the lesion with the:

a. **Greatest FFR**
b. **Lowest FFR**
c. **Greatest gradient**
d. **Lowest gradient**

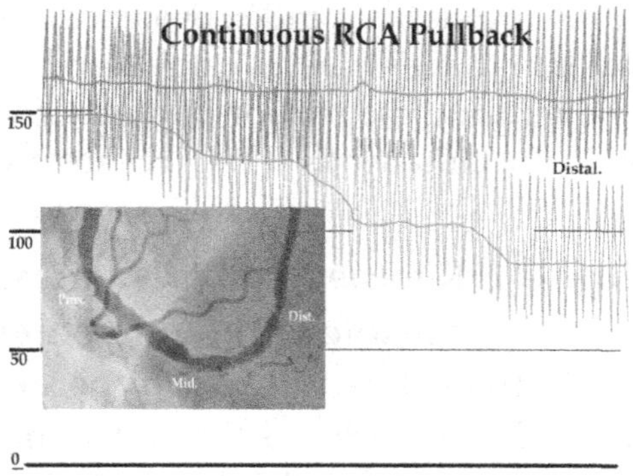

Answer: c. Greatest gradient. In significant serial lesions with a combined FFR <0.8, look at the pullback tracing and select the lesion showing the highest gradient to stent 1st. In this sample pullback there are 3 distinct pressure drops. The middle lesion shows a gradient of about 30 mmHg whereas the others are only 20 mmHg. Treat the middle lesion first.

Bhatt says, "when there is more than one significant lesion in the same epicardial vessel, each lesion blunts maximal flow (i.e., produces submaximal flow) and therefore results in an inaccurate individual lesion FFR. The extent to which both stenoses influence each other is somewhat unpredictable. However, the simple FFR can assess the summed result of any group of stenoses."

"Serial lesion assessment involves the following five steps:
1. Pass the pressure wire beyond the last lesion. Measure the FFR (total) across all lesions with IV adenosine in standard fashion. For example, if the FFR = 0.84 then none of the lesions would need treatment and nothing further needs to be done.
2. If the summed FFR in step 1 is <0.80 then perform a pressure pullback during IV adenosine hyperemia.
3. Determine which of the lesions produces the biggest pressure gradient. Do NOT measure separate lesion FFR values; it is the pressure gradient (ΔP) that will be used to decide which lesion to treat first.
4. Stent the lesion with the largest ΔP.
5. After treating the first lesion, reassess the remaining lesion(s) repeating the standard FFR technique. If the FFR is <0.80, then stent the next lesion. (If more than two lesions, and FFR remains abnormal, then stent the lesion with the next largest ΔP)." See: Bhatt, chapter on FFR

518. Which intracoronary pressure wire protocol does not require an adenosine infusion?

a. **FFR**
b. **iFFR**
c. **FFR pullback**
d. **CFVR**

ANSWER: b. iFFR is the instantaneous Fractional Flow Reserve. The iFFR can be computed from the Pd/Pa ratio automatically from pressures measured during the last phase of diastole without adenosine. It is reported to be as accurate as the adenosine FFR but does not cause the patient the discomfort or risk of an adenosine administration. The coronary flow velocity reserve (CFVR) requires distal and aortic hyperemic flow measures using a Doppler tipped guidewire.

Bhatt says, "Recently, the instantaneous wave-free ratio (iFR) index was developed, a pressure-derived index of stenosis severity that is not dependent on administration of a hyperemic agent. iFR is calculated by measuring the resting pressure gradient across a lesion during the portion of diastole when microvascular resistance is low and stable." See: Beck, Instantaneous wave-free ratio versus fractional flow reserve to guide PCI, ACC, 2017

519. How is iFR measured with a pressure wire across a stenosis?

- **a. In diastole without hyperemia**
- **b. In systole without hyperemia**
- **c. In diastole with hyperemia (adenosine)**
- **d. In systole with hyperemia (adenosine)**

ANSWER: a. In diastole without hyperemia. Instantaneous Flow Reserve is measured during the last part of diastole, starting at 75% of the time into the pressure wave. It can be automatically calculated and reported on screen at rest, with no adenosine administration. It is reported to be as accurate as the standard FFR which uses adenosine for hyperemia. But, it uses a higher cut point for revascularization, 0.89 instead of the 0.80 for standard FFR.

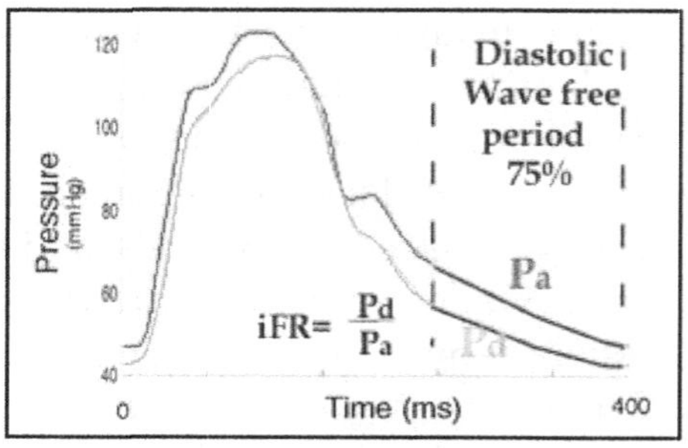

Philips/Volcano says, "The Hybrid iFR-FFR approach has been proposed as method of minimizing patient exposure to adenosine or other vasodilators. In this approach, an iFR can be measured, and stenoses with an iFR >0.93 may be deferred while those with an iFR <0.86 can be treated by revascularization. Stenoses with an iFR between 0.86-0.93 can undergo an FFR assessment to guide therapy. This range can be changed by the physician according to how closely they want to match an FFR-classification of lesions. Using this typical range, almost 60% of stenoses can be spared from needing vasodilator infusion." See: http://www.usa.philips.com/healthcare/product/HC85900P

IVUS

520. There are 2 types of IVUS transducers, supported by two different companies. Which type of transducer is most flexible, uses multiple transducers, and allows for color identified blood flow and tissue characterization?

- **a. Phased array by Boston Scientific**
- **b. Phased array by Volcano**
- **c. Mechanical by Boston Scientific**
- **d. Mechanical by Volcano**

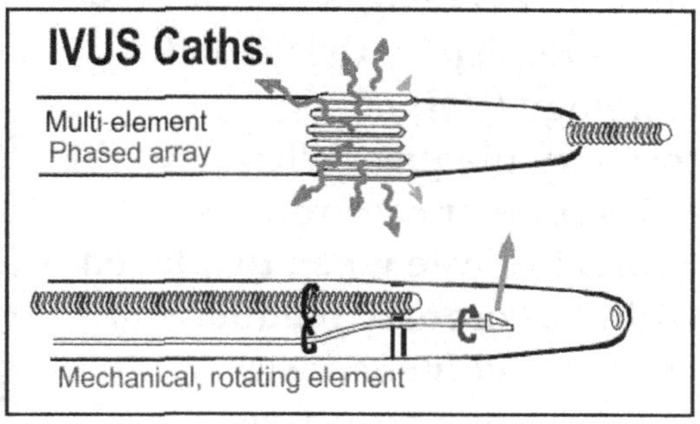

ANSWER b. Phased array by Volcano. Cardiologyhd.com says, "2 types of IVUS catheters: Mechanical and Phased Array. A mechanical catheter has a central drive-shaft and a single transducer mounted at the catheter tip which quickly rotates (1800 rpm) to visualize the entire vessel in cross section. Mechanical transducers provide excellent image quality. However, the disadvantages of the central drive-shaft is diminished flexibility and image distortion termed NURD (Non Uniform Rotational Distortion). Boston Scientific utilizes mechanical catheter technology."

"Phased array catheters consist of multiple transducer elements permanently mounted along the circumference of the catheter tip. Because this catheter has no moving parts or central drive-shaft there is greater flexibility, no NURD, and may be used in the carotids. Volcano utilizes phased array technology for their Eagle Eye Gold catheter." Volcano also makes a mechanical single crystal transducer. See: http://cardiologyhd.com/?s=technological+advancements+in+lesion+assessment

521. What is the typical resonant frequency of a cardiac ultrasound transducer used for ultrasound studies to best image the area labeled #1 (2D Intracardiac ICE) in the box?

a. 2.5 - 3.0 MHZ
b. 5 - 10 MHZ
c. 20 - 30 MHZ

* 1. 2D Intracardiac ICE
2. Adult transthoracic heart
3. Intravascular IVUS

ANSWER b. 5 - 10 MHZ. The higher the frequency of a transducer the finer the resolution, but the less the penetration. So the closest images with IVUS (1-5 mm - within vessels) require very small and high frequency transducers. ICE piezoelectric transducers are fixed to resonate at higher frequencies than adult transducers, because they are inside to the heart and withing 50 mm of the image. While, the adult transthoracic echo transducer needs to focus much further away and penetrate the adult chest wall- about 100 mm from the transducer.

STANDARD TRANSDUCER FREQUENCIES ARE:

1. 2D Adult transthoracic = 2.5 - 3.0 MHZ (Farfield frequency is ~ 4x slower)
2. 2D Intracardiac ICE = 5-10 MHZ (this is mid-range)
3. Intravascular IVUS = 20-30 MHZ (Near field frequency is ~ 4x faster)

Remember the higher the frequency the higher the resolution so the nearer it will image. So, remember the midrange ICE frequency, the near and Farfield frequencies a factor of four times slower for faster, as shown.

See: Curry, Chapter on "Ultrasound." Keywords: ultrasound frequencies

522. **Some IVUS images use colored pixels to display the virtual histology (VH) of coronary plaques. What does the red color (here around the white) indicate when displayed within a coronary plaque?**

- **a. Calcium deposit (strong reflective regions)**
- **b. Necrotic core (soft, lipid-like dead cells, foam cells and trapped blood cells)**
- **c. Fibrofatty plaque (loosely packed collagen, foam cells, thrombus)**
- **d. Fibrous plaque (no lipid)**

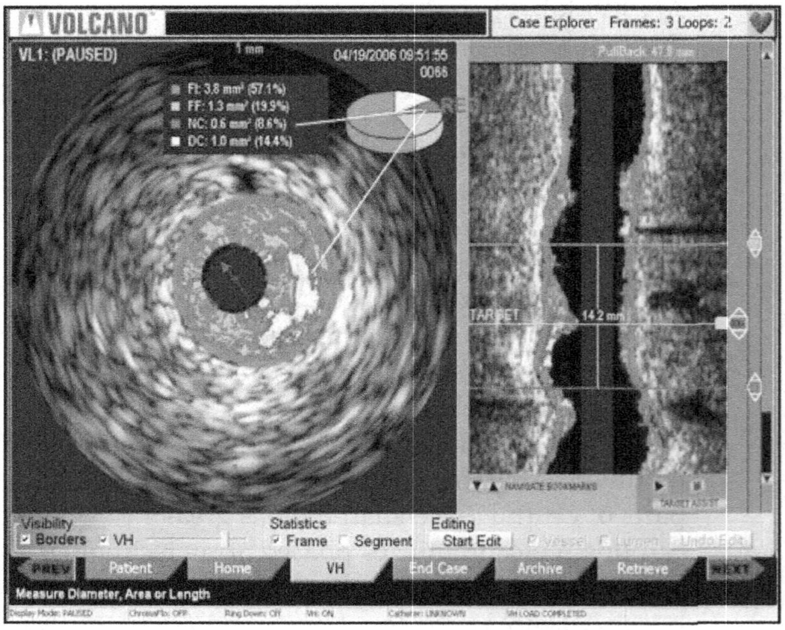

Virtual Histology IVUS image, pullback & pie chart
Color image available on CD, image from Volcanocorp.com

ANSWER b. Necrotic core (soft, lipid-like dead cells, foam cells and trapped blood cells) This tissue is found in unstable plaques, which may rupture. The 4 colors, difficult to see in black & white, are:

1. Dark green= fibrous plaque
2. Light green= fibrofatty plaque
3. Red= necrotic core
4. White= calcium

Murray says, "Plaque components are grouped into four basic tissue types during IVUS-VH imaging. These components are displayed on the image as different colour pixels. This technique is based on advanced radiofrequency analysis of reflected ultrasound signals in a frequency domain analysis and displays the reconstructed colour-coded tissue map of plaque composition superimposed on cross-sectional images of the coronary artery obtained by greyscale IVUS. "See: "Murray, et al. Contemporary Coronary Imaging from Patient to Plaque Part 1: IVUS-derived Virtual Histology" May 2010 Br J Cardiol 2010;17:129-32 Keywords: Virtual histology IVUS colors

523. **IVUS is often used post stent placement because it can best demonstrate:**

- **a. Thrombus and acute closure**
- **b. Coronary dissection**
- **c. Dog boning effect**
- **d. Suboptimal stent deployment**

ANSWER d. Suboptimal stent deployment. Grossman says: "In the early 1990's, Colombo and colleagues, using intravascular ultrasound (IVUS), demonstrated that the majority of stents were inadequately expanded despite excellent angiographic appearance. By employing routine high-pressure adjunctive dilation, he and other European investigators showed that such an optimal stenting reduced the incidence of stent thrombosis to less than 1% to 2% using only aspirin and a second antiplatelet agent, ticlopidine, ... " See: Grossman chapter on "Coronary Stenting" Keyword: IVUS best demonstrates suboptimal stent deployment

THIS IVUS IMAGE IS USED FOR THE NEXT 2 QUESTIONS.

524. How would you evaluate this coronary vessel?
- a. **Normal vessel**
- b. **Calcified eccentric plaque**
- c. **Mixed concentric plaque**
- d. **Ulcerated plaque**

525. In this IVUS image measure the total vessel diameter (Plaque + Media) is.
- a. **1.5 mm**
- b. **2.9 mm**
- c. **3.5 mm**
- d. **4.1 mm**

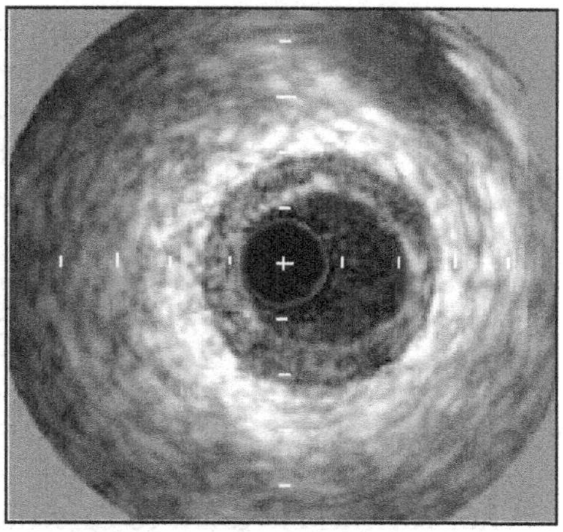
#524. IVUS with 1 mm markers

BOTH ANSWERS LISTED CONSECUTIVELY

524. ANSWER c. Mixed concentric plaque because of the few bright calcium speckles (seen around 12 o'clock) mixed with soft plaque material and the even plaque thickness all around the lumen. Concentric plaques like this are rare in CAD patients. Most plaques are irregular and eccentric. See: Baim, Chapter on Intravascular Ultrasound Imaging Keywords: IVUS concentric plaque

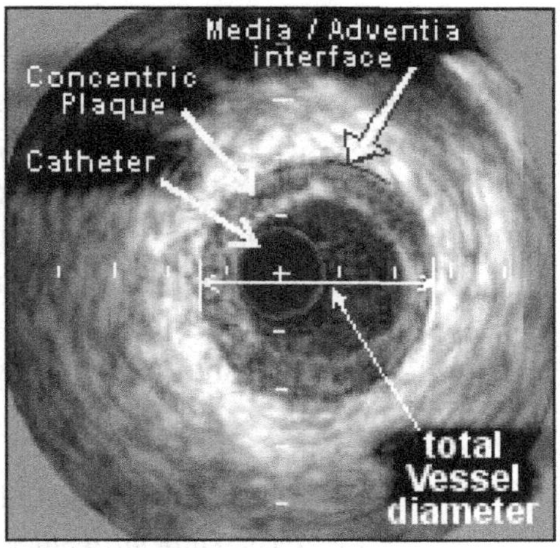

IVUS with 1 mm markers

525. ANSWER d. 4.1 mm. At the center of the grid is the small catheter/transducer ring. Outside this is the lumen of the artery filled with blood speckles. Outside this is the enlarged intima or plaque, which is 0.7 mm thick. Use the grid lines to measure this total vessel diameter. This vessel averages 4.2 mm in diameter. This area is comprised of the media, intima and plaque which are indistinguishable from each other. So they are termed the total vessel area. The concentric plaque surrounding the lumen is grey with speckles of calcium. If the lumen is not round, the average diameter is the average of the widest and narrowest diameters. See: Baim, Chapter on Intravascular Ultrasound Imaging Keywords: **IVUS diameter measurements**

526. **Which vessel structures does IVUS visualize? (Select 3)**

a. **Intima**
b. **Lumen**
c. **Media**
d. **Adventia**

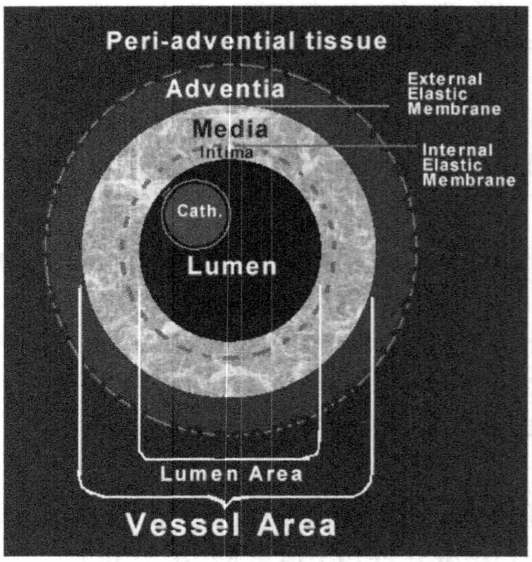

ANSWERS: a, b, & c. Intima, Lumen, and Media. Adventia is NOT usually distinguishable from the other peri-advential structures. The external elastic membrane (EEM) is the border between media and adventia, and it is the most visible border within the vessel wall. All the closer elements are well seen, containing the media, intima, plaque, and the vessel lumen. You often see other nearby structures such as coronary veins, pericardium, etc.

527. **What formula is used to calculate "plaque burden?" (note: TVA = Total Vessel Area, LA= Lumen Area)**

a. **PB = LA/TVA**
b. **PB = (TVA-LA) / LA**
c. **PB = (TVA-LA) / TVA**
d. **PB = (pi/2) x LA^2**

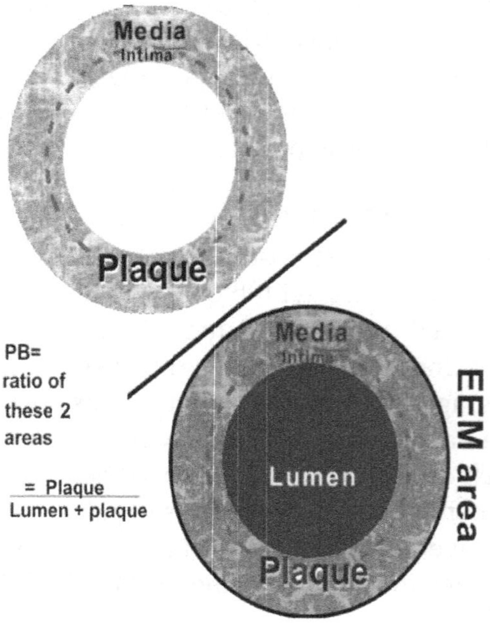

ANSWER c. PB = (TVA-LA) / TVA. The difference between Total Vessel Area and Lumen Area (TVA-LA) is the area of plaque (usually plaque + media). TVA is also termed EEM or External Elastic Membrane area. This important measurement is also termed Percent Plaque area shown as the upper circle in the diagram.

Baim says:

> "*the major ultrasound parameter that appears to correlate with subsequent restenosis is the percent plaque burden, viz., the ratio of the area of the plaque to the total vessel area (area within the media/adventia border).*"

DiMario says:

> "*As the adventia imperceptibly merges with the surrounding perivascular tissue, for the purpose of intracoronary ultrasound measurements the total cross-sectional area of the vessel is taken to mean the area enclosed by the outermost definable interface, i.e. the well delimited interface between the media and*

adventia coinciding with the position of the external elastic lamina. This is also referred to as the external elastic lamina area."

This calculation PB = (TVA-LA) / TVA is similar to calculating ejection fraction. Because EF = (EDV - ESV) / EDV is analogous to saying the largest area minus the smallest area divided by the largest area. Both are usually expressed as a percent, by multiplying the ratio by 100%. See: Baim, Chapter on Intravascular Ultrasound Imaging

USE THIS DIAGRAM FOR THE NEXT 2 QUESTIONS.

528. What is the dark line at #2 on this IVUS?

- a. **Media**
- b. **Adventia**
- c. **External Elastic Membrane**
- d. **Internal Elastic Membrane**

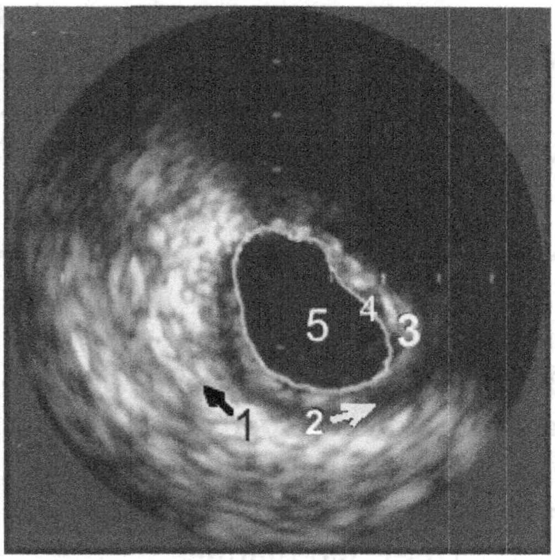

529. How would you evaluate this coronary vessel?

- a. **Normal vessel**
- b. **Calcified eccentric plaque**
- c. **Mixed concentric plaque**
- d. **Ulcerated plaque**

528. ANSWER c. External Elastic Membrane. This is the outer border of the plaque, and the division line between media and adventia. Structures shown are:

1. **Adventia**
2. **External elastic membrane**
3. **Media**
4. **Intima**
5. **Lumen**

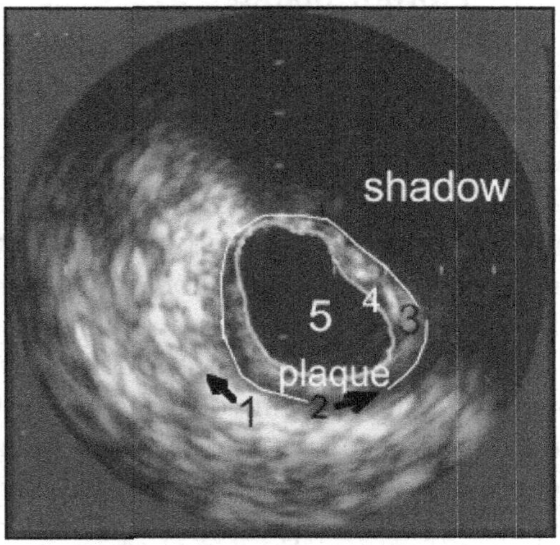

IVUS with 1 mm markers

529. ANSWER b. Calcified eccentric plaque. It is not a circular vessel and the plaque surrounding the lumen varies in thickness, making it eccentric plaque. There is calcium from 12 to 3 o'clock with shadowing behind.

530. On a grayscale IVUS image of a coronary artery where is the External Elastic Membrane is located?

- a. **Outside of the adventia**
- b. **Between media and adventia**
- c. **Between media and intima**
- d. **Inside of the intima**

Answer: b. Between media and adventia is also termed the "external elastic lamina" or the "tunica media" is the border between the arterial media and adventia. The External Elastic Membrane is usually seen as a dark line beneath the dark media and the brighter adventia. This is normally the only distinguishing line within arterial IVUS images, and one you will be expected to identify. The EEM is the line normally drawn within the vessel wall to separate normal artery from intimal/medial plaque. Incorrect answers are, Endothelium (the inner lining of a vessel or intima), and epithelium which is an outer lining.

Pandian says, "The external elastic membrane [EEM] is shorthand for the border between the hypoechoic media and the hyperechoic adventitia." See: Pandian N, Kreis A, et al. Ultrasound angioscopy: real-time, two-dimensional, intraluminal ultrasound imaging of blood vessels. Am J Cardiol 1988;62:493–4.

IVUS Pathology

531. In an IVUS image, bright reflections on the vessel wall with shadowing beyond the vessel (as shown from 12:00 to 3:00 o'clock) usually indicates a/an:

a. Calcium deposit
b. Atheromatous streak
c. Dissected plaque
d. Fibrotic plaque

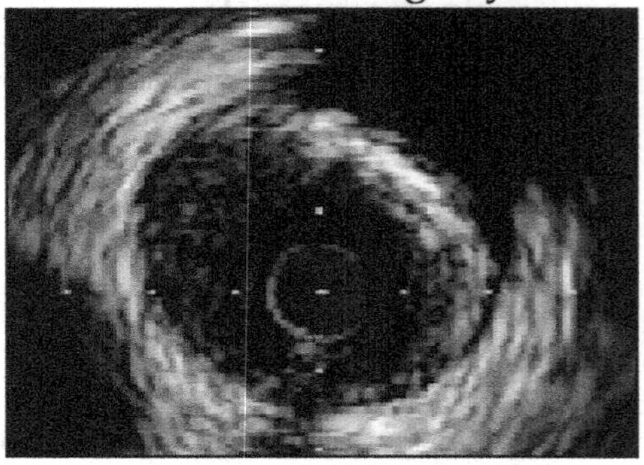

Coronary artery IVUS

ANSWER a. Calcium deposit.
Note the bright crescent from 12 to 3 o'clock on this IVUS image. The bright area indicates calcific plaque which is very echo-reflective. The dark area above and behind it is "shadowing." Shadowing occurs because the ultrasound cannot penetrate dense calcium deposits. Fibrous plaques may also appear bright, but do not block as much ultrasound as Ca and thus do not show shadowing behind the plaque.

Yock says: "Areas of calcification within plaque give a characteristic appearance on the ultrasound image, with a bright initial acoustic interface and then shadowing of the deeper tissue structures beyond the calcium . . . These calcium deposits are the single most important predictor of the way a particular lesion will respond to catheter interventions such as balloon angioplasty."

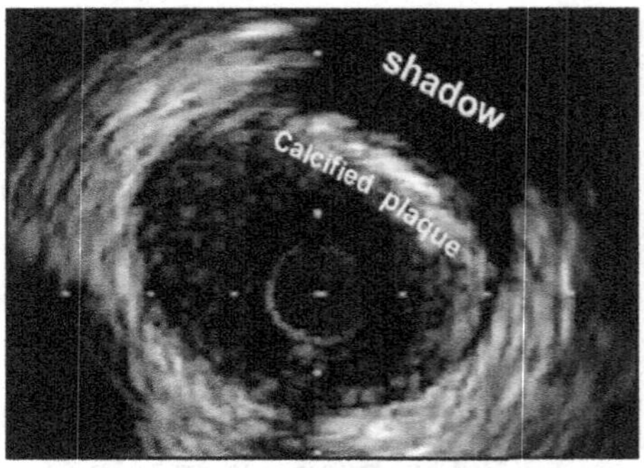

Calcific plaque from 12 - 3 o'clock shows shadowing behind

Metal stent struts will also appear bright on IVUS images and show shadowing like calcium.
See: Yock, Fitzherald & Popp, Chapter on "Intravascular Ultrasound" in Scientific American, Science and Medicine
Keywords: Calcium on IVUS image

532. In IVUS images, shadowing and ultrasound reverberations may be seen behind:

a. **Thrombus**
b. **Lipid pools**
c. **Dissected plaque**
d. **Calcium deposits**

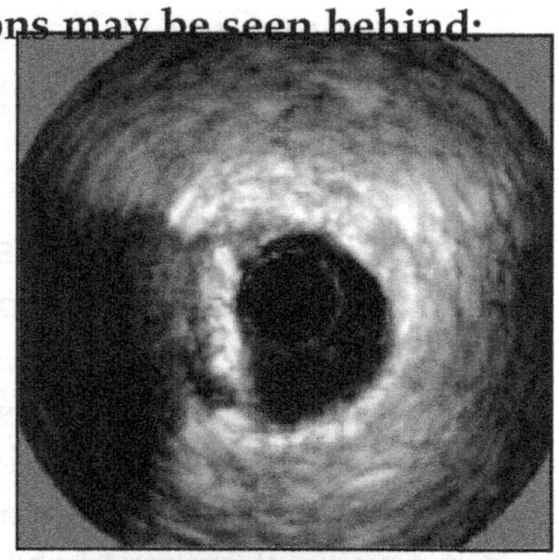

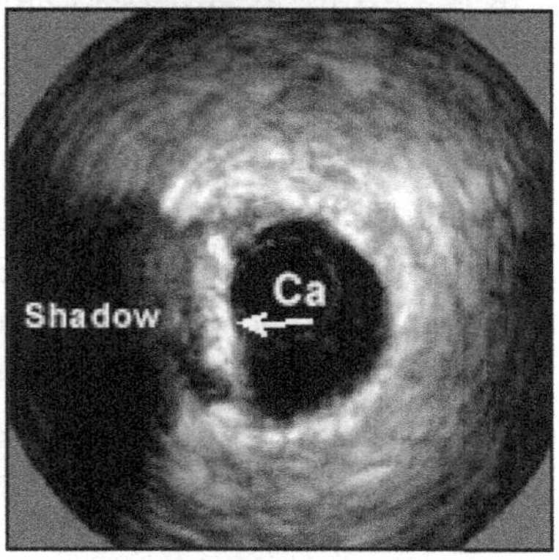

Calcific plaque from 7 - 10 o'clock shows shadowing behind

ANSWER d. Calcium deposits

Baim says: "*The easiest tissue type to identify- and the most significant clinically - is calcific plaque. A calcific deposit is recognized by its bright reflection with shadowing of all deeper tissue structures due to failure of the beam to penetrate beyond the calcified plaque. In some images, the shadowing will be accompanied by "reverberations," or ghost images of the calcium spaced in concentric arcs beyond the real calcium interface. Because of the shadowing, it is not possible to determine the depth of a calcific deposits or to define the vessel architecture beyond the calcium . . .* " See: Baim chapter on "Evaluation of Myocardial Blood Flow and Metabolism" Keywords: Calcium - bright reflective areas that cast a shadow

533. This IVUS image shows:

a. **Adequate stent apposition**
b. **Incomplete stent apposition**
c. **Side-branch occlusion**
d. **Disarticulated stent**

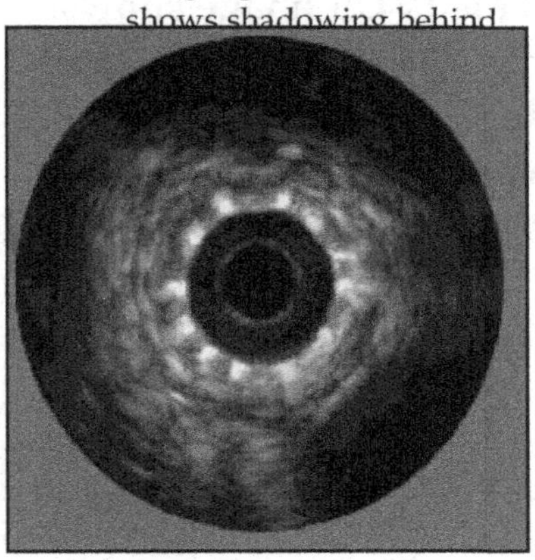

After Endosonics.com

ANSWER a. Adequate stent apposition. This important use of IVUS determined that many struts were not fully expanded into the vessel wall, leading to wider use of high pressure balloons to expand them.

In the diagram, the bright spots are the metal struts of a balloon inflated stent. All struts touch the vessel wall. This indicates the stent is fully deployed. If there were some distance between the stent and the vessel wall it is termed "incomplete apposition" and should be further expanded with a high pressure balloon.

See: Baim chapter on "Evaluation of Myocardial Blood Flow and Metabolism" Keywords: incomplete stent apposition

534. This chromaflow IVUS image shows:

- a. **Adequate stent apposition**
- b. **Incomplete stent apposition**
- c. **Side-branch occlusion**
- d. **Disarticulated stent**

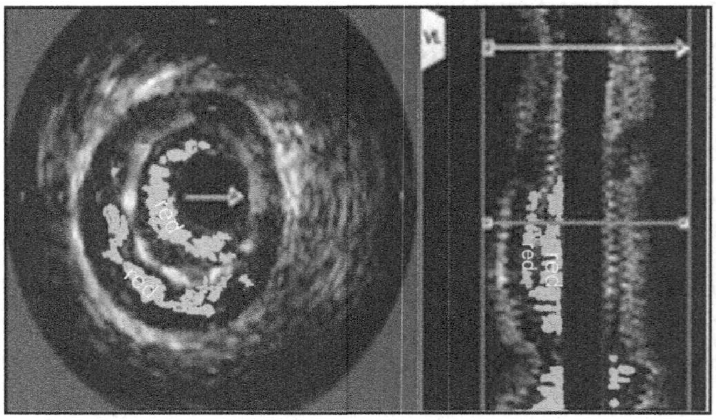

IVUS with Chromaflow

ANSWER b. Incomplete stent apposition with blood flowing around the stent. The stent appears in the pullback with red chromaflow around the lower half. "Because IVUS transducers ...are not forward looking but send pulses perpendicular to the catheter tip, the Doppler shift principle cannot be applied. So, IVUS color flow only "looks" like a Doppler image....The advantage of colorized flow is the ability to recognize more readily the true lumen by verifying the existence of circulating blood flow." See: Seminars in Vascular Surgery, Vol. 19, Issue 3 (Sept 2006) Diethrich, et al.

535. This IVUS image shows:

- a. **Intimal dissection**
- b. **Calcified stent**
- c. **Thrombosed stent**
- d. **Incomplete stent apposition**

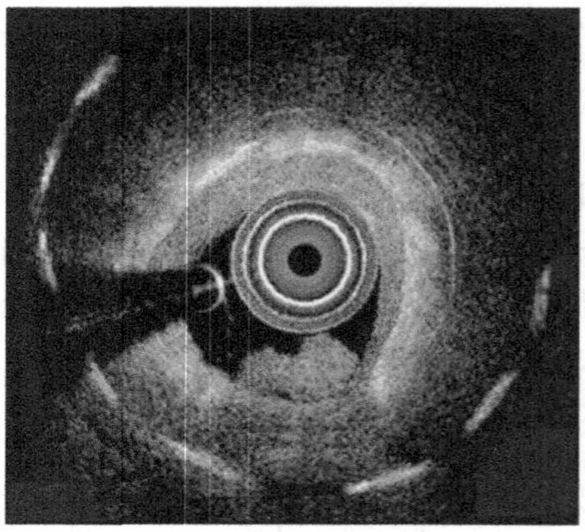

ANSWER c. Thrombosed stent with homogeneous layering on the top half with propagation of thrombus at 6:00 o'clock. This may be from a ruptured cap below the discrete clot, where lipids spilled into the lumen, causing thrombosis. Note several layers of thrombus with possible lipid core in the dark area at top of the image. The struts can be seen on lower half of the image. The guide wire is blocking the ultrasound at 8:00 o'clock causing shadowing. See: J.M. Hodgson, Technology Intravascular Ultrasound, An interactive Learning Tool With CME Credit, Solutions Group, Ltd., Ed. Div.

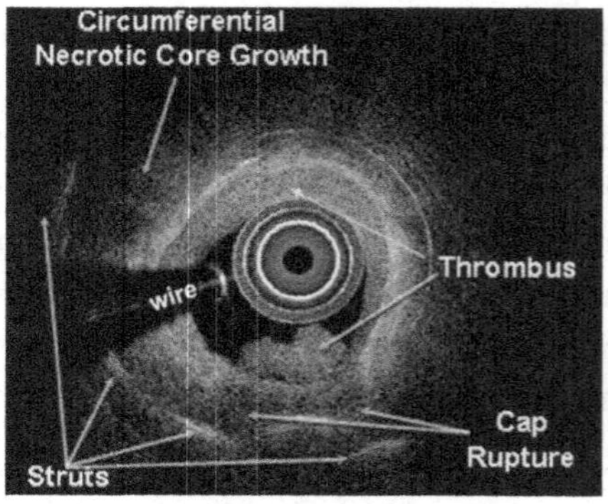

IVUS of Thrombosed stent

536. On this IVUS coronary image identify #D.
- a. IVUS catheter
- b. Lumen
- c. Eccentric plaque
- d. Media

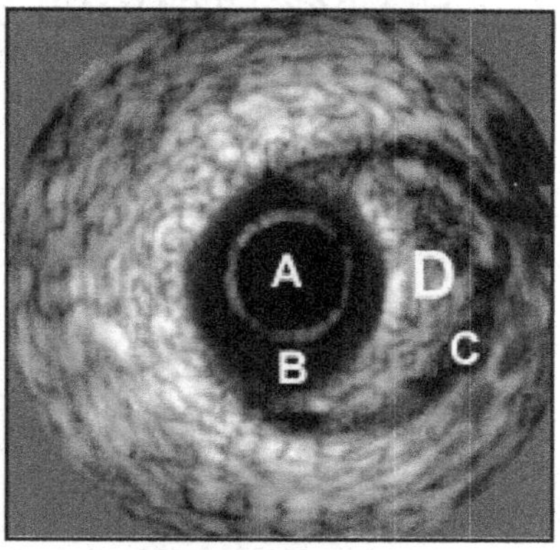

#538. Coronary IVUS

ANSWER c. Eccentric plaque is seen from 1 o'clock to 6 o'clock. It is clearly separated from the media at #C.
Correctly matched letters are:
A. IVUS catheter
B. Artery Lumen
C. Media, between plaque and adventia
D. Eccentric plaque of mixed fibrous and low density material
See: Baim chapter on "Evaluation of Myocardial Blood Flow and Metabolism"

537. What is seen on this post-angioplasty IVUS image at #D?
- a. Intimal proliferation
- b. Coronary perforation
- c. Dissected plaque
- d. Acute thrombus formation
- e. IVUS catheter

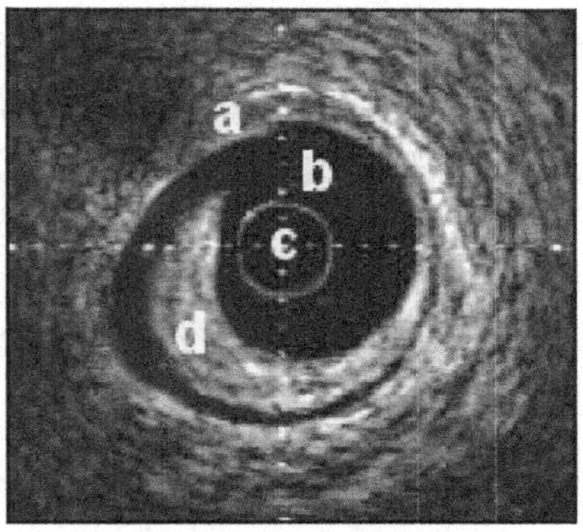

#537. Intracoronary IVUS

ANSWER c. Dissected plaque. Note the tear extending from 11 o'clock to 5 o'clock behind the "C" shaped plaque. Such dissections may be plastered back against the medial wall by stenting.
Baim say:

> *"Ultrasound has confirmed that tearing or dissection is a frequent and important concomitant of balloon angioplasty, occurring in 60 to 80% of cases. Less than half of these tears are seen by angiography. . . . Tearing is associated with a greater acute gain (initial increase in lumen diameter following the procedure) than is seen in plaques where there is no evident tearing."*

See: Baim, Chapter on Intravascular Ultrasound Imaging Keywords: IVUS saline flush

THE NEXT 3 QUESTIONS ARE FROM THE SAME PATIENT:

538. This patient has a positive stress test. This angiographic injection RAO caudal view shows a probable:

a. Left main stenosis
b. LAD - Circ. bifurcation stenosis
c. 1st diagonal bifurcation stenosis
d. Stenosis at origin of obtuse marginal

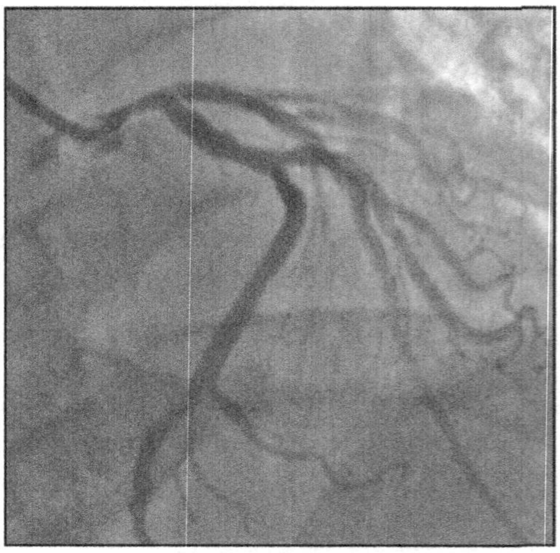

RAO caudal coronary angio.

ANSWER: a. Left main stenosis. The left main should be larger than the other arteries. The orifice is tight with diffuse disease along the length of the left main. Evaluate with FFR. The large circumflex is viewed to the left and below. The straighter LAD seen on the right. An FFR test would clarify the hemodynamic significance of this lesion.

539. This IVUS image was taken on the lesion seen in the patient above. What does it show at #4?

a. Eccentric calcified plaque
b. Eccentric fibrous plaque
c. Concentric calcified plaque
d. Concentric fibrous plaque

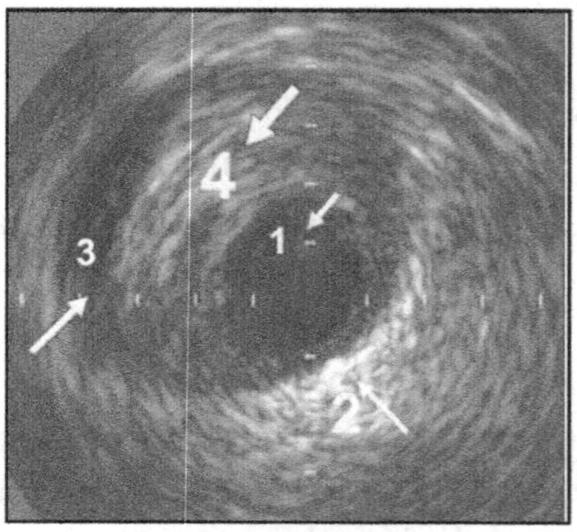

Intracoronary IVUS

540. What is seen on the above IVUS image at #3?

a. Lipid pool
b. Fibrous plaque
c. Dissected plaque
d. Internal elastic membrane

BOTH ANSWERS LISTED TOGETHER BELOW.
539. ANSWER b. Eccentric fibrous plaque seen at #4. This lumen (#1) is very eccentric to the crescent shaped plaque. This illustrates one of the best uses of IVUS, where left main stenosis does not show up well on angio.

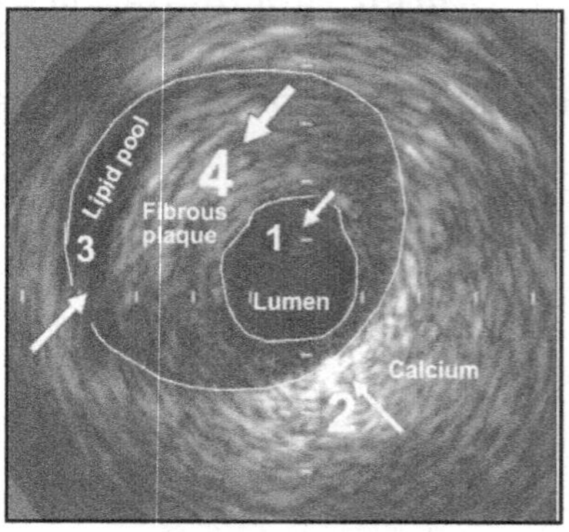

Intracoronary IVUS

540. ANSWER a. Lipid pool. The dark area in the media suggests a collection of soft runny fat. This fatty area creates a plane that is easy to shear off and may lead to plaque rupture and thrombosis. It is termed an echolucent core and is associated with vulnerable plaque. It's like spreading butter on a wood surface before gluing it. The

glue won't stick. Labeled areas are:

1. Lumen
2. Calcium spots
3. Lipid pool
4. Firbrous plaque

See: Baim, Chapter on Intravascular Ultrasound Imaging Keywords: Lipid pool

541. What is the appearance of lipid pools on a grayscale IVUS image?

a. Echo dense or black

b. Echo dense or bright white

c. Echo lucent or black

d. Echo lucent or bright white

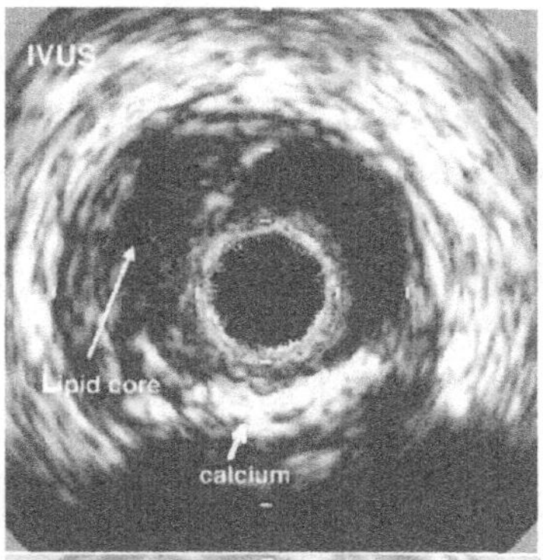

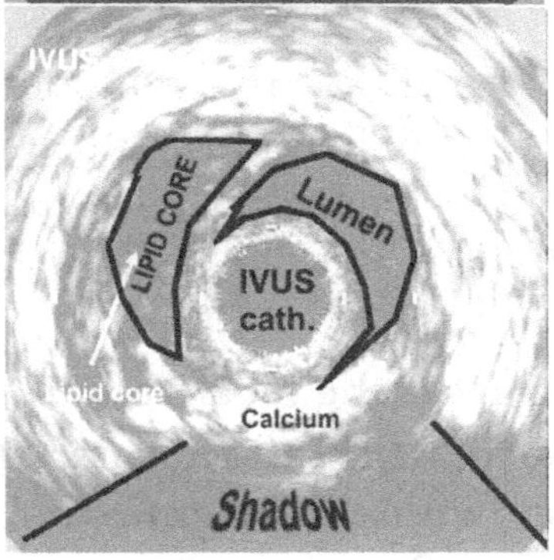

ANSWER: c. Echo lucent or black. Lucent means transparent, something that does not reflect ultrasound like fat. Lipid pools found in plaque are usually homogenous and echolucent showing as black. When a thin plaque covers one of these pools it is termed a thin-cap fibroatheroma (TCFA). They are liable to break open exposing the lipid or necrotic tissue to the lumen. This may cause clot formation and STEMI. Because they are so thin TCFA's are best seen on VH-IVUS (Virtual Histology) or OCT.

Calcium appears the opposite on IVUS. Ca is echodense and highly reflective showing as white, but leaving a dark shadow behind it. Note the appearance of these opposite tissues in this IVUS image shown.

Bhatt says: "Plaques rich in lipid are typically echolucent, whereas echodense ones are typically rich in fibrous tissue and calcification. Calcified lesions are usually very dense and have a back shadow due to the complete absorption of the ultrasound beam. Using the adjacent adventitia as a visual reference, echodensity indicates a plaque is "bright" or "brighter" than adventitia (closer to the white end of the grayscale), while echolucency refers to plaques that appear "darker" than adventitia (closer to the black end of the grayscale.)"

"TCFA is defined as a lipid-rich plaque (>10% confluent lipid core) with a very thin cap (<100 μm in thickness, not visible by VH) and with an area stenosis that is usually >40%. These plaques frequently contain speckles of calcification and are more prevalent in patients presenting with acute coronary syndromes, even in nonculprit segments." See, Bhatt, chapter on IVUS, Guidelines for Use and Appropriate Indications

542. Identify 5 IVUS characteristics associated with culprit lesions.

- a. **Ulceration**
- b. **Eccentricity**
- c. **Thrombosis**
- d. **Calcification**
- e. **Echo-opaque (Lipid) white core**
- f. **Positive remodeling**

ANSWERS: a, b, c, d, & f. Echo-opaque (Lipid) white core is NOT correct. It is an **echo-lucent** core, which appears dark and nonreflective or echogenic as in the previous question. Lipids appear opposite to calcium. Instead of being bright and reflective with shadowing, fat is dark, non-reflective and transmits the ultrasound. "Culprit lesions" are the ones that cause the patient's symptoms. According to DeMaria, IVUS characteristics of culprit lesions include:

1. Ulceration
2. Eccentricity
3. Thrombosis
4. Calcification
5. Positive remodeling (vessel wall expands)
6. Echo-lucent (Lipid) black core

See: DeMaria, "Imaging Vulnerable Plaque by Ultrasound" J Am Coll. Cardiol, 2006; 47:32-39, doi:10.1016/j.jacc.2005.11.047

543. What is the most valuable procedure in a successful intracoronary IVUS protocol, shown on the right panel of this IVUS image?

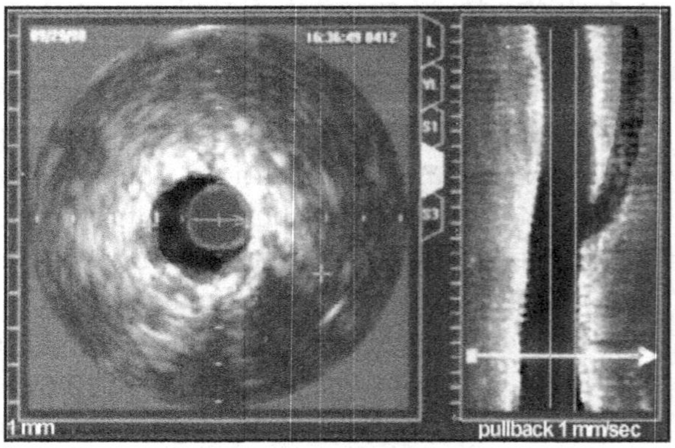

Normal Coronary IVUS

- a. **Careful real time scans back and forth over the stenosis**
- b. **Recording and analyzing a pullback scan through the area of stenosis**
- c. **Imaging the lesion pre and post adenosine**
- d. **Frequent flushing of the catheter to remove air bubbles**

ANSWER b. Recording and analyzing a pullback scan through the area of stenosis assures that the entire area is inspected, because many dangerous lesions are not in the areas of greatest narrowing. This diagram shows a cross section and scan of a normal artery. The arrow on the right indicates where the cross sectional view is taken, and corresponds to the image on the left. Note the vessel branching off the main artery on the right. Baim says:

> "*The single most critical procedural factor in the success of intracoronary imaging is following a well-defined imaging protocol. Because the morphology of a diseased artery can change dramatically over a very short distance, it is essential to perform a systematic scan of the artery rather than engage in a haphazard, "look and see" examination. A systemic scan*

is best accomplished by initially delivering a transducer well beyond the region of interest, and then slowly pulling the catheter (or, with the CVIS catheters, pulling the imaging core within the catheter) back through the artery."

See: Baim, Chapter on ICE Imaging Keywords: IVUS pullback protocol

544. This is an IVUS pullback from the LAD / Circumflex bifurcation - into the aorta. It shows:

- a. **LAD calcification**
- b. **Circ. calcification**
- c. **Coronary aneurysm**
- d. **Left main ostial stenosis**
- e. **Stent in left main**

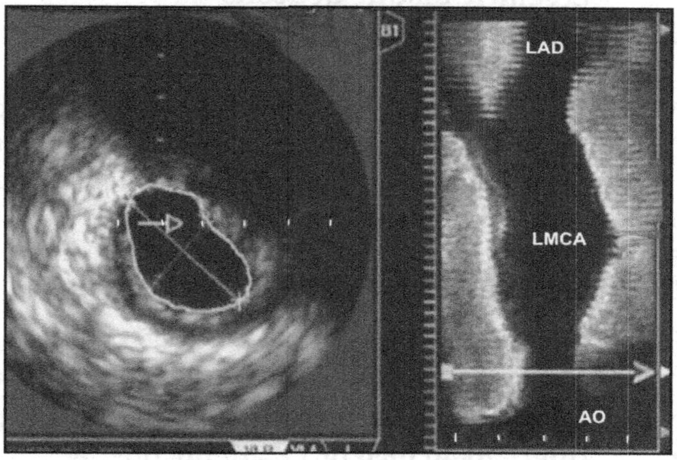

IVUS cross section & pullback. 1 mm markers

ANSWER: d. Left main ostial stenosis. The arrow on the right is where the cross section image was taken. You see the LAD & Circumflex bifurcation in the upper part of the pullback image. Note the narrowest diameter is under 2 mm. Cross sectional area was 6 mm^2 indicating significant left main disease. "One particular use of IVUS in the coronary anatomy is in the quantification of left main disease in cases where routine coronary angiography gives equivocal results. Many studies in the past have shown that significant left main disease can increase mortality, and that intervention (either coronary artery bypass graft surgery or percutaneous coronary intervention) to reduce mortality is necessary when the left main stenosis is significant."

"When using IVUS to determine whether an individual's left main disease is clinically significant, in terms of the desirability of physical intervention, the two most widely used parameters are the degree of stenosis and the minimal lumen area. A cross sectional area of =7 mm^2 in a symptomatic individual or =6 mm^2 in an asymptomatic individual is considered to be clinically significant and warrants intervention to improve one-year mortality"

545. What is the normal rate of travel for an automated IVUS pullback?

- a. **0.01-0.1 mm/sec**
- b. **0.5-1 mm/sec**
- c. **2-5 mm/sec**
- d. **5-10 mm/sec**

Answer: b. 0.5-1 mm/sec are available on current pullback devices.

Grossman says, "It is generally best to advance the imaging element distal to the area of interest and perform a systematic examination during pullback. Automated pullback devices withdraw the imaging element at a steady rate of 0.5 or 1.0 mm/second, which allows accurate axial registration of each cross section and thus, precise longitudinal distance measurements." Volcano, has several pullback devices which ensure a smooth, accurate pullback rate: 0.5 mm/sec or 1.0 mm/sec. See: Intracoronary Ultrasound, Gary

Mintz and www.volcanocorp.com Keywords: IVUS pullback 0.5-1 mm/sec

546. This IVUS image shows:

- **a. Adequately deployed stent**
- **b. Underdeployed stent**
- **c. Eccentric plaque deposits**
- **d. Concentric plaque deposits**

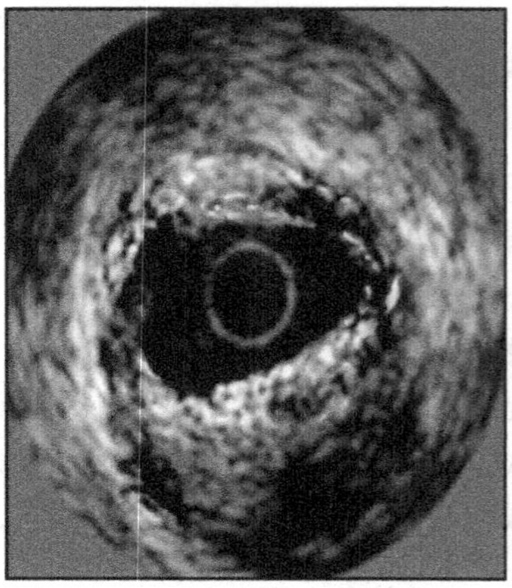

After www.cardiologyhd.com

ANSWER: c. Eccentric plaque deposits from 3 to 7 o'clock. This is eccentric or irregularly shaped. There is bright reflective calcium in the wall and on the plaque. Shadowing occurs from 4 to 6 o'clock. See: www.cardiologyhd.com And Grossman, chapter on "Intravascular Imaging Techniques" Keywords: IVUS eccentric plaque

547. Prior to inserting an IVUS imaging catheter into the coronary artery assure full anticoagulation and:

- **a. Inject 20-40 mcg of IV adenosine**
- **b. Inject 100-200 mcg IC verapamil**
- **c. Inject 100 - 300 ug of IC nitroglycerin**
- **d. Start drip of 180 mcg/kg Integrilin IV**

ANSWER: c. Inject 100 - 300 ug of IC nitroglycerin to reduce the irritation to the coronary artery. Grossman says, "The technique for delivering IVUS catheters is generally similar to that used for standard angioplasty/stent catheters. Prior to IVUS imaging, an intravenous injection of 5000 to 10000 unit heparin or equivalent anticoagulation should be administered, as well as intracoronary nitroglycerin (100-300 ug) to reduce the potential for spasm." See Grossman, chapter on "Intravascular Imaging Techniques"

548. The outside wall of a stenosed coronary artery often undergoes "positive remodeling." This is seen on IVUS as a:

- **a. Enlarged total vessel area**
- **b. Reduced total vessel area**
- **c. Enlarged lumen**
- **d. Reduced lumen**

ANSWER a. Enlarged total vessel area as seen by increased diameter of the external elastic lamina, which separates the adventitia and media.
Yock says:

> *"Remodeling is nature's way of maintaining blood flow as plaque builds up inside an artery. The wall of the artery expands as the plaque accumulates, so that the lumen is kept open as long as possible. The reverse of this process, negative remodeling, can happen after angioplasty, with a contraction of the treated segment leading to an accelerated renarrowing or 'restenosis.'"*

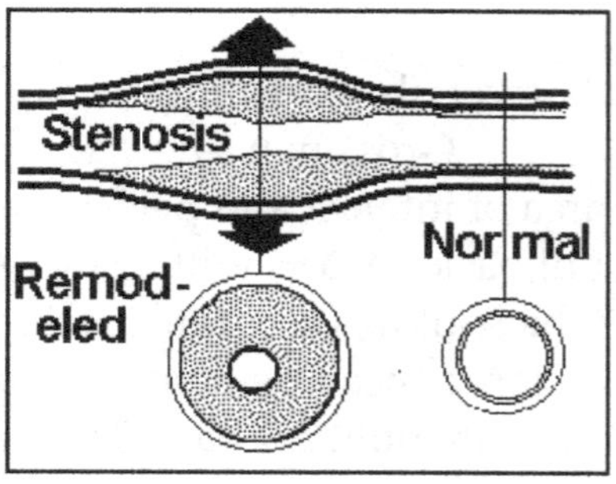

So, positive remodeling helps blood flow, but negative remodeling reduces flow. This remodeling response was described by the pathologist Glagov in 1995. So, this effect is sometimes termed the "Glagov effect." Although the stenosed lumen area is reduced the outer vessel enlarges; this defines remodeling.
See: Yock, Fitzherald & Popp, Chapter on "Intravascular Ultrasound" in Scientific American, Science and Medicine Keywords: Remodeling

549. In IVUS imaging of stenotic lesions, what lumen diameter reduction is considered to be hemodynamically significant and generally should be stented? (Compare stenotic lumen diameter to adjacent normal lumen diameter.)

a. >50 %
b. >70%
c. >80%
d. >90%

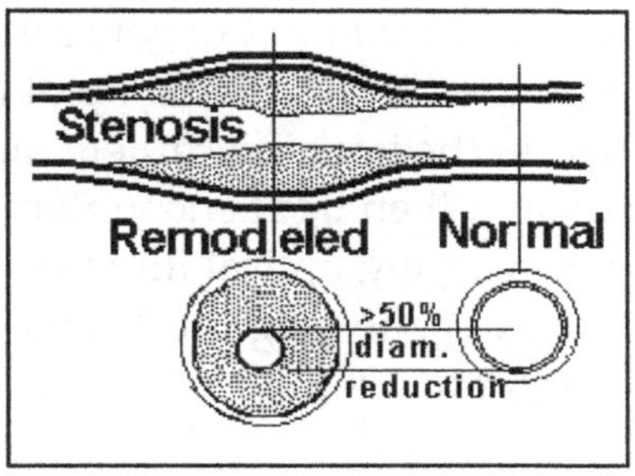

ANSWER a. >50% lumen reduction or 70% area diameter reduction.
Baim says:

> *"A 70% area stenosis (equivalent to a 50% diameter stenosis) is considered to constitute a hemodynamically significant obstruction."*

In this example, note the difference between the plaque burden and the % stenosis. Angiographic percent stenosis compares the stenotic lumen area to the area of an adjacent normal lumen. In this example, when the stenotic lumen is compared to a normal lumen (at the right) it yields a 50% diameter or 75% area stenosis. Note that in angiography, a 75% stenosis is usually considered hemodynamically significant. But, in angio we do not see the remodeled vessel wall.

Note in the cross sectional IVUS diagram the normal lumen to vessel diameter ratio is 50%, which is the same as a 70% area reduction (pi x r^2). The remodeled area shows the plaque burden. But, the stenosed lumen diameter must be referenced to a normal adjacent vessel lumen diameter to evaluate the lumen stenosis as shown.
See: Baim, Chapter on Intravascular Ultrasound Imaging Keywords: IVUS >70% area Hemodynamically significant, also see SCAI standards

550. Many cath labs do routine coronary angiography and IVUS imaging on heart transplant patients. They are usually looking for:

a. Cardiac Allograft Vasculopathy (CAV) with intimal thickening
b. Cardiac Allograft Vasculopathy (CAV) with adventitia thickening
c. Cardiac Heterograft Vasculopathy (CHV) with intimal thickening
d. Cardiac Heterograft Vasculopathy (CHV) with adventitia thickening

ANSWER: a. Cardiac Allograft Vasculopathy (CAV) with intimal thickening. In the incorrect answers, note that heterografts are transplanted from a different species, like a pig heart valve. Most coronary disease thickens the intima of the vessel not the adventia.

Weis says, "Cardiac allograft vasculopathy (CAV) remains a troublesome long-term complication of heart transplantation. It is manifested by a unique and unusually accelerated form of coronary disease affecting both intramural and epicardial coronary arteries and veins. CAV is characterized by vascular injury induced by a variety of noxious stimuli, including the immune system response to the allograft,... The obstructive vascular lesions are thought to progress through repetitive endothelial injury followed by repair response." See: Weis, Cardiac Allograft Vasculopathy, A Review, Circulation 1997

551. What type of radiation is used to image intravascular anatomy using Optical Coherence Tomography (OCT)?

a. **White light**
b. **Ultraviolet**
c. **Ultrasound**
d. **Near infra-red**

ANSWER: d. Near infra-red light.

Bhatt says, "OCT utilizes optical interference of near-infrared light to generate images. Near-infrared light is emitted from a distal tip of an optical fiber located within the imaging catheter and directed at the target tissue. When light encounters a boundary between objects with varying optical impedances, a portion of the light is backscattered. The OCT catheter measures the magnitude and echo time delay of the backscattered light signal." See: Bhatt, chapter on OCT

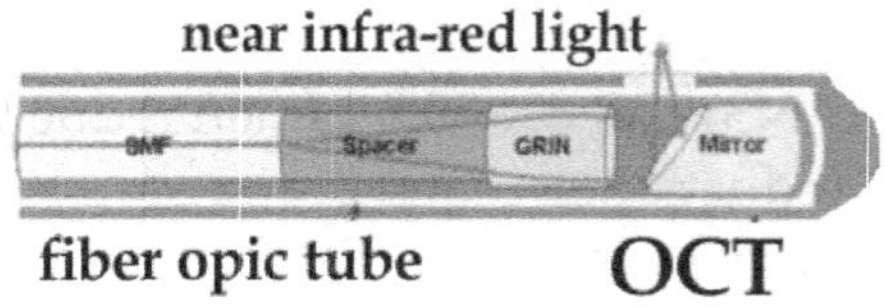

552. The chief advantage of Optical Coherence Tomography (OCT) imaging compared to IVUS imaging is:

a. **Increased resolution**
b. **Combined Doppler flow probe**
c. **Increased depth of penetration**
d. **Increased thrombus identification**

ANSWER a. Increased resolution (Is 10 times finer than for IVUS.)

Baim says, "Optical coherence tomography (OCT) generates real-time tomographic images from back-scattered reflection of infrared light.... The greatest advantage of this light-based imaging technology is its significantly higher resolution (10 times or greater) than that of conventional pulse-echo, ultrasound-based approaches....Thus, OCT has the advantage of being able to image through calcium without shadowing, as seen with IVUS. On the other hand, signal penetration through the diseased arterial wall is generally more limited (no more than 2 mm with current OCT devices)" In the

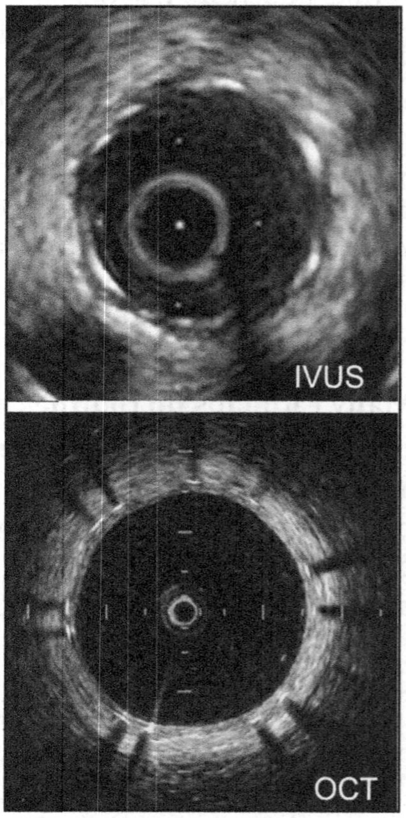

Stent imaging comparison

lower diagram, note the beautiful fine detail in the OCT image compared to the IVUS. This technology shows great promise for coronary imaging. Note the stent strut bright spots and shadows. See: Baim, Chapter on Intravascular Ultrasound Imaging Keywords: Angioscopy best to ID thrombus

553. Which intravascular diagnostic modality requires intracoronary contrast or Lactate Ringers injection during imaging?

- a. **Grayscale IVUS**
- b. **Virtual Histology IVUS**
- c. **Fractional Flow Reserve (FFR)**
- d. **Optical Coherence Tomography (OCT)**

ANSWER: d. Optical Coherence Tomography (OCT). Because OCT uses a near infra-red light source the blood must be flushed from the artery to see the vessel wall.

Bhatt says about OCT imaging, "Blood is displaced by continuous injection of iso-osmolar contrast or mixture of dextran and lactated Ringer's through the guiding catheter by manual injection or automated injection."
See: Bhatt, chapter on IVUS, Guidelines for Use and Appropriate Indications

Intracardiac Echocardiography - ICE

554. What types of cath lab cases commonly use intracardiac echo (ICE)?

- a. **Evaluating coronary stent apposition**
- b. **ICD and biventricular lead implant**
- c. **Transseptal catheterization and PFO closure**
- d. **LIMA or radial artery graft anastomoses during coronary bypass surgery**

ANSWER: c. Transseptal catheterization and PFO closures - often use intracardiac echocardiogram (ICE) catheters. Watson says, "ICE has been used for electrophysiologic procedures, guiding radio frequency ablations, trans-septal punctures, evaluating aortic aneurysms and aortic stent-graft procedures. Most recently, the technology has been applied to aiding complex pediatric and congenital procedures, such as atrial septal defect and patent foramen ovale closures. ICE allows superior imaging to transesophageal echocardiography by allowing a larger field of view, optimal soft-tissue contrast and more precise evaluation of the anatomy and defects." For viewing coronary stents, IVUS or OCT is preferred. See: Watson, chapter on "Invasive Ultrasound: Beyond Angiography" Keywords: ICE for transseptal and PFO

555. A major advantage to using intracardiac echocardiography (ICE) verses TEE is:

a. **Three dimensional images**
b. **General anesthesia is not needed**
c. **Tissue characterization (4 color images)**
d. **It is disposable**

ANSWER: b. General anesthesia is not needed, only the local anesthetic that is used in standard percutaneous entry -no anesthesiologist, no complications due to anesthetic, less time for induction, and less discomfort to the patient. The diagram shows 3 types of phased array echo transducers used in cardiology. All produce a pie-shaped sector scan. Being disposable is not an advantage, due to added expense. See: Watson, chapter on "Invasive Ultrasound" Keywords: ICE, no general anesthesia

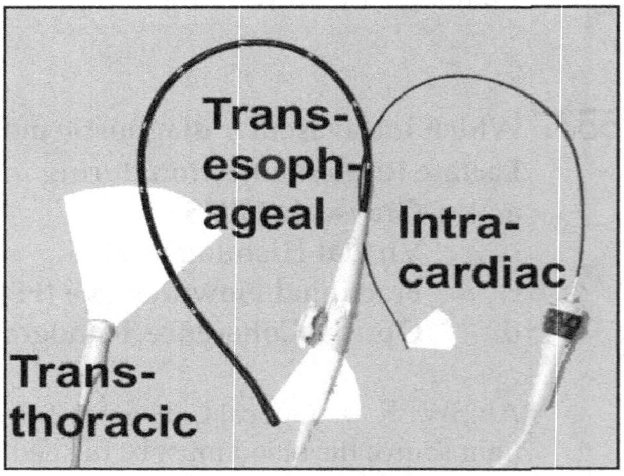

Three phased array ultrasound transducers (TTE, TEE, & ICE)

556. Intracardiac echocardiography uses ____ as an injectable contrast agent to view shunts or distinguish the right heart from the left heart chambers.

a. **Agitated saline**
b. **Doppler shifted plasma**
c. **Radio-isotope tagged red cells**
d. **Low osmolar angiographic contrast**

ANSWER: a. Agitated saline or doing a "bubble study looks like a dust storm in the chamber where they are injected as each bubble reflects ultrasound. Agitated saline, or doing a "bubble study," looks like a dust storm in the chamber where they are injected as each bubble reflects ultrasound. The technique uses a saline solution which is agitated by mixing it back and forth quickly between two syringes connected via a stopcock. This creates very small bubbles in the saline. When the saline is injected intravenously into the arm, these bubbles can be seen as they pass through the heart's chambers and they can be followed in the heart ultrasonically to determine if any bubbles do not follow the normal blood flow pathways. It is also termed a "contrast-enhanced ultrasound" (CEUS). The bubbles are filtered out in the lungs, and produce no ill effects. Some labs mix the saline with small amounts of blood for slightly better visualization.

557. **This patient is asked to do a Valsalva maneuver while agitated saline is injected into his arm vein. What pathology does this concurrent ICE image suggest?**

a. **VSD**
b. **PFO**
c. **PDA**
d. **ASD with Left to right shunt**

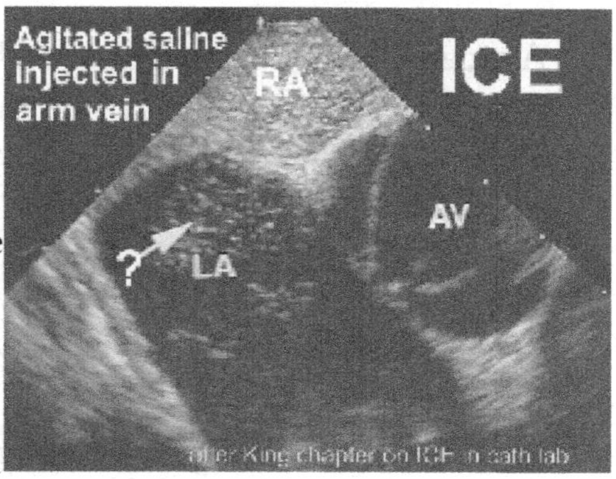

ANSWER: b. PFO or Patent Foramen Ovale with Rt. - Lt. shunting across the atrial septum. Note the bubbles at the arrow tip; these should not be present. They should normally be filtered out by the lungs. You can see the white cloud of bubbles in the RA and some bubbles appearing in the LA indicating a Right-to-Left shunt. The Valsalva maneuver or coughing increases right sided pressure to force right to left shunting if there is an atrial septal defect. A PFO like this with shunting is dangerous because it may allow passage of venous thrombi to pass into the left heart resulting in TIA or stroke. Agitating saline induces microbubbles that when injected act as a contrast agent easily seen on ultrasound. In the diagram LA = Left atrium, & AV = Aortic Valve.

King says, "Imaging from the mid-RA saline contrast (Bubbles) with Valsalva maneuver demonstrating passage of right-to-left contrast consistent with PFO." See: King, chapter on "ICE in the cath lab"

558. **What structure is seen at #3 on this ICE image taken from the Hi RA (#1)?**

a. **Coronary Sinus**
b. **LA appendage**
c. **RV trabeculations**
d. **RV moderator band**

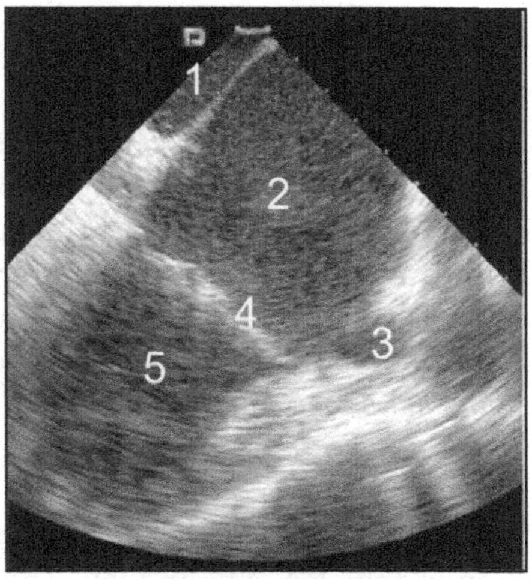

#558. ICE

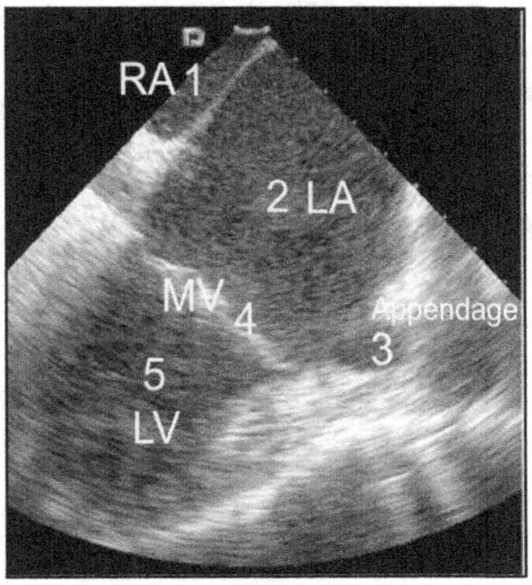

Hi RA ICE sector scan

ANSWER b. LA appendage. This is view #4 from the illustrated ICE views in question #551. The coronary sinus might have shown up on the left below the RA. Of course, in real time you can see the mitral valve opening and closing, which helps identify structures. See: Practical Intracardiac Echocardiography in Electrophysiology, by Jian-Tang Ren, et. al.

THESE 4 ICE IMAGES ARE FOR THE NEXT 2 QUESTIONS.

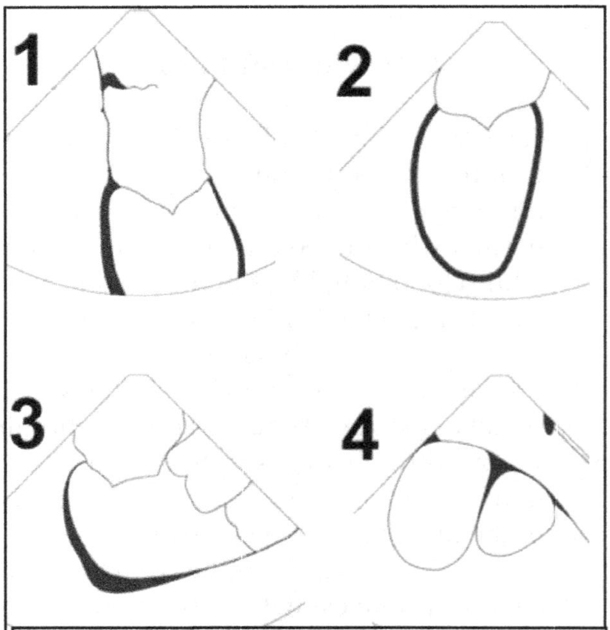

559. **A steerable sector scanning ICE transducer is in the RA. Of the four ICE drawings shown, identify the view labeled #1.**

- a. **AO & PA**
- b. **RA home view**
- c. **Intra-atrial septum & SVC**
- d. **Eustachian & tricuspid valve**

560. **Which of the 4 images above is the HOME or starting view for an ICE exam?**

- a. **#1**
- b. **#2**
- c. **#3**
- d. **#4**

BOTH ANSWERS LISTED CONSECUTIVELY

559. ANSWER: d. Eustachian & tricuspid valve. #1 is the eustachian ridge, remnant of the eustachian valve, and tricuspid valve isthmus. Withdraw the catheter to the inferior RA. The isthmus is between the eustachian ridge and the TV. *Remember an isthmus is a piece of land between 2 land masses, like the isthmus of Panama connects N. & S. America.*

560. Answer b. #2 is the "RA Home view" showing the RA, TV, and RV. The scan plane is facing anteriorly in a neutral position. This is where you always start.
#3 is the RA, TV, RV, AO & PA, where the transducer is rotated slightly clockwise from the anterior home view.
#4. Is the IAS & SVC with the catheter withdrawn to the inferior RA, tilted posteriorly with slight right rotation.

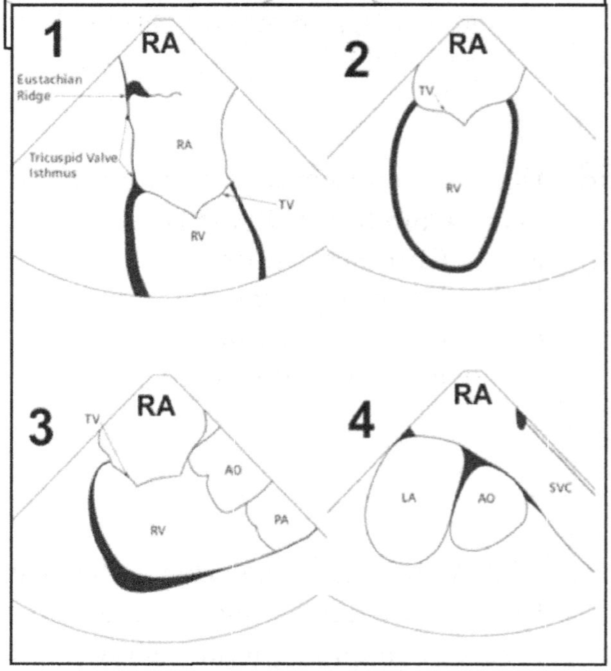

ICE views from RA - after Siemens online booklet

561. A steerable sector scanning ICE transducer is in the right heart. Of the four ICE drawings shown, identify the view labeled #1.

a. LV short axis
b. LV Long axis
c. Coronary sinus ostium
d. LA & LA appendage, MV, LV

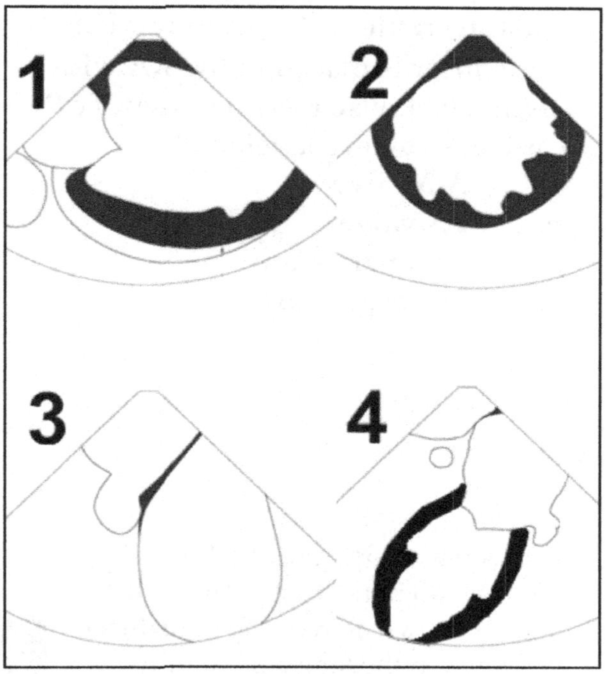

ICE views from RA - after Siemens online booklet

BE ABLE TO IDENTIFY ALL VIEWS AND STRUCTURES LISTED BELOW.

Answer: #1 is b. LV Long axis view. Advance the ICE catheter into the RV and rotate clockwise to see the intra-ventricular septum. LV is on the other side.
#2. Is the LV short axis view. From the LV long axis view tilt the steering knob until the circular LV and papillary muscles are seen.
#3. Is the Coronary Sinus Ostium seen from the RA by rotating clockwise and looking inferiorly.
#4. Is the LA appendage, mitral valve and LV view. Rotate clockwise past the AO/PA view with some left tilt. See: Siemens.com

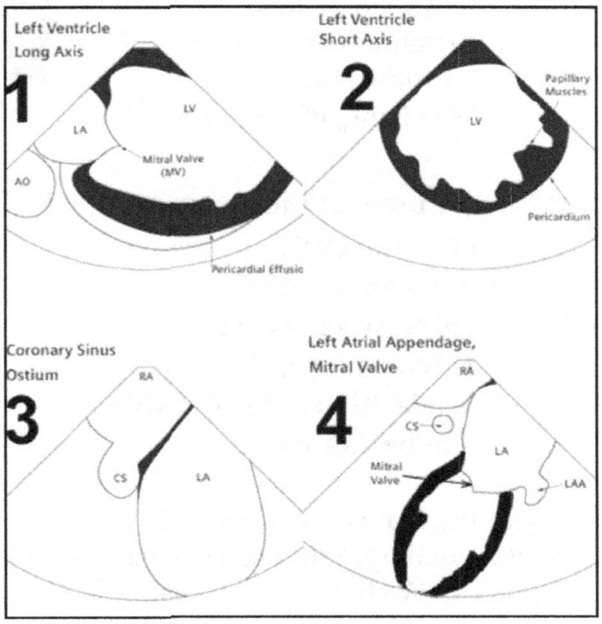

ICE views from RA - after Siemens online booklet

562. This steerable sector scanning ICE transducer is placed in the RA with slight clockwise rotation. Identify the cardiac structure labeled #3.

a. AO valve
b. PA valve
c. Coronary sinus
d. Tricuspid valve

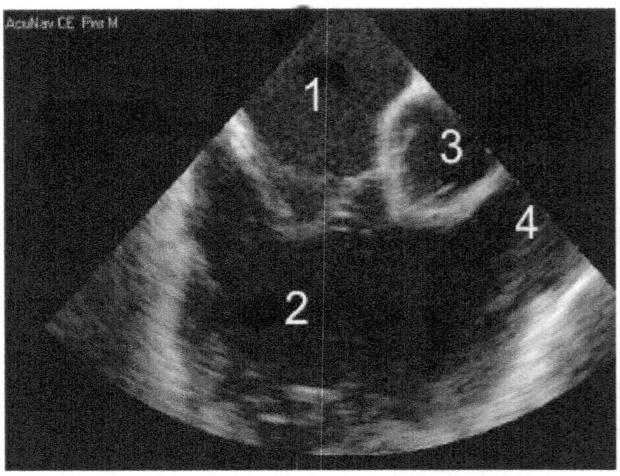

ICE view from RA *from Medscape.com*

Answer: a. AO valve at #3. This is the view #3 in the first group of ICE images shown above. The transducer is rotated in the long axis slightly clockwise from the anterior home view. The ICE image is rotated 90 degrees to orient it to the heart drawing. Structures shown are:

1. RA
   Tricuspid valve
2. RV
3. Ao root/valve
4. Pulmonary valve & outflow track

See: King, chapter on ICE

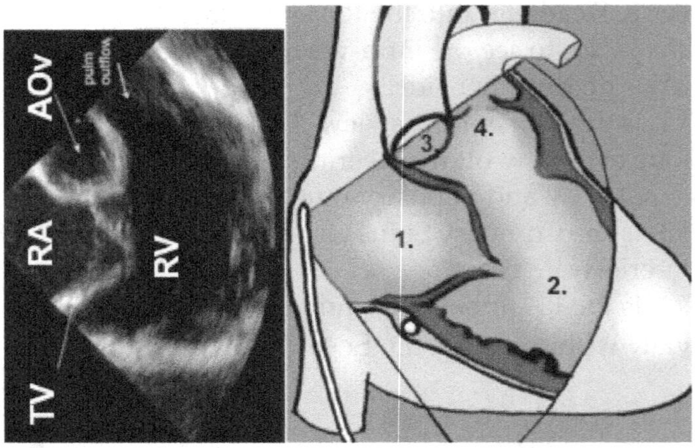

ICE view from RA *after King chapter on "ICE"*

563. What is shown at the arrow on this ICE image in the RA "home view" just superior to the IVC?

a. Tricuspid valve
b. Inferior vena cava
c. Interatrial septum
d. Eustachian ridge & valve
e. Thebesian valve

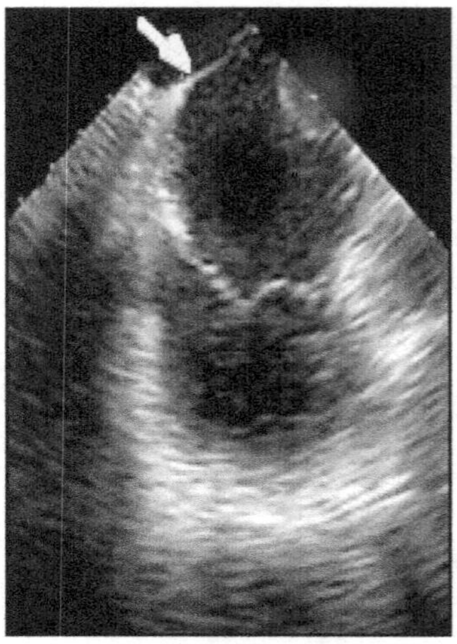
ICE Home View

ANSWER: d. Eustachian ridge & valve as seen from the default position in the RA. In this view we also see the RA, tricuspid valve and RV chamber. The eustachian ridge and valve are a remnant venous valve over the IVC. The Thebesian valve (not shown) is also a remnant valve over the coronary sinus. These valves can become obstacles to catheter placement during EP studies.

The valve of the inferior vena cava (eustachian valve) lies at the junction of the inferior vena cava and right atrium. In fetal life, the eustachian valve helps direct the flow of oxygen-rich blood through the right atrium into the left atrium via the foramen ovale (preventing blood flowing into the right ventricle). While the eustachian valve persists in adult life, it essentially does not have a specific function. Most commonly, it is a crescentic fold of endocardium arising from the anterior rim of the IVC orifice. The lateral horn of the crescent tends to meet the lower end of the crista terminalis, while the medial horn joins the thebesian valve, a semicircular valvular fold at the orifice of the coronary sinus. See: King, chapter on "Intracardiac Echocardiography in the Catheterization and Laboratory" and Keywords: Eustachian ridge & valve

564. What is shown on this ICE image?

- a. **Swan Ganz in RA**
- b. **ASD occluder placement**
- c. **Catheter in coronary sinus**
- d. **Transseptal sheath tenting**
- e. **MitraClip intervention**

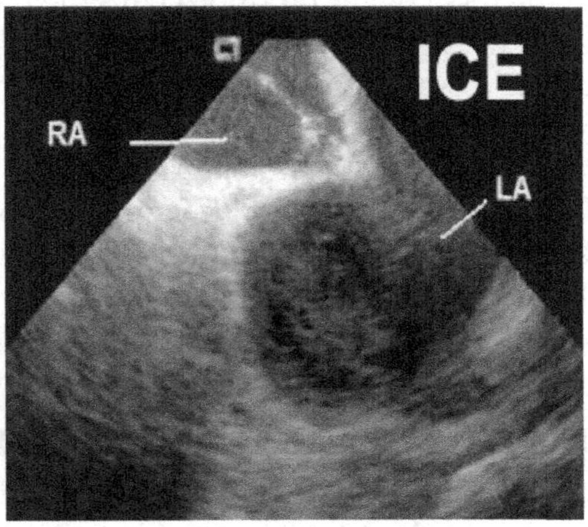

ANSWER: d. Transseptal sheath tenting, which is a sheath and long needle pushing against the fossa ovalis and deforming it. It creates a V shape as this force is applied to the septum, like pushing on a tent canvas with a tent pole, thus the term "tenting." This V shape indicates you are at the necessary thin part of the septum - the fossa ovalis. Then as the needle and sheath are advanced it pops through the septum into the LA. The sheath can then be advanced over the long Brockenbraugh needle into the LA. The needle is removed, a guidewire advanced through the sheath, and specialized catheters can then be advanced over the wire. Transseptal catheterization is common in many left heart interventions.

Russo says, "when advanced in the right atrium, the echocardiographic catheter provides a cross-sectional view of the FO [Foramen Ovale], which allows the position of both the needle and the sheath to be checked in the middle of the FO. This helps to determine the exact position of the needle by looking for tenting of the membranous septum at the time of the puncture." See: Russo, et al, Role of Intracardiac Echocardiography in Atrial Fibrillation Ablation, vein., jafib, 2013 online at: http://www.jafib.com/published.php?type=pdf&id=786

565. These ICE images from the RA show placement of:
- **a. Amplatzer ASD occluder**
- **b. Double clamshell septal umbrella**
- **c. Transseptal needle through ductus arteriosus**
- **d. Transseptal needle through fossa ovalis**

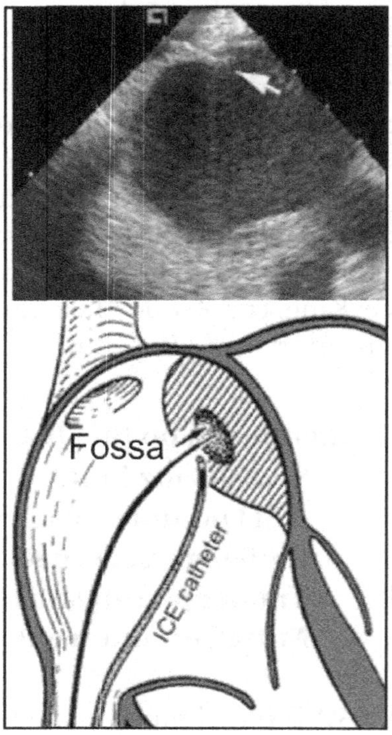

Answer: d. Transseptal needle through fossa ovalis. The drawing shows a transseptal needle beginning to puncture the fossa ovalis. Note how the ICE catheter is placed close to the fossa ovalis on fluoro with the transseptal catheter in view. The upper ICE images show the catheter pushing on the fossa which causes a "tenting" indentation. In the lower image the needle is seen passing through the interatrial septum and entering the LA. See: Mitchel, Intracardiac Ultrasound Imaging During Transseptal Catheterization, Chest, July 1995 Keywords: IVUS, Transseptal needle in Fossa Ovalis

566. This ultrasound image is from the RA during transseptal puncture. What type of ultrasound system is used here?
- **a. IVUS through IV septum**
- **b. Duplex scan of IV septum**
- **c. Mechanical ICE catheter**
- **d. Phased array ICE catheter**

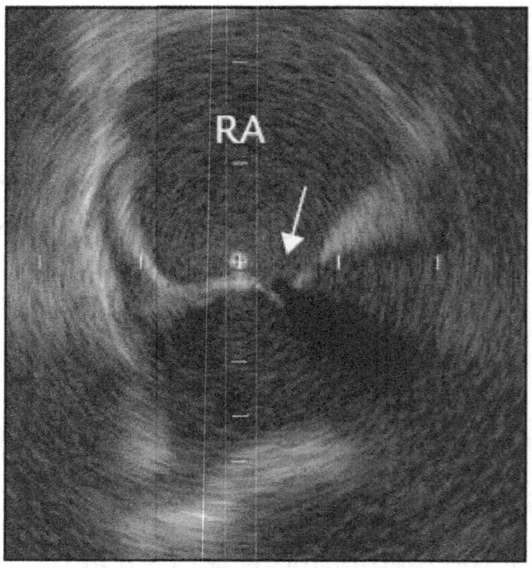

Ultrasound view from RA

ANSWER: c. Mechanical ICE catheter. The entire RA is seen in a 360 degree view with the mechanical ICE catheter at the center of the image. The Boston Scientific mechanical scanners show an entire 360 degree plane. Although it yields a larger view this mode has no Doppler capability and uses a relatively inflexible catheter. The phased array catheters in the previous questions always show as a pie-shaped sector-scan.

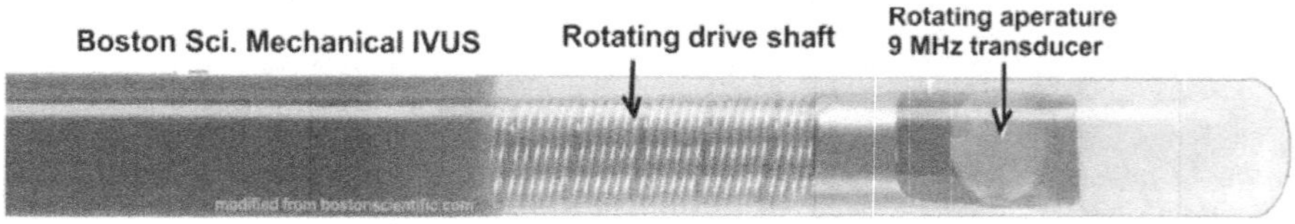

At the arrow note the black spot and shadowing below the transseptal catheter which is pushing on the fossa ovalis. The lower chamber is the LA. The Mullins catheter pushes on the fossa causing a reassuring "tenting" indentation of the thin fossa ovalis in the septum. You know you are in the right place, so the needle can be advanced. Remember the ICE frequency is 5-10MHz - that's midrange..

Liang says, "The [transseptal] intervention is simplified by positioning the

echocardiography catheter at the fossa ovalis and using this as a reference point for fluoroscopic monitoring of the progress of the Brockenbrough needle. (See previous question.) The optimal puncture site can be assessed by simultaneous detection of the characteristic downward jump of the transseptal needle onto the fossa ovalis by intracardiac ultrasound and fluoroscopy." These authors prefer the mechanical ICE system for transseptal puncture because it is cheaper and shows the entire RA. See: Liang, et. al., "Comparisons of Mechanical Versus Phase-array..." Nantou, Taiwan, 2010 http://homepage.vghtpe.gov.tw/~jcma/73/9/471.pdf
Keywords: Mechanical ICE catheter image showing "tenting" of fossa ovalis

567. This patient presented with acute mitral regurgitation. This ICE image in the LV long axis view shows a small bright vibrating structure in systole suggesting:

a. RA myxoma
b. Transseptal needle tip
c. Thrombus in LA appendage
d. Ruptured mitral papillary muscle

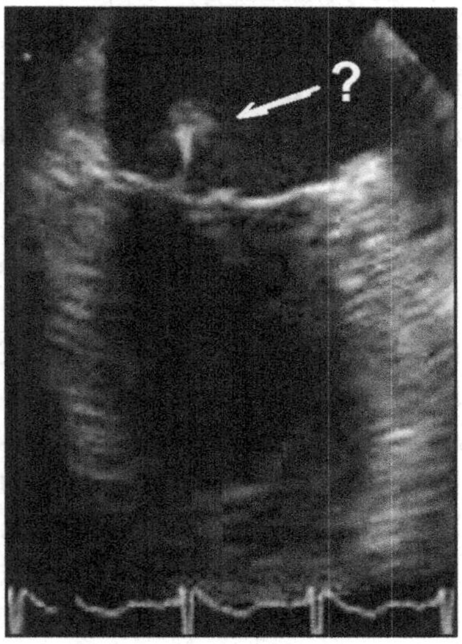

LV Long Axis ICE view

ANSWER: d. Ruptured mitral papillary muscle flailing back into the LA in systole. There is mitral regurgitation which blows the loose chordae tendinea back like a flag in the wind. When seen real time, it vibrates in the regurgitant stream. This can happen post MI as a papillary muscle becomes infarcted and tears loose from the LV wall. See: King, chapter on "ICE in the Catheterization Laboratory"
Keywords: ruptured papillary muscle

568. These fluoro and ICE images from the RA show placement of a/an:

a. Amplatz ASD septal occluder
b. Percutaneous AO valve
c. Distal protection basket
d. IVC filter

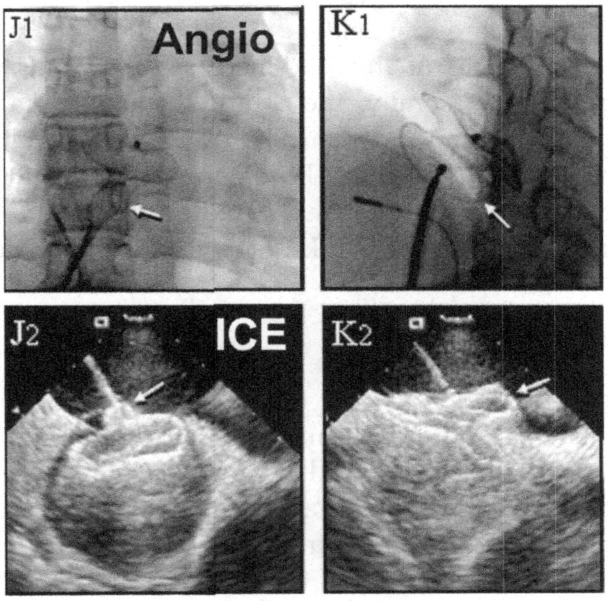

ICE view from RA *after King chapter on "ICE"*

ANSWER: a. Amplatz ASD septal occluder. This shows fluoro and ICE images as an Amplatzer septal occluder is placed across an ASD. The ICE catheter is in the RA with resulting images shown in the lower pictures. Note how clearly the inter-atrial septum shows up, for accurate expansion of the nitinol discs, that cannot be seen on fluoro. Arrows point to the RA portion of the occluder which is expanded in pictures K1 & K2.

Transseptal puncture is simplified by positioning the echocardiography

catheter at the fossa ovalis and using this as a reference point for fluoroscopic monitoring of the progress of the Brockenbrough needle. The optimal puncture site can be assessed by simultaneous detection of the characteristic downward jump of the transseptal needle onto the fossa ovalis by intracardiac ultrasound and fluoroscopy. See: online article, Rigatelli, *Intracardiac Echocardiography in CV Catheter-Based Interventions, Jn. Inv. Cardiology, online, 2006* online at:
www.invasivecardiology.com/articles/intracardiac-echocardiography-cardiovascular-catheter-based-interventions-different-devices

569. What pathology is shown on this ICE image with transducer in RV?

- a. **LV hypertrophy**
- b. **Pericardial effusion**
- c. **Ruptured chordae tendinea**
- d. **Mitral calcification and stenosis**

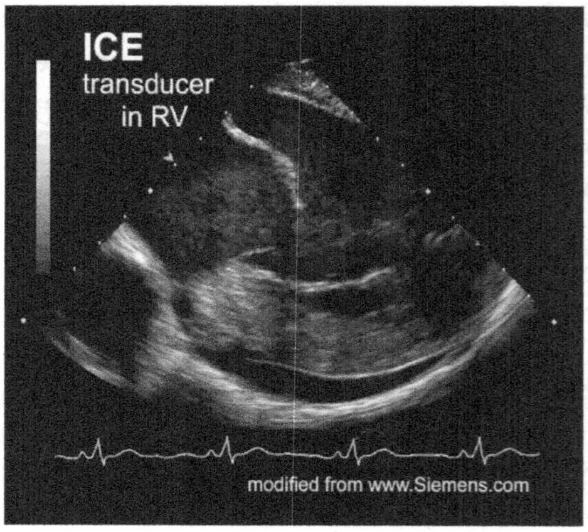

ANSWER: b. Pericardial effusion is seen as a black fluid filled space below the posteriorbasal LV wall. This is a beautiful ICE image of the long axis LV, mitral valve, and the pericardial effusion. Although effusion is not a major use of ICE, it will show the same pathology as seen on 2D echo and TEE. Note, labeled image below.

Braunwald says, "Because of their convenience, M-mode and two-dimensional Doppler echocardiography remain the standard noninvasive diagnostic methods for detection of pericardial effusion and tamponade. A pericardial effusion appears as a lucent separation between parietal and visceral pericardium. With a true effusion, separation is present for the entire cardiac cycle. Small effusions are first evident over the posterobasal left ventricle. As the fluid increases, it spreads anteriorly, laterally, and behind the left atrium, where its limit is demarcated by the visceral pericardial reflection. Ultimately, the separation becomes circumferential." See: Braunwald chapter on Pericardial Effusion and Tamponade

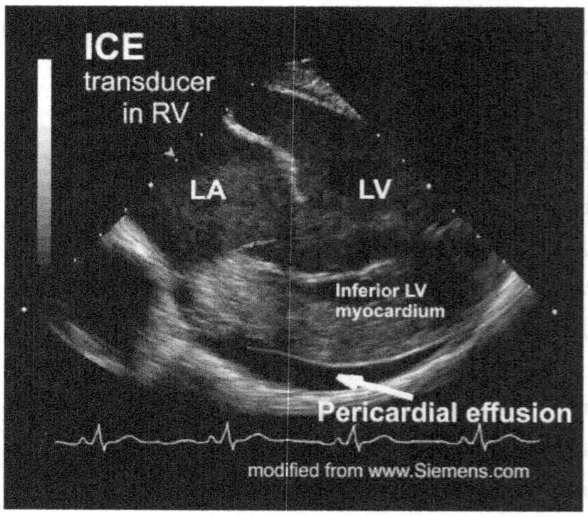

REFERENCES:

Baim, D. S. and Grossman W., *Cardiac Catheterization, Angiography, and Intervention,* 7th Ed., Lea and Febiger, 2006

Beck, Instantaneous wave-free ratio versus fractional flow reserve to guide PCI, ACC, 2017

Bhatt, Cardiovascular Intervention, A Companion to Braunwald's Heart Disease, Elsevier Inc., 2016

Braunwald, et. al. Ed., *Heart Disease, a Textbook of CV Medicine*, 9th Ed., Saunders, 2012

Pappano & Wier., *Cardiovascular Physiology*, 6th Ed., Mosby Year Book, 2013
Curry, Dowdey, and Murry, Christensen's Introduction to the Physics of Diagnostic Radiology, 3rd Ed., Lea & Febiger Publishers
Freed, Grines, and Safian, The New Manual of Interventional Cardiology 2nd printing, Physicians Press, 1996
Kern, M. J., Ed., *The Cardiac Catheterization Handbook*, 6th Ed., Mosby-Year Book, Inc., 2016
Kern, M. J., Ed., SCAI Interventional Cardiology Board Review Book, Lippincott, 2006
King, Spencer B., *Interventional Cardiology*, McGraw-Hill Inc., 2007
RADI Medical Systems, Inc., *Coronary Pressure Measurement CD*, featuring PressureWire™, http: www.radi.se, 1995
Reynolds, Terry, RDCS, BS, ULTRASOUND PHYSICS, A Registry Exam Preparation Guide, School of Cardiac Ultrasound, Arizona Heart Institute Foundation, Phoenix, AZ 1996
St. Jude Medical, FFR Fundamentals online
Topol, Textbook of Interventional Cardiology, chapter by Serreys, DiMario, and Kern, on "Intracoronary Doppler"
Vogel J.H.K. and King, S.B., *The Practice of Interventional Cardiology,* 2nd Ed., Mosby Year Book Co., 1993
Watson, Sandy, Ed., Invasive Cardiology, A manual for Cath Lab Personnel, 2nd Ed., Physicians Press, 2005

Doppler REFERENCES:

Pappano & Wier., *Cardiovascular Physiology*, 10th Ed., Mosby Year Book, 2013
Curry, Dowdey, and Murry, Christensen's Introduction to the Physics of Diagnostic Radiology, 3rd Ed., Lea & Febiger Publishers
Nguyen, & Colombo, et all., Practical Handbook of Advanced Interventional Cardiology, 3rd Ed., Blackwell Futura, 2009
Reynolds, Terry, RDCS, BS, ULTRASOUND PHYSICS, A Registry Exam Preparation Guide, School of Cardiac Ultrasound, Arizona Heart Institute Foundation, Phoenix, AZ 1996
Kern, M. J., Ed., *The Cardiac Catheterization Handbook*, 9th Ed., Mosby-Year Book, Inc., 2016
Topol, Textbook of Interventional Cardiology, chapter by Serreys, DiMario, and Kern, on "Intracoronary Doppler"
Vogel J.H.K. and King, S.B., *The Practice of Interventional Cardiology,* 2nd Ed., Mosby Year Book Co., 1993

IVUS & ICE References:

DiMario, et. al., "Clinical application and image interpretation in intracoronary ultrasound" in European Heart Journal, 1998
Endosonics Company Literature and
http://www.onlinejacc.org/content/accj/45/2/204.full.pdf
Intravascular Ultrasound, An interactive Learning Tool With CME Credit, J.M. Hodgson, Senior Editor, Technology Solutions Group, Ltd., Ed. Div.
King, & Yeung, Interventional Cardiology, McGraw-Hill Co., 2007
Yock, Fitzgerald, and Popp, Intravascular Ultrasound in Scientific American, Science and Medicine, 1995
"Murray, et. Al. Contemporary coronary imaging from patient to plaque part 1:

IVUS-derived virtual histology" May 2010 Br J Cardiol 2010;17:129-32
Nantou, Taiwan, 2010 http://homepage.vghtpe.gov.tw/~jcma/73/9/471.pdf
Siemens.com AcuNav instruction manual online,
https://www.medical.siemens.com/siemens/en_US/gg_us_FBAs/files/brochures/AcuNav/Instructional_Guide.pdf
Yock, Fitzherald & Popp, Chapter on "Intravascular Ultrasound" in Scientific American, Science and Medicine

OUTLINE: Coronary Artery Hemodynamics

1. Doppler Principles
    a. Piezoelectric Transducer
        i. Sends and receives ultrasound
        ii. Single crystal transducer
        iii. Frequency = 12-15 MHZ.
    b. Doppler Principle
    c. Doppler Target = RBCs
2. CORONARY PHYSIOLOGY AND FLOW
    a. Predominantly diastolic flow
    b. RCA may have slow steady flow
    c. Normal Coronary Velocity = same in all normal vessels & branches
3. DOPPLER CORONARY FLO-WIRE
    a. CFR = Coronary Flow Reserve
        i. Measures increased coronary flow with vasodilation
        ii. Formula for CFR = Maximal flow/ basal flow
        iii. Measure CFR
    b. Hyperemic agents
        i. Dipyridamole, Papaverine
        ii. Nitrates
        iii. Adenosine (drug of choice)
            (1) RCA 8-18 μg IC
            (2) LCA 10-12 μg IC
            (3) IV 140 ug/Kg/min
4. PRESSURE WIRE
    a. Fractional Flow Reserve (FFR)
    b. Normal hyperemic pressure response
    c. FFR = 1.0 indicates an artery with normal blood flow
    d. FFR> .80 indicates that narrowing is unlikely to cause ischemia
    e. FFR< .80 indicates that narrowing is responsible for ischemia
    f. FFR = Pd/Pa
    g. Culprit Pd waveform =Ventricularization
    h. Measure FFR from hyperemic pressures
    i. FAME study: FFR saves $, lower MACE
    j. Post-stent expect FFR>.96
    k. Diffuse disease use IV adenosine 140 mcg/Kg/min
5. IVUS
    a. 2 types of IVUS transducers
        i. Mechanical
        ii. Phased array
    b. Suboptimal stent deployment
        i. Thrombosed stent
    c. Eccentric - concentric lesions
    d. On IVUS identify:
        i. Intima
        ii. Lumen
        iii. Media
        iv. External elastic membrane
    e. Plaque bourdon
        i. Formula = plaque/lumen area
        ii. Dissected plaque
    f. Calcium & shadowing
    g. Culprit coronary lesions show:
        i. Ulceration
        ii. Eccentricity
        iii. Thrombosis
        iv. Calcification
        v. Positive remodeling
        vi. Echo-lucent (Lipid) black core
    h. IVUS Pullbacks
    i. Positive remodeling
    j. Virtual histology - Tissue characterization
        i. Dark green= fibrous plaque
        ii. Light green= fibrofatty plaque
        iii. Red= Necrotic core
        iv. White= Calcium
        v. Chromaflow
    k. Optical Coherence Tomography
        i. High resolution images
        ii. Infrared light reflected
    l. Angioscopy best for thrombus
        i. Fiber optic bundle
6. ICE- Intracardiac Echocardiography
    a. ICE equipment
            (1) 2D
            (2) 3D
            (3) mechanical
            (4) phased array
            (5) linear array
            (6) Bubble study/ contrast
    b. ID CE views
        i. AO & PA
        ii. RA home view
        iii. Intra-atrial septum & SVC
        iv. Eustachian & Tricuspid valve
        v. LV short axis
        vi. LV Long axis
        vii. Coronary sinus ostium
        viii. LA & LA app., MV, LV
    c. In ICE images identify:
        i. Cardiac Chambers
        ii. Cardiac structures
        iii. Cardiac valves
    d. Identify uses of ICE
        i. Amplatzer placement
        ii. Transseptal
            (1) tenting
        iii. Uptured papillary uscle
        iv. PFO amplatzer placement
        v. Pericardial effusion

HEMODYNAMIC FORMULAS I

PRESSURES: (Chapter E1-E5)

◆Mean BP : mean BP ≅ CO x SVR
or estimated by mean BP ≅ (Syst. + 2x Diast) / 3
◆Pk. to pk. gradient : Pk. to pk. gradient = LV systolic - AO systolic
◆Pulse Pressure : AO Pulse Pr. = AO Systolic - AO Diastolic

FICK CARDIAC OUTPUT (Chapter D6)

◆Hgb. O2 Content : CaO2 =1.36 x Hgb x O2 Sat/100
◆Hgb. O2 Capacity : O2 Cap. =1.36 x 100% Sat x Hgb
◆% O2 Saturation : O2 Content / O2 Capacity x 100%

◆Oxygen Consumption (assumed) : VO_2 = BSA x 125 ml O_2/BSA/ M^2
◆Oxygen Consumption (measured) : VO_2 = minute ventilation$_{\text{corr. STPD ml/min}}$ x (Room air O_2 %- Expired air O_2%) / 100%
◆Fick CO : Fick CO = $\dfrac{O_2\text{ Consumption}}{(\text{a - v dif.}) \times 10} = \dfrac{O_2\text{ Consumption}}{(\text{AO - PA}) \times 10}$
◆Cardiac Index : CI = CO / BSA
◆Systemic Blood Flow: SBF = Q_s = O_2 cons / [(SA - SV) x1.36 x Hgb x 10)]
◆Pulmonary Blood Flow: PBF = Q_p= O_2 cons / [(PV - PA) x1.36 x Hgb x 10)]
◆Shunt Flow : L-R shunt flow = PBF - SBF = Q_p - Q_s.
◆Shunt Ratio : Q_p/Q_s = (SA% - SV%) / (PV% - PA%) using % O_2 Sat.
Q_p/Q_s = (AO% - SVC%) / (PV% - PA%) = PBF / SBF
◆Flamm Equation (in ASD): RA O2 Sat. = (3 x SVC Sat. + IVC Sat.) / 4
Bidirectional Shunt : Q_{eff} = O_2 consumption / [(PV - SV) x 10]
: R-L shunt$_{\text{bidir.}}$ = Q_s - Q_{eff}
: L-R shunt$_{\text{bidir.}}$ = Q_p - Q_{eff}

THERMODILUTION CO: (Chapter E7)

Thermo. CO : CO = K V_i (T_b - T_i) / ∫Area under curve x C
◆ Normal CO : TDCO = Fick CO = LVMF = PBF = SBF
(unless shunt or regurgitation present)

QUANTITATIVE LV ANGIOGRAPHY (Chapter E8)

◆Stroke Volume : SV = EDV - ESV
◆ : SV = CO/HR
◆ : SV = EF x EDV

◆Ejection Fraction : EF = SV/EDV
: EF = (EDV - ESV)/ EDV
: EF = 1 - (ESV/EDV)
EF (single plane) : EF = 1 - [$(Aes)^2$ (Led)]/ [$(Aed)^2$ (Les)]
◆LVMF (Angio CO) : LVMF = SV x HR = Left Ventricular Minute Flow
LV Volume (single plane): LV Vol. = [(0.682 A^2 CF^3)/ L] + 2 cc

◆ Indicates important formulas

HEMODYNAMIC FORMULAS II

REGURGITATION (Chapter E8)

◆Forward CO : Fd. CO = Fick CO

◆Total CO : Total CO = LVMF

◆Forward SV : Fd. SV = Fick CO/ HR

◆Total Stroke Volume: $TSV = SV_{angio} = (EDV - ESV)$

◆Total EF = SV_{angio}/EDV: EF = 100% (EDV - ESV) / EDV (also termed global EF)

◆Regurgitant flow : Regurgitant flow = Total Angio CO - Forward CO

Regurgitation/min = LVMF - (Fick or thermo CO)

◆Regurgitant Fraction: RF = 100% (Regurgitation/min) / (LVMF)

: $RF = 100\% \times (SV_{angio} - SV_{Fick}) / SV_{angio}$

Advanced LV Angio. Formulas:

Volume of ellipse (single plane): $Vol_{ellipse} = (\pi/6)\, L \times M \times N$

Volume of ellipse (bi- plane): $Vol_{ellipse} = (8/3\pi)\, (A_{RAO}\, A_{LAO} / L_{min})$

VASCULAR RESISTANCE: (Chapter E9)

◆Absolute Resistance Units : Absolute resistance = 80 x Hybrid resistance

◆Systemic Vascular Resistance: $SVR = (\overline{AO} - \overline{RA}) / SBF$

SVR = (mean AO - mean RA pressure) / Systemic blood flow

◆Pulmonary Vascular Resistance: $PVR = (\overline{PA} - \overline{PAW}) / PBF$

PVR = (mean PA - mean PAWP) / Pulmonary blood flow

◆Ohm's Law (fluid) : $R = (P_i - P_o) / Q$ = Pressure drop/blood flow

◆Indexed Systemic Vascular Resistance: SVRI = SVR x BSA

◆Indexed Pulmonary Vascular Resistance: PVRI = PVR x BSA

Poiseuille's Resistance : $R = 8(\text{Viscosity})(\text{Length}) / (\pi)(\text{radius})^4$

or $R = (P_i - P_o) / Q$ (revised Ohm's law)

VALVE AREA (Chapter E10)

◆Heart Rate : HR = 60/ r-r interval

◆Heart Rate : $HR\ (\text{bts./min}) = \dfrac{60\ (\text{sec/min}) \times \text{paper speed} \times (\text{mm/sec})}{\text{r-r interval (mm)}}$

◆Diastolic Filling Period : DFP (sec) = dfp (cm) / paper speed (cm/sec)

◆Systolic Ejection Period : SEP (sec) = sep (cm) / paper speed (cm/sec)

◆Aortic Flow (Gorlin) : AO Flow = CO / (SEP x HR)

◆Mitral Flow (Gorlin) : Mitral Flow = CO / (DFP x HR)

◆Mitral VA formula (Gorlin): $MVA = \text{Flow} / 38 \sqrt{\text{Mean gradient}}$

◆AO VA formula (Gorlin) : $AO\ VA = \text{Flow} / 44.5 \sqrt{\text{Mean gradient}}$

Aortic valve resistance : AO Valve Resistance = Mean gradient / (CO / SEP)

◆VA formula (Hakki) : $AO\ \text{valve area} = CO / \sqrt{(\text{Peak - peak gradient})}$

CORONARY HEMODYNAMICS (Chapter E11)

Doppler Shift : $Vel._{Doppler} = [\,(F_1 - F_0) \times C\,] / (2 F_0 \cos\varphi)$

◆Fractional Flow Reserve : FFR = Pd/Pa

◆ Plaque Burdon : PB = (TVA-LA) / TVA

◆ Indicates important formulas

PHYSICAL PRINCIPLES *(Review Book I, Chapters B)*

***Distance : D = V x t**

Distance = Velocity x time

Acceleration : A = V / t = Velocity / time = D / t^2

Graham's Law Diffusion: $$D = \frac{\Delta P \times A \times S}{d \times \sqrt{MW}}$$

D = rate of diffusion, ΔP = Pressure gradient
A = Area, S = Solubility, d = density, MW = Molecular Weight

Henry's Law Gases :S = C x P / t =Sol. coef. x Partial Pr. / temp.

Dalton's Law Gases: $P_t = P_1 + P_2 + \ldots P_n$ = Sum of partial pressures

ULTRASOUND : *(Review Book I, Chapters C)*

***Period = 1/ frequency**

***Wavelength = propagation speed / frequency**

Wavelength = propagation speed x Period

***(note: in soft tissue propogation speed = 1540 M/sec)**

PHYSIOLOGY *(Review Book I, Chapters B)*

Ohm's Law (fluid) : R = (Pi - Po) / Q = Pressure drop/blood flow

Continuity Eqn. : Q = V x A = Velocity x Area

Poisieulle's Law :

$$Q = \frac{\pi(P_i - P_o)r^4}{8\eta l}$$

Q = flow, P_i= Pressure in, *r*= radius, *η*=viscosity, *l* = length
or since R = $(P_i - P_o)$ / Q

Poiseuille's Resistance: R= 8(Viscosity)(Length) / (π)$(\text{radius})^4$
=(revised Ohm's law)

Laplace Law : T = P x R Tension = Pressure x radius

Kinetic Energy : $\frac{1}{2}mv^2$ = 1/2 mass x velocity ^{2}

Potential Energy : mgh = mass x gravity x height

Bernoulli Eqn. : K = $1/2mv^2$ + mgh

Starling's Eqn. : Fluid Movement = $k(P_c+\pi_i) - (P_i+\pi_p)$.
where k = constant
π_p = plasma protein oncotic pressure
P_c = hydrostatic capillary pressure

Cardiovascular Review Books

PERFECT TO:

Self Study at home or in the cath lab.
Help staff pass the Cath Lab Registry Exams.
Resource for in-service educators.
Assess your cath lab knowledge and skills.
Text to accompany CV Review CD

ORDER TODD's CV REVIEW BOOKS

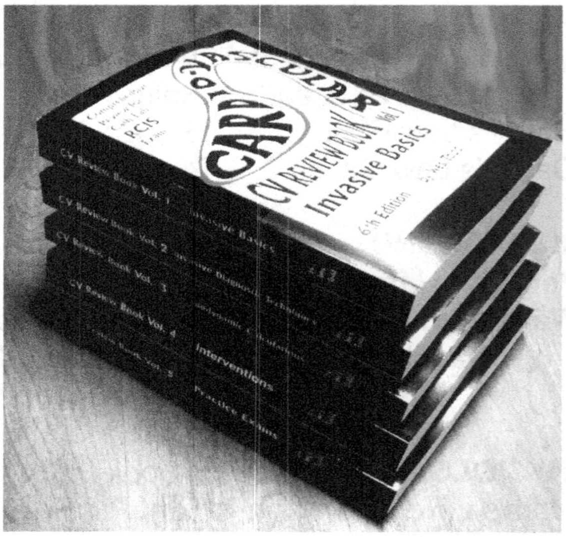

5 Vol. Book Set

- Vol. I: Invasive Basics **Includes Pt. Care, A&P, Pathology**
- Vol. II: Cath Lab **Diagnostic Techniques**
- Vol. III: Cath Lab **Hemodynamics**
- Vol. IV: Cath Lab **Interventions**
- Vol. V, Practice Exams, Includes **8 Invasive Mock Exams**

Recommended for all cath lab staff, Invasive students, Cath lab nurses & Technicians.

We recommend that your prepare for your exam with all our instructional materials.

Together they complement each other.

Order from www.Amazon.com Or www.westodd.com

More information at http://www.westodd.com
Or Email info@westodd.com

Made in United States
North Haven, CT
10 November 2026

22088881R00193